I0066525

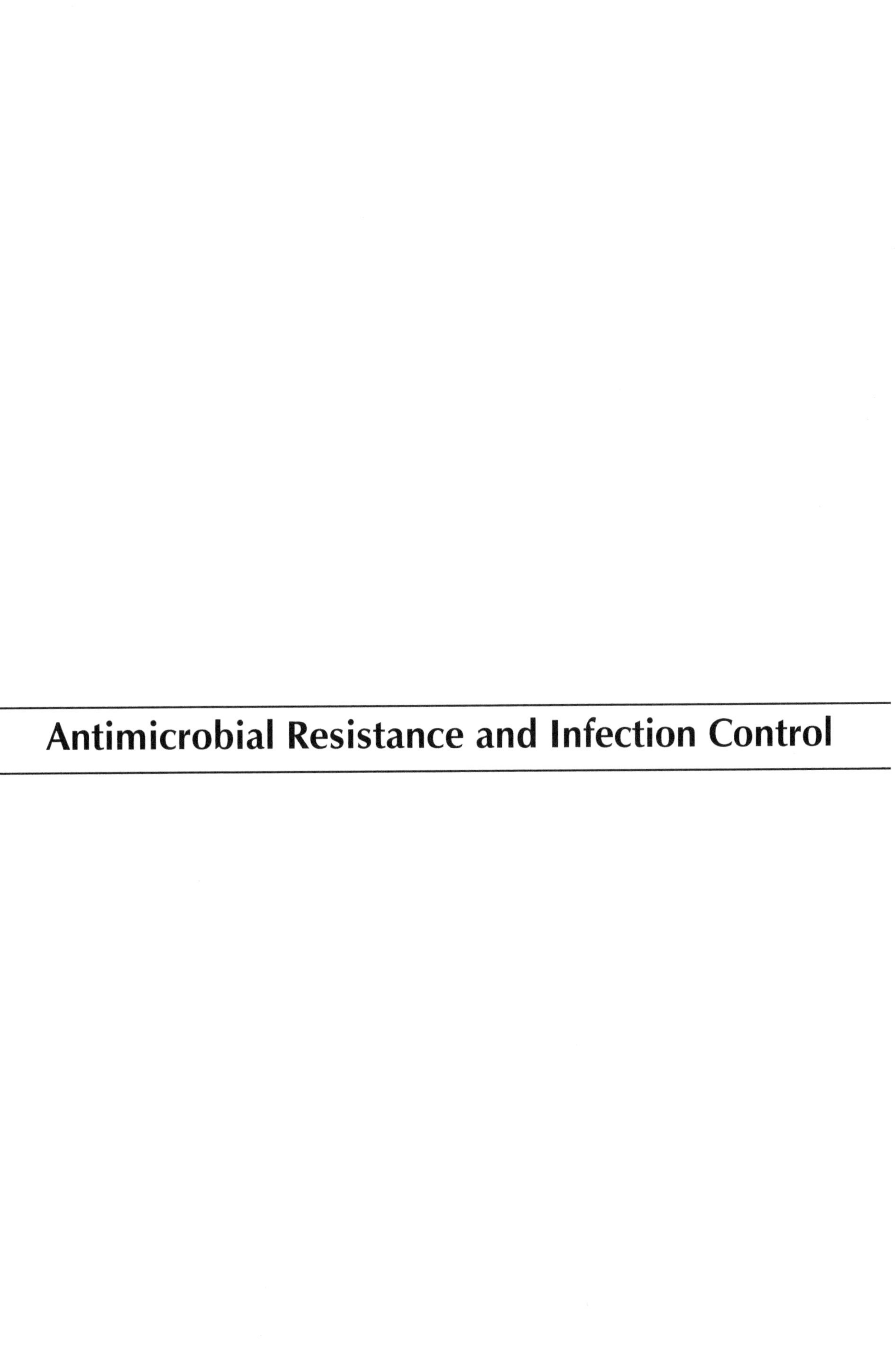

Antimicrobial Resistance and Infection Control

Antimicrobial Resistance and Infection Control

Editor: Ralph Allen

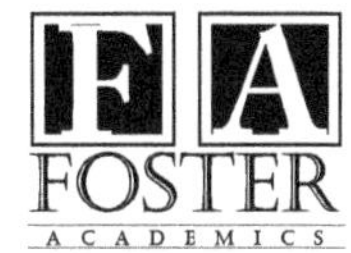

www.fosteracademics.com

www.fosteracademics.com

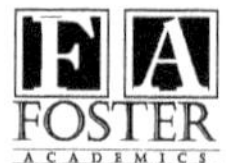

Cataloging-in-publication Data

Antimicrobial resistance and infection control / edited by Ralph Allen.
p. cm.
Includes bibliographical references and index.
ISBN 978-1-63242-690-1
1. Drug resistance in microorganisms. 2. Anti-infective agents. 3. Infection--Treatment.
4. Drug resistance. I. Allen, Ralph.
QR177 .A58 2019
616.904 1--dc23

Foster Academics,
118-35 Queens Blvd., Suite 400,
Forest Hills, NY 11375, USA

ISBN 978-1-63242-690-1 (Hardback)

Antimicrobial Resistance and Infection Control

Editor: Ralph Allen

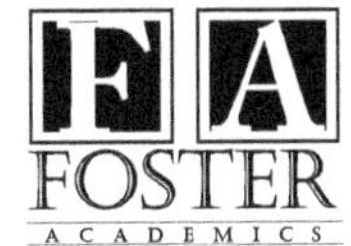

www.fosteracademics.com

www.fosteracademics.com

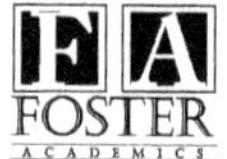

Cataloging-in-publication Data

Antimicrobial resistance and infection control / edited by Ralph Allen.
p. cm.
Includes bibliographical references and index.
ISBN 978-1-63242-690-1
1. Drug resistance in microorganisms. 2. Anti-infective agents. 3. Infection--Treatment.
4. Drug resistance. I. Allen, Ralph.
QR177 .A58 2019
616.904 1--dc23

Foster Academics,
118-35 Queens Blvd., Suite 400,
Forest Hills, NY 11375, USA

ISBN 978-1-63242-690-1 (Hardback)

Contents

Preface

This book has been an outcome of determined endeavour from a group of educationists in the field. The primary objective was to involve a broad spectrum of professionals from diverse cultural background involved in the field for developing new researches. The book not only targets students but also scholars pursuing higher research for further enhancement of the theoretical and practical applications of the subject.

Antimicrobial resistance (AMR) refers to the ability of a microbe to resist the effects of medication aimed to kill it. Antibiotic resistance is a form of AMR. Some microbes can be resistant to multiple antimicrobials. They are called multidrug resistant microbes. Resistant microbes are difficult to treat and require higher doses of antimicrobials or alternative medications. Resistance typically occurs through genetic mutation, natural resistance or by acquiring resistance from another species. Proper sanitation and hygiene maintenance can minimize the spread of infections. Another strategy for achieving this is using narrow-spectrum antibiotics over broad-spectrum antibiotics. The field of infection control addresses all factors related to the spread of infections within the healthcare setting. This book unravels the recent studies in antimicrobial resistance and infection control. It will provide interesting topics for research, which interested readers can take up. The extensive content herein provides the readers with a thorough understanding of the subject.

It was an honour to edit such a profound book and also a challenging task to compile and examine all the relevant data for accuracy and originality. I wish to acknowledge the efforts of the contributors for submitting such brilliant and diverse chapters in the field and for endlessly working for the completion of the book. Last, but not the least; I thank my family for being a constant source of support in all my research endeavours.

Editor

1

Mupirocin-resistant *Staphylococcus aureus* in Africa

Adebayo O. Shittu[1*], Mamadou Kaba[2,3], Shima M. Abdulgader[2], Yewande O. Ajao[1], Mujibat O. Abiola[1] and Ayodele O. Olatimehin[1]

Abstract

Background: Mupirocin is widely used for nasal decolonization of *Staphylococcus aureus* to prevent subsequent staphylococcal infection in patients and healthcare personnel. However, the prolonged and unrestricted use has led to the emergence of mupirocin-resistant (mupR) *S. aureus*. The aim of this systematic review was to investigate the prevalence, phenotypic and molecular characteristics, and geographic spread of mupR *S. aureus* in Africa.

Methods: We examined five electronic databases (EBSCOhost, Google Scholar, ISI Web of Science, MEDLINE, and Scopus) for relevant English articles on screening for mupR *S. aureus* from various samples in Africa. In addition, we performed random effects meta-analysis of proportions to determine the pooled prevalence of mupR *S. aureus* in Africa. The search was conducted until 3 August 2016.

Results: We identified 43 eligible studies of which 11 (26%) were obtained only through Google Scholar. Most of the eligible studies (28/43; 65%) were conducted in Nigeria (10/43; 23%), Egypt (7/43; 16%), South Africa (6/43; 14%) and Tunisia (5/43; 12%). Overall, screening for mupR *S. aureus* was described in only 12 of 54 (22%) African countries. The disk diffusion method was the widely used technique (67%; 29/43) for the detection of mupR *S. aureus* in Africa. The *mupA*-positive *S. aureus* isolates were identified in five studies conducted in Egypt ($n = 2$), South Africa ($n = 2$), and Nigeria ($n = 1$). Low-level resistance (LmupR) and high-level resistance (HmupR) were both reported in six human studies from South Africa ($n = 3$), Egypt ($n = 2$) and Libya ($n = 1$). Data on mupR-MRSA was available in 11 studies from five countries, including Egypt, Ghana, Libya, Nigeria and South Africa. The pooled prevalence (based on 11 human studies) of mupR *S. aureus* in Africa was 14% (95% CI =6.8 to 23.2%). The proportion of *mupA*-positive *S. aureus* in Africa ranged between 0.5 and 8%. Furthermore, the frequency of *S. aureus* isolates that exhibited LmupR, HmupR and mupR-MRSA in Africa were 4 and 47%, 0.5 and 38%, 5 and 50%, respectively.

Conclusions: The prevalence of mupR *S. aureus* in Africa (14%) is worrisome and there is a need for data on administration and use of mupirocin. The disk diffusion method which is widely utilized in Africa could be an important method for the screening and identification of mupR *S. aureus*. Moreover, we advocate for surveillance studies with appropriate guidelines for screening mupR *S. aureus* in Africa.

Keywords: Africa, Prevalence, Meta-analysis, Mupirocin, *Staphylococcus aureus*, Systematic review

* Correspondence: bayo_shittu@yahoo.com
[1]Department of Microbiology, Obafemi Awolowo University, Ile-Ife, Osun State 22005, Nigeria
Full list of author information is available at the end of the article

Background

Staphylococcus aureus is a well-recognized human pathogen that is implicated in a wide array of superficial, invasive and toxigenic infections [1]. Meta-analyses of published studies have provided evidence that *S. aureus* nasal carriage is an important risk factor for subsequent infection among patients with surgical site infections and atopic dermatitis [2, 3]. Other high-risk groups include patients colonized with methicillin-resistant *Staphylococcus aureus* (MRSA) undergoing dialysis, and patients admitted in the intensive care unit [4, 5]. Consequently, infection prevention strategies such as nasal decolonization are employed to minimize the occurrence of staphylococcal infection and reduce the risk of transmission in healthcare settings [6, 7]. Mupirocin (2%) nasal ointment alone or in combination with 4% chlorhexidine (CHG) based body wash is considered as the main decolonization strategy for *S. aureus* carriage [8, 9]. Mupirocin is a naturally occurring antibiotic produced by *Pseudomonas fluorescens* that interferes with protein synthesis by competitive inhibition of the bacterial isoleucyl-tRNA synthetase (IRS) [10, 11]. It gained prominence in the mid-1990s for the eradication of *S. aureus* nasal carriage due to its effectiveness, safety and cost [12].

Mupirocin-resistant (mupR) *S. aureus* was first reported in the United Kingdom in 1987 [13]. Since then, it has been reported in several countries worldwide [14–17]. The emergence of mupR *S. aureus* has been associated with unrestricted policies and use of mupirocin for long periods in health care settings [8, 18]. Decolonization failure in patients with *S. aureus* carriage is associated with high-level mupirocin resistance (HmupR - minimum inhibitory concentration [MIC]: ≥512 μg/ml), while that of low-level mupirocin resistance (LmupR – MIC: 8-64 μg/ml) is still unclear [7, 19]. LmupR is mediated through point mutation (largely V588F and V631F) in the native isoleucyl-tRNA synthetase (*ileS*) gene [20]. In contrast, HmupR is mainly attributed to the acquisition of plasmids with the *mupA* (or *ileS2*) gene encoding an additional IRS with no affinity for mupirocin [11, 21]. Another determinant for HmupR is the acquisition of a plasmid-mediated *mupB* gene [22].

There is no data summarizing reports on screening, prevalence, characterization, and geographic spread of mupR *S. aureus* in Africa. This systematic review evaluated published articles that assessed for mupirocin resistance in African *S. aureus* isolates. The findings from this systematic review highlight the need to develop an early warning system, including harmonized strategies for the prompt screening and identification of mupR *S. aureus* in Africa.

Methods

Literature search strategy

The relevant English articles from human and animal investigations were retrieved by three authors (YA, SA, and AS) from five electronic databases (EBSCOhost, Google Scholar, ISI Web of Science, MEDLINE, and Scopus). The search terms for each database are reported in Table 1. The literature search was concluded on 3 August 2016.

Eligible article identification

The identification of the eligible articles was conducted according to the guidelines for preferred reporting items for systematic reviews and meta-analyses (PRISMA) [23]. We defined an eligible article as a peer-reviewed publication that (i) included mupirocin in the antibiotic susceptibility testing of *S. aureus* isolates, and (ii) employed phenotypic ((disc diffusion, E-test, minimum inhibitory concentration (MIC), VITEK and other automated methods)), and/or molecular ((conventional or real-time polymerase chain reaction (PCR)) techniques. International multicentre studies that included African countries were also eligible for inclusion.

Data extraction and analysis

The relevant data were extracted from each of the eligible articles included in this systematic review. A study that analysed *S. aureus* isolates from another investigation but answered a different research question were both considered as one study (Table 2). We performed three levels of analysis (Fig. 1). First, to understand the characteristics and geographic spread of mupR *S. aureus* in Africa, studies that included mupirocin in the antibiotic susceptibility testing and employed phenotypic and/or molecular techniques were identified. Secondly, the prevalence of *S. aureus* with the *mupA* gene, isolates that expressed LmupR and HmupR, and mupR-MRSA in Africa were derived from each eligible study as follows:

$$\textit{MupA}\text{-positive } S.\ aureus = \frac{\text{Number of } \textit{MupA}\text{-positive } S.\ aureus \text{ isolates}}{\text{Total number of isolates screened with mupirocin}}$$

$$S.\ aureus \text{ that expressed LmupR} = \frac{\text{Number of } S.\ aureus \text{ isolates with LmupR}}{\text{Total number of isolates screened with mupirocin}}$$

$$S.\ aureus \text{ that expressed HmupR} = \frac{\text{Number of } S.\ aureus \text{ isolates with HmupR}}{\text{Total number of isolates screened with mupirocin}}$$

$$\text{MupR-MRSA} = \frac{\text{Number of mupR-MRSA isolates}}{\text{Total number of isolates screened with mupirocin}}$$

Thirdly, to estimate the prevalence of mupR *S. aureus* in humans, studies that employed at least one of the screening methods with defined breakpoint for mupirocin resistance were included in the meta-analysis. The StatsDirect

Table 1 Keywords used to identify eligible studies available in five biomedical databases

Database	Search period	Search strategy
MEDLINE via PubMed EBSCOhost via Academic Search premier, Africa-Wide information and CINAHL ISI Web of Science	1974 - August 2016 1982 - August 2016 1950 - August 2016	(Staphylococcus aureus OR S. aureus) AND (Mupirocin) AND (Algeria OR Angola OR Benin OR Botswana OR Burkina Faso OR "Burkina Faso" OR Burkina Fasso OR Upper Volta OR "Upper Volta" OR Burundi OR Cameroon OR Cape Verde OR "Cape Verde" OR Central African Republic OR Chad OR Comoros OR "Iles Comores" OR Iles Comores OR Comoro Islands OR "Comoro Islands" OR Congo OR Democratic Republic Congo OR "Democratic Republic of the Congo" OR Zaire OR Djibouti OR Egypt OR Equatorial Guinea OR "Equatorial Guinea" OR Eritrea OR Ethiopia OR Gabon OR Gambia OR Ghana OR Guinea OR Guinea Bissau OR "Guinea Bissau" OR Ivory Coast OR "Ivory Coast" OR Cote d'Ivoire OR "Cote d'Ivoire" OR Kenya OR Lesotho OR Liberia OR Libya OR Libia OR Jamahiriya OR Jamahiryia OR Madagascar OR Malawi OR Mali OR Mauritania OR Mauritius OR Ile Maurice OR "Ile Maurice" OR Morocco OR Mozambique OR Moçambique OR Namibia OR Niger OR Nigeria OR Rwanda OR Sao Tome OR "Sao Tome" OR Senegal OR Seychelles OR Sierra Leone OR "Sierra Leone" OR Somalia OR South Africa OR "South Africa" OR Sudan OR South Sudan OR "South Sudan" OR Swaziland OR Tanzania OR Tanganyika OR Zanzibar OR Togo OR Tunisia OR Uganda OR Western Sahara OR "Western Sahara" OR Zambia OR Zimbabwe OR Africa OR Africa* OR Southern Africa OR West Africa OR Western Africa OR Eastern Africa OR East Africa OR North Africa OR Northern Africa OR Central Africa OR Sub Saharan Africa OR Subsaharan Africa OR Sub-Saharan Africa) NOT (Guinea pig* OR "Guinea pig*" OR Aspergillus niger OR "Aspergillus niger" OR Europe* OR America* OR Asia*)
Scopus from SciVerse	1982 - August 2016	(Staphylococcus aureus OR S. aureus) AND (Mupirocin) AND (Africa)[a]
Google Scholar**		(Staphylococcus aureus OR S. aureus) AND (Mupirocin) AND (Name of each African country) Examples (Staphylococcus aureus OR S. aureus) AND (Mupirocin) AND (Algeria) (Staphylococcus aureus OR S. aureus) AND (Mupirocin) AND (Zimbabwe)

[a]The African countries were manually selected (as recommended by Scopus database) to exclude studies from other continents
**The Google Scholar search was conducted between July-September 2015

statistical software version 3.0.165 (England: StatsDirectLtd.2016) was utilized to assess the heterogeneity of the eligible studies included in the meta-analysis (Cochran Q-test) [24], and to ascertain the inconsistency across the studies (I2 statistic) [25]. The random effects model was used to determine the pooled prevalence of mupR *S. aureus* in Africa. The criterion for statistical significance for heterogeneity was set at alpha = 0.05. The risk of publication bias was assessed and visualized by a Funnel plot [26, 27].

Results

Eligible studies from electronic database search

We identified 43 reports (Table 1) of which 34 studies investigated only human samples. The remaining nine studies assessed samples from only animals (n = 5), human and environmental sources (n = 2), human and animal sources (n = 1), and cockroaches (n = 1). Most of the eligible studies (32/43; 74%) were obtained from EBSCOhost, ISI Web of Science, MEDLINE, and Scopus. The remaining studies (11/43; 26%) were obtained only through Google Scholar and consisted of studies conducted in Egypt [28–31], South Africa [32–34], Nigeria [35, 36], Ethiopia [37] and Kenya [38].

Screening and identification of mupR *S. aureus* in Africa

Only 12 of the 54 (22%) African countries reported data on screening for mupR *S. aureus* (Fig. 2). The first published article indicated that mupirocin had been in use in Africa, at least from the late 1980s [39]. Most of these studies (28/43; 65%) were conducted in Nigeria (10/43; 23%), Egypt (7/43; 16%), South Africa (6/43; 14%) and Tunisia (5/43; 12%) (Fig. 2). MupR *S. aureus* was mainly identified through the disk diffusion method (29/43; 67%). The guidelines by the Clinical and Laboratory Standards

Table 2 Characteristics of the 43 eligible studies on screening for mupirocin resistance in *Staphylococcus aureus* from various sources in Africa

Region	Country	Study Period	Setting	Sample		Method for testing resistance to mupirocin	Guideline (year of publication)	Published reports for detection of mupR *S. aureus*	Number of *S. aureus* isolates screened with mupirocin	Mupirocin resistant isolates				Reference
				Source	Type					Number (%)	Number MRSA (%)	Number LmupR/ HmupR	Number *mupA* gene + LMupR/HmupR (Method)	
North Africa	Algeria	2005–2007	C & H	Human	Pus, venous catheter, tracheal aspirate, punction fluid, blood, urine	Disk diffusion VITEK-2	CLSI (NA)	–	19	0 (0)	0 (0)	–	–	[47]
	Egypt	2005–2006	C & H	Human	NA	Disk diffusion	NCCLS (2003)	–	64	0 (0)	0 (0)	–	–	[28]
	Egypt	2008–2009	C & H	Human	Skin and soft tissue, post-operative wound swab	Disk diffusion	CLSI (2007)	–	386	1 (0.3)	NA	NA	–	[29]
	Egypt	2007–2008	C	Human	Pus, sputum, catheter, blood, urine, wound abscess	Broth dilution	CLSI (2005)	–	21	0 (0)	0 (0)	–	–	[58]
	Egypt	2010	H	Human	Sputum, blood, catheter, traumatic wound, urine	E-test	–	Kresken et al., (2004)	86	30 (34.9)	30 (34.9)	25/5	2/3 (PCR)	[30]
	Egypt	2012	H	Human	Wound discharge, blood, body fluid aspirate, urine, faeces, sputum, nasal, throat, ear and genital swab	Disk diffusion Agar dilution	CLSI (2007)	–	150	0 (0)	0 (0)	–	–	[40]
	Egypt	2012–2013	H	Human	Nasal swab	Disk diffusion	CLSI (2011)	–	39	3 (7.7)	3 (3.7)	NA	–	[31]
	Egypt	2013–2015	H	Human	Pus & Wound swab	Agar dilution	CLSI (2011)	–	73	13 (17.8)	13 (17.8)	5/8	0/6 (PCR)	[52]
	Libya	NA	H	Human	Skin swab	Disk diffusion	NA	–	40	0 (0)	NA	–	–	[61]
	Libya	2008–2009	H	Human & Environment	NA	Disk diffusion	BSAC (2008)	–	86	13 (15.1)	13 (8.1)	NA	–	[56]
	Libya	2009	H	Human	Nasal swab	Disk diffusion Agar dilution	BSAC (2008)	–	109	5 (4.6)	5 (4.6)	4/1	–	[57]
	Morocco	2008-	H	Human	Nasal swab	Disk diffusion	CA-SFM (2007)	–	81	0 (0)	0 (0)	–	–	[62]
	Tunisia	2008–2009	C	Human	Nasal swab	Disk diffusion	CLSI (2008)	–	55	0 (0)	0 (0)	–	–	[41]

Table 2 Characteristics of the 43 eligible studies on screening for mupirocin resistance in *Staphylococcus aureus* from various sources in Africa *(Continued)*

Region	Country	Study Period	Setting	Sample		Method for testing resistance to mupirocin	Guideline (year of publication)	Published reports for detection of mupR *S. aureus*	Number of *S. aureus* isolates screened with mupirocin	Mupirocin resistant isolates				Reference
				Source	Type					Number (%)	Number MRSA (%)	Number LmupR/ HmupR	Number *mupA* gene + LMupR/HmupR (Method)	
	Tunisia	2003–2005	C	Human	Pus, blood, articular puncture, venous catheter	Phoenix Automated Microbiology System	CA-SFM (2006)	–	64	NA	NA	–	–	[59]
	Tunisia	2013	H	Human	Wound abscess	Disk diffusion	CA-SFM (2013)	–	8	NA	NA	–	–	[60]
	Tunisia	2010	C	Animal (Sheep)	Nasal swab	Disk diffusion	CLSI (2010)	–	73	0 (0)	0 (0)	–	–	[42]
	Tunisia	2010	C	Animal (Donkeys)	Nasal swab	Disk diffusion	CLSI (2010)	–	50	0 (0)	0 (0)	–	–	[43]
West Africa	Ghana	2011–2012	H	Human	Nasal swab	Disk diffusion	EUCAST (2012)	–	105	1 (0.9)	0 (0)	0/1	–	[54]
	Ghana	2011–2012	C	Human	Nasal swab	Disk diffusion	EUCAST (2012)	–	124	0 (0)	0 (0)	–	–	[67]
	Ghana	2010–2013	C & H	Human	NA	Broth microdilution	EUCAST (NA)	–	30	4 (13.3)	4 (13.3)	4/0	0/0 (DNA microarray)	[55]
	Ghana	2012–2013	C	Human	Nasal & Wound swab	VITEK-2	EUCAST (NA)	–	91	0 (0)	0 (0)	–	–	[68]
	Nigeria*	NA	NA	Human	NA	Disk diffusion	NA	–	1	0 (0)	0 (0)	–	–	[80]
	Nigeria*	2002–2004	H	Human	Wound, blood, ear, eye, urine	Disk diffusion	–	Udo et al., (1999)	200	1 (0.5)	0 (0)	0/1	0/1 (PCR)	[53]
	Nigeria	2006	C	Human	Nasal swab	Disk diffusion	CLSI (2005)	–	101	12 (11.9)	NA	NA	–	[44]
	Nigeria	2007	H	Human	NA	Disk diffusion	CLSI (NA)	–	96	0 (0)	0 (0)	–	–	[48]
	Nigeria*	NA	H	Human	Wound swab, blood, urine, endotracheal aspirate	Disk diffusion E-test	NCCLS (2003)	–	1	1	0 (0)	0/1	0/1 (PCR)	[45]
	Nigeria	2009	H	Human	Wound, sputum, semen, nasal swab	Broth microdilution	DIN 58940 (2004)	–	68	0 (0)	0 (0)	–	–	[63]
	Nigeria	2010	H	Human	NA	VITEK-2	–	–	51	0 (0)	0 (0)	–	–	[64]
	Nigeria	2009–2011	H	Human	Aspirate, blood, ear, eye, vaginal discharge, sputum, wounds, urine, nasal swab	Disk diffusion	CLSI (NA)	–	62	0 (0)	0 (0)	–	–	[49]

Table 2 Characteristics of the 43 eligible studies on screening for mupirocin resistance in *Staphylococcus aureus* from various sources in Africa *(Continued)*

Region	Country	Study Period	Setting	Sample		Method for testing resistance to mupirocin	Guideline (year of publication)	Published reports for detection of mupR *S. aureus*	Number of *S. aureus* isolates screened with mupirocin	Mupirocin resistant isolates				Reference
				Source	Type					Number (%)	Number MRSA (%)	Number LmupR/ HmupR	Number *mupA* gene + LMupR/HmupR (Method)	
	Nigeria	2010–2011	H	Human	NA	VITEK-2	EUCAST (NA)	–	290	0 (0)	0 (0)	–	–	[65]
	Nigeria	2008–2010	C	Animal (Bats)	Faecal swab	Disk diffusion	–	Udo et al., (1999)	107	0 (0)	0 (0)	–	–	[66]
	Nigeria	2006–2007	C & H	Animal (Bovine) & (Ovine)	Nasal & skin swab	Disk diffusion	–	Udo et al., (1999)	173	0 (0)	0 (0)	–	–	[35]
	Nigeria	2012	C	Human Animal	Nasal swab Milk	Disk diffusion	CLSI (2006)	–	10 Humans 77 Animals	33 (37.9)	NA	0/33	–	[36]
Central Africa	Gabon	2009	C & H	Human	Nasal, axillae, inguinal swab	VITEK-2	–	–	5	0 (0)	0 (0)	–	–	[69]
	São Tomé & Príncipe	2010–2012	H	Human	Nasal swab	Disk diffusion	BSAC (NA)	–	55	0 (0)	0 (0)	–	–	[70]
East Africa	Ethiopia	NA	H & R	Cockroach	Cockroach Body surface/Gut	Disk diffusion	–	Jorgenson et al., (1999)	17	17 (100)	NA	NA	–	[37]
	Kenya	2011	H	Human	Nasal and axillary skin swab	VITEK-2	CLSI (2012)	–	86	0 (0)	0 (0)	–	–	[71]
	Kenya	2011–2013	H	Human	Pus, blood, urine	VITEK-2	CLSI (2010)	–	731	0 (0)	0 (0)	–	–	[72]
	Kenya	NA	C	Animal (Camel)	Raw camel milk	Disk diffusion Broth microdilution	CLSI (2008)	–	47	0 (0)	0 (0)	–	–	[38]
South Africa	South Africa	1996	H	Human	Wound, urine, skin and blood	Disk diffusion	NCCLS (2000)	–	236	5 (2.1)	NA	NA	–	[46]
	South Africa**	2001–2003	H	Human	Wound, sputum, blood	Disk diffusion	–	Udo et al., (1999)	227	16 (7.0)	15 (6.6)	14/2	0/2 (PCR)	[50]
	South Africa	2005–2006	H	Human	Blood, pus & skin wound, cerebrospinal fluid	Disk diffusion E-test	–	Udo et al., (2006)	248	123 (49.6)	123 (49.6)	117/6	–	[32]
	South Africa**	NA	H	Human	Wound swab, blood, urine, endotracheal aspirate	Disk diffusion E-test	NCCLS (2003)	–	16	16 (100)	14 (87.5)	14/2	0/2 (PCR)	[45]
	South Africa	2013	H	Human	Tissue, blood, cerebrospinal fluid, wound swab	Disk diffusion VITEK-2	CLSI (2012)	–	997	277 (27.8)	NA	43/234	0/5 (Real time PCR)	[33]

Table 2 Characteristics of the 43 eligible studies on screening for mupirocin resistance in *Staphylococcus aureus* from various sources in Africa *(Continued)*

Region	Country	Study Period	Setting	Sample		Method for testing resistance to mupirocin	Guideline (year of publication)	Published reports for detection of mupR *S. aureus*	Number of *S. aureus* isolates screened with mupirocin	Mupirocin resistant isolates				Reference
				Source	Type					Number (%)	Number MRSA (%)	Number LmupR/ HmupR	Number *mupA* gene + LMupR/HmupR (Method)	
	South Africa	2010–2012	H	Human	Blood	Microscan (MIC Panel Type 33)	CLSI (2015)	–	2709	236 (8.7)	202 (7.5)	NA	–	[51]
	South Africa	2009–2010	H	Human & Environment	Nasal & hand swab, dialysate fluid, surface swab, air samples	VITEK-2	–	–	13	4 (30.8)	4 (30.8)	0/4	–	[34]

KEY: mupR *S. aureus*: mupirocin resistant *Staphylococcus aureus*; *LmupR* low-level mupirocin resistance, *HmupR* high-level mupirocin resistance, *mupA* mupirocin resistance gene, *MIC* Minimum inhibitory concentration, *BSAC* British Society for Antimicrobial Chemotherapy, *CA-SFM* Comité de l'Antibiogramme de la Société Française de Microbiologie, *CLSI* Clinical and Laboratory Standards Institute, *DIN 58940* Deutsches Institut für Normung DIN 58940, *EUCAST* European Committee on Antimicrobial Susceptibility Testing, *NCCLS* National Committee for Clinical Laboratory Standards, *PCR* Polymerase Chain Reaction; – Not determined, *NA* Not available, *H* Hospital, *C* Community, *R* Restaurant

*Separate reports that analyzed the same isolates but answered different questions (considered as one single study) in Nigeria; **: Separate reports that analyzed the same isolates but answered different questions (considered as one single study) in South Africa.

Reference [45] is recorded in Nigeria and South Africa, but the isolates were derived from studies in Nigeria [53] and South Africa [50], respectively

Other published reports applied for the detection of mupR *S. aureus* in Africa

1. Jorgenson JH, Turnidge JD, Washington JA. Dilution and disc diffusion method. In: Murray PR, Baron EJ, Pfaller MA, Tenover FC, Yolken RH, editors. Manual of Clinical Microbiology, 7th edition. American Society for Microbiology, Washington DC, 1999. p. 1526–1543. Adapted from NCCLS: National Committee for Clinical Laboratory Standards 1997. Approved Standard M2-A6; National Committee for Clinical Laboratory Standards 1999. Approved Standard M100-S9.
2. Kresken M, Hafner D, Schmitz FJ, Wichelhaus TA. Prevalence of mupirocin resistance in clinical isolates of *Staphylococcus aureus* and *Staphylococcus epidermidis*. Results of the antimicrobial resistance surveillance study of the Paul-Ehrlich Society for Chemotherapy, 2001. Int J Antimicrob Agents, 2004, 23:577–81. The widely accepted breakpoints: ≤4 mg/l (susceptible), 8–256 mg/l (low-level resistance) and ≥ 512 mg/l (high-level resistance) was utilized in this study.
3. Udo EE, Farook VS, Mokadas EM, Jacob LE, Sanyal SC. Molecular fingerprinting of mupirocin-resistant methicillin-resistant *Staphylococcus aureus* from a burn unit. Int J Infect Dis, 1999,3:82–7. Growth within a 14-mm zone of inhibition with the 5 μg mupirocin disk detected low-level resistance, while growth to the edge of the 200 μg mupirocin disk indicated high-level resistance.
4. Udo EE, Al-Sweih N, Mokaddas E, Johny M, Dhar R, Gomaa HH, Al-Obaid I, Rotimi VO. Antibacterial resistance and their genetic location in MRSA isolated in Kuwait hospitals, 1994–2004. BMC Infect Dis, 2006;6:168. The widely accepted breakpoints:≤4 mg/l (susceptible), 8–256 mg/l (low-level resistance) and ≥ 512 mg/l (high-level resistance) was utilized in this study.

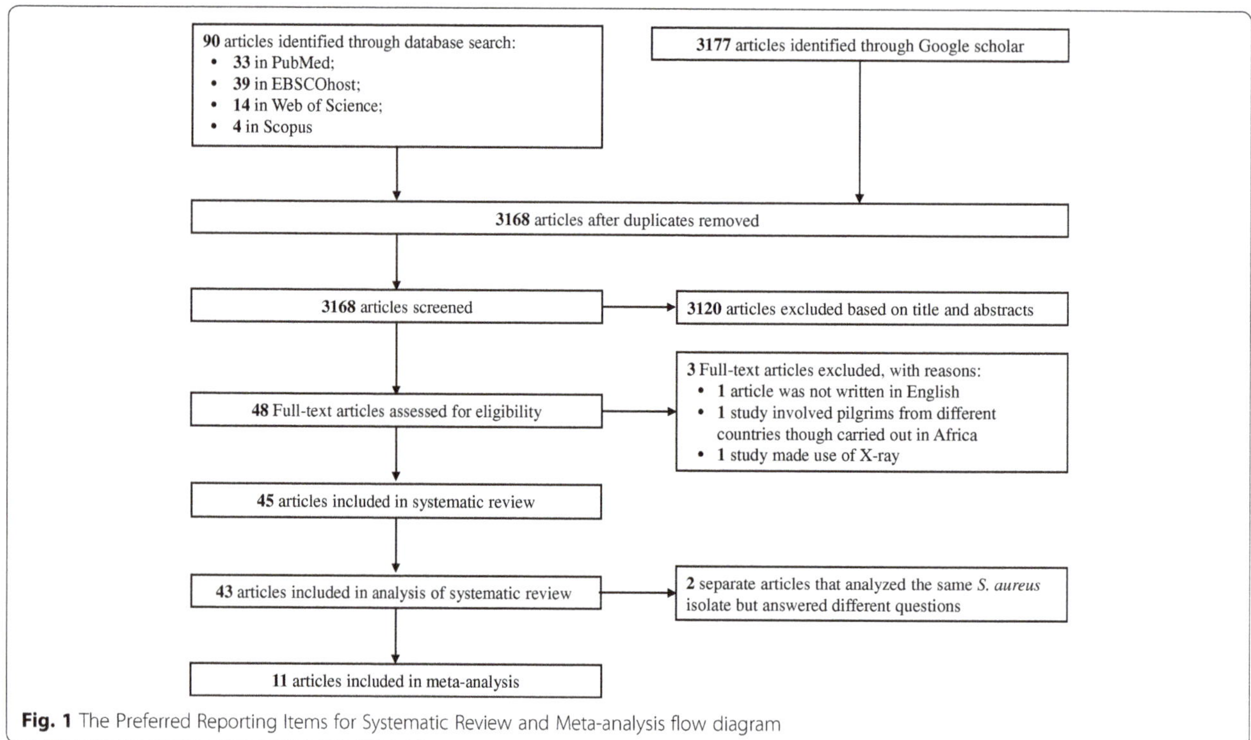

Fig. 1 The Preferred Reporting Items for Systematic Review and Meta-analysis flow diagram

Institute (CLSI), previously known as National Committee for Clinical Laboratory Standards (NCCLS), were broadly used in Africa (Table 2). However, a number of studies [28, 29, 31, 33, 36, 40–46] utilized the disk diffusion method with CLSI guidelines that had no zone diameter breakpoint for mupirocin. Moreover, some studies [47–49] did not provide information on the year of publication of the CLSI guidelines. MupR *S. aureus* was reported in six African countries including South Africa [32–34, 46, 50, 51], Egypt [29–31, 52], Nigeria [36, 44, 53], Ghana [54, 55], Libya [56, 57] and Ethiopia [37] (Fig. 2; Table 2). The *mupA*-positive *S. aureus* was detected in five studies from Egypt [30, 52], South Africa [33, 50] and Nigeria [53]. LmupR and HmupR were both reported in six human studies conducted in South Africa [32, 33, 50], Egypt [30, 52] and Libya [57]. The

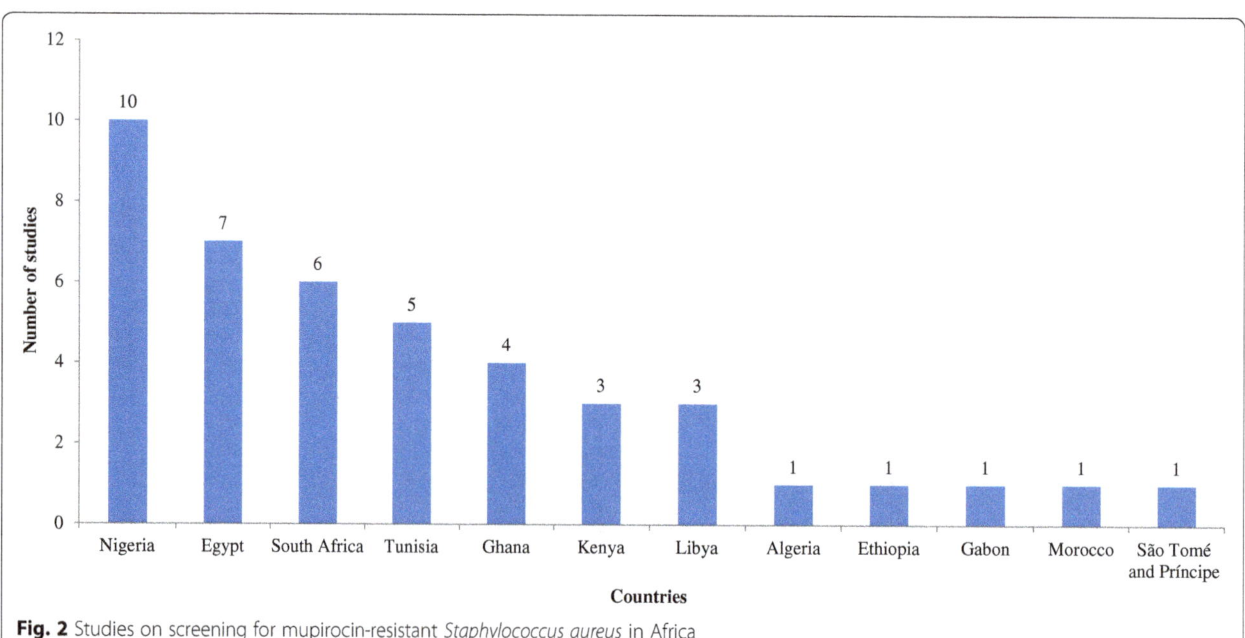

Fig. 2 Studies on screening for mupirocin-resistant *Staphylococcus aureus* in Africa

Table 3 Prevalence of mupirocin-resistant *S. aureus* from various sources in Africa based on phenotypic and molecular methods

Mupirocin resistance	Country	Source	Number positive/Total tested (%)	Phenotypic						Molecular		Guidelines or reports				Reference
				Agar Dilution	Broth microdilution	Disk diffusion	E-test	Microscan system	VITEK	PCR	Micro array	BSAC	CLSI	EUCAST	Other reports	
MupA-positive *S. aureus*	Egypt	Human	5/86 (5.8)	–	–	–	√	–	–	√	–	–	–	–	√[a]	[30]
	Egypt	Human	6/73 (8.2)	√	–	–	–	–	–	√	–	–	√	–	–	[52]
	Nigeria	Human	1/200 (0.5)	–	–	√	–	–	–	√	–	–	–	–	√[b]	[53]
	South Africa	Human	2/227 (0.9)	–	–	√	–	–	–	√	–	–	–	–	√[b]	[50]
	South Africa	Human	NA	–	–	√	–	–	√	√	–	–	√	–	–	[33]
LmupR *S. aureus*	Egypt	Human	25/86 (29.1)	–	–	–	√	–	–	√	–	–	–	–	√[a]	[30]
	Egypt	Human	5/73 (6.8)	√	–	–	–	–	–	√	–	–	√	–	–	[52]
	Ghana	Human	4/30 (13.3)	–	√	–	–	–	–	–	√	–	–	√	–	[55]
	Libya	Human	4/109 (3.7)	√	–	√	–	–	–	–	–	√	–	–	–	[57]
	South Africa	Human	14/227 (6.2)	–	–	√	–	–	–	–	–	–	–	–	√[b]	[50]
	South Africa	Human	117/248 (47.2)	–	–	√	√	–	–	–	–	–	–	–	√[c]	[32]
	South Africa	Human	43/997 (4.3)	–	–	√	–	–	√	–	–	–	√	–	–	[33]
	South Africa	Human & Environment	4/13 (30.8)	–	–	–	–	–	√	–	–	–	–	–	–	[34]
HmupR *S. aureus*	Egypt	Human	5/86 (5.8)	–	–	–	√	–	–	√	–	–	–	–	√[a]	[30]
	Egypt	Human	8/73 (11)	√	–	–	–	–	–	√	–	–	√	–	–	[52]
	Ghana	Human	1/105 (1.0)	–	–	√	–	–	–	–	–	–	–	√	–	[54]
	Libya	Human	1/109 (0.9)	√	–	√	–	–	–	–	–	√	–	–	–	[57]
	Nigeria	Human	1/200 (0.5)	–	–	√	–	–	–	√	–	–	–	–	√[b]	[53]
	Nigeria	Human	12/101 (11.9)	–	–	√	–	–	–	–	–	–	√	–	–	[44]
	Nigeria	Human & Animal	33/87 (37.9)	–	–	√	–	–	–	–	–	–	√	–	–	[36]
	South Africa	Human	2/227 (0.9)	–	–	√	–	–	–	√	–	–	–	–	√[b]	[50]
	South Africa	Human	6/248 (2.4)	–	–	√	√	–	–	–	–	–	–	–	√[c]	[32]
	South Africa	Human	234/997 (23.5)	–	–	√	–	–	√	–	–	–	√	–	–	[33]
mupR-MRSA	Egypt	Human	30/86 (34.9)	–	–	–	√	–	–	√	–	–	–	–	√[a]	[30]
	Egypt	Human	3/39 (7.7)	–	–	√	–	–	–	–	–	–	√	–	–	[31]
	Egypt	Human	13/73 (17.8)	√	–	–	–	–	–	√	–	–	√	–	–	[52]
	Ghana	Human	4/30 (13.3)	–	√	–	–	–	–	–	√	–	–	√	–	[55]
	Libya	Human	13/86 (15.1)	–	–	√	–	–	–	–	–	√	–	–	–	[56]
	Libya	Human	5/109 (4.6)	√	–	√	–	–	–	–	–	√	–	–	–	[57]
	Nigeria	Human & Animal	33/87 (37.9)	–	–	√	–	–	–	–	–	–	√	–	–	[36]
	South Africa	Human	15/227 (6.6)	–	–	√	–	–	–	√	–	–	–	–	√[b]	[50]

Table 3 Prevalence of mupirocin-resistant *S. aureus* from various sources in Africa based on phenotypic and molecular methods *(Continued)*

Mupirocin resistance	Country	Source	Number positive/Total tested (%)	Phenotypic						Molecular		Guidelines or reports				Reference
				Agar Dilution	Broth microdilution	Disk diffusion	E-test	Microscan system	VITEK	PCR	Micro array	BSAC	CLSI	EUCAST	Other reports	
	South Africa	Human	123/248 (49.6)	–	–	√	√	–	–	–	–	–	–	–	√[c]	[32]
	South Africa	Human	202/2709 (7.5)	–	–	–	–	√	–	–	–	–	√	√	–	[51]
	South Africa	Human & Environment	4/13 (30.8)	–	–	–	–	–	√	–	–	–	–	–	–	[34]

KEY: *BSAC* British Society for Antimicrobial Chemotherapy, *CLSI* Clinical and Laboratory Standards Institute, *EUCAST* European Committee on Antimicrobial Susceptibility Testing, *NA* Not Available, *PCR* Polymerase Chain Reaction, √: test was performed. -: test was not performed

[a]The widely accepted breakpoints: ≤4 mg/l (susceptible), 8–256 mg/l (low-level resistance) and ≥ 512 mg/l (high-level resistance) was utilized in this study: Kresken M, Hafner D, Schmitz FJ, Wichelhaus TA. Prevalence of mupirocin resistance in clinical isolates of *Staphylococcus aureus* and *Staphylococcus epidermidis*. Results of the antimicrobial resistance surveillance study of the Paul-Ehrlich Society for Chemotherapy, 2001. Int J Antimicrob Agents, 2004, 23:577–81. [b]Growth within a 14-mm zone of inhibition with the 5 μg mupirocin disk detected low-level resistance, while growth to the edge of the 200 μg mupirocin disk indicated high-level resistance according to: Udo EE, Farook VS, Mokadas EM, Jacob LE, Sanyal SC. Molecular fingerprinting of mupirocin-resistant methicillin-resistant *Staphylococcus aureus* from a burn unit. Int J Infect Dis, 1999,3:82–7.

[c]The widely accepted breakpoints: ≤4 mg/l (susceptible), 8–256 mg/l (low-level resistance) and ≥ 512 mg/l (high-level resistance) was utilized in this study: Udo EE, Al-Sweih N, Mokaddas E, Johny M, Dhar R, Gomaa HH, Al-Obaid I, Rotimi VO. Antibacterial resistance and their genetic location in MRSA isolated in Kuwait hospitals, 1994–2004. BMC Infect Dis, 2006;6:168

mupR-MRSA isolates were identified in South Africa [32, 34, 50, 51], Egypt [30, 31, 52], Libya [56, 57], Ghana [55] and Nigeria [36] (Table 3). MupR-MRSA was not reported from MRSA isolates recovered from studies conducted in Egypt [28, 58], Tunisia [59, 60] and Algeria [47].

An assessment of data on mupR *S. aureus* at the regional level is described as follows (Fig. 3).

North Africa

Seventeen eligible studies were recorded from this region, including Egypt [28–31, 40, 52, 58], Tunisia [41–43, 59, 60], Libya [56, 57, 61], Algeria [47] and Morocco [62]. MupR *S. aureus* was reported in six studies conducted in two North African countries: Egypt [29–31, 52] and Libya [56, 57]. PCR detection of the *mupA* gene was performed in only two studies conducted in Egypt [30, 52]. In addition, one of the reports identified two *mupA* positive MRSA that exhibited LmupR [30]. MupR *S. aureus* was not detected in Tunisia [41–43, 59, 60], Algeria [47], and Morocco [62].

West Africa

S. aureus resistance to mupirocin was investigated in Nigeria [35, 36, 44, 48, 49, 53, 63–66] and Ghana [54, 55, 67, 68]. Only two studies from Ghana reported on mupR *S. aureus* [54, 55]. In Nigeria, three studies (including two from only human sources and one from both animal and human samples, respectively) reported on *S. aureus* isolates that demonstrated HmupR [36, 44, 53].

Central Africa

MupR *S. aureus* was not detected in studies conducted in Gabon [69], and São Tomé and Príncipe [70].

East Africa

In this review, we identified four eligible studies conducted in Kenya [38, 71, 72] and Ethiopia [37]. A report on the role of cockroaches as potential vectors of foodborne pathogens in Ethiopia identified 17 mupR *S. aureus* isolates [37]. All the *S. aureus* isolates (one animal and two human studies) from Kenya were susceptible to mupirocin [38, 71, 72].

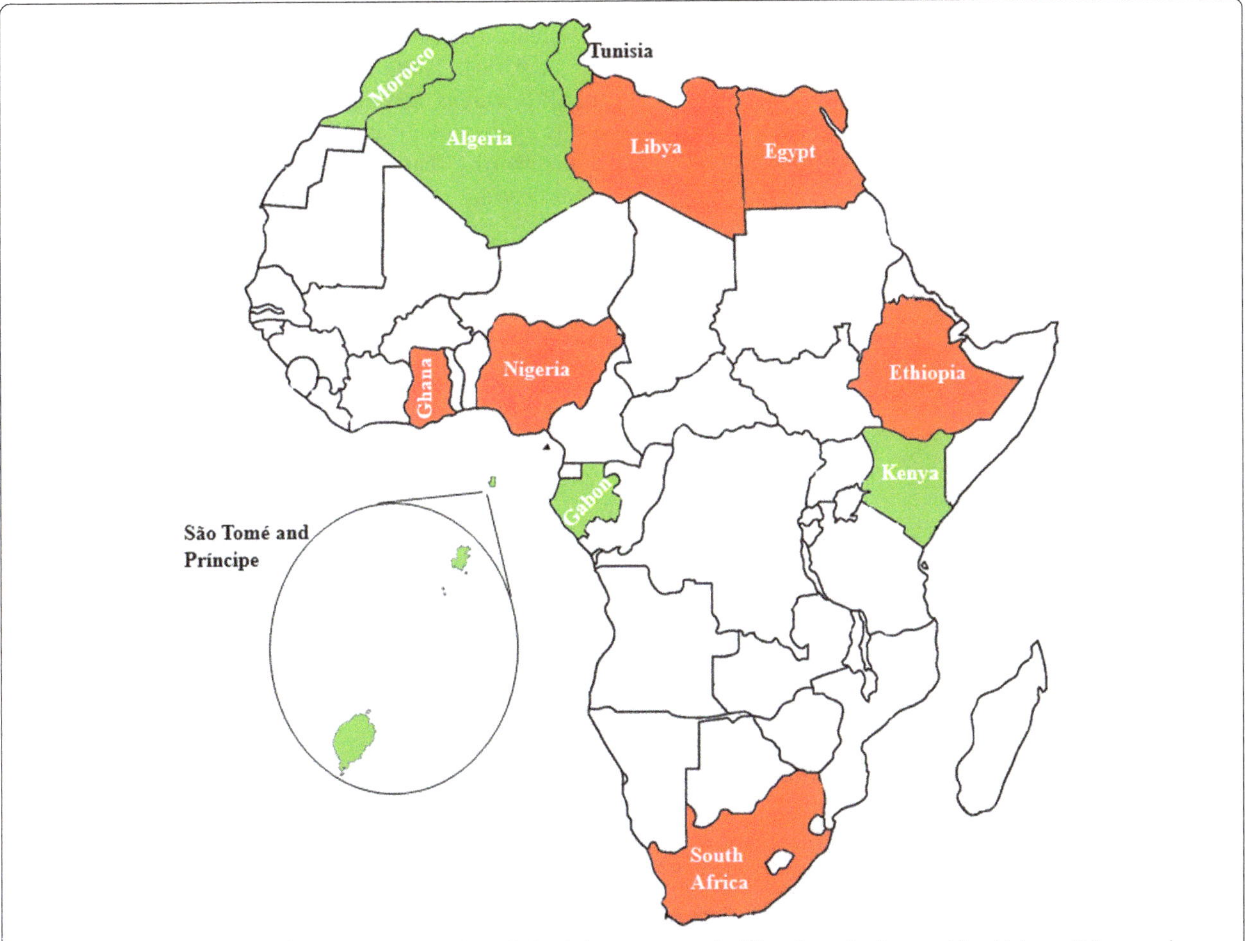

Fig. 3 Geographic distribution of mupirocin-resistant (mupR) *Staphylococcus aureus* in Africa. Countries (in green) in which mupR *S. aureus* have been investigated but not reported. Countries (in red) in which mupR *S. aureus* have been investigated and reported

Southern Africa

The six studies reported in this geographical area were from South Africa and consisted of two single centre studies [34, 46] and four multicenter studies [32, 33, 50, 51]. MupR *S. aureus* was identified in all the reports, while *mupA*-positive *S. aureus* isolates were noted in only two studies [33, 50].

Prevalence of mupR *S. aureus* in Africa

The random-effects pooled prevalence of mupR *S. aureus* in Africa is 14% (95% CI =6.8 to 23.2%). This was calculated based on 11 heterogeneous human studies (Figs. 4 and 5) conducted in South Africa [32, 33, 50, 51], Ghana [54, 55], Egypt [30, 52], Libya [56, 57] and Nigeria [53]. In Africa, the proportion of *S. aureus* isolates with the *mupA* gene, and those that expressed LmupR and HmupR ranged between 0.5 and 8%, 4 and 47%, 0.5 and 38%, respectively. The frequency of mupR-MRSA isolates ranged between 5 and 50% (Table 3).

Association of MupR *S. aureus* with mupirocin use in Africa

There is no data on the use of mupirocin as an agent for *S. aureus* decolonization and its association with mupR *S. aureus* in Africa.

MupR *S. aureus* and biofilm production

A report from Egypt noted that mupR-MRSA were moderate to strong biofilm producers [52].

MupR *S. aureus* and co-resistance to other antibiotics

In this systematic review, two studies (conducted in Egypt and South Africa) showed that mupR *S. aureus* was associated with multi-drug resistance [30, 33].

Molecular characterization of mupR *S. aureus* in Africa

Only three studies provided molecular data on mupR *S. aureus* in Africa [45, 54, 55]. A report provided evidence of a 35 kb (non-conjugative) and 41.1 kb (conjugative) plasmid encoding *mupA* in *S. aureus* isolates from Nigeria and South Africa [45]. It also described an MRSA clone that demonstrated LmupR in South Africa. LmupR was also identified among MRSA isolates assigned with ST36, ST88, and ST789 in Ghana [55]. A cross-sectional *S. aureus* study identified a methicillin susceptible *S. aureus* (MSSA) strain with HmupR from a 51-year-old hospital staff in Ghana [54]. Molecular characterization indicated that the strain (*spa* type t4805) was PVL-positive.

Discussion

This is the first systematic review on mupR *S. aureus* in Africa and clearly showed the paucity of data on the continent. Nevertheless, this study indicated a high prevalence ((14% (95% CI =6.8 to 23.2)) of mupR *S. aureus* in Africa. These observations support the need for mupR *S. aureus* surveillance data to provide information on its epidemiology and clinical significance in Africa. It is noteworthy that Google Scholar was valuable in the identification of several eligible studies [28–38]. We

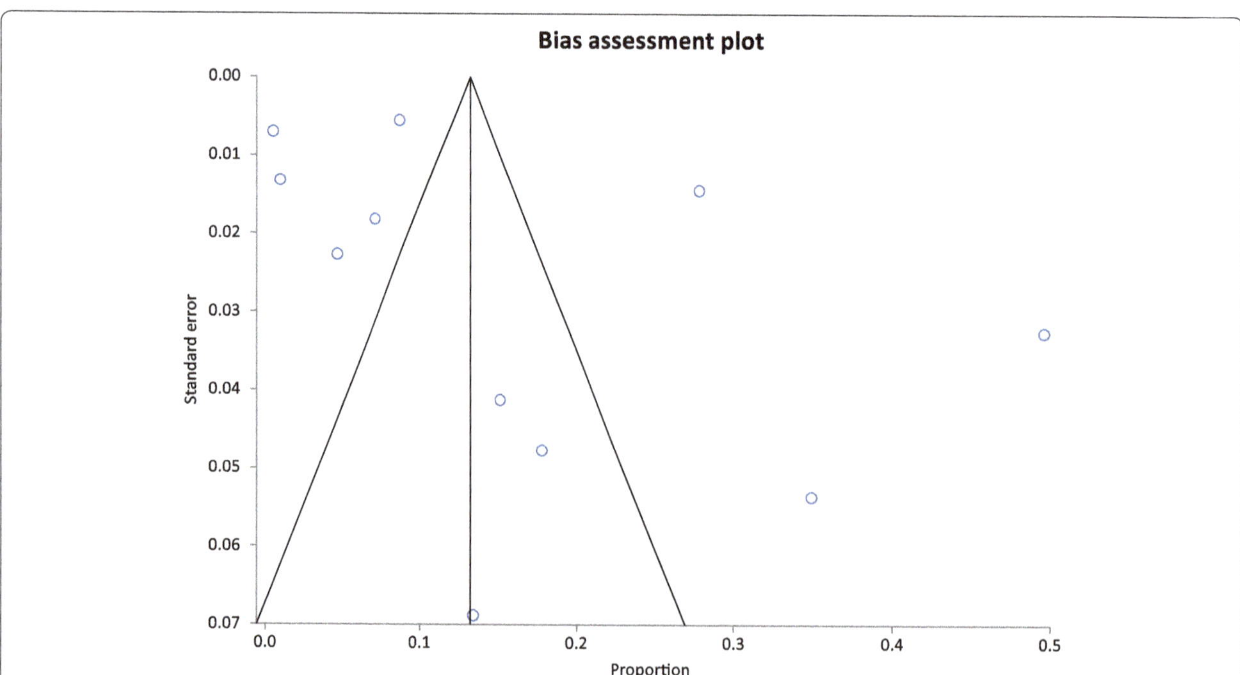

Fig. 4 Bias assessment (Funnel) plot for studies assessing rates of mupirocin-resistant *Staphylococcus aureus* in Africa. Random effects (DerSimonian-Laird). Pooled proportion = 0.139303 (95% CI = 0.067511 to 0.23165). Bias indicators, Begg-Mazumdar: Kendall's tau = 0.2 $P = 0.4454$, Egger: bias = 4.771137 (95% CI = −2.517874 to 12.060148) $P = 0.1728$, Harbord: bias = 2.014783 (92.5% CI = −5.90181 to 9.931377) $P = 0.6208$

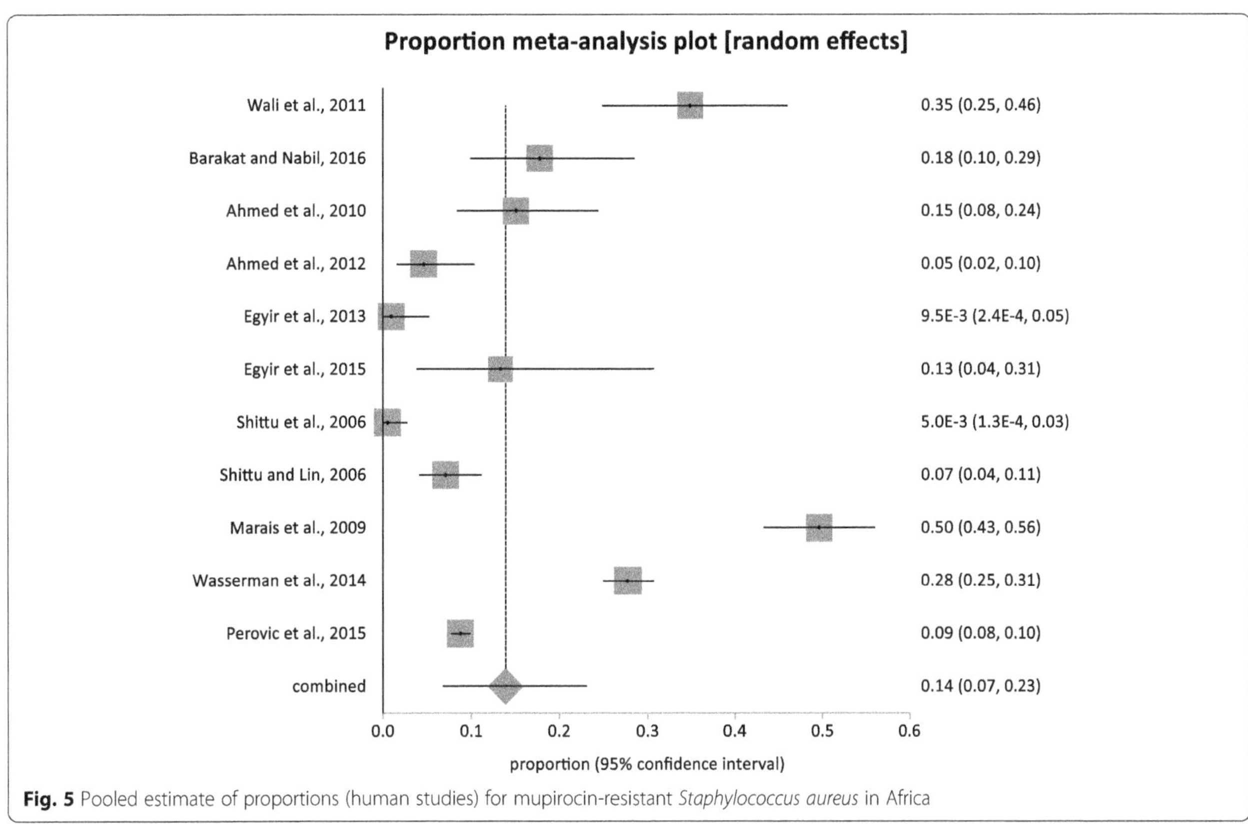

Fig. 5 Pooled estimate of proportions (human studies) for mupirocin-resistant *Staphylococcus aureus* in Africa

observed that 26% (11/43) of the eligible studies were identified from African journals which were not indexed in commonly used electronic databases. Google Scholar has been considered as a useful supplement with other electronic databases for systematic review search [73] including recent meta-analyses of published studies on *S. aureus* in Africa [74, 75].

The phenotypic methods for the screening and identification of mupR *S. aureus* include disc diffusion (two-disc strategy: 5 μg and 200 μg), agar dilution, broth micro-dilution and E-test [19]. In this study, the disk diffusion method and the CLSI (formerly NCCLS) guidelines were strategies mainly applied to detect mupR *S. aureus* in Africa. However, we observed certain inconsistencies [28, 29, 31, 33, 36, 40–49]. For instance, a number of studies [28, 29, 31, 33, 36, 40–42, 44–46] applied the disk diffusion method with the CLSI guidelines that had no breakpoint values for mupirocin. The 2017 CLSI guidelines recommend the use of the 200 μg disk to differentiate between HmupR and the absence of HmupR (i.e. no zone = HmupR; any zone = absence of HmupR) [76]. The 200 μg disk with a different breakpoint (Susceptible ≥30 mm, Resistance < 18 mm) is also endorsed for the differentiation between HmupR and the absence of HmupR in the latest versions (accessed 28th May, 2018) of the European Committee for Antimicrobial Susceptibility Testing (EUCAST) and Comité de l'antibiogramme de la Société Française de Microbiologie (CA-SFM) [77, 78]. The breakpoint values for the detection of LmupR and differentiation from HmupR are not provided in these documents (CA-SFM, CLSI, and EUCAST). Despite this limitation, the disk diffusion method in conjunction with any of these guidelines could at least be valuable for the preliminary screening and identification of HmupR *S. aureus* in Africa. MRSA decolonization failure is of clinical significance as it is often attributed to persistence or re-colonization associated with isolates exhibiting HmupR, while that of LmupR is not clear [7, 19, 79]. In this review, the prevalence of *S. aureus* that exhibited LmupR, HmupR and mupR-MRSA in Africa was predicated on a range of methods using different guidelines. We suggest that surveillance data from Africa is established on harmonized guidelines to enhance quality assurance and comparison at the continental and global level.

We noted a prevalence of mupR-MRSA ranging between 5 and 50% in Africa (Table 3). This is of serious concern. Specifically, the relationship between mupirocin resistance and MRSA has important consequences on infection control measures and effectiveness of decolonization strategies [8]. MupR-MRSA could limit the choices available for the control and prevention of healthcare-associated MRSA infections (7, 8). Therefore, surveillance studies are important to investigate the emergence and spread of mupirocin resistance in hospital settings in Africa. This is important among patients at high risk of MRSA infections, including patients in the dermatology, dialysis and the Intensive Care Units. In addition, there is the need for more data on the molecular characterization of mupR *S. aureus* in Africa [45, 54, 55]. For instance, whole genome sequencing (WGS) will assist in understanding the transmission dynamics of mupR *S. aureus* in Africa. Moreover, WGS data will allow comprehensive investigation of the genetic basis for LmupR mutation (which is largely due to V588F and V631F in the native gene (*ile*S)) and *mupB*-positive *S. aureus* in Africa.

Language bias was the main limitation of this systematic review as we did not include studies published in French, Portuguese, Arabic and Spanish.

Conclusions

This study showed the need for more epidemiological data to understand the transmission, burden and risk factors associated with mupR *S. aureus* in Africa. In addition, there is a need for data on administration and use of mupirocin in community and hospital setting in Africa. This is important in antibiotic stewardship to mitigate the emergence and spread of mupR *S. aureus* in Africa. Finally, this systematic review highlighted the need for harmonized guidelines to facilitate the comparison of data on mupR *S. aureus* from Africa.

Abbreviation

HmupR: High-level mupirocin resistance; LmupR: Low-level mupirocin resistance; MIC: Minimum inhibitory concentration; MRSA: Methicillin-resistant *Staphylococcus aureus*; MSSA: Methicillin-susceptible *S. aureus*; mupR: Mupirocin-resistant; PCR: Polymerase chain reaction; PVL: Panton Valentine Leucocidin; *S. aureus*: *Staphylococcus aureus*; ST: Sequence type

Acknowledgments

SMA was supported by the Organization for Women in Science in the Developing World (OWSD). AOS received funding through the Deutscher Akademischer Austausch Dienst (DAAD award) Staff Exchange Programme (2016). MK was a Wellcome Trust (UK) Fellow (102429/Z/13/Z). His research is currently supported by the Carnegie Corporation of New York (USA) early-career fellowship, the CIHR CTN International Fellowship (Canada), and the US National Institutes of Health (1R01HD093578-01). We appreciate the kind assistance of Oluwafemi Daramola in the preparation of the manuscript.

Funding

This review received support through the Deutscher Akademischer Austausch Dienst (DAAD award) Staff Exchange Programme (2016). However, the opinions expressed in this review are that of the authors.

Authors' contributions

AOS conceived the project. YOA, SMA and AOS extracted the data and reviewed the articles. MOA and AOO wrote the initial draft of the manuscript. AOS, SMA, YOA, and MK wrote the subsequent draft. All the authors reviewed and agreed on the final version of the manuscript before submission for publication.

Consent for publication

Not applicable.

Competing interests

The authors declare that there are no competing interests.

Author details

[1]Department of Microbiology, Obafemi Awolowo University, Ile-Ife, Osun State 22005, Nigeria. [2]Division of Medical Microbiology, Department of Pathology, Faculty of Health Sciences, University of Cape Town, Cape Town, South Africa. [3]Institute of Infectious Disease and Molecular Medicine, Faculty of Health Sciences, University of Cape Town, Cape Town, South Africa.

References

1. Lowy FD. *Staphylococcus aureus* infections. N Engl J Med. 1998;339:520–32.
2. Levy PY, Ollivier M, Drancourt M, Raoult D, Argenson JN. Relation between nasal carriage of *Staphylococcus aureus* and surgical site infection in orthopedic surgery: the role of nasal contamination. A systematic literature review and meta-analysis. Orthop Traumatol Surg Res. 2013;99:645–51. https://doi.org/10.1016/j.otsr.2013.03.030.
3. Totté JE, van der Feltz WT, Hennekam M, van Belkum A, van Zuuren EJ, Pasmans SG. Prevalence and odds of *Staphylococcus aureus* carriage in atopic dermatitis: a systematic review and meta-analysis. Br J Dermatol. 2016;175:687–95. https://doi.org/10.1111/bjd.14566.
4. Zacharioudakis IM, Zervou FN, Ziakas PD, Mylonakis E. Meta-analysis of methicillin-resistant *Staphylococcus aureus* colonization and risk of infection in dialysis patients. J Am Soc Nephrol. 2014;25:2131–41. https://doi.org/10.1681/ASN.2013091028.
5. Ziakas PD, Anagnostou T, Mylonakis E. The prevalence and significance of methicillin-resistant *Staphylococcus aureus* colonization at admission in the general ICU setting: a meta-analysis of published studies. Crit Care Med. 2014;42:433–44. https://doi.org/10.1097/CCM.0b013e3182a66bb8.
6. Wertheim HF, Melles DC, Vos MC, van Leeuwen W, van Belkum A, Verbrugh HA, Nouwen JL. The role of nasal carriage in *Staphylococcus aureus* infections. Lancet Infect Dis. 2005;5:751–62. https://doi.org/10.1016/S1473-3099(05)70295-4.
7. Septimus EJ, Schweizer ML. Decolonization in prevention of health-care associated infections. Clin Microbiol Rev. 2016;29:201–22. https://doi.org/10.1128/CMR.00049-15.
8. Poovelikunnel T, Gethin G, Humphreys H. Mupirocin resistance: clinical implications and potential alternatives for the eradication of MRSA. J Antimicrob Chemother. 2015;70:2681–92. https://doi.org/10.1093/jac/dkv169.
9. Global Guidelines for the prevention of surgical site infection. World Health Organization, Geneva. 2016. http://www.who.int/gpsc/ssi-prevention-guidelines/en/ Accessed 15 June 2017.
10. Fuller AT, Mellows G, Woolford M, Banks GT, Barrow KD, Chain EB. Pseudomonic acid: an antibiotic produced by *Pseudomonas fluorescens*. Nature. 1971;234:416–7.
11. Gilbart J, Perry CR, Slocombe B. High-level mupirocin resistance in *Staphylococcus aureus*: evidence for two distinct isoleucyl-tRNA synthetases. Antimicrob Agents Chemother. 1993;37:32–8.
12. Perl TM, Golub JE. New approaches to reduce *Staphylococcus aureus* nosocomial infection rates: treating *S. aureus* nasal carriage. Ann Pharmacother. 1998;32:S7–16.
13. Rahman M, Noble WC, Cookson B. Mupirocin resistant *Staphylococcus aureus*. Lancet. 1987;330:387–8. https://doi.org/10.1016/S0140-6736(87)92398-1.
14. Hughes J, Stabler R, Gaunt M, Karadag T, Desai N, Betley J, Ioannou A, Aryee A, Hearn P, Marbach H, Patel A, Otter JA, Edgeworth JD, Tosas AO. Clonal variation in high- and low-level phenotypic and genotypic mupirocin resistance of MRSA isolates in south-East London. J Antimicrob Chemother. 2015;70:3191–9. https://doi.org/10.1093/jac/dkv248.

15. Boswihi SS, Udo EE, Al-Sweih N. Shifts in the clonal distribution of methicillin-resistant *Staphylococcus aureus* in Kuwait hospitals: 1992-2010. PLoS One. 2016;11:e0162744. https://doi.org/10.1371/journal.pone.0162744.
16. Hayden MK, Lolans K, Haffenreffer K, Avery TR, Kleinman K, Li H, Kaganov RE, Lankiewicz J, Moody J, Septimus E, Weinstein RA, Hickok J, Jernigan J, Perlin JB, Platt R, Huang SS. Chlorhexidine and mupirocin susceptibility of methicillin-resistant *Staphylococcus aureus* isolates in the REDUCE-MRSA trial. J Clin Microbiol. 2016;54:2735–42.
17. Gostev V, Kruglov A, Kalinogorskaya O, Dmitrenko O, Khokhlova O, Yamamoto T, Lobzin Y, Ryabchenko I, Sidorenko S. Molecular epidemiology and antibiotic resistance of methicillin-resistant *Staphylococcus aureus* circulating in the Russian Federation. Infect Genet Evol. 2017;53:189–94. https://doi.org/10.1016/j.meegid.2017.06.006.
18. Hetem DJ, Bonten MJ. Clinical relevance of mupirocin resistance in *Staphylococcus aureus*. J Hosp Infect. 2013;85:249–56. https://doi.org/10.1016/j.jhin.2013.09.006.
19. Swenson JM, Wong B, Simor AE, Thomson RB, Ferraro MJ, Hardy DJ, Hindler J, Jorgensen J, Reller LB, Traczewski M, McDougal LK, Patel JB. Multicenter study to determine disk diffusion and broth microdilution criteria for prediction of high- and low-level mupirocin resistance in *Staphylococcus aureus*. J Clin Microbiol. 2010;48:2469–75. https://doi.org/10.1128/JCM.00340-10.
20. Antonio M, McFerran N, Pallen MJ. Mutation affecting the Rossman fold of isoleucyl-tRNA synthetase are correlated with low-level mupirocin resistance in *Staphylococcus aureus*. Antimicrob Agents Chemother. 2002;46:438–42. https://doi.org/10.1128/AAC.46.2.438-442.2002.
21. Hodgson JE, Curnock SP, Dyke KG, Morris R, Sylvester DR, Gross MS. Molecular characterization of the gene encoding high-level mupirocin resistance in *Staphylococcus aureus* J2870. Antimicrob Agents Chemother. 1994;38:1205–8. https://doi.org/10.1128/AAC.38.5.1205.
22. Seah C, Alexander DC, Louie L, Simor A, Low DE, Longtin J, Melano RG. MupB, a new high-level mupirocin resistance mechanism in *Staphylococcus aureus*. Antimicrob Agents Chemother. 2012;56:1916–20. https://doi.org/10.1128/AAC.05325-11.
23. Moher D, Liberati A, Tetzlaff J, Altman DG, PRISMA group. Preferred reporting items for systematic reviews and meta-analyses: the PRISMA statement. PLoS Med. 2009;6:e1000097. https://doi.org/10.1371/journal.pmed.1000097.
24. Cochran WG. The combination of estimates from different experiments. Biometrics. 1954;10:101–29.
25. Huggins JPT, Thompson SG, Deeks JJ, Altman DG. Measuring inconsistency in meta-analyses. BMJ. 2003;327:557–60. https://doi.org/10.1136/bmj.327.7414.557.
26. Egger M, Smith GD, Schneider M, Minder C. Bias in meta-analysis detected by a simple, graphical test. BMJ. 1997;315:629–34. https://doi.org/10.1136/bmj.315.7109.629.
27. Sterne JA, Sutton AJ, Ioannidis JP, Terrin N, Jones DR, Lau J, Carpenter J, Rücker G, Harbord RM, Schmid CH, Tetzlaff J, Deeks JJ, Peters J, Macaskill P, Schwarzer G, Duval S, Altman DG, Moher D, Higgins JP. Recommendations for examining and interpreting funnel plots assymettry in meta-analysis of randomised control trials. BMJ. 2011;342:1–8. https://doi.org/10.1136/bmj.d4002.
28. Salama MF. Comparative molecular analysis of community or health care associated methicillin-resistant *Staphylococcus aureus*. Egypt J Med Microbiol. 2006;15:371–80.
29. Taher S, Roshdy H. Prevalence of Panton-Valentine Leukocidin genes among *Staphylococcus aureus* isolates in Mansoura University hospitals. Egypt J Med Microbiol. 2009;18:97–108.
30. Wali I, Ouda N, El-Seidi E. Mupirocin resistance among methicillin resistant *Staphylococcus aureus* isolates in an Egyptian hospital. Egypt J Med Lab Sci. 2011;20:1–11.
31. Melake N, Zakaria AS, Ibrahim NH, Salama M, Mahmoud AZ. Prevalence of *agr* specificity groups among in vitro biofilm forming methicillin resistant *Staphylococcus aureus* strains isolated from nasal carriers. Int J Microbiol Res. 2014;5:76–84. https://doi.org/10.5829/idosi.ijmr.2014.5.2.83184.
32. Marais E, Aithma N, Perovic O, Oosthuyen WF, Musenge E, Dusé AG. Antimicrobial susceptibility of methicillin-resistant *Staphylococcus aureus* isolates from South Africa. S Afr Med J. 2009;99:170–3.
33. Wasserman E, Orth H, Senekal M, Harvey K. High prevalence of mupirocin resistance associated with resistance to other antimicrobial agents in *Staphylococcus aureus* isolated from patients in private health care, Western Cape. South Afr J Infect Dis. 2014;29:126–32.
34. Swe Swe K, Naidoo N, Jaglal P. Molecular epidemiology of a suspected methicillin-resistant *Staphylococcus aureus* outbreak in a renal unit of a central academic hospital in KwaZulu-Natal, South Africa. South Afr J Infect Dis. 2015;30:6–10.
35. Bamaiyi PH, Aniesona AT. Prevalence and antimicrobial susceptibility patterns of bovine and ovine *Staphylococcus aureus* isolates in Maiduguri, Nigeria. Adv Anim Vet Sci. 2013;1:59–64.
36. Mai-siyama IB, Okon KO, Adamu NB, Askira UM, Isyaka TM, Adamu SG, Mohammed A. Methicillin-resistant *Staphylococcus aureus* (MRSA) colonization rate among ruminant animals slaughtered for human consumption and contact persons in Maiduguri, Nigeria. Afr J Microbiol Res. 2014;8:2643–9. https://doi.org/10.5897/AJMR2014.6855.
37. Tachbele E, Erku W, Gebre-Michael T, Ashenafi M. Cockroach-associated food-borne bacterial pathogens from some hospitals and restaurants in Addis Ababa, Ethiopia: Distribution and antibiograms. JRTPH. 2006;5:34–41.
38. Njage PMK, Dolci S, Jans C, Wangoh J, Lacroix C, Meile L. Phenotypic and genotypic antibiotic resistance patterns of *Staphylococcus aureus* from raw and spontaneously fermented camel milk. BJAST. 2013;3(3):87–98.
39. Rode H, Hanslo D, de Wet PM, Millar AJW, Cywes S. Efficacy of mupirocin in methicillin-resistant *Staphylococcus aureus* burn wound infection. Antimicrob Agents Chemother. 1989;33:1358–61.
40. Salem-Bekhit M. Phenotypic and genotypic characterization of nosocomial isolates of *Staphylococcus aureus* with reference to methicillin resistance. Trop J Pharm Res. 2014;13:1239–46. https://doi.org/10.4314/tjpr.v13i8.7.
41. Ben Slama K, Gharsa H, Klibi N, Jouini A, Lozano C, Gómez-Sanz E, Zarazaga M, Boudabous A, Torres C. Nasal carriage of *Staphylococcus aureus* in healthy humans with different levels of contact with animals in Tunisia: genetic lineages, methicillin resistance, and virulence factors. Eur J Clin Microbiol Infect Dis. 2011;30:499–508. https://doi.org/10.1007/s10096-010-1109-6.
42. Gharsa H, Slama KB, Lozano C, Gomez-Sanz E, Klibi N, Sallem RB, Gomez P, Zarazaga M, Boudabous A, Torres C. Prevalence, antibiotic resistance, virulence traits and genetic lineages of *Staphylococcus aureus* in healthy sheep in Tunisia. Vet Microbiol. 2012;156:367–73. https://doi.org/10.1016/j.vetmic.2011.11.009.
43. Gharsa H, Sallem RB, Slama KB, Gomez-Sanz E, Lazano C, Jouini A, Klibi N, Zarazaga M, Boudabous A, Torres C. High diversity of genetic lineages and virulence genes in nasal *Staphylococcus aureus* isolates from donkeys destined to food consumption in Tunisia with predominance of the ruminant associated CC133 lineage. BMC Vet Res. 2012;8:203. https://doi.org/10.1186/1746-6148-8-203.
44. Olonitola OS, Inabo HI, Olayinka BO, Bugo ID. Nasal carriage of methicillin-resistant *Staphylococcus aureus* by primary school pupils in a university staff school, Zaria, Nigeria. Int J Bio. Chem Sci. 2007;1:71–5. https://doi.org/10.4314/ijbcs.v1i1.39701.
45. Shittu AO, Udo EE, Lin J. Phenotypic and molecular characterization of *Staphylococcus aureus* isolates expressing low- and high-level mupirocin resistance in Nigeria and South Africa. BMC Infect Dis. 2009;9:10. https://doi.org/10.1186/1471-2334-9-10.
46. Zinn CS, Westh H, Rosdahl VT. SARISA study group. An international multicenter study of antimicrobial resistance and typing of hospital *Staphylococcus aureus* isolates from 21 laboratories in 19 countries or states. Microb Drug Resist. 2004;10:160–8. https://doi.org/10.1089/1076629041310055.
47. Ouchenane Z, Smati F, Rolain J-M, Raoult D. Molecular characterization of methicillin-resistant *Staphylococcus aureus* isolates in Algeria. Pathol Biol (Paris). 2011;59:e129–32. https://doi.org/10.1016/j.patbio.2009.11.004.
48. Okon KO, Basset P, Uba A, Lin J, Oyawoye B, Shittu AO, Blanc DS. Co-occurrence of predominant Panton-Valentine Leukocidin-positive sequence type (ST) 152 and multidrug-resistant ST 241 *Staphylococcus aureus* clones in Nigerian hospitals. J Clin Microbiol. 2009;47:3000–3. https://doi.org/10.1128/JCM.01119-09.
49. Raji A, Ojemhen O, Umejiburu U, Ogunleye A, Blanc D, Basset P. High genetic diversity of *Staphylococcus aureus* in a tertiary care hospital in Southwest Nigeria. Diagn Microbiol Infect Dis. 2013;77:367–9. https://doi.org/10.1016/j.diagmicrobio.2013.08.030.
50. Shittu AO, Lin J. Antimicrobial susceptibility patterns and characterization of clinical isolates of *Staphylococcus aureus* in KwaZulu-Natal province, South Africa. BMC Infect Dis. 2006;6:125. https://doi.org/10.1186/1471-2334-6-125.
51. Perovic O, Iyaloo S, Kularatne R, Lowman W, Bosman N, Wadula J, Seetharam S, Duse A, Mbelle N, Bamford C, Dawood H, Mahabeer Y, Bhola P, Abrahams S, Singh-Moodley A. Prevalence and trends of *Staphylococcus*

aureus bacteraemia in hospitalized patients in South Africa, 2010-2012: laboratory-based surveillance mapping of antimicrobial resistance and molecular epidemiology. PLoS One. 2015;10:e0145429. https://doi.org/10.1371/journal.pone.0145429.
52. Barakat GI, Nabil YM. Correlation of mupirocin resistance with biofilm production in methicillin-resistant *Staphylococcus aureus* from surgical site infections in a tertiary Centre, Egypt. J Glob Antimicrob Resist. 2016;4:16–20. https://doi.org/10.1016/j.jgar.2015.11.010.
53. Shittu A, Lin J, Kolawole D. Antimicrobial susceptibility patterns of *Staphylococcus aureus* and characterization of MRSA in southwestern Nigeria. Wounds. 2006;18:77–84.
54. Egyir B, Guardabassi L, Nielsen SS, Larsen J, Addo KK, Newman MJ, Larsen AR. Prevalence of nasal carriage and diversity of *Staphylococcus aureus* among inpatients and hospital staff at Korle Bu teaching hospital, Ghana. J Glob Antimicrob Resist. 2013;1:189–93. https://doi.org/10.1016/j.jgar.2013.05.006.
55. Egyir B, Guardabassi L, Monecke S, Addo KK, Newman MJ, Larsen AR. Methicillin-resistant *Staphylococcus aureus* strains from Ghana include USA300. J Glob Antimicrob Resist. 2015;3:26–30. https://doi.org/10.1016/j.jgar.2014.11.006.
56. Ahmed MO, Abuzweda AR, Alghazali MH, Elramalli AK, Amri SG, Aghila ES, Abouzeed YM. Misidentification of methicillin-resistant *Staphylococcus aureus* (MRSA) in hospitals in Tripoli, Libya. Libyan J Med. 2010;5:5230. https://doi.org/10.3402/ljm.v5i0.5230.
57. Ahmed MO, Elramalli AK, Amri SG, Abuzweda AR, Abouzeed YM. Isolation and screening of methicillin-resistant *Staphylococcus aureus* from health care workers in Libyan hospitals. EMHJ. 2012;18:37–42.
58. Enany S, Yaoita E, Yoshida Y, Enany M, Yamamoto T. Molecular characterization of Panton-Valentine Leukocidin-positive community-acquired methicillin-resistant *Staphylococcus aureus* isolates in Egypt. Microbiol Res. 2010;165:152–62. https://doi.org/10.1016/j.micres.2009.03.005.
59. Ben Nejma MB, Mastouri M, Jrad BBH, Nour M. Characterization of ST80 Panton-Valentine Leukocidin-positive community-acquired methicillin-resistant *Staphylococcus aureus* clone in Tunisia. Diagn Microbiol Infect Dis. 2013;77:20–4. https://doi.org/10.1016/j.diagmicrobio.2008.02.010.
60. Ben Nejma MB, Merghni A, Mastouri M. Genotyping of methicillin resistant *Staphylococcus aureus* strains isolated from hospitalized children. Int J Pediatr. 2014;2014:314316. https://doi.org/10.1155/2014/314316.
61. Ferghani NEL. An open study of mupirocin in Libyan patients with skin infections. J Int Med Res. 1995;23:508–17. https://doi.org/10.1177/030006059502300615.
62. Souly K, Ait el Kadi M, Lhmadi K, Biougnach H, Boughaidi A, Zouhdi M, Benasila S, Elyoussefi Z, Bouattar T, Zbiti N, Skalli Z, Rhou H, Ouzeddoun N, Bayahia R, Benamar L. Epidemiology and prevention of *Staphylococcus aureus* nasal carriage in hemodialyzed patients. Med Mal Infect. 2011;41: 469–74. https://doi.org/10.1016/j.medmal.2011.05.005.
63. Shittu AO, Okon K, Adesida S, Oyedara O, Witte W, Strommenger B, Layer F, Nübel U. Antibiotic resistance and molecular epidemiology of *Staphylococcus aureus* in Nigeria. BMC Microbiol. 2011;11:92. https://doi.org/10.1186/1471-2180-11-92.
64. Shittu A, Oyedara O, Abegunrin F, Okon K, Raji A, Taiwo S, Ogunsola F, Onyedibe K, Elisha G. Characterization of methicillin-susceptible and -resistant staphylococci in the clinical setting: a multicentre study in Nigeria. BMC Infect Dis. 2012;12:286. https://doi.org/10.1186/1471-2334-12-286.
65. Ayepola OO, Olasupo NA, Egwari LO, Becker K, Schaumburg F. Molecular characterization and antimicrobial susceptibility of *Staphylococcus aureus* isolates from clinical infection and asymptomatic carriers in Southwest Nigeria. PLoS One. 2015;10:e0137531. https://doi.org/10.1371/journal.pone.0137531.
66. Akobi B, Aboderin O, Sasaki T, Shittu A. Characterization of *Staphylococcus aureus* isolates from faecal samples of the Straw-Coloured Fruit Bat (*Eidolon helvum*) in Obafemi Awolowo University (OAU), Nigeria. BMC Microbiol. 2012;12:279. https://doi.org/10.1186/1471-2180-12-279.
67. Egyir B, Guardabassi L, Esson J, Nielsen SS, Newman MJ, Addo KK, Larsen AR. Insights into nasal carriage of *Staphylococcus aureus* in an urban and a rural Community in Ghana. PLoS One. 2014;9:e96119. https://doi.org/10.1371/journal.pone.0096119.
68. Amissah NA, Glasner C, Ablordey A, Tetteh CS, Kotey NK, Prah I, van der Werf TS, Rossen JW, van Dijl JM, Stienstra Y. Genetic diversity of *Staphylococcus aureus* in Buruli ulcer. PLoS Negl Trop Dis. 2015;9:e0003421. https://doi.org/10.1371/journal.pntd.0003421.
69. Ngoa UA, Schaumburg F, Adegnika AA, Kösters K, Möller T, Fernandes JF, Alabi A, Issifou S, Becker K, Grobusch MP, Kremsner PG, Lell B. Epidemiology and population structure of *Staphylococcus aureus* in various population groups from a rural and semi-urban area in Gabon, Central Africa. Acta Trop. 2012;124:42–7. https://doi.org/10.1016/j.actatropica.2012.06.005.
70. Conceição T, Silva IS, de Lencastre H, Aires-de-Sousa M. *Staphylococcus aureus* nasal carriage among patients and health care workers in São Tomé and Príncipe. Microb Drug Resist. 2014;20:57–66. https://doi.org/10.1089/mdr.2013.0136.
71. Aiken AM, Mutuku IM, Sabat AJ, Akkerboom V, Mwangi J, Scott JAG, Morpeth SC, Friedrich AW, Grundmann H. Carriage of *Staphylococcus aureus* in Thika level 5 hospital, Kenya: a cross-sectional study. Antimicrob Resist Infect Control. 2014;3:22. https://doi.org/10.1186/2047-2994-3-22.
72. Omuse G, Kabera B, Revathi G. Low prevalence of methicillin resistant *Staphylococcus aureus* as determined by an automated identification system in two private hospitals in Nairobi, Kenya: a cross sectional study. BMC Infect Dis. 2014;14:669. https://doi.org/10.1186/s12879-014-0669-y.
73. Haddaway NR, Collins AM, Coughlin D, Kirk S. The role of Google scholar in evidence reviews and its applicability to Grey literature searching. PLoS One. 2015;10:e0138237. https://doi.org/10.1371/journal.pone.0138237.
74. Eshetie S, Tarekegn F, Moges F, Amsalu A, Birhan W, Huruy K. Methicillin resistant *Staphylococcus aureus* in Ethiopia: a meta-analysis. BMC Infect Dis. 2016;16:689. https://doi.org/10.1186/s12879-016-2014-0.
75. Deyno S, Fekadu S, Astatkie A. Resistance of *Staphylococcus aureus* to antimicrobial agents in Ethiopia: a meta-analysis. Antimicrob Resist Infect Control. 2017;6:85. https://doi.org/10.1186/s13756-017-0243-7.
76. Clinical and Laboratory Standard Institute (CLSI). Performance standards for antimicrobial susceptibility testing: 27th edition. CLSI supplement M100. Wayne CLSI. 2017.
77. The European Committee on Antimicrobial Susceptibility Testing. Breakpoint tables for interpretation of MICs and zone diameters. Version 8.1, 2018. http://www.eucast.org. Accessed 28th May, 2018.
78. Comite de l'antibiogramme de la Societe Francaise de Microbiologie – recommendations 2018 v.1.0 mai. http://www.sfm-microbiologie.org. Accessed 28th May, 2018.
79. Hurdle JG, O'Neill AJ, Mody L, Chopra I, Bradley SF. In vivo transfer of high-level mupirocin resistance from *Staphylococcus epidermidis* to methicillin-resistant *Staphylococcus aureus* associated with failure of mupirocin prophylaxis. J Antimicrob Chemother. 2005;56:1166–8.
80. Shittu AO, Lin J, Morrison D, Kolawole DO. Isolation and molecular confirmation of a multiresistant catalase-negative *Staphylococcus aureus* in Nigeria. J Infect. 2003;46:203–4. https://doi.org/10.1053/jinf.2002.1106.

2

Prevalence of methicillin resistant *Staphylococcus aureus*, multidrug resistant and extended spectrum β-lactamase producing gram negative bacilli causing wound infections at a tertiary care hospital of Nepal

Narbada Upreti[1*], Binod Rayamajhee[2,3*], Samendra P. Sherchan[4], Mahesh Kumar Choudhari[5] and Megha Raj Banjara[1]

Abstract

Background: Treatment and prevention of wound infection continues to be a challenging issue in clinical settings of Nepal especially in the context of globally growing problem of antimicrobial resistance. Study on opportunistic pathogens and sensitivity to commonly prescribed local antimicrobial agents are cardinal to reduce the disease burden of wound infections. The aim of this study was to determine the prevalence and antimicrobial susceptibility pattern of methicillin resistant *Staphylococcus aureus* (MRSA) and extended spectrum β-lactamase (ESBL) producing bacteria from wound infections of patients at a tertiary care hospital in Nepal.

Methods: Pus specimens were processed using standard microbiological procedures. Antimicrobial susceptibility test was performed following the modified Kirby Bauer disc diffusion technique. Clinical information of patients was obtained from preformed questionnaire and hospital record.

Results: One hundred eighty two pus specimens from wounds of different body parts: leg, hand, backside, abdominal part, foot, breast and chest, head and neck region were collected and analyzed; 113 bacterial isolates were isolated showing the overall bacterial growth rate of 62%, where the highest rate was among patients of ≤10 years age group (82.1%). A higher rate (68.5%) of bacterial isolates were from inpatients ($p < 0.05$). Among 116 bacterial isolates, *Staphylococcus aureus* was the most predominant bacteria (56.9%) followed by *Escherichia coli* (8.6%), coagulase negative staphylococci (7.8%), *Acinetobacter* spp. (5.2%), *Klebsiella pneumoniae* (5.2%), *Pseudomonas aeruginosa* (4.3%), *Enterococcus* spp. (4.3%), *Citrobacter freundii* (2.6%), *Proteus vulgaris* (1.6%) and *P. mirabilis* (0.9%). Both Gram positive (73.3%) and negative (78.8%) isolates showed high frequency of sensitive to gentamycin.

Conclusion: Among *S. aureus* isolates, 60.6% were MRSA strains, whereas 40% of *K. pneumoniae* and 33.3% of *C. freundii* were ESBL producing bacteria followed by *E. coli* (25%). It is thus paramount to address the burden of silently and speedily increasing infections caused by drug resistant strains of MRSA and ESBL in Nepal.

Keywords: Wound infection, Methicillin resistant *Staphylococcus aureus*, ESBL, Multidrug resistant, Nepal

* Correspondence: upreti.naru@gmail.com; rayamajheebinod@gmail.com
[1]Central Department of Microbiology, Tribhuvan University, Kirtipur, Nepal
[2]National College (Tribhuvan University), Khusibu, Kathmandu, Nepal
Full list of author information is available at the end of the article

Background

Wound infections result after the active interactions that takes place between a host, a potential pathogen and the surrounding extrinsic factors. The intensity of wound infections may range from a simple self-healing to a severe and life threatening [1]. Tissue invasion by bacterial pathogens is determined by the location of wound [2]. The common bacterial pathogens isolated from wound infections are *Staphylococcus aureus, S. epidermidis, S. pyogenes,* coagulase negative staphylococci (CoNS), *Acinetobacter* spp., *Pseudomonas* spp., *Escherichia coli, Klebsiella* spp., *Proteus* spp., *Enterobacter* spp., *Citrobacter* spp., and anaerobes such as *Clostridium* spp. and *Peptostreptococcus* spp. [3, 4]. Acquisition of drug resistance by these pathogenic strains has posed serious challenges for the remedy and management of wound infections around the world [5]. Wound infections can be monomicrobial or polymicrobial [6]. The presence of bacterial pathogens in wound infections is not uncommon but all wounds do not support the same range and number of species [7]. Hospital-acquired wound infections are the leading cause of morbidity hence, proper management of wound infection in clinical settings is paramount [8]. The treatment of wound infections is being more challenging due to methicillin resistant *S. aureus* (MRSA), involvement of polymicrobial flora and fungi [9]. In addition, antimicrobial resistance (AMR) is creating a serious problem in all clinical settings and AMR has become the biggest public health threat globally [10].

MRSA, a leading strain of wound infections, involves significant areas of skin or deeper soft tissues like abscesses, cellulitis, burns or infected deep ulcers [11]. Extended spectrum β- lactamase (ESBL) producing Enterobacteriaceae are also in frontline of wound infections. In ESBL, positive strains plasmid mediated AmpC enzymes, and carbapenem hydrolyzing β- lactamase (carbapenemases) conferred resistance to the newer β- lactam antimicrobials [12]. ESBL have been reported most frequently in *Escherichia coli* and *Klebsiella* spp. including other bacterial species such as *Salmonella enterica, P. aeruginosa*, and *Serratia marcescens* [13]. This surge in antimicrobial resistance further delays wound healing and the infection becomes more worst which increases hospital stay, prolongs trauma care, and high medical costs [14]. On the other hand, most of the clinical laboratories in underdeveloped countries are not equipped with testing facilities to detect ESBL producing bacteria. In Nepal, there is scanty data on the prevalence of ESBL-producing bacteria causing wound infections. The goal of this study was to determine the prevalence of MRSA, multidrug resistant and ESBL producing Gram negative bacilli from wound infections of patients visiting KIST Medical College and Teaching Hospital, Lalitpur, Nepal. Early reporting of drug resistant pathogens and evidence-based treatment algorithm can control the wound infections.

Methods

Study site and population

A descriptive cross-sectional study was designed and carried out to determine the bacteriological profile of wound infections. MRSA, MDR and ESBL producing bacteria were identified from the pus samples of patients with wound infection visiting KIST Medical College and Teaching Hospital, Kathmandu, Nepal from November 2014 to August 2015. A total of 182 pus and Fine Needle Aspirate specimens were collected from patients with clinical features of wound infection like patients with pain, complaints of regular discharge, foul smelling and red swelling. During the study, patients of all age groups and both genders from out-patients (39/182) and in-patients (143/182) were included. Patients who were admitted in the hospital for more than 3 days and/or in prior antibiotic treatment and anaerobic wound infections were excluded from this study.

Sampling procedure

Pus specimens were collected from elective surgery wounds of hospital wards [surgical, post- operative, trauma, orthopedic, ENT (eye-nose-throat), gynecology wards], open and dressed wounds. Sterile cotton swabs and fine needle syringes (FNS) were used to collect pus samples from open wounds then each sample was labeled properly with date/time of sample collection, collection method and the patient's details. Swabs from open wounds were aseptically collected after cleaned off while pus from dressed wounds were collected after removing the dressing items. The information of each patient was recorded such as site of infection, signs and symptoms, other underlying diseases, and prior antibiotics administration. Before collecting the sample, the area was rinsed with sterile normal saline and then a sterile cotton swab was gently rolled over the surface of the wound. The swab with pus was kept in a sterile test tube with cap where details was labeled properly. For the collection of pus sample from deep wounds, FNS was used. Specimens were collected from wounds of different body parts: leg, hand, back part of body, abdominal part, foot region, breast and chest part, head and neck region. Amies transport medium was used to transport the collected specimens. For Fine Needle Aspiration Cytology (FNAC), the syringe was properly capped, labeled and dispatched to the laboratory immediately.

Processing of samples

Macroscopic examination of samples

Among 182 pus specimens collected, 56 (30.8%) were from the leg region, 43 (23.6%) from hand, 15 (8.2%)

from back part of body, 14 (7.8%) from abdominal part, 15 (8.2%) from foot region, 6 (3.3%) from breast and chest part, and 33 (18.1%) were from head and neck region wounds. All the specimens were visually examined for consistency, color, turbidity, presence or absence of blood depending upon the type and site of wound. Additionally, pus swabs were observed whether they were labeled correctly or not.

Microscopic examination of samples

After transportation of specimens to the laboratory, Gram staining of each specimens was performed [15].

Culture of specimens and identification of isolated bacteria

Pus specimens were inoculated into Chocolate agar, Blood agar, MacConkey agar, Nutrient agar and Potato Dextrose agar plates as per the clinical laboratory guidelines [16]. The preliminary identification of the isolated bacteria was done based on colony form, size, shape, pigmentation, margin, and elevation. The isolated organisms were identified by performing different biochemical tests and Gram staining then antimicrobial susceptibility tests were performed. In case of no growth after 24 h of incubation further incubation was done up to 48 h at 37 C. After proper incubation period, the culture plates were examined for microbial growth. In every case, each plate was carefully observed. Then, biochemical tests were performed in sterile media for the identification of bacterial isolates. Identification of Staphylococci spp. was done by Gram staining, catalase test, slide coagulase and tube coagulase test. Similarly, Gram negative strains were identified based on result of different biochemical tests; Oxidase, Catalase, Methyl Red (MR), Voges Proskauer (VP), Citrate utilization, Urea Hydrolysis, Triple Sugar Iron agar (TSI), Sulfide Motility and Indole test. Colony morphology and microscopic observation were taken in account for identification of *Candida* spp.

Examination of antimicrobial susceptibility pattern of isolated organism

Antimicrobial susceptibility pattern was performed for isolated and identified bacteria from pus samples following the modified Kirby Bauer disc diffusion technique. A dilution of the identified organism was prepared comparing with the standard 0.5 McFarland turbidity which was used to swab over the Mueller Hinton agar (MHA) medium for the antimicrobial susceptibility test (AST). Discs of antibiotic used for Gram positive bacteria were ampicillin (10 μg), cefotaxime (30 μg), gentamycin (10 μg), ciprofloxacin (5 μg), trimethoprim + sulfamethoxazole (25 μg), cefoxitin (30 μg), amikacin (30 μg) and tetracycline (30 μg) whereas antibiotics used for Gram negative organisms were ampicillin (10 μg), trimethoprim + sulfamethoxazole (25 μg), gentamycin (10 μg), ciprofloxacin (5 μg), cefazolin (30 μg), ceftriaxone (30 μg), cefotaxime (30 μg), amikacin (30 μg), piperacillin (100 μg), tobramycin (10 μg), imipenem (10 μg), and meropenem (10 μg). After 24 h of incubation period at 37 C, the zone of inhibition (ZOI) was measured then the results were analyzed according to the guidelines issued by the Clinical Laboratory Standard Institute (CLSI - M100-S25, 2015) [16]. Isolates resistant to two or more antimicrobial classes were reported as multi drug resistant (MDR) strains. Antimicrobials and their doses were selected based on prescription frequency by physician and availability in the study setting. Minimum inhibitory and bactericidal concentration (MIC and MBC) of used antimicrobials were not determined due to unavailability of all antimicrobials powder at the time of study period.

Screening and confirmation for ESBL producers

Enterobacteriaceae isolates were screened for possible ESBL producing bacteria using antibiotic discs of cefotaxime (30 μg), ceftazidime (30 μg), ceftriaxone (30 μg) and aztreonam (30 μg) [17]. According to the guidelines, bacterial isolates showing ceftazidime < 22 mm, and cefotaxime < 27 mm are the possible ESBL producer. The suspected ESBL producer strains were subjected to double disc synergy test (DDST) for the confirmation of ESBL producing Enterobacteriaceae [18].

Statistical analysis

All data were examined using iBM SPSS version 21.0. Frequencies were calculated for categorical variables. Chi-square test was calculated to analyze significant difference at 95% of confidence level, p value of < 0.05 was considered significant, unless otherwise noted.

Quality control

All prepared biochemical and streaking media were checked for their sterility. Strains of *E. coli* ATCC 25922 and *S. aureus* ATCC 25923 were used as reference strains for quality control of AST and biochemical tests. The same strain of *E. coli* was also considered as a negative control during the screening and phenotypic confirmation (DDST) tests of ESBL producing Gram-negative bacilli.

Results

Bacterial growth

A total of 182 samples were collected and examined from hospital patients with clinical features of wound infection, 113 (62%) specimens were positive for aerobic bacterial growth. Out of 116 bacterial isolates obtained from 113 positive samples, 83 (71.6%) bacterial isolates were Gram positive and 33 (28.4%) isolates were Gram negative. Among processed specimens, 64% (100/156) of pus swabs and 50% (13/26) of aspirated pus specimens have shown aerobic bacterial growth (Fig. 1). Out of 113

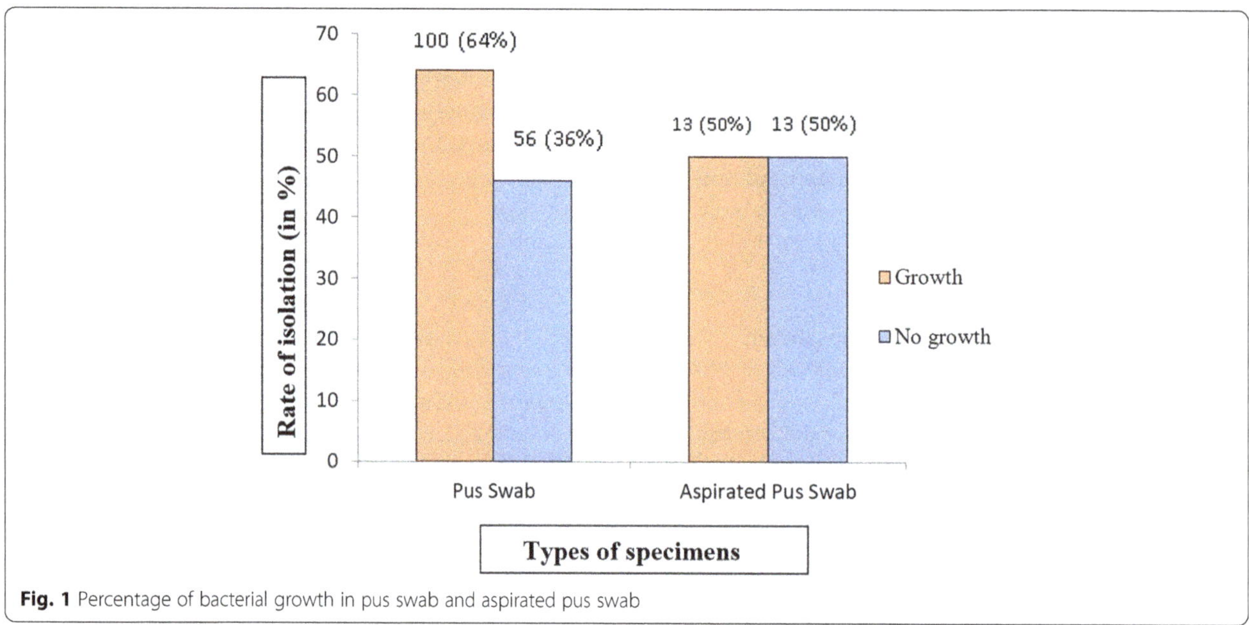

Fig. 1 Percentage of bacterial growth in pus swab and aspirated pus swab

specimens positive for aerobic bacterial culture, polymicrobial growth was observed in 3 (2.7%) specimens where combinations of *S. aureus* - *Acinetobacter* spp., *S. aureus* - *Citrobacter freundii* and *Enterococcus* spp. - *Candida* spp. were reported. High incidence of MRSA 60.6% (40/66), MDR (80% of *E. coli*, 68.2% of *S. aureus*, 80% of *P. aeruginosa*, 77.7% of CoNS and 50% of *Proteus* spp.) and ESBL (25% of *E. coli*, 40% of *K. pneumoniae*, and 33.3% of *C. freundii*) producing isolates were reported in this study.

Sixty two (34.1%) specimens processed were collected from the leg, 36 (19.8%) from hand, 16 (8.8%) from backside, 15 (8.2%) from abdominal, 22 (12.1%) from foot, 13 (7.1%) from breast and chest, 18 (9.9%) from head and neck part. Majority of patients (86%) were presented with fever, lethargy and muscle pain at the time of sample collection. None of the patients were reported with any underlying diseases. Patients who had other infections and antibiotic treatment were excluded from the study subject.

Wound infection in relation with demographic characteristics of the patients

Eighty one (44.5%) samples were from male patients and among them 45 (55.5%) samples showed aerobic bacterial growth, while 101 (55.5%) samples were from female patients, and 68 (68.3%) samples were positive for aerobic bacterial growth but there was no significant difference in between aerobic bacterial growth and gender of patients ($p > 0.05$) (Table 1). Highest rate of wound infection was observed among patients of age group ≤10 years (82.1%), followed by patients of age group 71–80 years (77.8%).

Growth pattern in outpatient and inpatient departments

One hundred forty three samples were from inpatient department (from different wards) and 39 samples were from outpatient department. Out of 143 samples from inpatient, 98 (68.5%) were positive and out of 39 samples from outpatient, 15 (38.5%) were positive for bacterial growth. Type of patients based on department had a positive correlation with aerobic bacterial growth ($p < 0.05$).

Pus specimens were collected from inpatient departments/wards (such as surgical wards, post- operative

Table 1 Socio-demographic features of the patients and ratio of wound infection

Demographic features	Infected [No. (%)]	Not infected [No. (%)]	Total [No. (%)]
Sex			
Male	45 (55.6)	36 (44.4)	81 (44.5)
Female	68 (67.3)	33 (32.7)	101 (55.5)
Total	113 (62.1)	69 (37.9)	182 (100)
Age in years			
≤ 10	23 (82.1)	5 (17.9)	28 (15.4)
11–20	18 (60.0)	12 (40.0)	30 (16.5)
21–30	12 (44.4)	15 (55.6)	27 (14.9)
31–40	21 (65.6)	11 (34.4)	32 (17.6)
41–50	9 (40.9)	13 (59.1)	22 (12.0)
51–60	15 (68.2)	7 (31.8)	22 (12.0)
61–70	8 (66.7)	4 (33.3)	12 (6.6)
71–80	7 (77.8)	2 (22.2)	9 (5.0)
Total	113 (62.00)	69 (38.00)	182 (100)

wards, orthopedic ward, ENT (eye-nose-throat), gynecology wards) and from outpatient department. Eighty nine (48.9%) specimens were from traumatic cases, followed by 57 (31.3%) specimens which were from postoperative cases. The most common bacterial isolate was *S. aureus* followed by *E. coli.* Out of 116 microbial isolates, 83 (71.6%) were Gram-positive and among them, *S. aureus* 66 (79.6%) was the most common isolate followed by CoNS 9 (10.8%), *Enterococcus* spp. 5 (6%) and *Candida* spp. 3 (3.6%). On the other hand, 33 (28.4%) were Gram-negative of which *E. coli* 10 (30.3%) was predominant isolate followed by *K. pneumoniae* 6 (18.2%), *Acinetobacter* spp. 6 (18.2%), *P. aeruginosa* 5 (15.1%), *C. freundii* 3 (9.1%), *P. vulgaris* 2 (6.1%) and *P. mirabilis* 1 (3%). In pus swab, *S. aureus* (58%) was the predominant isolate followed by *E. coli* (10%) and CoNS (9%). Similarly, in case of aspirates pus samples, *S. aureus* (50%) was the highest followed by *K. pneumoniae* (18.7%) (Table 2 and Additional file 1).

Antibiogram result of gram negative bacteria isolated from patients at KIST Hospital, November 2014 to august 2015

A total of 10 *E. coli* were isolated from wound specimens and 80% (8/10) of isolates were sensitive to gentamicin, 60% were sensitive to ciprofloxacin, 50% were sensitive to cefotaxime and 40% were sensitive to cotrimoxazole. All isolates of *E. coli* (100%) were resistant to ampicillin followed by cefazolin (80%) and ceftriaxone (70%). All the isolates of *P. aeruginosa* (100%) were susceptible to amikacin, tobramycin and imipenem while 80% of the *P. aeruginosa* isolates were sensitive to ciprofloxacin. In contrast, 40% and 60% of *P. aeruginosa* isolates were resistant to ceftazidime and piperacillin respectively. Similarly, 83.3% (6/5) of *K. pneumoniae* were sensitive to meropenem while 66.7% of isolates were susceptible to ciprofloxacin, gentamycin and amikacin. A total of 50% of the *K. pneumoniae* isolates were sensitive to cotrimoxazole and ceftriaxone. All the isolates (100%) of both *Proteus vulgaris* and *P. mirabilis* were susceptible to cefotaxime and amikacin. There was 100% resistant of *P. mirabilis* to cotrimoxazole and cefazolin while 50% and 100% of *P. vulgaris* isolates were resistant to cotrimoxazole and cefazolin respectively. All isolates (100%) of *C. freundii* were resistant to ampicillin and cefazolin while 33.3% (1/3) were sensitive to ciprofloxacin, cotrimoxazole, cefotaxime, gentamycin and ceftriaxone (Table 3).

Table 2 Pattern of microbial isolates in wound samples

Type of organism	Type of Specimens				Total	
	Pus swab		Aspirated pus			
	No.	%	No.	%	No.	%
S. aureus	58	58	8	50	66	56.9
E. coli	10	10	–	–	10	8.6
P. aeruginosa	5	5	–	–	5	4.3
CoNS	9	9	–	–	9	7.8
Acinetobacter spp.	6	6	–	–	6	5.2
Enterococcus spp.	3	3	2	12.5	5	4.3
C. freundii	1	1	2	12.5	3	2.6
K. pneumoniae	3	3	3	18.7	6	5.2
P. vulgaris	2	2	–	–	2	1.6
P. mirabilis	1	1	–	–	1	0.9
Candida spp.	2	2	1	6.3	3	2.6
Total	100	100	16	100	116	100

Antibiogram result of gram positive S. aureus, CoNS, and Enterococcus species

Among total isolated *S. aureus*, 77.3% of *S. aureus* were susceptible to gentamycin, where 75.8% of the isolates were susceptible to cefotaxime. Similarly, 45.5% of *S. aureus* were susceptible to ciprofloxacin while 39.4% of *S. aureus* isolates were susceptible to cefoxitin. Eighty percent of *Enterococcus* spp. were sensitive to tetracycline. (Table 4). Among 66 *S. aureus* isolated from pus swab and aspirated pus, 40 (60.6%) isolates of *S. aureus* were MRSA.

ESBL producers among Enterobacteriaceae isolates

Among 10 isolates of *E. coli*, 2 (25%) were positive for ESBL and among 6 isolates of *K. pneumoniae*, 2 (40%) were positive for ESBL. Additionally, among 3 isolates of *C. freundii*, 1 (33.3%) was ESBL positive whereas *Proteus* spp. were negative for ESBL (Table 5).

Antibiogram result of isolates

Eighty percent (80%) of *E. coli* and 68.2% of *S. aureus* were MDR (resistant to two or more than two antimicrobial classes) strains. Similarly, 80% of *P. aeruginosa* and 77.7% of CoNS were MDR strains. Additionally, 83.3% of *K. pneumoniae* isolates were resistant to at least two different classes of used antibiotics. In this study, 50% of *Proteus* spp. isolates were MDR (Table 6).

Discussion

Aerobic bacteria causing wound infections were isolated and identified from pus specimens by series of biochemical tests and their antimicrobial susceptibility patterns to commonly used antibiotics in study area were examined. Enterobacteriaceae isolates were further processed for confirmation of ESBL producer. In this study, 60.4% of culture positive specimens showed monomicrobial growth, 1.7% showed polymicrobial and 37.9% were negative for aerobic bacterial growth. This finding is consistent with previous studies conducted by Egbe et al. and Kumari et al. [19, 20]. Bhatta et al., [21] have reported 60% of bacterial wound infection from Nepal in 2008. Out of 182 non-repeated samples analyzed, 143 (78.6%) samples were from inpatients, where 98 (68%) were positive for aerobic

Table 3 Antibiotic susceptibility test result of Gram negative bacteria isolated from pus specimens

Isolates		Antimicrobial agents								
	RXN	AMP	AK	CIP	COT	GEN	CTX	CTR	CZ	MRP
E.. coli (10)	S	0	Nt	6 (60)	4 (40)	8 (80)	5 (50)	3 (30)	2 (20)	Nt
	R	10 (100)	Nt	4 (40)	6 (60)	2 (20)	5 (50)	7 (70)	8 (80)	Nt
P. aeruginosa (5)	S	Nt	5 (100)	4 (80)	Nt	Nt	Nt	Nt	Nt	Nt
	R	Nt	0	1 (20)	Nt	Nt	Nt	Nt	Nt	Nt
K. pneumoniae (6)	S	Nt	4 (66.7)	4 (66.7)	3 (50)	4 (66.7)	Nt	3 (50)	Nt	5 (83.3)
	R	Nt	2 (33.3)	2 (33.3)	3 (50)	2 (33.3)	Nt	3 (50)	Nt	1 (16.7)
P. vulgaris ($n = 2$)	S	0	2 (100)	1 (50)	1 (50)	Nt	2 (100)	Nt	0	Nt
	R	2 (100)	0	1 (50)	1 (50)	Nt	0	Nt	2 (100)	Nt
P. mirabilis ($n = 1$)	S	1 (100)	1 (100)	1 (100)	0	Nt	1 (100)	Nt	0	Nt
	R	0	0	0	1 (100)	Nt	0	Nt	1 (100)	Nt
C. freundii (3)	S	0	Nt	1 (33.3)	1 (33.3)	1 (33.3)	1 (33.3)	1 (33.3)	0	Nt
	R	3 (100)	Nt	2 (66.7)	2 (66.7)	2 (66.7)	2 (66.7)	2 (66.7)	3 (100)	Nt
Acinetobacter spp. ($n = 6$)	S	2 (33.3)	4 (66.7)	4 (66.7)	3 (50)	4 (66.7)	3 (50)	Nt	3 (50)	Nt
	R	4 (66.7)	2 (33.3)	2 (33.3)	3 (50)	2 (33.3)	3 (50)	Nt	3 (50)	Nt
		Antimicrobial agents								
	RXN	AMP	AK	CIP	CAZ	TOB	IMP	PI	CZ	MRP
P. aeruginosa (5)	S	Nt	5 (100)	4 (80)	2 (40)	5 (100)	5 (100)	3 (60)	Nt	Nt
	R	Nt	0	1 (20)	3 (60)	0	0	2 (40)	Nt	Nt
Total ($n = 38$)	S	3 (13.6)	21 (84)	25 (65.7)	14 (42.4)	22 (73.3)	17 (63)	10 (41.7)	5 (22.7)	5 (83.3)
	R	19 (86.4)	4 (16)	13 (34.3)	19 (57.6)	8 (26.7)	10 (37)	14 (58.3)	17 (77.3)	1 (16.7)

Nt not tested, *S* Sensitive, *R* Resistant, *RXN* Reaction, *AMP* Ampicillin, *AK* Amikacin, *CIP* Ciprofloxacin, *COT* trimethoprim + sulfamethoxazole (cotrimoxazole), *GEN* Gentamicin, *CTX* Cefotaxime, *Caz* Ceftazidime, *TOB* Tobramycin, *IMP* Imipenem, *PI* Piperacillin, *CTR* Ceftriaxone, *CZ* Cefazolin, *MRP* Meropenem

bacterial growth. Our finding shows higher rate of wound infection in inpatients (68%) as compare to outpatients (39%) and the result was statistically significant ($p < 0.05$). Similar finding was reported by Stephen et al. [19]. Among 182 specimens collected, 156 (85.7%) were pus swabs with 64% (100/156) aerobic bacterial growth and 26 (14.3%) were aspirated pus where 13 (50%) were positive for aerobic bacterial growth. Shrestha et al., [21] have found the similar prevalence rate in Nepal before. Pus aspiration is generally taken as sample of choice from deep seated and closed wound infections [22, 23].

Eighty one (44.5%) pus specimens were collected from male patients, while 101 (55.5%) specimens were from female patients and the result was statistically insignificant ($p > 0.05$). In this study, female patients outnumbered the male patients [24] but other studies showed wound

Table 4 Antibiotic susceptibility test result of Gram positive bacteria isolated from pus specimens

Isolates		Antimicrobial agents							
	RXN	AMP	AK	CIP	COT	GEN	CTX	CX	TE
S. aureus ($n = 66$)	S	5 (7.6)	Nt	37 (56.1)	26 (39.4)	54 (81.8)	53 (80.3)	26 (39.4)	29 (43.9)
	R	61 (92.4)	Nt	29 (43.9)	40 (60.6)	12 (18.2)	13 (19.7)	40 (60.6)	37 (56.1)
CoNS ($n = 9$)	S	1 (11.1)	Nt	3 (33.3)	4 (44.4)	6 (66.7)	2 (22.2)	4 (44.4)	5 (55.6)
	R	8 (88.9)	Nt	6 (66.7)	5 (55.6)	3 (33.3)	7 (77.8)	5 (55.6)	4 (44.4)
Enterococcus spp. ($n = 5$)	S	3 (60)	2 (40)	3 (60)	3 (60)	3 (60)	3 (60)	Nt	4 (80)
	R	22 (40)	3 (60)	2 (40)	2 (40)	2 (40)	2 (40)	Nt	1 (20)
Total ($n = 80$)	S	9 (11.25)	2 (40)	43 (53.75)	33 (41.25)	63 (78.75)	58 (72.5)	30 (40)	38 (47.5)
	R	71 (88.75)	3 (60)	37 (46.25)	47 (58.75)	17 (21.25)	22 (27.5)	45 (60)	42 (52.5)

Nt not tested, *S* Sensitive, *R* Resistant, *RXN* Reaction, *AMP* Ampicillin, *AK* Amikacin, *CIP* Ciprofloxacin, *COT* trimethoprim + sulfamethoxazole (cotrimoxazole), *GEN* Gentamicin, *CTX* Cefotaxime, *CX* Cefoxitin, *TE* Tetracycline

Table 5 ESBL producers among Enterobacteriaceae

Bacterial isolates	Total	ESBL producer	
		No.	%
E. coli	10	2	25.0
K. pneumoniae	6	2	40.0
P. vulgaris	2	0	0
P. mirabilis	1	0	0
C. freundii	3	1	33.3

infection was higher in male as compared to female [25, 26]. In our study, lower number of male patients (44.5%) might be due to small sample size as compared to other studies. In this study, monomicrobial growth (97.3%) was higher than polymicrobial growth (2.7%) both in pus swab and aspirated pus. Multiple studies carried out in wound infections have shown higher rate of monomicrobial infection than polymicrobial infection [27]. Similarly a high rate (86–100%) of monomicrobial wound infection was reported from different states of India [28, 29].

Among different age groups, the prevalence of wound infections was highest among age group ≤10 years (82.1%) followed by age group 70–80 years (77.8%). This is in agreement with study carried by Lakhey et al. where higher prevalence of wound infection was reported among patients of age group 60–80 years [20]. Similarly, in a study done by Mohammedaman et al., [5] in South Ethiopia, 87.5% wound infection was in patients with age ≥ 60 years. Since old individuals and children have weak immunity, that might be the reason for them being more prone to wound infections. Ranjan et al. have reported more pathogenic strains from patients of age group 21–40 years in post-operative wound infections in India [30].

Among 116 bacterial isolates, 11 different species were identified. *S. aureus* (56.9%) was the most common isolate followed by *E. coli* (8.6%) and CoNS (7.8%). Other identified bacteria from pus specimens included *P. aeruginosa* (4.3%), *Acinetobacter* spp. (5.2%), *Enterococcus* spp. (4.3%), *C. freundii* (2.6%), *K. pneumoniae* (5.2%), *P. vulgaris* (1.6%), and *P. mirabilis* (0.9%). The predominance of *S. aureus* in wound infection is supported by different studies [21, 30]. As being a normal flora of human skin, it can get access into the wound easily. Kansakar et al., [32] have reported that 82.5% of bacterial growth in pus samples and 13 different bacterial species were isolated where *S. aureus* was predominant (57.7%) species followed by *E. coli* (11%) and CoNS (3%). According to Mumtaz et al., [33] *S. aureus* was the most common bacteria (49%) found in wound infections followed by *E. coli* (25.9%), *Klebsiella* spp. (9.5%), *P. aeruginosa* (8.6%), *Proteus* spp. (4%) and *Acinetobacter* (2.7%) spp. *S. aureus* is the most common strain (25%) as a commensal organism of human skin and nasal passage. Hence, most frequent isolation of *S. aureus* from pus specimens might also be due to contamination of collected specimens with skin normal flora [31]. Contribution of multidrug resistant *Acinetobacter* spp. to nosocomial infections has increased over the past decade, and many outbreaks involving this bacterium have been reported worldwide [32].

Table 6 Antibiogram result of isolates

Isolated organisms	Antibiogram				Total MDR [N(%)]
	No. (%) of resistance				
	R2	R3	R4	R5	
Gram positive					
S. aureus ($n = 66$)	20 (30.3)	18 (27.3)	3 (4.5)	4 (6.1)	45 (68.2)
CoNS ($n = 9$)	4 (44.4)	1 (11.1)	2 (22.2)	0	7 (77.7)
Enterococcus spp. ($n = 5$)	3 (60)	0	1 (20)	0	4 (80)
Total ($n = 80$)	27 (33.75)	19 (23.75)	6 (7.5)	4 (5)	56 (70)
Gram negative					
E. coli ($n = 10$)	6 (60)	1 (10)	0	1 (10)	8 (80)
P. aeruginosa ($n = 5$)	2 (40)	1 (20)	1 (20)	0	4 (80)
Acinetobacter spp. ($n = 6$)	2 (33.3)	1 (16.7)	1 (16.7)	0	4 (66.7)
C. freundii ($n = 3$)	2 (66.7)	0	0	0	2 (66.7)
K. pneumoniae ($n = 6$)	2 (33.3)	1 (16.7)	0	2 (33.3)	5 (83.3)
P. vulgaris ($n = 2$)	1 (50)	0	0	0	1 (50)
P. mirabilis ($n = 1$)	1 (50)	0	0	0	1 (50)
Total ($n = 33$)	10 (30.3)	3 (9.1)	2 (6.1)	2 (6.1)	17 (51.5)

R2-R5 number of antibiotics class where an isolate was resistant

Shrestha et al., [21] have found that 85% of *S. aureus* isolates were sensitive to ciprofloxacin, 83% and 82% were sensitive to cephalexin and cotrimoxazole respectively. In this study, 60.6% of Staphylococci isolates were resistant to cefoxitin. *S. aureus* which was resistant to cefoxitin antibiotic was reported as MRSA species. Rajbhandari et al., [36] have also reported 61.6% of MRSA prevalence in wound infection. The second common isolate of this study was *E. coli* where 80%, 60%, 50% and 40% of the isolates were susceptible to gentamycin, ciprofloxacin, cefotaxime and cotrimoxazole respectively. All the isolates of *E. coli* (100%) were resistant to ampicillin where 30% and 20% were resistant to ceftriaxone and cefazolin respectively. Similarly, 60% and 40% of *E. coli* isolates were susceptible to ciprofloxacin and cotrimoxazole respectively. This study showed low sensitivity rate as compared to other studies [33]. Hence, increased antimicrobial resistant rate of *E. coli* depicts its important role in nosocomial infections.

All the isolates of *P. aeruginosa* (100%) were sensitive to amikacin, tobramycin and imipenem while 80% and 60% were sensitive to ciprofloxacin and piperacillin respectively. Only 40% of the *P. aeruginosa* were susceptible to the antibiotic ceftazidime. In a study conducted by Shrestha et al., [21] 93% of isolates were sensitive to amikacin and 66.7% of isolates were sensitive to ciprofloxacin. Our finding in this context is similar with other results where *P. aeruginosa* isolated from pus samples has shown least resistance to ciprofloxacin (6.2–24%) [34]. More prevalence of antimicrobial resistant *P. aeruginosa* in wound infection is being a challenging issue especially in resource limited countries [26].

K. pneumoniae was most sensitive to meropenem (83.3%) and 66.7% of *K. pneumoniae* isolates were equally resistant to gentamycin, ciprofloxacin, and amikacin where 50% of isolated *K. pneumoniae* were resistant to cotrimoxazole and ceftriaxone. In a study reported by Mohammedaman et al., [5] 35.7% of *K. pneumoniae* were resistant to ciprofloxacin and doxycycline. Furthermore, Rajput et al., [24] had reported that 45.5% and 80% of *K. pneumoniae* strains were resistant to ciprofloxacin and cotrimoxazole respectively. All isolates (100%) of *P. vulgaris* were susceptible to amikacin, and cefotaxime but 100% of *P. vulgaris* isolates were resistant to ampicillin and cefazolin while 50% of isolated *P. vulgaris* were resistant to ciprofloxacin and cotrimoxazole. All isolates (100%) of *P. mirabilis* were sensitive to ciprofloxacin, amikacin and cefotaxime whereas 100% were resistant to ampicillin, cotrimoxazole and cefazolin. This result is comparable with study carried by Bhatta et al. [20].

Among Enterobacteriaceae isolates, 25% of *E. coli*, 40% of *K. pneumoniae* and 33.3% of *C. freundii* were ESBL producer. But none of the *Proteus* species were ESBL producer. Chander et al., [35] have reported 13.51% and 16.55% of *E. coli* and *K. pneumoniae* as ESBL producer respectively. The prevalence rate may vary based on sample collection method, site of sample collection, microbial detection technique, antimicrobial agents used, and geographical location. In this study, 68.2% of *S. aureus* and 80% of *E. coli* isolates were MDR strains. The highest rate (83.3%) of MDR was observed in *K. pneumoniae*. This finding is in agreement with the study conducted in South-West Ethiopia by Mohammedaman et al. [5]. Most of the Gram negative isolates were resistant to ampicillin (86.4%) and cefazolin (77.3%) while 88.6% and 60% of Gram positive bacteria were resistant to ampicillin and amikacin respectively. In Nepal, oral administration of antibiotics is common practice which may reduce absorption of antibiotics by blood stream. Long term use of antibiotics via oral route could contribute to bacteria developing resistance.

Wound infection is a burning public health issue especially in developing countries. Severe wound infection can cause great loss including higher rate of morbidity and mortality; longer hospital stays, delay in wound healing, increase economic burden and increase discomfort which in turn increases disease burden significantly. Wound infection is being a common nosocomial infections which accounts for 0–80% of patient's mortality [35, 36].

Modernization in control and prevention of infections has not completely controlled wound infection due to increasing problem of antimicrobial resistance [37]. As compared to previous studies, antimicrobial resistance pattern is increasing at high rate. Multiple factors may contribute to rapid development of antimicrobial resistance by pathogens including misuse, overuse, and underuse of antimicrobials by both clinicians and patients. In Nepal, people purchase antimicrobials without physician's prescription, which is a common practice. This leads to misuse of antimicrobials that contributes to the emergence and spread of antimicrobial resistant strain. MRSA and ESBL producing bacteria are creating a serious problem in wound treatment in different parts of the country.

Conclusion

In this study, the most common isolate was *S. aureus* in pus specimens. Among *S. aureus* isolates, 60.6% were MRSA strains, whereas 40% of *K. pneumoniae* and 33.3% *C. freundii* were ESBL producer followed by *E. coli* (25%). Eighty percent (80%) of *E. coli*, *P. aeruginosa*, and 68.2% of *S. aureus* were MDR strains. This study emphasizes the importance of strict nosocomial infection control strategies and careful prescription of antimicrobials should be implemented by the health care centres. It should be mandatory to screen out ESBL, MRSA, and MDR pathogens and regular monitoring of their antimicrobial susceptibility pattern for prevention and control of wound infections. Early reporting of drug resistant pathogens and evidence-based treatment algorithm can control the wound infections. Research on AMR is in its infancy stage in Nepal, but it is paramount to establish surveillance programs to reduce burden of wound infections.

Abbreviations

AMR: Antimicrobial resistance; AST: Antibiotic susceptibility test; ATCC: American type culture collection; CDC: Centers for disease control and prevention; CLSI: Clinical laboratory standard institute; CoNS: Coagulase negative Staphylococci; DDST: Double disc synergy test; ENT: Eye-Nose-Throat; ESBL: Extended spectrum β-lactamase; FNAC: Fine needle aspiration cytology; MDR: Multi-drug resistant; MHA: Mueller Hinton agar; MRSA: Methicillin resistant *Staphylococcus aureus*; SPSS: Statistical package for the social sciences; WHO: World health organization; ZOI: Zone of inhibition; µg: Micro gram

Acknowledgements

We would like to acknowledge KIST Medical College and Teaching Hospital, and all the staff of pathology department for guiding the study and Hi Media Pvt. Ltd., India- who provided antibiotic discs for the antimicrobial susceptibility tests.

Authors' contributions

First author: NU is primary author who designed the study methodology, performed laboratory investigations and prepare the manuscript. Second authors: MRB and MKC helped for design the study, analysis of results, proof reading of article, manage necessary arrangements during laboratory investigations and supervised the complete study. BR and SS edited, proof read, helped in data analysis and revised the complete manuscript for submission. All authors approved the final manuscript before submission to the Antimicrobial Resistance & Infection Control.

Consent for publication

Not applicable.

Competing interests

The authors declare they do not have any competing interests.

Author details

[1]Central Department of Microbiology, Tribhuvan University, Kirtipur, Nepal. [2]National College (Tribhuvan University), Khusibu, Kathmandu, Nepal. [3]Department of Infectious Diseases and Immunology, Kathmandu Research Institute for Biological Sciences (KRIBS), Lalitpur, Nepal. [4]Department of Global Environmental Health Sciences, School of Public Health and Tropical Medicine, Tulane University, New Orleans, LA, USA. [5]KIST Medical College and Teaching Hospital, Imadole, Lalitpur, Nepal.

References

1. Moet GJ, Jones RN, Biedenbach DJ, Stilwell MG, Fritsche TR. Contemporary causes of skin and soft tissue infections in North America, Latin America, and Europe: report from the SENTRY antimicrobial surveillance program (1998–2004). Diagn Microbiol Infect Dis. 2007;57(1):7–13.
2. Oluwatosin OM. Surgical wound infection: a general overview. Ann Ibadan Postgrad Med. 2005;3(2):26–31.
3. Collier M. Wound-bed management: key principles for practice. Professional nurse (London, England) 2002;18(4):221–225.
4. Forbes BA, Sahm DF, Weissfeld AS. Overview of bacterial identification methods and strategies. Bailey and Scott's Diagnostic Microbiology. 12. Mosby Elsevier, Missouri. 2007:216–247.
5. Mama M, Abdissa A, Sewunet T. Antimicrobial susceptibility pattern of bacterial isolates from wound infection and their sensitivity to alternative topical agents at Jimma University specialized hospital, south-West Ethiopia. Ann Clin Microbiol Antimicrob. 2014;13(1):14.
6. Brook IT, Frazier EH. The aerobic and anaerobic bacteriology of perirectal abscesses. J Clin Microbiol. 1997;35(11):2974–6.
7. Liu SS, Richman JM, Thirlby RC, Wu CL. Efficacy of continuous wound catheters delivering local anesthetic for postoperative analgesia: a quantitative and qualitative systematic review of randomized controlled trials. J Am Coll Surg. 2006;203(6):914–32.
8. Centers for Disease Control and Prevention (CDC). Soft tissue infections among injection drug users-San Francisco, California, 1996-2000. MMWR Morb Mortal Wkly Rep. 2001;50(19):381.
9. Steed LL, Costello J, Lohia S, Jones T, Spannhake EW, Nguyen S. Reduction of nasal *Staphylococcus aureus* carriage in health care professionals by treatment with a nonantibiotic, alcohol-based nasal antiseptic. Am J Infect Control. 2014;42(8):841–6.
10. Cohen ML. Changing patterns of infectious disease. Nature. 2000;406(6797):762.
11. Weigelt J, Itani K, Stevens D, Lau W, Dryden M, Knirsch C. Linezolid CSSTI study group. Linezolid versus vancomycin in treatment of complicated skin and soft tissue infections. Antimicrob Agents Chemother. 2005;49(6):2260–6.
12. Jacoby GA. AmpC β-lactamases. Clin Microbiol Rev. 2009;22(1):161–82.
13. Bush K. Extended-spectrum β-lactamases in North America, 1987–2006. Clinical Microbiology and Infection. 2008;14:134–43.
14. Magiorakos AP, Srinivasan A, Carey RB, Carmeli Y, Falagas ME, Giske CG, Harbarth S, Hindler JF, Kahlmeter G, Olsson-Liljequist B, Paterson DL. Multidrug-resistant, extensively drug-resistant and pandrug-resistant bacteria: an international expert proposal for interim standard definitions for acquired resistance. Clin Microbiol Infect. 2012;18(3):268–81.
15. Smith, A.C., Hussey, M.A., 2005. Gram stain protocols.
16. Wayne PACLSI. Performance standards for antimicrobial susceptibility testing; twenty-fifth informational supplement. CLSI document M100-S25. In: Clinical and laboratory standards institute; 2015.
17. Wayne PA. Clinical and laboratory standards institute. Performance standards for antimicrobial susceptibility testing, vol. 17; 2007.
18. Harwalkar A, Sataraddi J, Gupta S, Yoganand R, Rao A, Srinivasa H. The detection of ESBL-producing *Escherichia coli* in patients with symptomatic urinary tract infections using different diffusion methods in a rural setting. J Infect Public Health. 2013;6(2):108–14.
19. Mshana SE, Kamugisha E, Mirambo M, Chakraborty T, Lyamuya EF. Prevalence of multiresistant gram-negative organisms in a tertiary hospital in Mwanza, Tanzania. BMC Res Notes. 2009;2(1):49.
20. Kumari K. Pattern of bacterial isolates and antibiogram from open wound infection among the indoor patients of Bir Hospital (Doctoral dissertation, M. Sc. Dissertation, Central Department of Microbiology, Tribhuvan University, Kirtipur, Kathmandu, Nepal).
21. CPa B, Mb L. The distribution of pathogens causing wound infection and their antibiotic susceptibility pattern. J Nepal Health Res Counc. 2008;5(1):22–6.
22. Parikh AR, Hamilton S, Sivarajan V, Withey S, Butler PE. Diagnostic fine-needle aspiration in postoperative wound infections is more accurate at predicting causative organisms than wound swabs. Ann R Coll Surg England. 2007;89(2):166–7.
23. Bowler PG, Duerden BI, Armstrong DG. Wound microbiology and associated approaches to wound management. Clin Microbiol Rev. 2001;14(2):244–69.
24. Rajput A, Singh KP, Kumar V, Sexena R, Singh RK. Antibacterial resistance pattern of aerobic bacteria isolates from burn patients in tertiary care hospital. Biomedical research. 2008;19(1). http://www.alliedacademies.org/biomedical-research/archive/aabmr-volume-19-issue-1-year-2008.html.
25. Gelaw A, Gebre-Selassie S, Tiruneh M, Mathios E, Yifru S. Isolation of bacterial pathogens from patients with postoperative surgical site infections and possible sources of infections at the University of Gondar Hospital, Northwest Ethiopia. J Environ Occup Sci. 2014;3(2): 103 8.

26. Goswami NN, Trivedi HR, Goswami AP, Patel TK, Tripathi CB. Antibiotic sensitivity profile of bacterial pathogens in postoperative wound infections at a tertiary care hospital in Gujarat, India. J Pharmacol Pharmacother. 2011;2(3):158.
27. Komolafe OO, James J, Kalongolera L, Makoka M. Bacteriology of burns at the queen elizabeth central hospital, Blantyre, Malawi. Burns. 2003;29(3):235–8.
28. Sanjay KR, Prasad MN, Vijaykumar GS. A study on isolation and detection of drug resistance gram negative bacilli with special importance to post operative wound infection. J Microbiol Antimicrob. 2011;3(9):68–75.
29. Lakshmidevi N. Surgical site infections: assessing risk factors, outcomes and antimicrobial sensitivity patterns. Afr J Microbiol Res. 2009;3(4):175–9.
30. Mulu W, Kibru G, Beyene G, Damtie M. Postoperative nosocomial infections and antimicrobial resistance pattern of bacteria isolates among patients admitted at Felege Hiwot referral hospital, Bahirdar, Ethiopia. Ethiop J Health Sci. 2012;22(1):7–18.
31. Adegoke AA, Komolafe AO. Nasal colonization of school children in Ile-Ife by multiple antibiotic resistant *Staphylococcus aureus*. Int J Biotechnol Allied Sci. 2008;3(1):317–22.
32. Forster, D.H. and Daschner, F.D., 1998. *Acinetobacter* species as nosocomial pathogens.
33. Biadglegne F, Abera B, Alem A, Anagaw B. Bacterial isolates from wound infection and their antimicrobial susceptibility pattern in Felege Hiwot referral Hospital North West Ethiopia. Ethiop J Health Sci. 2009;19(3):173–177.
34. Manyahi J. Bacteriological spectrum of post operative wound infections and their antibiogram in a Tertiary Hospital, Dar Es Salaam, Tanzania (Doctoral dissertation, Muhimbili University of Health and Allied Sciences).
35. Gottrup F, Melling A, Hollander DA. An overview of surgical site infections: aetiology, incidence and risk factors. EWMA J. 2005;5(2):11–5.
36. Howell-Jones RS, Wilson MJ, Hill KE, Howard AJ, Price PE, Thomas DW. A review of the microbiology, antibiotic usage and resistance in chronic skin wounds. J Antimicrob Chemother. 2005;55(2):143–9.
37. Heinzelmann M, Scott M, Lam T. Factors predisposing to bacterial invasion and infection. Am J Surg. 2002;183(2):179–90.

3

The effect of antibiotic stewardship interventions with stakeholder involvement in hospital settings: a multicentre, cluster randomized controlled intervention study

Jannicke Slettli Wathne[1,2,3*], Lars Kåre Selland Kleppe[4], Stig Harthug[1,2], Hege Salvesen Blix[5], Roy M. Nilsen[6], Esmita Charani[7], The Bergen Intervention Teams and Ingrid Smith[8*]

Abstract

Background: There is limited evidence from multicenter, randomized controlled studies to inform planning and implementation of antibiotic stewardship interventions in hospitals.

Methods: A cluster randomized, controlled, intervention study was performed in selected specialities (infectious diseases, pulmonary medicine and gastroenterology) at three emergency care hospitals in Western Norway. Interventions applied were audit with feedback and academic detailing. Implementation strategies included co-design of interventions with stakeholders in local intervention teams and prescribers setting local targets for change in antibiotic prescribing behaviour. Primary outcome measures were adherence to national guidelines, use of broad-spectrum antibiotics and change in locally defined targets of change in prescribing behaviour. Secondary outcome measures were length of stay, 30-day readmission, in-hospital- and 30-day mortality.

Results: One thousand eight hundred two patients receiving antibiotic treatment were included. Adherence to guidelines had an absolute increase from 60 to 66% for all intervention wards ($p = 0.04$). Effects differed across specialties and pulmonary intervention wards achieved a 14% absolute increase in adherence ($p = 0.003$), while no change was observed for other specialties. A pulmonary ward targeting increased use of penicillin G 2 mill IU × 4 for pneumonia and COPD exacerbations had an intended increase of 30% for this prescribing behaviour ($p < 0.001$).

Conclusions: Pulmonary wards had a higher increase in adherence, independent of applied intervention. The effect of antibiotic stewardship interventions is dependent on how and in which context they are implemented. Additional effects of interventions are seen when stakeholders discuss ward prescribing behaviour and agree on specific targets for changes in prescribing practice.

Keywords: Antibiotic stewardship, Intervention, cRCT, Audit with feedback, Academic detailing, Hospital, Goal setting

Background

Globally, the overuse and misuse of antibiotics, especially broad-spectrum agents, has accelerated the development and selection of resistant bacteria [1–3]. The increase in broad-spectrum antibiotic prescribing cannot be explained by increased antibiotic resistance alone [4].

* Correspondence: jannicke.slettli.wathne@sav.no; ismith@who.int
[1]Department of Clinical Science, University of Bergen, Bergen, Norway
[8]Innovation, Access and Use, Department of Essential Medicines and Health Products, World Health Organization (WHO), Avenue Appia 20, 1211 Geneva 27, Switzerland
Full list of author information is available at the end of the article

Antibiotic stewardship programs have been introduced to hospitals worldwide to promote more prudent antibiotic use [5, 6]. The basis of stewardship programs are evidence based clinical guidelines for antibiotic prescribing to ensure effective treatment for individual patients, while minimizing development of antimicrobial resistance (AMR). Adherence to antibiotic guidelines varies among countries and institutions [6]. Interventions like audit with feedback, providing a summary of clinical performance over time and educational outreach through academic detailing have been shown to be effective in increasing adherence. However, the need for studies addressing cultural, contextual and behavioural determinants when developing, implementing and reporting stewardship interventions has been highlighted [6–9]. There is also a need for more studies that apply behaviour change theory to investigate effect on antibiotic use across hospitals, specialties and diagnoses to help identify the most effective means of implementing interventions that are transferable and generalizable [6, 10, 11]. We report here the findings of a multicentre, cluster randomized controlled intervention study, investigating the effect of behaviour change interventions with stakeholder involvement and local target setting for change in antibiotic prescribing [12].

Methods

Definitions

Substances of ATC-group J01 (Antibacterials for systemic use), metronidazole tablets (P01AB01) and vancomycin tablets (A07AA09) were included in the definition of antibiotics for this study [13]. Broad-spectrum antibiotics were defined as penicillins with enzyme inhibitor (J01CR), 2. and 3. generation cephalosporins (J01D C-D), carbapenems (J01DH) and quinolones (J01MA), the five groups targeted in the National Action Plan Against Antibiotic Resistance in Health Services [14, 15].

Study design

This prospective, cluster randomized, controlled intervention study was performed within three specialties at three emergency care and teaching hospitals as a parallel group study with three arms (Table 1).

Participants and data collection

Eligible clusters were wards within one of the medical specialties; infectious diseases, pulmonary medicine and gastroenterology at hospital A, B and C in Western Norway. Specialties were selected based on infectious diseases and pulmonary medicine having the highest consumption of antibiotics in the included hospitals. Gastroenterology was included since hospital B had a joint medication storage area for the ward of pulmonary medicine and the ward of gastroenterology. Hospital A and B were tertiary care hospitals with 1100 and 600 beds, respectively. Hospital C was a secondary care hospital with 160 beds. For description of case mix, see Table 2.

Patients who received antibiotics during hospitalization and were discharged from the study wards in the time period from 10th of February to 11th of July 2014 were eligible for inclusion in the study. Patients who received antibioticprophylaxis, had orthopaedic prosthesis infections, or had a hospital stay < 24 h or > 21 days were excluded. Patients whose indication for treatment was not in the antibiotic guideline or whose antibiotics were discontinued at day 1, was excluded. Only the first stay of readmitted patients was included. Patients were included consecutively. Patient data were collected manually from electronic medical records. Data collected included patient demographics, indication for antibiotic treatment, antibiotic prescribing, microbiological test results, estimated glomerular filtration rate (eGFR) on admission, length of stay, 30-day readmission, in-hospital and 30-day mortality and admittance from- or discharge to other hospitals or nursing homes. Indications for antibiotic treatment were registered as documented in the medical record and not assessed for validity.

Broad-spectrum antibiotic use for study wards in the period 2013–2015 was collected from the hospital pharmacies sales statistics and adjusted per 100 patient bed days.

Interventions

The primary intervention aim was to increase adherence to The National Guidelines for Antibiotic Use in Hospitals (hereafter guidelines), across diagnoses [16]. Each hospital assigned local intervention teams of 1–2 physicians and 1 pharmacist to co-design and implement the interventions. Authors I.S and J.S.W developed initial intervention concepts, which were discussed in a regional meeting with all project participants. Each intervention team then refined the interventions to fit their local context. A common presentation template was prepared for all intervention sessions with information about antibiotic resistance, the national antibiotic guideline, local antibiotic sales statistics and principals of antibiotic dosing. All intervention teams modified this material to fit the individual wards. Academic detailing sessions focused on recently admitted infectious diseases patients, including cases with treatment both adherent and non-adherent to guidelines. The teams' selection of patient cases decided the focus in wards receiving academic detailing.

Audit with feedback wards had predefined target areas of pneumonia and COPD exacerbations, as these patients were frequently admitted to both intervention wards. Fifty patients with these diagnosis were included consecutively from February to April 2014 to get a reasonable overview of prescribing practice over the given time period, without excessive workload for the intervention teams. For the audit data, intervention teams assessed adherence. The level of detail and focus in the feedback was at the discretion of the teams and varied between the two feedback wards.

Intervention ward physicians were invited to academic detailing- or audit with feedback- group sessions in May 2014, led by local intervention teams. No specific threshold for acceptable attendance was defined, but more than one meeting was held if the intervention team considered the attendance at the first meeting to be too low. Physicians present at the main session at each ward were invited to identify one or two specific challenges to be addressed as local targets for improvement of antibiotic prescribing based on discussions during the session. Specific actions to

Table 1 Overview of implemented interventions

Intervention	Hospital	Specialty	Intervention sessions	Attendance consultants/ residents (estimated)	Performed by	Special features of each intervention	Common features of intervention sessions for both audit with feedback and academic detailing
Audit with feedback	A	Pulmonary medicine	16.05.14	70%	Local pharmacist + study ward consultant	Focus areas: Pneumonia (CAP) COPD exacerbations - > Adherence to guideline (50 patients) Use of broad-spectrum antibiotics - > Indication for treatment (50 patients)	1. Verbal presentation including: - Antibiotic resistance - Antibiotic guideline - Dosing of antibiotics - Ward antibiotic sales statistics 2. Discussion among ward physicians: - Ward prescribing practice - Challenges - Target setting (1–2 targets)
	B	Infectious diseases	20.05.14 27.05.14	100%			
Academic detailing	A	Gastro-enterology	14.05.14	90%	Local ID-physician	Case discussions on recently discharged patients with infectious diseases. Variety of diagnoses, chosen by ID-physician	
	B	Pulmonary medicine	13.05.14 23.05.14	100%			
	C	Infectious diseases	20.05.14 21.05.14	70%			
Control	A	Infectious diseases					
	B	Gastro-enterology					
	C	Pulmonary medicine					

Table 2 Patient characteristics and patient outcome pre- and post-implementation of interventions, per intervention group and specialty

	Pulmonary medicine Period			Infectious diseases Period			Gastroenterology Period			Audit with feedback Period			Academic detailing Period			Control (all three specialities) Period		
	Pre $N = 427$ n (%)	Post $N = 162$ n (%)	*p*-value	Pre $N = 424$ n (%)	Post $N = 153$ n (%)	*p*-value	Pre $N = 78$ n (%)	Post $N = 39$ n (%)	*p*-value	Pre $N = 478$ n (%)	Post $N = 182$ n (%)	*p*-value	Pre $N = 451$ n (%)	Post $N = 172$ n (%)	*p*-value	Pre $N = 350$ n (%)	Post $N = 169$ n (%)	*p*-value
Age (mean - years)	69.6	68.99	0.66	67.5	64.4	0.10	68.9	64.8	0.35	67.1	66.1	0.51	70.2	67.1	0.05	63.2	65.7	0.22
Sex																		
Female	213 (49.9)	88 (54.3)	0.34	180 (42.5)	80 (52.3)	**0.04**	37 (47.4)	16 (41.0)	0.51	221 (46.2)	101 (55.5)	**0.03**	209 (46.3)	83 (48.3)	0.67	167 (47.7)	80 (47.3)	0.94
Male	214 (50.1)	74 (45.7)		244 (57.5)	73 (47.7)		41 (52.6)	23 (59)		257 (53.8)	81 (44.5)		242 (53.7)	89 (51.7)		183 (52.3)	89 (52.7)	
Admitted from hospital/nursing home	55 (12.9)	15 (9.3)	0.23	68 (16.0)	30 (19.7)	0.30	14 (18.0)	3 (7.7)	0.14	67 (14.0)	20 (11.0)	0.30	70 (15.5)	28 (16.4)	0.79	51 (14.6)	23 (13.6)	0.75
Indication for antibiotic treatment																		
Pneumonia	136 (31.9)	63 (38.9)	0.20	115 (27.1)	45 (29.6)	0.06	11 (14.1)	3 (7.7)	0.16	162 (33.9)	67 (36.8)	**0.01**	100 (22.2)	44 (25.7)	0.15	65 (18.7)	23 (13.6)	0.31
COPD exacerbation, infectious	183 (42.9)	63 (38.9)		59 (13.9)	7 (4.6)		1 (1.3)	2 (5.1)		132 (27.6)	34 (18.7)		111 (24.6)	38 (22.2)		25 (7.2)	15 (8.9)	
LRTI - Other	23 (5.4)	9 (5.6)		16 (3.7)	6 (3.95)		6 (7.7)	2 (5.1)		19 (4.0)	4 (2.2)		26 (5.8)	13 (7.6)		22 (6.3)	7 (4.1)	
Sepsis	40 (9.4)	17 (10.5)		61 (14.4)	24 (15.8)		16 (20.5)	5 (12.8)		57 (11.9)	26 (14.3)		60 (13.3)	20 (11.7)		73 (21.0)	50 (29.6)	
Skin and soft tissue	3 (0.7)	2 (1.2)		62 (14.6)	33 (21.7)		9 (11.5)	6 (15.4)		31 (6.5)	25 (13.7)		43 (9.5)	16 (9.4)		58 (16.7)	22 (13.0)	
Gastrointestinal tract	1 (0.2)	0 (0)		9 (2.12)	4 (2.6)		9 (11.5)	11 (28.2)		6 (1.3)	2 (1.1)		13 (2.8)	13 (7.6)		35 (10.1)	14 (8.3)	
Urinary tract	9 (2.1)	5 (3.1)		75 (17.7)	21 (13.8)		17 (21.8)	9 (23.1)		31 (6.5)	16 (8.8)		70 (15.5)	19 (11.1)		36 (10.3)	19 (11.2)	
Other	32 (7.5)	3 (1.9)		27 (6.4)	12 (7.9)		9 (11.5)	1 (2.6)		40 (8.4)	8 (4.4)		28 (6.2)	8 (4.7)		34 (9.8)	19 (11.2)	
Antibiotic allergies	62 (14.5)	28 (17.3)	0.41	35 (8.3)	19 (12.4)	0.13	8 (10.3)	4 (10.3)	0.99	59 (12.3)	26 (14.3)	0.51	46 (10.2)	25 (14.5)	0.13	25 (7.2)	17 (10.1)	0.18
Patient outcomes Δ																		
Length of stay (days)	7.2	6.9	0.40	6.5	6.5	0.99	7.0	6.1	0.30	7.2	6.5	**0.04**[Δ]	6.5	6.8	0.41	7.5	6.8	0.11
In-hospital mortality	30 (7.0)	7 (4.3)	0.23	12 (2.8)	4 (2.61)	0.89	3 (3.9)	2 (5.13)	0.76	28 (5.9)	9 (5.0)	0.65	17 (3.8)	4 (2.3)	0.37	13 (3.7)	3 (1.8)	0.23
30-day mortality	53 (12.4)	11 (6.8)	0.05	30 (7.1)	8 (5.3)	0.44	3 (3.9)	4 (10.3)	0.17	50 (10.5)	12 (6.6)	0.13	36 (8.0)	11 (6.4)	0.51	24 (6.9)	6 (3.6)	0.13
30-day readmission	117 (29.3)	38 (24.5)	0.26	78 (19.1)	18 (12.2)	0.06	16 (21.3)	6 (17.1)	0.61	111 (24.6)	36 (20.9)	0.33	100 (23.1)	26 (15.7)	**0.04**[Δ]	58 (17.5)	30 (18.6)	0.75

***p*-values are obtained by chi-square test (categorical variables) and t-test (continuous variables) per group**

Δ Patient outcomes were also tested for interaction between intervention groups/specialty and period using linear and logistic regression. *p*-value interaction length of stay = 0.080. *p*-value interaction 30-day readmission = 0.105

achieve targets were not included in the target discussions. For details of interventions, see Table 1.

Outcomes

Primary outcome measures

1) Adherence to guidelines was assessed on the second day of treatment to allow sufficient time for patients to be reviewed by study ward physicians and measured as percentage of correctly prescribed empiric treatment (choice of active substance) before and after interventions [16]. CRB-65 was not routinely documented, so pneumonia and severe pneumonia was assessed together (both empiric treatments assessed as adherent). All hospitals were committed to use the national guideline, as recommendations were appropriate with regards to local antibiotic resistance patterns.
2) Use of broad-spectrum antibiotics was assessed as DDD/100 bed days in time series before and after intervention. Broad-spectrum antibiotic use was selected as an outcome measure because the guidelines mainly recommend narrow-spectrum antibiotics as empiric treatment and a shift towards guideline adherent prescribing was expected to cause a reduction in broad-spectrum antibiotic use.
3) Change in locally targeted prescribing behaviour was assessed according to the defined targets and compared before and after interventions.

Secondary outcome measures were length of stay, 30-day readmission and mortality (all cause in-house and 30-day mortality). Patient outcomes were measured to ensure that the interventions did not have any negative consequences for patient treatment.

Sample size

As baseline adherence to guidelines was unknown in Norway, calculation of the sample size prior to the study was challenging. According to the original research protocol, we assumed an absolute 20% improvement in adherence from 50% pre-intervention to 70% post-intervention for each cluster. Given a power of 80% and a type 1 error of 5%, the smallest number of subjects needed to detect this difference was 93 both before and after the intervention. Although this was sufficient for the current study, we calculated at least 155 patients before and after intervention to answer additional research questions listed in the original protocol. However, the sample size calculations did not include intra-cluster correlation coefficient (ICC) or comparison with a control group. Based on pre-intervention data of adherence to guideline, ICC coefficient for this outcome was 0.012 with 95% CI (0.003, 0.053).

Randomization

Authors I.S and J.S.W. performed randomization and assigned clusters to interventions by drawing lots of hospital and intervention groups per specialty. Across the hospitals, infectious diseases and pulmonary medicine received both academic detailing and audit with feedback and had a control group. Only two of the hospitals had specific gastroenterology wards, so this specialty received only one intervention and had a control group (Table 1).

Blinding

Prescribing physicians at the wards were not informed about the study being performed during the baseline period and were at that point blinded to intervention group, with the exception of the physicians assigned to the project teams. Control ward physicians were blinded throughout the study period.

Assessment of adherence to guidelines was performed blinded to the intervention- or treatment group, by using syntax in SPSS. An adherence variable was generated, combining the variable indication for treatment with the variable for prescribed treatment. First choice of empiric therapy was coded as adherent. Manual adjustment of adherence of antibiotic prescriptions was made in patients with antibiotic allergies or kidney failure.

Statistical analysis

Analyses were performed both per intervention group and per specialty, but due to fewer patients than expected in the post-intervention period, analysis per cluster was not performed. Differences in study group characteristics pre- and post-interventions were tested using Pearson's chi-square test for categorical data and independent two-sample t-test for continuous data. Pearsons chi-square test was also applied to test adherence to guidelines pre- and post-interventions for individual intervention groups and specialties. To test whether percentage of adherence to guidelines or patient outcomes in intervention and specialty groups changed differently over time compared with the control group, we evaluated the group-by-period interaction term in simple logistic or linear regression models, as appropriate. Adherence to guideline or patient outcome were dependent variables, with group of intervention (audit vs control/academic detailing vs control) or specialty (e.g. pulmonary medicine vs control/infectious diseases vs control) and period (before-after) were independent variables together with the interaction term. The level – and trend effect of broad-spectrum antibiotic use (sales statistics) pre- and post-intervention was estimated with the Interrupted Times Series (ITS) analysis method described by the Cochrane Effective Practice and Organisation of Care (EPOC) group [17]. All tests were two-sided and p-values < 0.05 was considered statistical significant for all analyses.

Statistical analysis was conducted using SPSS for Windows, version 24 and Stata SE for Windows, version 15.

Results

Patients

Two thousand four hundred five admissions were eligible for inclusion. After applying exclusion criteria, 1802 unique patients were included in analysis, 1279 and 523 patients in the pre- and post-intervention periods respectively (Table 2). The study period was fixed due to time-limited allocation of project resources and mandatory information of included patients. Interventions were conducted later than originally planned due to practical considerations at the study wards. This caused skewness in data with two thirds of the patients included pre-interventions (Table 2). Patient characteristics were similar pre- and post-interventions, except for some differences in distribution of diagnoses in the audit with feedback group (Table 2).

Primary outcomes

Adherence to guidelines

Across all intervention wards, adherence to guideline increased from 60% to 66% ($p = 0.04$), but when compared with the control group, this was not significant (Table 3). The effect of interventions differed largely between the specialties. Infectious diseases and gastroenterology wards displayed no effect of interventions on adherence, while pulmonary medicine wards displayed significant effect of interventions compared to the control group (Table 3). Academic detailing and audit with feedback increased total adherence to guideline by 14% and 13% respectively (absolute increase), in the pulmonary wards (not shown in tables).

The audit with feedback intervention specifically targeted pneumonia and COPD exacerbations. For these diagnoses, the pulmonary medicine ward increased adherence by 12% and infectious diseases ward by 2% (not shown in tables).

Use of broad-spectrum antibiotics

Interrupted time series analysis showed that the overall trend of activity-adjusted broad-spectrum antibiotic use pre- and post-interventions was significantly improved, as was the level at 12 and 18 months post intervention for the audit with feedback group (Appendix: Table 5 and Fig. 1). The gastroenterology intervention ward had a significant decrease in the use of broad-spectrum antibiotics at 3 and 6 months, but it increased thereafter (Appendix: Table 5 and Fig. 1). No significant change in broad-spectrum antibiotic use was seen at the intervention wards receiving academic detailing, the control group and for other intervention wards per specialty (Appendix: Table 5 and Fig. 1).

Local targets

Intervention wards were invited to set local targets for follow up after the intervention sessions (Table 4). The pulmonary ward at Hospital A had a significant and intended 30% increase in the targeted use of Penicillin G 2 mill IU × 4 for patients with pneumonia and COPD exacerbations post intervention ($p < 0.001$). The use of Ciprofloxacin at the ward of gastroenterology was reduced at all time points following the intervention, though not statistically significant (Appendix: Table 6). The other study wards either [a)] did not reach consensus on targets [b)] did not identify any targets or [c)] the identified target was not evaluable.

Secondary outcome measures

When analysed per intervention, there was a decrease of 0.7 days in the mean length of stay for patients in the audit with feedback group ($p = 0.037$) (Table 2). In the academic detailing group, 30-days readmission had an absolute decrease of 7.4% ($p = 0.044$). Compared with

Table 3 Percentage of adherence to antibiotic guidelines in periods before and after interventions were implemented

Group	Group description	N Before/after	Period		Absolute Change %	P for change[a]	P for Interaction[b]
			Before n (%)	After n (%)			
Intervention							
Control	All specialties	350/169	174 (50)	84 (50)	0	0.998	
Interventions	All specialties	929/354	556 (60)	234 (66)	6	**0.04**	0.252
Academic detailing	All specialties	451/172	265 (59)	111 (65)	6	0.188	0.353
Audit with feedback	Infectious diseases + Pulmonary medicine	478/182	291 (61)	123 (68)	7	0.111	0.265
Specialty							
Pulmonary medicine	Both interventions	427/162	249 (58)	116 (72)	14	**0.003**	**0.034**
Infectious diseases	Both interventions	424/153	268 (63)	99 (65)	2	0.741	0.857
Gastroenterology	Academic detailing	78/39	39 (50)	19 (49)	-1	0.896	0.556

[a]By chi-square test per group
[b]By logistic regression of given group vs control wards (all specialties), giving the p-value for the interaction between group and period
P-values < 0.05 are given in boldface

Table 4 Local targets set by study intervention wards and outcome for targeted change in prescribing practice

Hospital	Ward	Intervention	Targets	Outcome
A	Pulmonary medicine	Audit with feedback	Increase the use of Penicillin G 2 mill IU × 4 to treat pneumonia (CAP) and infectious COPD exacerbations	30% increase ($p < 0.001$)[a]
A	Gastro enterology	Academic detailing	Reduce ciprofloxacin use for inflammatory bowel disease, and shift to Co-trimoxazol *(indication outside national antibiotic guideline)*	Too few patients with targeted indication to assess outcome by indication. Assessed by use of sales statistics. Reduction in use of Ciprofloxacin at 3, 6, 12 and 18 months following the intervention (not significant)[b] (Appendix Table 6).
B	Pulmonary medicine	Academic detailing	Target areas discussed: - Reevaluation of initiated treatment on arrival to ward and - after 48–72 h - Increase use of CRB-65 and antibiotic guideline	*Consensus on 1–2 targets not achieved*
B	Infectious diseases	Audit with feedback	Target areas discussed: - Increase use of Penicillin G 2 mill × 4 to treat infectious COPD exacerbations - Reassess length of iv-antibiotics for patients with osteomyelitis - Increase consultants presence in the emergency room to increase guidelines adherence on admission - Reevaluation of treatment during the patient stay	*Consensus on 1–2 targets not achieved*
C	Infectious diseases	Academic detailing	*No target area identified.*	*No target area identified*

[a]By chi-square test [b]By Interrupted time series analysis (Appendix Table 6)

the control group, these findings were not statistically significant. In-hospital death, 30-day mortality, 30-day readmission and length of stay for the other groups were not significantly changed (Table 2).

Discussion

This study highlights the effect of engaging local stakeholders (physicians) in setting specific targets for change in antibiotic prescribing behaviours. A specific target area, which is easy to remember and act upon, makes it possible to achieve change within a short timeframe, as observed in the pulmonary ward at Hospital A where adherence to targeted behaviour increased by 30%. Another finding was how the effect of interventions differed across specialties. Both interventions were more effective at the pulmonary wards, than wards of infectious diseases and gastroenterology.

Interventions to improve antibiotic prescribing practices have shown a 15% average increase in adherent prescribing in intervention wards, however the effect depends on how they are designed and implemented [6, 18]. When Schouten et al. tailored interventions to each intervention hospital; they achieved an average 14% increase in adherence to guidelines for empiric treatment of lower respiratory tract infections (LRTI). The level of change was very similar for all the intervention hospitals, although it was not stated how the patients were distributed across the wards of internal- and pulmonary medicine [19]. Their results are comparable to our findings at the pulmonary wards, with a 14% absolute change in adherence to guidelines, while it differs substantially from effects seen across infectious diseases and gastroenterology wards. A single site Norwegian study focusing on pneumonia and COPD exacerbations within pulmonary medicine, added a pocket guideline to their audit with feedback intervention [20]. From a baseline adherence of 62%, similar to our study, adherence was increased by 22%.

Involving clinicians in identifying challenges, finding solutions and setting local targets is both reasonable and recommended and has previously proven effective in increasing compliance to target behaviour [6, 21–23]. Jobson et al. increased the timeliness of antibiotics for febrile patients with central lines presenting in the ED from 63 to 99% [23]. They exceeded their goal of 90% timeliness through active engagement of the caregiving staff and the use of multiple plan-study-do-act-cycles (PDSA-cycles) [24]. At the pulmonary ward at hospital A, the audit data made it easy for clinicians to identify local challenges and set a specific, measureable, attractive and realistic target for change in prescribing behaviour and we found a similar change of 30% increase in target behaviour.

The wards receiving audit with feedback had different case-mix. In infectious diseases, 41% of patients were treated for pneumonia and COPD exacerbations, compared to 71% in the pulmonary ward. This could partly explain the lack of effect seen in the infectious disease ward, as pneumonia and COPD exacerbations were the selected focus for the feedback sessions. Empirical therapy according to guidelines across diagnoses was the main outcome measure for all intervention wards. Pre-audits at every intervention ward would have made it easier to identify each ward's prescribing challenges, and tailor the interventions to context specific improvement areas for each ward. As this study is intervening in the very heart of ID-specialists' area of expertise, it may also be a bigger challenge to advocate a shift in prescribing practice towards general antibiotic guidelines, limiting the autonomy of the prescriber [25].

The national guideline was published approximately 6 months prior to study initiation and some wards had already started promoting its use [16]. A previous study by Skodvin et al. showed that interns and residents heavily relied on guidelines when initiating antibiotic treatment [26]. This could have caused a positive shift in prescribing practice already, decreasing the potential for absolute effect of interventions. Including physicians mainly working in the emergency room in interventions could have given increased effects, but intervention and control wards at the same hospital would then be challenging because of spill over effects between the wards.

Champions can play a powerful role in behaviour change [25, 26]. Special emphasis was made on using local champions for developing and implementing interventions as they are familiar to the ward physicians, know possible barriers and facilitators and could tailor the presentations to the ward's needs. Local involvement could also increase the chance of continuous work within the area after study completion. An example of tailoring is adding information about a previous local outbreak of Vancomycin-resistant enterococci (VRE) to the audit with feedback session at the pulmonary ward at Hospital A, to increase local ownership. At the gastroenterology ward, academic detailing was performed by an ID-physician. During evaluation, he suggested that including a physician from the gastroenterology ward could have increased the ownership of the intervention and the identified target. Interventions were only applied at one time-point during the study period. Adding more intervention sessions could probably have increased the effects seen [6].

We aimed to achieve responsible antibiotic prescribing practice in a complex hospital setting. This study is a "real-life" study, including the most common infections treated at hospitals in the western world and three specialties in three separate hospitals where patterns of prescribing may differ, as will patient mix. All three hospitals and specialties contributed both to the intervention and control groups, reducing the potential for confounding and increasing external validity of the findings. The study was initiated in a "normal" clinical situation and not as a response to an outbreak. Random time effects should therefore be reduced. Seasonality is likely, but the inclusion of control groups within the same time period allow us to control for the effects. Findings should be generalizable to other hospital wards within the same specialties and in settings with a similar, relatively flat organizational structure.

The short post-intervention period and skewness of data between pre- and post-intervention periods is the major limitation to this study, caused by the fixed date for study period when applying for study approval and the substantial workload for manual data collection of individual prescription data. This also led to insufficient power to look at intervention effect on adherence at each cluster. Activity-adjusted antibiotic sales statistics for broad-spectrum antibiotics provides however the opportunity to assess change in levels and trends of broad-spectrum antibiotic use, indicating prescribing behaviour over longer periods of time.

In our study we found that the context we implemented interventions in were even more important than the type of intervention selected. Tailoring the interventions to the local context and challenges of each study ward and more focus on using SMART[1] goals during the planning and implementation of interventions, could increase the possibility to get the desired outcomes. LRTIs are common in stewardship intervention studies [6, 18]. It is a wise place to start optimization of antibiotic prescribing, because the volume of patients secures great impact on total antibiotic use. More severe diagnoses, like infections in immunocompromised patients may be a bigger challenge to target in behaviour change. Especially inexperienced physicians may feel the need to secure adequate coverage with broad-spectrum antibiotics at treatment initiation and the thought of "never change a winning team" may lead to lack of re-evaluation and focusing treatment [26].

When designing behavioural change interventions in antibiotic stewardship programs, we need careful planning. Attention should be paid to local barriers and facilitators for change and we should have in-depth knowledge of local antibiotic prescribing practices and case mix to guide the focus of interventions.

Conclusions

Pulmonary intervention wards had an increase in adherence, independent of applied intervention, while no effect was seen at wards of infectious diseases and gastroenterology. This shows that the context in which interventions are implemented is important and may also indicate that pulmonary wards may be a good place to start when changing antibiotic prescribing behavior in similar hospital settings. We also showed that when ward physicians were actively involved in the process of discussing their own prescribing behavior and could identify and agree on specific targets for change in prescribing practice, great change was achieved within a short timeframe.

Endnotes

[1]SMART: Specific, Measurable, Attractive, Realistic and Time-bound

Appendix

Appendix show results for interrupted time series analysis of the use of broad- spectrum antibiotics for intervention groups and specialties:

Table 5 Interrupted time series analysis of the use of broad-spectrum antibiotics in defined daily doses per 100 bed days for intervention and control groups from 2013 to 2015

		Audit with feedback (Intervention wards)			Academic detailing (Intervention wards			Pulmonary medicine (Intervention wards)			Infectious diseases (Intervention wards)			Gastroenterology (Intervention ward)			Control (all specialties)		
		Estimate	SE	*p*-value	Estimate	SE	*p*-value	Estimate	SE	*p*-value	Estimate	SE	*p*-value	Estimate	SE	*p*-value	Estimate	SE	*p*-value
DDD per 100 bed days	Const	70.288	5.854	0.000	103.078	8.415	0.000	84.736	5.056	0.000	60.371	7.407	0.000	27.605	1.592	0.000	87.691	5.387	0.000
	AR	−0.495	0.326	0.172	−0.247	0.370	0.525	−0.429	0.348	0.257	−0.239	0.372	0.542	−0.796	0.203	0.006	−0.512	0.323	0.157
Pre-slope		4.332	1.523	**0.025**	−2.903	2.181	0.225	−2.292	1.312	0.124	3.985	1.926	0.077	−0.075	0.411	0.861	1.002	1.404	0.498
Difference between pre- and post-slope		−6.789	2.028	**0.012**	2.920	2.985	0.360	−0.669	1.770	0.717	−5.753	2.615	0.064	2.472	0.545	**0.003**	−1.033	1.863	0.597
Level effect																			
3 months		−8.971	7.809	0.288	−3.162	11.053	0.783	8.314	6.686	0.254	−10.360	9.839	0.327	−11.157	2.082	**0.001**	1.407	7.191	0.850
6 months		−15.761	8.313	0.100	−0.242	11.823	0.984	7.646	7.131	0.319	−16.112	10.503	0.169	−8.685	2.220	**0.006**	0.374	7.672	0.962
12 months		−29.338	10.490	**0.027**	5.599	15.115	0.722	6.308	9.052	0.508	−27.617	13.357	0.077	−3.740	2.811	0.225	−1.691	9.694	0.866
18 months		−42.916	13.561	**0.016**	11.439	19.708	0.580	4.971	11.751	0.685	−39.122	17.355	0.059	1.205	3.640	0.750	−3.757	12.525	0.773

Broad-spectrum antibiotics were defined as penicillins with enzyme inhibitor, 2. and 3. generation cephalosporins, carbapenems and quionolones

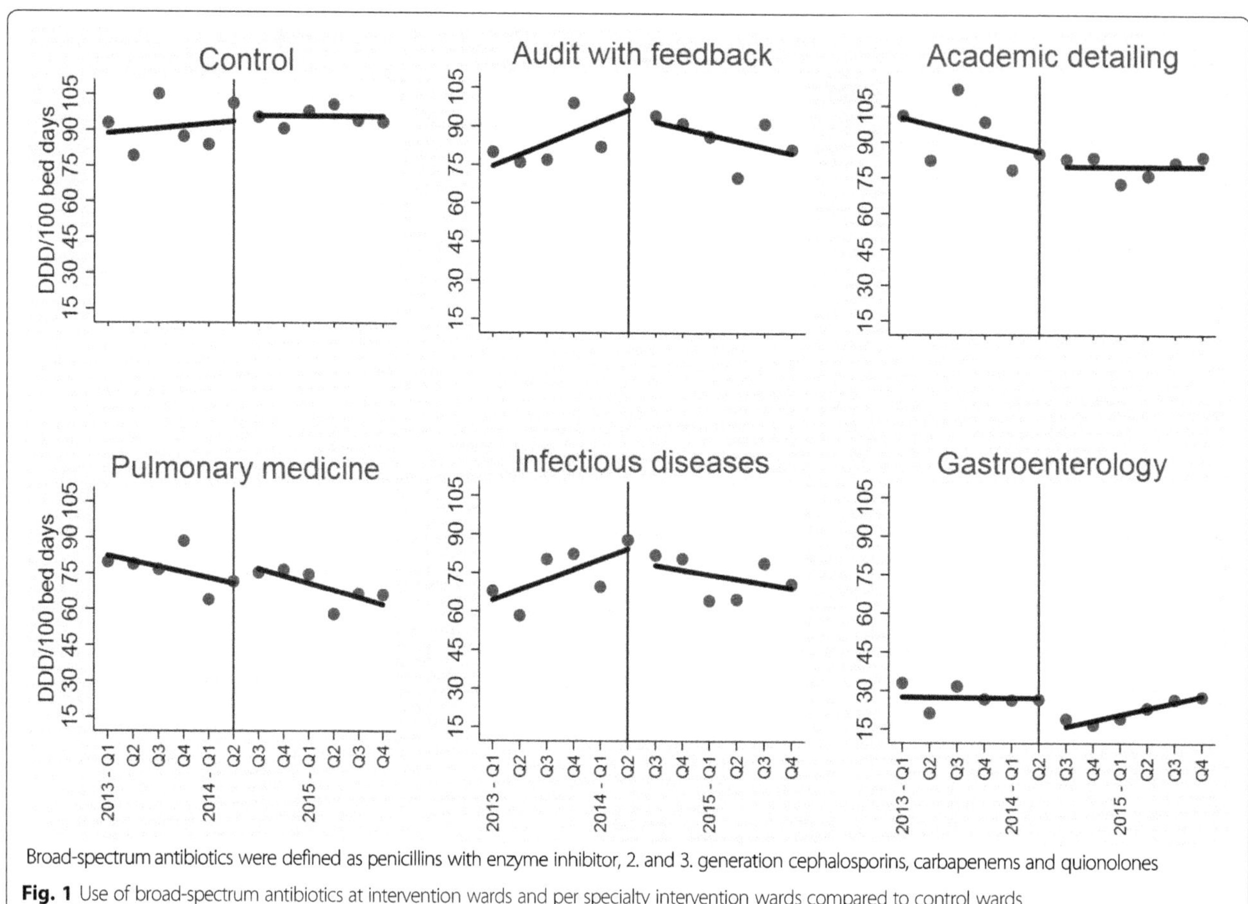

Broad-spectrum antibiotics were defined as penicillins with enzyme inhibitor, 2. and 3. generation cephalosporins, carbapenems and quionolones

Fig. 1 Use of broad-spectrum antibiotics at intervention wards and per specialty intervention wards compared to control wards

Table 6 Interrupted Time Series analysis of the use of Ciprofloxacin at the ward of Gastroenterology, Hospital A, from 2013 to 2015

		Estimate	SE	*p*-value
Ciprofloxacin DDD per 100 bed days	Constant	10.291	1.283	0.000
	AR	−0.090	0.520	0.868
Pre-slope		−0.169	0.341	0.636
Difference between pre- and post-slope		−0.106	0.461	0.825
Level effect				
3 months		−4.254	1.905	0.061
6 months		−4.360	1.956	0.061
12 months		−4.571	2.343	0.092
18 months		−4.783	2.975	0.152

Use of Ciprofloxacin is measured as quarterly sales of Ciprofloxacin, adjusted for bed days

Abbreviations

COPD: Chronic obstructive pulmonary disease; CRB-65: Score of community acquired pneumonia assessing: Confusion – Respiratory rate – Blood pressure – Age (65-years of age or older); eGFR: estimated Glomerular Filtration Rate; EPOC: Cochrane Effective Practice and Organization of Care; ITS: Interrupted time series; LRTI: Lower respiratory tract infection; SMART goals: Specific – Measurable – Achievable/Attractive – Realistic – Time-bound

Acknowledgements

[Δ]Bergen Intervention Teams.
Dagfinn Lunde Markussen[1] dagfinn.lunde.markussen@helse-bergen.no, Andreas Thelle[2] andreas.thelle@helse-bergen.no, Marion Neteland[3] marion.iren.neteland@helse-bergen.no, Ottar Hope[4] ottarhope@gmail.com
[1] Department of Emergency Medicine, Haukeland University Hospital, Bergen, Norway.
[2] Department of Pulmonary Medicine, Haukeland University Hospital, Bergen, Norway.
[3] Norwegian Advisory Unit for Antibiotic Use in Hospitals, Department of Research and Development, Haukeland University Hospital, Bergen, Norway.
[4] Department of Internal Medicine, Haraldsplass Deaconess Hospital, Bergen, Norway.

We would also like to thank Dr. Eli Leirdal Hoem at Haraldsplass Deaconess Hospital and pharmacist Anne Kathrine Horvei at Stavanger Hospital Pharmacy who also participated in the intervention teams with development and implementation of interventions, Brita Skodvin for data collection and validation, Torhild Vedeler for data collection, Torbjørn Smith and Vegard Smith for data plotting. We thank all physicians, managers and secretaries at the participating wards at Haukeland University Hospital, Stavanger University Hospital and Haraldsplass Deaconess Hospital.

Funding

This work was supported by Haukeland University Hospital, The Hospital Pharmacies Enterprise in Western Norway, Stavanger University Hospital and Haraldsplass Deaconess Hospital through the participation of all members of the project team and by The Western Regional Health Authority by a 3-month grant in Patient Safety Research for preparation of the manuscript (HV1199 to J.S.W.). E.C. is funded by the National Institute for Health Research, UK Department of Health (HPRU-2012-10047) in partnership with Public Health England and the Economic and Social Science Research Council (ESRC).

Authors' contributions

Study design and initial concept of interventions: JSW, IS. Development and implementation of interventions: JSW, IS, LKSK, AT, MIN, DLM, OH. Data collection and validation: JSW, IS, LKSK, MIN. Data analysis: JSW, RMN, IS, SH. Interpretation of data: JSW, IS, SH, HSB, LKSK, AT, DLM, EC. Writing of manuscript: JSW, IS. Critical assessment and approval of manuscript: IS, LKSK, SH, HSB, EC, RMN, AT, DLM, OH, MIN. All authors read and approved the final manuscript.

Consent for publication

Not applicable

Competing interests

J.S.W received a 3-month grant in patient safety research for preparation of the manuscript, but the funder has not played any role in the design, execution, analysis or reporting of the research. Competing interests for other authors: None to declare.

Author details

[1]Department of Clinical Science, University of Bergen, Bergen, Norway. [2]Norwegian Advisory Unit for Antibiotic Use in Hospitals, Department of Research and Development, Haukeland University Hospital, Jonas Lies vei 65, N-5021 Bergen, Norway. [3]Department of Quality and Development, Hospital Pharmacies Enterprise in Western Norway, Bergen, Norway. [4]Department of Infectious Diseases and Unit for Infection Prevention and Control, Department of Research and Education, Stavanger University Hospital, Stavanger, Norway. [5]Department of Drug Statistics, Norwegian Institute of Public Health, Oslo, Norway. [6]Faculty of Health and Social Sciences, Western Norway University of Applied Sciences, Bergen, Norway. [7]NHIR Health Protection Research Unit in Healthcare Associated Infections and Antimicrobial Resistance, Imperial College, London, UK. [8]Innovation, Access and Use, Department of Essential Medicines and Health Products, World Health Organization (WHO), Avenue Appia 20, 1211 Geneva 27, Switzerland.

References

1. Bronzwaer SL, Cars O, Buchholz U, Molstad S, Goettsch W, Veldhuijzen IK, et al. A European study on the relationship between antimicrobial use and antimicrobial resistance. Emerg Infect Dis. 2002;8(3):278–82.
2. Austin DJ, Kristinsson KG, Anderson RM. The relationship between the volume of antimicrobial consumption in human communities and the frequency of resistance. Proc Natl Acad Sci U S A. 1999;96(3):1152–6.
3. Frank U, Kleissle EM, Daschner FD, Leibovici L, Paul M, Andreassen S, et al. Multicentre study of antimicrobial resistance and antibiotic consumption among 6,780 patients with bloodstream infections. Eur J Clin Microbiol Infect Dis. 2006;25(12):815–7.
4. Haug JB, Berild D, Walberg M, Reikvam A. Increased antibiotic use in Norwegian hospitals despite a low antibiotic resistance rate. J Antimicrob Chemother. 2011;66(11):2643–6.
5. Barlam TF, Cosgrove SE, Abbo LM, MacDougall C, Schuetz AN, Septimus EJ, et al. Implementing an antibiotic stewardship program: guidelines by the Infectious Diseases Society of America and the Society for Healthcare Epidemiology of America. Clin Infect Dis. 2016;62(10):e51–77.
6. Davey P, Marwick CA, Scott CL, Charani E, McNeil K, Brown E, et al. Interventions to improve antibiotic prescribing practices for hospital inpatients. Cochrane Database of Systematic Reviews. 2017 Issue 2. Art.nr.: CD003543; doi:https://doi.org/10.1002/14651858.
7. Hulscher ME, Grol RP, van der Meer JW. Antibiotic prescribing in hospitals: a social and behavioural scientific approach. Lancet Infect Dis. 2010;10(3):167–75.
8. French SD, Green SE, O'Connor DA, McKenzie JE, Francis JJ, Michie S, et al. Developing theory-informed behaviour change interventions to implement evidence into practice: a systematic approach using the theoretical domains framework. Implement Sci. 2012;7:38.
9. Davey P, Peden C, Charani E, Marwick C, Michie S. Time for action-improving the design and reporting of behaviour change interventions for antimicrobial stewardship in hospitals: early findings from a systematic review. Int J Antimicrob Agents. 2015;45(3):203–12.
10. de Kraker MEA, Abbas M, Huttner B, Harbarth S. Good epidemiological practice: a narrative review of appropriate scientific methods to evaluate the impact of antimicrobial stewardship interventions. Clin Microbiol Infect. 2017;23(11):819–25.
11. Stenehjem E, Hersh AL, Buckel WR, Jones P, Sheng X, Evans RS, et al. Impact of implementing antibiotic stewardship programs in 15 small hospitals: a cluster-randomized intervention. Clin Infect Dis. 2018; https://doi.org/10.1093/cid/ciy155.
12. Wathne JS, Kleppe LK, Harthug S, Blix HS, Nilsen RM, Thelle A, et al., editors. The effect of antibiotic stewardship interventions with stakeholder involvement in multispecialty settings: a multicentre, cluster randomized controlled intervention study. ECCMID 2018, accepted abstract (Oral presentation O0846); 2018 23.04.2018; Madrid; 2018.
13. WHO Collaborating Centre for Drug Statistics Methodology. ATC Index with DDDs. Norwegian Insitute of Public Health. 2017. https://www.whocc.no/atc_ddd_index/. Accessed 15 Dec 2017.

14. NORM/NORM-VET. Usage of Antimicrobial Agents and Occurrence of Antimicrobial Resistance in Norway 2016. Tromso/Oslo: Norwegian surveillance system for antibiotic resistance in microbes (NORM), Norwegian Veterinary Institute, Norwegian Institute of Public Health, . 2017. https://unn.no/Documents/Kompetansetjenester,%20-sentre%20og%20fagråd/NORM%20-%20Norsk%20overvåkingssystem%20for%20antibiotikaresistens%20hos%20mikrober/Rapporter/NORM%20NORM-VET%202016.pdf. Accessed 5 Dec 2017.
15. Norwegian Ministry of Health and Care Services. Action plan against antibiotic resistance in health care. 2015. https://www.regjeringen.no/contentassets/915655269bc04a47928fce917e4b25f5/handlingsplan-antibiotikaresistens.pdf. Accessed 21 Mar 2016.
16. Norwegian Directorate of Health. Norwegian National Clinical Guideline for Antibiotic Use in Hospitals. 2013. https://helsedirektoratet.no/retningslinjer/antibiotika-i-sykehus. Accessed 3 Jan 2016.
17. Cochrane Effective Practice and Organisation of Care (EPOC). Interrupted time series (ITS) analyses. EPOC Resources for review authors. 2017. http://epoc.cochrane.org/sites/epoc.cochrane.org/files/public/uploads/Resources-for-authors2017/interrupted_time_series_analyses.docx. Accessed 13 Oct 2017.
18. Hulscher M, Prins JM. Antibiotic stewardship: does it work in hospital practice? A review of the evidence base. Clin Microbiol Infect. 2017;23(11):799–805.
19. Schouten JA, Hulscher ME, Trap-Liefers J, Akkermans RP, Kullberg BJ, Grol RP, et al. Tailored interventions to improve antibiotic use for lower respiratory tract infections in hospitals: a cluster-randomized, controlled trial. Clin Infect Dis. 2007;44(7):931–41.
20. Hogli JU, Garcia BH, Skjold F, Skogen V, Smabrekke L. An audit and feedback intervention study increased adherence to antibiotic prescribing guidelines at a Norwegian hospital. BMC Infect Dis. 2016;16(1):96.
21. Weinberg M, Fuentes JM, Ruiz AI, Lozano FW, Angel E, Gaitan H, et al. Reducing infections among women undergoing cesarean section in Colombia by means of continuous quality improvement methods. Arch Intern Med. 2001;161(19):2357–65.
22. Volpe D, Harrison S, Damian F, Rachh P, Kahlon PS, Morrissey L, et al. Improving timeliness of antibiotic delivery for patients with fever and suspected neutropenia in a pediatric emergency department. Pediatrics. 2012;130(1):e201–10.
23. Jobson M, Sandrof M, Valeriote T, Liberty AL, Walsh-Kelly C, Jackson C. Decreasing time to antibiotics in febrile patients with central lines in the emergency department. Pediatrics. 2015;135(1):e187–95.
24. Associates in Process Improvement. Model for Improvement. 2018. http://www.apiweb.org/. Accessed 19 Feb 2018.
25. Charani E, Castro-Sanchez E, Sevdalis N, Kyratsis Y, Drumright L, Shah N, et al. Understanding the determinants of antimicrobial prescribing within hospitals: the role of "prescribing etiquette". Clin Infect Dis. 2013;57(2):188–96.
26. Skodvin B, Aase K, Charani E, Holmes A, Smith I. An antimicrobial stewardship program initiative: a qualitative study on prescribing practices among hospital doctors. Antimicrob Resist Infect Control. 2015;4:24.
27. World Medical Association. World medical association declaration of Helsinki: ethical principles for medical research involving human subjects. JAMA. 2013;310(20):2191–4.

4

Migrant and refugee populations: a public health and policy perspective on a continuing global crisis

Mohamed Abbas[1*], Tammam Aloudat[2], Javier Bartolomei[3], Manuel Carballo[4], Sophie Durieux-Paillard[5], Laure Gabus[6], Alexandra Jablonka[7,8], Yves Jackson[9,10], Kanokporn Kaojaroen[11], Daniel Koch[12], Esperanza Martinez[13], Marc Mendelson[14], Roumyana Petrova-Benedict[15], Sotirios Tsiodras[16,17], Derek Christie[18], Mirko Saam[19], Sally Hargreaves[20,21] and Didier Pittet[1]

Abstract

The 2015–2017 global migratory crisis saw unprecedented numbers of people on the move and tremendous diversity in terms of age, gender and medical requirements. This article focuses on key emerging public health issues around migrant populations and their interactions with host populations. Basic needs and rights of migrants and refugees are not always respected in regard to article 25 of the Universal Declaration of Human Rights and article 23 of the Refugee Convention. These are populations with varying degrees of vulnerability and needs in terms of protection, security, rights, and access to healthcare. Their health status, initially conditioned by the situation at the point of origin, is often jeopardised by adverse conditions along migratory paths and in intermediate and final destination countries. Due to their condition, forcibly displaced migrants and refugees face a triple burden of non-communicable diseases, infectious diseases, and mental health issues. There are specific challenges regarding chronic infectious and neglected tropical diseases, for which awareness in host countries is imperative. Health risks in terms of susceptibility to, and dissemination of, infectious diseases are not unidirectional. The response, including the humanitarian effort, whose aim is to guarantee access to basic needs (food, water and sanitation, healthcare), is gripped with numerous challenges. Evaluation of current policy shows insufficiency regarding the provision of basic needs to migrant populations, even in the countries that do the most. Governments around the world need to rise to the occasion and adopt policies that guarantee universal health coverage, for migrants and refugees, as well as host populations, in accordance with the UN Sustainable Development Goals. An expert consultation was carried out in the form of a pre-conference workshop during the 4th International Conference on Prevention and Infection Control (ICPIC) in Geneva, Switzerland, on 20 June 2017, the United Nations World Refugee Day.

Keywords: Migrant populations, Refugees, Crisis, Global health, Public health policy, Infectious diseases

Background

The current global refugee crisis peaked in 2015–2016, and by late 2017 the number of people attempting to cross borders globally – although still high – was receding. The highest levels of forced displacement since World War II were observed in 2015, with a dramatic increase in the numbers of refugees, asylum-seekers and internally displaced people (IDPs) across the world – from Africa to the Middle East and South Asia. "Desperate" migration towards Europe became increasingly seaborne – with over one million migrants arriving by boat in Greece and Italy in 2015. Such operations are highly risky; in the Mediterranean, several thousand migrants have drowned every year since 2014. At the global level, at least 60′000 migrants have died or gone missing over the past 20 years [1]. Although statistics on migration are difficult to collect, it is necessary to avail oneself of the available data which should be viewed as estimates (Fig. 1) [2].

* Correspondence: mohamed.abbas@hcuge.ch
[1]Infection Control Programme and WHO Collaborating Centre on Patient Safety, Faculty of Medicine, University of Geneva Hospitals, Geneva, Switzerland
Full list of author information is available at the end of the article

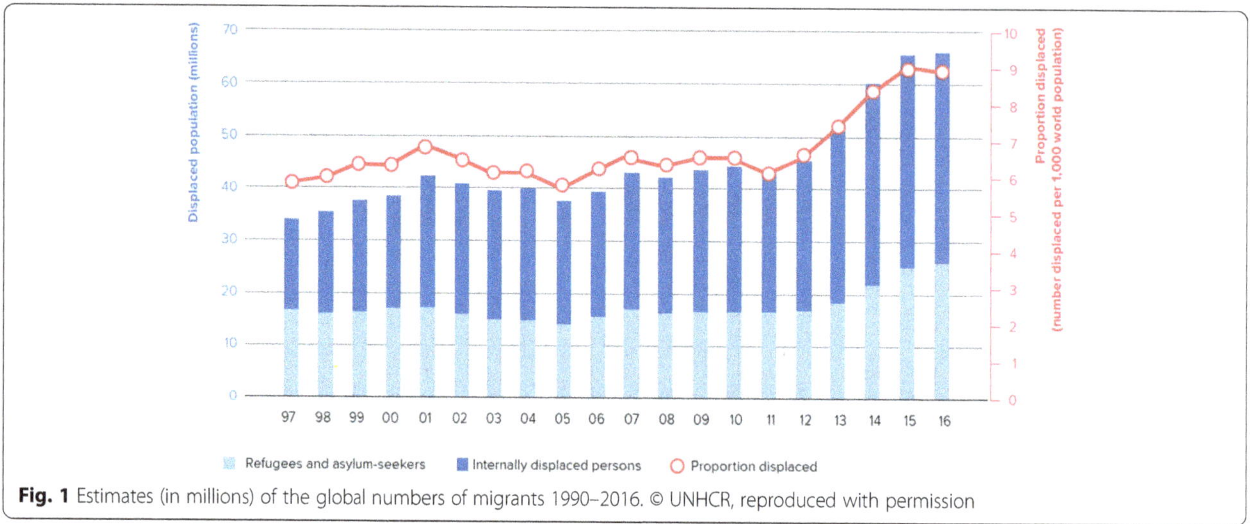

Fig. 1 Estimates (in millions) of the global numbers of migrants 1990–2016. © UNHCR, reproduced with permission

For purposes of ease of reading, and because we believe that the current nomenclature is arbitrary, in this paper we will use the International Organization for Migration's (IOM) definition, and refer to a migrant as "any person who is moving or has moved across an international border or within a State away from his/her habitual place of residence, regardless of (1) the person's legal status; (2) whether the movement is voluntary or involuntary; (3) what the causes for the movement are; or (4) what the length of the stay is." [3] We will use the term interchangeably with the words refugees and asylum-seekers, whether documented or not.

A hallmark of global migration patterns is that IDPs are the highest in number, and low and middle-income countries host most of the world's refugees. In 2016, Turkey had more than 3 million refugees and asylum-seekers on its soil, including 2.7 million Syrians; Lebanon had the highest number relative to its population, nearly one in five inhabitants is a refugee. Of this, the United Nations (UN) Secretary General, António Guterres, said "It is so inspiring to see countries with the least often doing the most for refugees" [4]. In this context, the so-called European "migrant crisis" pales in comparison, and perhaps a change in perspective is required, as in Natalie Nougayrède's words:

> "If there was a crisis in 2015, it had less to do with the refugees – who knew what they were fleeing and where they wanted to go – and much more to do [*sic*] with European governments and societies who did not all step up to the plate. In fact, Europe isn't confronted with a refugee and migrant crisis. It's the refugees and migrants who are confronted with a crisis of Europe. The scandal is that, in the Mediterranean, they have been paying with their lives." [5]

The reasons for forced migration and displacement are increasingly varied, but stem from fragility of states, due to armed conflict and civil unrest, extreme poverty, crime, persecution (including political discrimination), failure of governance, or climate change [6–8]. Over half of the refugees globally come from three countries: Syria, Afghanistan and Somalia; yet refugees are the tip of the iceberg, when one considers the number of IDPs. Altogether, more than 1.5 billion people live in the 56 fragile states that engender refugees [9].

On the occasion of the UN World Refugee Day, 20 June 2017, we conducted an expert consultation in the form of a pre-conference workshop during the 4th International Conference on Prevention and Infection Control (ICPIC) in Geneva.

Basic needs and rights

The 1951 Refugee Convention guarantees basic rights such as liberty, security, right to family life, protection, and freedom of movement [10]. Refugees are therefore not to be returned to their home country against their will. Other basic needs include the right to education and justice. Also, article 23 of the Refugee Convention guarantees the right of refugees to public relief, that is, to access physical and mental health services at the same level as other residents. This fundamental right is also guaranteed by article 25 of the Universal Declaration of Human Rights [11].

In the present crisis, these basic rights have not always been met. While there have been some advances in the form of migrant-friendly hospitals, health systems overall are not sufficiently responsive to migrants, to diversity, or to specific medical and psychosocial care. A needs-based approach is required to address these issues.

Beyond basic needs, migrants, like all humans, aspire to self-actualisation, have hopes and dreams, and demand dignity (Figs. 2 and 3). They need to be considered as human beings, beyond the stereotypes entertained by certain host populations, and to be freed from any form of discrimination, as indeed assumptions and prejudice inform many political decisions. The humanitarian response in the field also needs to take into account the importance of maintaining communication with those left behind, because of its strong links to psychosocial health and well-being. The first thing that many look for when they have survived a sea-crossing is wireless local area networking ("WiFi") – to inform and obtain news from loved ones [12]. Social isolation is also a reality, with over two-thirds of migrants stating that needs for social contact were unmet, and this has direct mental health consequences [13, 14].

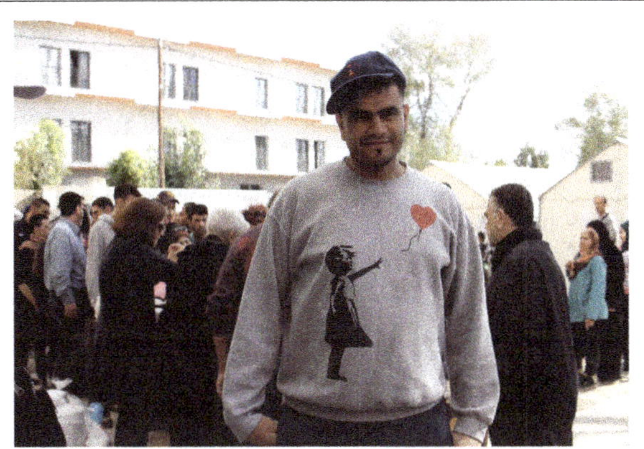

Fig. 3 Man posing in the refugee camp during the Sunday meal distribution organized by Leros' residents. He has just received new clothes, distributed by mutual aid associations. On his jumper, a Bansky drawing. Most smugglers ask migrants to get rid of their luggage before crossing the Aegean Sea so as not to weigh down the inflatable boat. © Laure Gabus

Universal health coverage

First recognised by the UN in 2010 [15], the commitment to universal health coverage was subsequently reinforced [16] and is a core component of sustainable development at the global level [17–19]. It requires that all people have access to health services – including prevention, treatment, rehabilitation and palliative care – without risk of financial hardship [20]. Its impact on migrants' health would be even more positive if this policy were embedded into a broader perspective of universal social rights coverage as put forward by the International Convention on the Protection of the Rights of All Migrant Workers and Members of Their Families adopted by United Nations General Assembly resolution 45/158 of 18 December 1990.

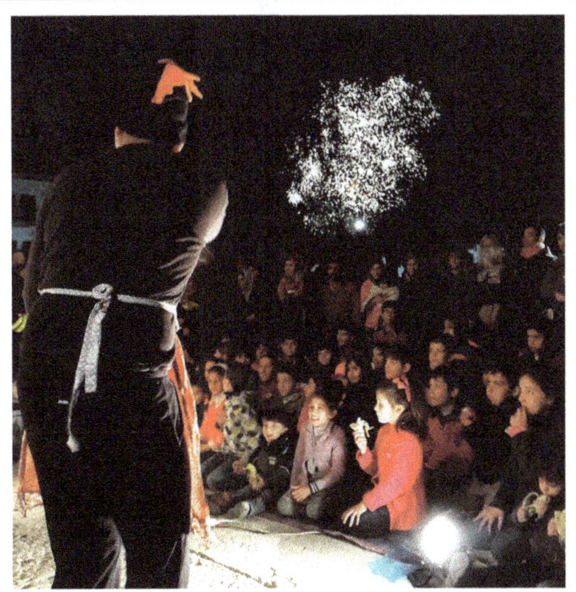

Fig. 2 A Greek theatre company gives a show in a refugee camp in Leros. The play, in Greek, is about a little black fish lost in the ocean. None of the spectators understand, but everyone is laughing. © Laure Gabus

For universal health coverage to occur, research and public health action must take place all along the migratory route, not just upon arrival in a host country. The health status and challenges of many migrating populations are insufficiently addressed until they arrive in a high-profile country. There is, therefore, a clear need to provide and improve healthcare along migration routes. This requires the alignment of the public health and humanitarian agendas, all the more so because health and social systems along the way are often weak.

Vulnerability

The unprecedented number of forcibly displaced migrants is compounded by increasing demographic, socio-economic, and medical complexity. For example, the global number of child refugees has reached alarming levels: at least 300,000 unaccompanied children moving across borders were registered over two years in 2015–2016, representing a nearly five-fold increase from 2010 to 2011 [21]. Proportions of pregnant women, the elderly and people with disabilities halve also increased in the past years. Migrants are more than ever a heterogeneous group, migrants in irregular status can often be averse to sharing personal details with any administration – including hospitals or medical services – out of fear and/or distrust. Their motivations or even their desired destination may change during the journey. This unprecedented diversity leads to an extended range of medical requirements [22, 23] as well as complex gender and social issues [24–26].

The "healthy migrant" hypothesis suggests that self-selection prior to migration leads to the observation that upon arrival, migrants tend to be younger and fitter than host (or origin) populations [27]. Emerging knowledge on the evolution of newcomers' health shows that this effect subsides over time, and that migrant health deteriorates after several years due to poverty, poor living conditions, and restricted access to healthcare [27, 28]. The healthy migrant effect may therefore be called into question, as has been suggested by several authors [27, 29, 30].

Violence is a key risk factor for forcibly displaced migrants. In studies in Médecins Sans Frontières (MSF) mental health clinics in Serbia, up to a third of migrants were found to have been victims of violent events [31]. Potentially traumatic events were experienced by 60% and 90% of migrants in their home country and during migration, respectively [32]. In Morocco, among 154 sub-Saharan migrants, 90% reported cases of multiple victimizations, 45% of which were sexual, predominantly gang rape; 79 respondents (51%) were personally victimized, and 27% were forced to witness relatives or co-migrants being victimized [33]. Prisons in all countries are prone to violence, and some administrative detention centres can be even more violent than civilian prisons, due to the absence of rights traditionally granted to prisoners [34], and failiure to follow the UN Standard Minimum Rules for the Treatment of Prisoners ("the Nelson Mandela" rules) [35]. The proportions of foreign inmates in prisons can be very high (e.g. 72% in Switzerland); some are undocumented migrants in administrative detention [36, 37]. Also, due to overcrowding, these are settings where the transmission of infectious diseases of public health interest can occur, especially tuberculosis and sexually transmitted diseases such as syphilis, HIV and hepatitis [38, 39].

In practice, clustering often occurs in migrant populations, with several diseases or conditions affecting the same individuals or groups. This is due to shared vulnerabilities, lack of financial resources, length and duration of the journey and many intermediate destinations, in addition to the epidemiological burden in the country of origin. There are specific risks for women, children (especially unaccompanied minors) and the elderly. Overcrowding and deficient water and sanitation in camps and reception facilities increase risks related to infectious diseases, e.g. vaccine-preventable diseases. Thereafter, restrictive policies in the destination country affect living conditions by limiting access and accessibility to healthcare, education, labour market as well as increasing language and other communication barriers [40].

The concept of syndemics (synergistic epidemics) can be useful to approach the clustering of certain risk factors or diseases, in certain populations and settings [41]. For example, in a context of migratory stress, synergy between infectious diseases, metabolic diseases and mental health would yield a worse outcome (Fig. 4). Syndemics such as SAVA (substance abuse, violence and AIDS) or VIDDA (violence, immigration, diabetes, depression and abuse) serve as pertinent examples [41].

Medical footprint and burden of disease

The *medical footprint* is a useful framework to understand each migrant's personal health capital and its evolution. Whenever a person decides to move, they bring with them a social, cultural and economic capital, which is liable to change during the trajectory of the individual through time and space. Each migrant also has a *personal health capital*, which will also evolve during their journey from their home country to an eventual destination. It is important to take into account migrants' health capital, and its evolution, the latter being impacted by social determinants of health, and advocate for enabling polices to maintain and develop it. This is important for health equity – universal coverage cannot be realised if certain populations are left aside – but also because there are interactions between migrant and host populations. This dynamic sequence of events can be divided into six stages, each characterised by shortages and medical implications (Table 1).

Even if, and it is hardly ever the case, healthcare may be available and relatively accessible when migrants arrive in a host country, this rarely compensates the months and years spent in either a risk-ridden and often prolonged transit phase, or at the point of origin [42]. For migrants, there usually is a succession of stressful incidents or phases: the experience of exile itself, followed by fear linked to life-threatening situations such as crossing the Mediterranean on an overcharged boat, and then administrative anguish as they wait for applications to be processed in a camp or underground shelter. A further stressor might be the uncertainty of their future in a potential host country. Moreover, exposure to conflict and war has a lasting impact on mental health. Due to these life events, the prevalence of psychiatric disorders in refugee populations is much higher than in those not forcibly displaced [14, 43–45]. The link between environmental and psychological stress and adverse health outcomes is well documented. Mental health conditions including anxiety and depression are associated with certain infectious diseases, as has been suggested in a recent review [46].

Forcibly displaced populations are increasingly facing the triple burden of chronic non-communicable diseases (e.g. diabetes, cardiovascular diseases, respiratory conditions and cancer), infectious diseases (e.g. tuberculosis, HIV, hepatitis), and psychiatric illnesses (e.g. post-traumatic stress disorder, depression). A recent survey of a Jordanian camp mainly populated by Syrian refugees indicated prevalence rates for hypertension of 21% and 52%, cardiovascular disease of 7.5% and 21%, diabetes of 12% and 32%, in the 40–59 and 60+ age groups, respectively [47]. Due to the increasing complexity and

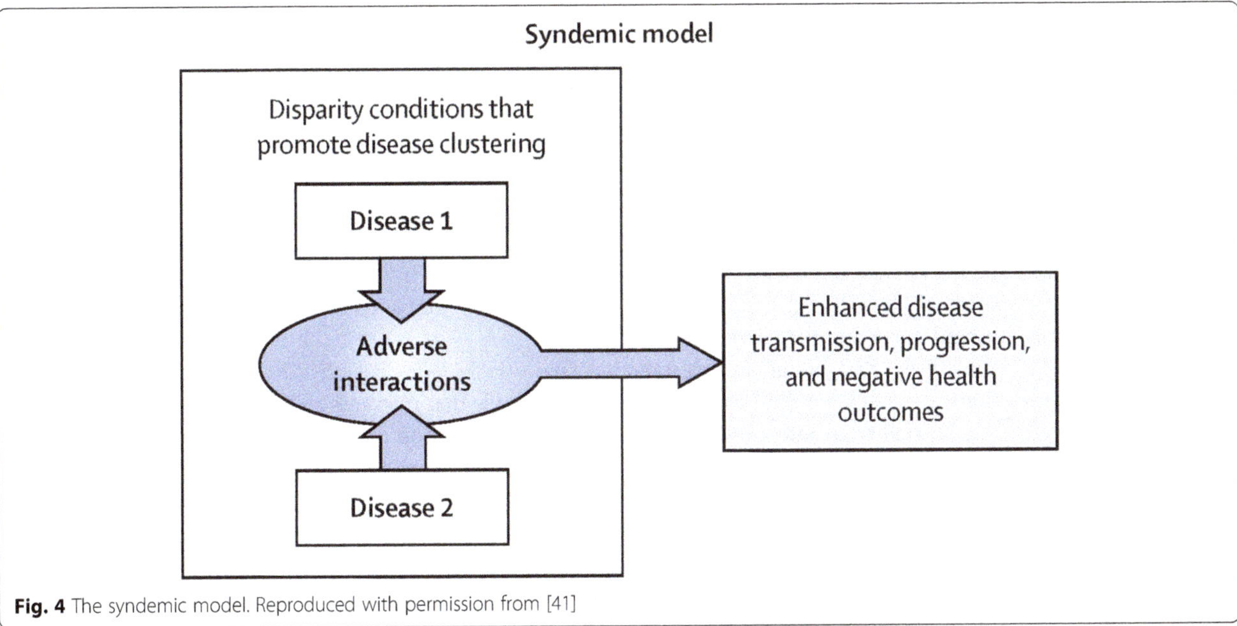

Fig. 4 The syndemic model. Reproduced with permission from [41]

diversity of migrant populations, there is also the problem of overlapping medical conditions further perplexing appropriate interventions. Increasingly, polymorbidity, often arising at a premature life stage, becomes a challenge among forced migrants in Europe [48]. The impact of community-acquired infections leading to admission to intensive care units seems much higher in refugees in host countries than in the autochthonous population [49, 50].

Infectious diseases

The prevalence of certain chronic parasitic diseases in asymptomatic migrants reflects, in general, the

Table 1 Key steps and health determinants of migrants' health – medical footprint

Step	Main problems/issues	Shortages
1. Pre-migration health experience	Local epidemiological situation and poverty, conflict and war	Diagnosis, vaccination, healthcare, clean water, adequate housing, personal safety
2. Transit health experience	Long in time and space, often worse than in country of origin	Water, nutrition, hygiene, sanitation, housing (overcrowding), social and sexual protection (hostility of resident populations, exploitation by criminal gangs). Exposure to new pathogens for which they have no immunity
3. Destination experience	Unfavourable and unhealthy. Lasting situations governed by the will to survive. Adverse weather conditions outdoors, or if indoors overcrowded conditions and risk of transmission of infectious diseases among migrants	Lack of appropriate clothes, shoes and personal belongings (often abandoned, lost or stolen before or during sea crossings), lack of psychosocial support
4, Healthcare access/use experience	Fear of the law, suspicion of giving out personal data and the general feeling of not being appreciated may affect the evaluation by migrants of their right to access healthcare and other services	Trained healthcare personnel
5. New transit experience	There are often several transit experiences, for instance through North Africa and Southern Europe; through Turkey and the Balkans; or through Central America and Mexico	Water, nutrition, hygiene, sanitation, housing (overcrowding), social and sexual protection (hostility of resident populations, exploitation by criminal gangs). Exposure to new pathogens for which they have no immunity
6. Final destination experience	If and when a migrant finds a job, it is often dirty, dangerous and degrading ("3 Ds"). It may also be illegal, with no insurance coverage and limited access to healthcare. These informal jobs are vitally important for the economies of high-income countries	Lack of appropriate clothes, shoes and personal belongings (often abandoned, lost or stolen before or during sea crossings), lack of psychosocial support

epidemiologic burden at the country of origin and may be high, up to 5.8%, 48.5%, and 56.1%, for schistosomiasis, Chagas disease, and strongyloidiasis respectively, according to one report [51]. Knowledge of such "tropical diseases", which may be a misnomer as they have become global, is imperative for proper patient management. Furthermore, more efforts should be undertaken to include migrants in programmes aiming to eradicate neglected tropical diseases [52]. The prevalence of chronic viral diseases, such as HIV, hepatitis C (HCV), and hepatitis B is also higher than in host populations and can be as high as 2.3%, 1.3%, and 14%, respectively, depending on country of origin [51]. Co-infections, e.g. between viral and parasitic infections increase susceptibility to infection, risk of transmission, as well as severity and progression of the disease [53–56]. This may be particularly concerning for chronic viral infections that lead to cancer, such as chronic hepatitis associated hepatocellular carcinoma, or human papillomavirus associated cervical precancerous and cancerous lesions [57]. Migration into Europe is changing the epidemiology of many diseases, including HCV. If the goal of HCV eradication is to be achieved, more inclusive policies and practices will be required [58].

Epidemiological screening is a legitimate tool to better study the profile of migrant populations and to understand their needs [59, 60]. In developing countries facing high rates of internal displacements, there is an urgent need to unify screenings and treatments, and to fight the as yet largely unaddressed problem of counterfeit medicines. In the more developed destination countries, screening of migrant populations seeking healthcare may also help to understand and control the inter-country spread of antibiotic resistance [61]. Health assessment on arrival is a useful way of gaining an initial understanding of the health of incident migrant populations. Screening can be systematic or performed on a case-to-case basis, whereupon arrival, each migrant obtains a personal consultation to describe their medical and transit history [59, 60]. Based on this information, the physician can decide whether to test the person for an array of medical conditions. One such EU-level initiative is the development of the electronic personal and health record, Re-Health (http://re-health.eea.iom.int/). A recent systematic review has estimated that approximately 3% of screened individuals have an infectious disease, but 15% have latent tuberculosis [62]. Furthermore, it was shown that not only is uptake of screening high by migrant populations, but that screening is an effective strategy with moderate/high cost-effectiveness [62]. Evidence also shows positive cost-effectiveness and public health effects of screening and providing early treatment to Latin American women of child-bearing age at risk of suffering and transmitting Chagas disease outside endemic countries [63, 64].

Vaccine-preventable diseases and vaccination

Screening can also include assessment of immunity to vaccine-preventable diseases. Several studies have shown that vaccination coverage of migrants on arrival is insufficient, although heterogeneity exists between different countries of origin [65–69]. A recent study in Denmark has shown that one third of asylum-seeking children were not immunised in accordance with the national guidelines [65]. This incomplete immunisation may have consequences in terms of outbreaks in refugee camps [70–72].

The WHO-UNHCR-UNICEF Joint Technical Guidance recommends that migrants should be immunized according to the immunisation schedule of the country in which they intend to stay for more than 1 week [73]. It also states that access should be "non-discriminatory and equitable", and that measles-mumps-rubella (MMR) and polio vaccines should be a priority [73]. A similar strategy is also endorsed by the ECDC [74]. Unfortunately, many countries in Europe have yet to put in place directives on immunisation of migrants [75]. Implementing this strategy, however, is not without challenges related to the migrant condition (lack of information on immunization status, high mobility of migrants, economic difficulties), and further efforts are required in order to harmonise practices and improve communication between host countries and/or agencies [69, 76].

Benefits of achieving adequate vaccine coverage include a decrease in the burden of infectious diseases, and prevention and/or termination of outbreaks; as such, there has recently been interest in the effects of vaccination in reducing AMR [77–80]. It has been previously shown that vaccination strategies against *Haemophilus influenzae* and *Streptococcus pneumoniae* have been associated with decreases in the incidence of infections with resistant pathogens [77–80]. Presumably, one of the several proposed mechanisms would be mediated by decreases in the overall incidence of disease, including that of resistant strains as well as decreases in transmission of antibiotic resistant strains, although further research is required in order to fully understand and develop models [80, 81].

Health risks: For us or for them?

It has been known for many years that human mobility is linked to transmission, but also susceptibility, to infectious diseases. Movement of people, animals and goods has allowed dissemination of infectious diseases at least since 1000 B.C. [82]. Often, the health risk for the host populations has been politicised by various political groups with an anti-immigration agenda (e.g. Front National in France, Alternative für Deutschland in Germany, Schweizerische Volkspartei in Switzerland) to create a climate of fear surrounding migration. To counter this, the European Centre for Disease Control and Prevention (ECDC) produced a technical document which states that newly-arrived migrants and refugees "do not represent a significant risk for EU/EEA populations" with regards to communicable diseases [83]. This document also states that the risk to refugees has increased due to overcrowding at reception facilities, with the potential for increased transmission of entities like meningococcal disease, measles, varicella and influenza.

Antimicrobial resistance may be considered an emerging infectious disease, and is clearly linked to human mobility [84, 85]. Prevalence of carriage of methicillin-resistant *Staphylococcus aureus* and multi-drug resistant *Enterobacteriaceae* in migrant populations may be as high as 27% [61, 85–87]. Migrants are also overrepresented in terms of multi-drug resistant tuberculosis compared to host populations [88]. A recent systematic review suggests that migrants might acquire antimicrobial-resistant pathogens during the migration process or once they have arrived in the host country; indeed, the prevalence of AMR in the latter would be a major determining factor in transmission to migrants [87]. This may have implications for infection control policies if migrants are hospitalised in low-endemicity settings, as is the case for returned travellers and repatriated patients. Epidemiological screening may be a legitimate tool to better study the profile of migrant populations and understand their needs, and may also help understand and control the spread of antibiotic resistance [61]. It should not, however, be used as a political tool.

Humanitarian response

Non-governmental partners such as MSF or the International Red Cross and Red Crescent Movement, as well as UN agencies such as UNHCR and IOM, are at the forefront of attempts to manage acute and lasting migratory flows, and are confronted with a considerable diversity of profiles and needs [89]. All too often, the humanitarian response is under such financial and time constraints that its only realistic objective is to help individuals and families survive the current trip and arrive at their next destination without an increase in their medical and psychosocial problems. A recurrent concern is that the international media only focus on migrants when they reach via dramatic journey a high-profile, and often high-income country. Obstacles to integration for regularly residing migrants need to be addressed as well, in the interest of public health and social cohesion. Furthermore, the vast majority of migrants are IDPs in Asia or Africa, where resources for vital interventions are often lacking. Proportionately, IDPs pay the highest burden for mortality, morbidity and malnutrition. Along the migratory pathways, there is a need to standardise diagnostic and treatment protocols, particularly because of chronic diseases requiring continuity of care. This has recently been a problem in many settings, from Lebanon to Ukraine.

The humanitarian response has had to handle many challenges that are either invisible or constantly overlooked, such as interpersonal violence or mental and sexual health. Other challenges include the safety of humanitarian and healthcare personnel [90]. If a hospital is attacked, beyond immediate victims, people will stop going there, which will engender more victims [90, 91]. The Health Care in Danger Project (part of the International Red Cross and Red Crescent Movement) has documented 1809 attacks against healthcare providers worldwide in 2012–2013, 40% of which were directed against healthcare facilities [92]. In the report, it was found that State armed and security forces (military and police) and armed non-State actors are equally involved in these attacks. Use of access to healthcare as a military strategy, known as the weaponisation of healthcare, as for example in Syria, is unacceptable [91]. Unfortunately, evidence suggests that these attacks may be increasing with time [90]. Warring parties and governments need to understand, respect and provide the basic provision of sanitation and health. Also, some migrants are not able or willing to wait for help to arrive: when a team comes to examine a group, it may have moved on, as was experienced by MSF in the Balkans in 2015–2016.

Focus on policy

The health strand of the Migration Integration Policy Index (MIPEX), collaboratively developed by IOM, has 38 indicators for health policy that can be measured and be addressed towards achieving health equity (health being one of eight sectors covered by MIPEX). Health indicators fall into four dimensions: entitlement to health services, policies to facilitate access, responsive health services and measures to achieve change. According to MIPEX, even well-performing host countries such as Germany or Sweden only achieve around 70% health equity [93].

Policies towards migrants in Europe and the United States tend to be volatile and election-dependent. They are also poorly coordinated with each other. A case in point is the so-called "Dublin Treaty" (the Dublin III Regulation Number 604/2013 came into force on 19 July 2013) which makes the first EU Member State where fingerprints are stored or an asylum claim is lodged, responsible for a person's asylum claim. This is one of the reasons why Italy and Greece have had to deal with so many migrants and have consistently felt let down by the international community. This policy, as well as its underlying assumptions, has been criticised in the past by UNHCR, and the Parliamentary Assembly of the Council of Europe [94–97].

Because of the Dublin Treaty, many migrants are sent back to the first European country where they were registered, which is often Italy or Greece. These countries have limited perspectives for the realisation of their dreams of economic opportunity. Deportation to the first "Dublin" country often leads to depression, suicidal thoughts or risky behaviour such as unprotected sex or substance abuse.

At the UN General Assembly in September 2016, Member States issued the New York Declaration for Refugees and Migrants, which is a set of commitments as well as an action plan to implement these commitments [98]. This has resulted not only in the Comprehensive Refugee Response Framework, the core elements of which have been agreed on, and which contains four key elements (easing pressure on host countries, enhancing refugee self-reliance, expanding third-country solutions, and supporting conditions in countries of origin for return in safety and dignity), but also the Global Compact on Refugees which will be presented by the High Commissioner for Refugees at the General Assembly in September 2018 [99].

Conclusion and way forward

Humanitarian problems require political solutions, therefore political commitment is sorely needed to try to reduce the number of uprooted people, and improve their conditions when they are on the move. There is a need to work in a concerted manner on points of origin, points of transit and final points of destination.

The improvement of health of populations, as set out in the UN Sustainable Development Goals, which includes for the first time a migration target (Goal 10), requires the medical and scientific community to understand the complex dynamics of migration. A better grasp of the forces involved is necessary, using a trans-disciplinary approach combining humanitarian, economic, sociological and public health approaches. Accessing and improving basic rights including healthcare along transit routes is a definite priority.

Academics also have a responsibility in lending their voice to the cause of bettering the condition of migrants, and indeed many have taken or called for action [100, 101]. Conducting research that sheds light on the plight of migrants, or on how policy can negatively affect their existence is valuable. Improving awareness of primary-care teams to specific migrant health issues as well as transcultural dimensions by training is another such example [102]. One of the aims of the UCL-*Lancet* Commission on Migration and Health, a multidisciplinary group of academics, policymakers, and health system experts, is to "articulate evidence-base approaches to inform public discourse and policy"and will produce a report set to coincide with the UN General Assembly in September 2018 [103].

This article lends support to recent calls for improved governance mechanisms to ensure the integration of migration within health systems, currently designed for resident populations [104]. Whereas there always seem to be sufficient funds for walls, borders or barriers to the movement of people, more investment is necessary to achieve universal health coverage. Research within Germany has shown that regions that invested less in healthcare for migrants have ended up spending more in the long run [105]. Likewise, a review of the resources invested by the UNHCR in 70 sites in 17 countries shows that increased spending on refugee populations is correlated with lower mortality, reflecting not only efficacy on the part of humanitarian action but also the considerable vulnerability and dependence of migrant populations on international aid [106].

Health equity and early access to healthcare appear as critical responses to the migratory crisis. The principles of public health equity mean that medicine must be used to assist human populations in distress. This commitment at a global level must be followed by concerted actions in the field, where migrants need assistance and protection. Too often, they are denied healthcare or health insurance. If universal health coverage is to be achieved, it cannot be conditioned upon the status of any person [107].

Another point is the opportunity to look at the positive aspects of migration. Global remittances from migrants to their countries of origin have been estimated by the World Bank to be $429 billion [108], which is higher than the "net official development assistance (ODA) flows from member countries of the Development Assistance Committee (DAC) of the OECD" of $135.2 billion in 2014 [109]. Also, a majority of adult migrants have skills that could be put to good use [110–112]. Among migrants and refugees are engineers and healthcare professionals who are able and willing to help, but often cannot do this due to administrative hurdles. It makes sense to find ways of employing these professionals, thus breaking their economic dependence, whilst giving them recognition, and increasing cost-efficiency and the overall well-being of both migrant and host populations, not to mention stopping the drain of human resources affecting low-to middle income countries. This was recognized by the EU when it launched the "science4refugees" initiative [113]. Finally, much of the healthcare provided to migrants during the 2015–2017 crisis was by volunteers. These dedicated people need to be supported by sufficiently strong healthcare, administrative and financial systems [114].

In the words of the UN High Commissioner for Refugees, Filippo Grandi, we must "ask ourselves what each of us can do to overcome indifference or fear and to embrace the idea of inclusion, to welcome refugees to our own communities, and counter narratives that would seek to exclude and marginalise refugees and other uprooted people" [115].

Authors' contributions
MA and DP were responsible for the organisation of the workshop, and were significantly assisted by SH. TA, JB, MC, SDP, LG, AJ, YJ, KK, DK, EM, MM, RPB, and ST were participants in the workshop and the round-table and either gave presentations, moderated the workshop. DC and MS wrote the first draft of the manuscript, which was significantly edited by MA. All authors read and approved the final manuscript.

Consent for publication
The persons who have been photographed have provided consent that the photographs taken of them will may be published, and may be freely available on the internet and may be seen by the general public. Oral consent was provided to the photographer, and a form was not signed. It was not possible to contact the photographed persons for the purposes of signing a consent form.

Competing interests
The authors declare that they have no competing interests.

Author details
[1]Infection Control Programme and WHO Collaborating Centre on Patient Safety, Faculty of Medicine, University of Geneva Hospitals, Geneva, Switzerland. [2]Médecins sans Frontières, Geneva, Switzerland. [3]CAPPI Servette, Department of Mental Health and Psychiatry, Geneva University Hospitals, Genève, Switzerland. [4]International Centre for Migration, Health and Development, Geneva, Switzerland. [5]Programme Santé Migrants, Department of Community Medicine, Primary Care and Emergency Medicine, Geneva University Hospitals, Geneva, Switzerland. [6]Geneva, Switzerland. [7]Department of Clinical Immunology and Rheumatology, Hannover Medical School, Hannover, Germany. [8]German Center for Infection Research (DZIF), PARTNER Site Hannover-Braunschweig, Hannover, Germany. [9]Division of Primary Care Medicine, Geneva University Hospitals, Geneva, Switzerland. [10]Institute of Global Health, Geneva University, Geneva, Switzerland. [11]Department of Service Delivery & Safety, World Health Organization, Geneva, Switzerland. [12]Division of Communicable Diseases, Federal Office of Public Health, Bern, Switzerland. [13]Health Unit, International Committee of the Red Cross (ICRC), Geneva, Switzerland. [14]Division of Infectious Diseases & HIV Medicine, Department of Medicine, Groote Schuur Hospital, University of Cape Town, Cape Town, South Africa. [15]International Organization for Migration (IOM), Migration Health Division (MHD), Regional office (RO), Brussels, Belgium. [16]4th Department of Medicine, Medical School, National and Kapodistrian University of Athens, Athens, Greece. [17]Hellenic Centre for Disease Control & Prevention, Athens, Greece. [18]Division of environmental health, Institute of Global Health, Faculty of Medicine, University of Geneva, Geneva, Switzerland. [19]Communication in Science, Geneva, Switzerland. [20]Section of Infectious Diseases and Immunity, Department of Medicine, Imperial College London, Hammersmith Hospital, London W12 0HS, UK. [21]The Institute for Infection and Immunity, St George's, University of London, London WC1E 7HU, UK.

References

1. International Organization for Migration. Missing Migrants Project. https://missingmigrants.iom.int/. Accessed 8 Sept 2017. 2017.
2. Dijstelbloem H. Migration tracking is a mess. Nature. 2017;543(7643):31–3.
3. International Organization for Migration. Who is a migrant? https://www.iom.int/who-is-a-migrant (accessed 01.03.2018).
4. Guterres A. World Refugee Day 2017 - Secretary-General Video Message. 20. 06.2017 2017. https://www.un.org/sg/en/content/sg/statement/2017-06-20/secretary-generals-message-world-refugee-day (accessed 01.10.2017).
5. Nougayrède N. Refugees aren't the problem. Europe's identity crisis is. The Guardian. 2016;31:10. https://www.theguardian.com/commentisfree/2016/oct/31/refugees-problem-europe-identity-crisis-migration. Accessed 1 June 2017.
6. Betts A. Survival Migration. Failed Governance and the Crisis of Displacement. Ithaca: Cornell University Press. 2013. http://www.jstor.org/stable/10.7591/j.ctt32b5cd.
7. Burkle FM. The politics of global public health in fragile states and ungoverned territories. PLoS Currents 2017; 9: ecurrents.dis.ba3beede71ca0746a972aa3837ed618.
8. Hayes S, Lundy BD, Hallward MC. Conflict-induced migration and the refugee crisis: global and local perspectives from Peacebuilding and development. Journal of Peacebuilding & Development. 2016;11(3):1–7.
9. OECD (2016), States of Fragility 2016: Understanding Violence, OECD Publishing, Paris. https://doi.org/10.1787/9789264267213-en.
10. World Health Organization. Office of the High Commissioner for human rights, International Organization for Migration. International migration, health and human rights. Geneva: International Organization for Migration; 2013.
11. da Costa R. Rights of refugees in the context of integration: legal standards and recommendations. Legal and protection policy research series. In: UNHCR; 2006.
12. Vernon A, Deriche K, Eisenhauer S. Connecting refugees. How Internet and Mobile Connectivity can Improve Refugee Well-Being and Transform Humanitarian Action. Geneva: UNHCR; 2016.
13. Gorst-Unsworth C, Goldenberg E. Psychological sequelae of torture and organised violence suffered by refugees from Iraq. Trauma-related factors compared with social factors in exile. Br J Psychiatry. 1998;172:90–4.
14. McColl H, Johnson S. Characteristics and needs of asylum seekers and refugees in contact with London community mental health teams - a descriptive investigation. Soc Psychiatry Psychiatr Epidemiol. 2006;41(10):789–95.
15. Kutzin J. Anything goes on the path to universal health coverage? No. Bull World Health Organ. 2012;90(11):867–8.
16. Ghebreyesus TA. All roads lead to universal health coverage. Lancet Glob Health. 2017;5(9):e839–e40.
17. Abiiro GA, De Allegri M. Universal health coverage from multiple perspectives: a synthesis of conceptual literature and global debates. BMC Int Health Hum Rights. 2015;15:17.
18. Fajardo-Dolci G, Gutierrez JP, Garcia-Saiso S. Effective access to health services: operationalizing universal health coverage. Salud publica de Mexico. 2015;57(2):180–6.
19. Chapman AR. Assessing the universal health coverage target in the sustainable development goals from a human rights perspective. BMC Int Health Hum Rights. 2016;16(1):33.
20. World Health Organization. Questions and answers on universal health coverage. http://www.who.int/healthsystems/topics/financing/uhc_qa. Accessed 8 Sept 2017.
21. UNICEF. A child is a child: protecting children on the move from violence. In: Abuse and exploitation; 2017.
22. International Organization for Migration. The push and pull factors of asylum-related migration: a literature review. 2016.
23. Newbold B, McKeary M. Investigating the diversity of Canada's refugee population and its health implications: does one size fit all? Int J Migr Health Soc Care. 2017;13(2):145–56.
24. Kristiansen M, Razum O, Tezcan-Guntekin H, Krasnik A. Aging and health among migrants in a European perspective. Public Health Rev. 2016;37:14.
25. Cheung SY, Phillimore J. Gender and refugee integration: a quantitative analysis of integration and social policy outcomes. J Soc Policy. 2017;46(2):211–30.
26. Shawyer F, Enticott JC, Block AA, Cheng IH, Meadows GN. The mental health status of refugees and asylum seekers attending a refugee health clinic including comparisons with a matched sample of Australian-born residents. Bmc Psychiatry. 2017;17:76.
27. Fennelly K. The "healthy migrant" effect. Minn Med. 2007;90(3):51–3.
28. Norredam M, Agyemang C, Hansen OKH, et al. Duration of residence and disease occurrence among refugees and family reunited immigrants: test of the 'healthy migrant effect' hypothesis. Tropical Med Int Health. 2014;19(8):958–67.
29. Hamilton TG. The healthy immigrant (migrant) effect: in search of a better native-born comparison group. Soc Sci Res. 2015;54:353–65.
30. Rubalcava LN, Teruel GM, Thomas D, Goldman N. The healthy migrant effect: new findings from the Mexican family life survey. Am J Public Health. 2008;98(1):78–84.
31. Arsenijevic J, Schillberg E, Ponthieu A, et al. A crisis of protection and safe passage: violence experienced by migrants/refugees travelling along the Western Balkan corridor to northern Europe. Confl Heal. 2017:11.

32. Crepet A, Rita F, Reid A, et al. Mental health and trauma in asylum seekers landing in Sicily in 2015: a descriptive study of neglected invisible wounds. Confl Heal. 2017:11.
33. Keygnaert I, Dialmy A, Manco A, et al. Sexual violence and sub-Saharan migrants in Morocco: a community-based participatory assessment using respondent driven sampling. Glob Health. 2014:10.
34. Esposito F, Ornelas J, Arcidiacono C. Migration-related detention centers: the challenges of an ecological perspective with a focus on justice. BMC Int Health Hum Rights. 2015;15.
35. United Nations. Standard Minimum Rules for the Treatment of Prisoners. 30 August 1995. http://www.refworld.org/docid/3ae6b36e8.html (accessed 7 Nov 2017).
36. Institute for Criminal Policy Research. World Prison Brief. http://www.prisonstudies.org/highest-to-lowest/foreign-prisoners?field_region_taxonomy_tid=14 (accessed 23.10.2017).
37. Aebi MF, Tiago MM, Burkhardt C. SPACE I – Council of Europe Annual Penal Statistics: prison populations. Survey 2015. Strasbourg: Council of Europe; 2016.
38. Kazi AM, Shah SA, Jenkins CA, Shepherd BE, Vermund SH. Risk factors and prevalence of tuberculosis, human immunodeficiency virus, syphilis, hepatitis B virus, and hepatitis C virus among prisoners in Pakistan. Int J Infect Dis. 2010;14:E60–E6.
39. Kamarulzaman A, Reid SE, Schwitters A, et al. Prevention of transmission of HIV, hepatitis B virus, hepatitis C virus, and tuberculosis in prisoners. Lancet. 2016;388(10049):1115–26.
40. International Organization for Migration. Summary report on the MIPEX health Strand and country reports. Geneva: International Organization for Migration; 2016.
41. Singer M, Bulled N, Ostrach B, Mendenhall E. Syndemics and the biosocial conception of health. Lancet. 2017;389(10072):941–50.
42. Rechel B, Mladovsky P, Devillé W, Rijks B, Petrova-Benedict R, McKee M. Migration and health in European Union. Maidenhead: McGraw Hill/Open University Press; 2011.
43. Bogic M, Ajdukovic D, Bremner S, et al. Factors associated with mental disorders in long-settled war refugees: refugees from the former Yugoslavia in Germany, Italy and the UK. Br J Psychiatry. 2012;200(3):216–23.
44. Gerritsen AAM, Bramsen I, Deville W, van Willigen LHM, Hovens JE, van der Ploeg HM. Physical and mental health of afghan, Iranian and Somali asylum seekers and refugees living in the Netherlands. Soc Psychiatry Psychiatr Epidemiol. 2006;41(1):18–26.
45. Fazel M, Wheeler J, Danesh J. Prevalence of serious mental disorder in 7000 refugees resettled in western countries: a systematic review. Lancet. 2005;365(9467):1309–14.
46. Coughlin SS. Anxiety and Depression: Linkages with Viral Diseases. Public Health Rev. 2012;34(2):92.
47. Doocy S, Lyles E, Roberton T, Akhu-Zaheya L, Oweis A, Burnham G. Prevalence and care-seeking for chronic diseases among Syrian refugees in Jordan. BMC Public Health. 2015;15.
48. Chauvin P, Parizot I, Simmonot N. L'accès aux soins de personnes sans autorisation de séjour dans 11 pays d'Europe. Paris: Observatoire Européen de l'accès aux soins de Médecins du Monde; 2009.
49. Turktan M, Ak O, Erdem H, et al. Community acquired infections among refugees leading to intensive care unit admissions in Turkey. Int J Infect Dis. 2017;58:111–4.
50. Jackson Y, Paignon A, Wolff H, Delicado N. Health of undocumented migrants in primary care in Switzerland. PLoS One. 2018;13(7):e0201313.
51. Monge-Maillo B, Lopez-Velez R, Norman FF, Ferrere-Gonzalez F, Martinez-Perez A, Perez-Molina JA. Screening of imported infectious diseases among asymptomatic sub-Saharan African and Latin American immigrants: a public health challenge. Am J Trop Med Hyg. 2015;92(4):848–56.
52. Errecaborde KM, Stauffer W, Cetron M. Neglected Tropical Disease Control and Elimination: Is Human Displacement an Achilles Heel. PLoS Negl Trop Dis. 2015;9(3):e0003535.
53. Mbabazi PS, Andan O, Fitzgerald DW, Chitsulo L, Engels D, Downs J. Examining the relationship between urogenital schistosomiasis and HIV infection. Tropical Med Int Health. 2013;18:55–6.
54. Kamal SM, Turner B, He Q, et al. Progression of fibrosis in hepatitis C with and without schistosomiasis: correlation with serum markers of fibrosis. Hepatology. 2006;43(4):771–9.
55. Siegel MO, Simon GL. Is Human Immunodeficiency Virus Infection a Risk Factor for Strongyloides stercoralis Hyperinfection and Dissemination. Plos Negl Trop Dis. 2012;6(7):e1581.
56. Sartori AMC, Ibrahim KY, Westphalen EVN, et al. Manifestations of Chagas disease (American trypanosomiasis) in patients with HIVAIDS. Ann Trop Med Parasitol. 2007;101(1):31–50.
57. Tornesello ML, Giorgi Rossi P, Buonaguro L, Buonaguro FM. Group HPVPIW. Human Papillomavirus Infection and Cervical Neoplasia among Migrant Women Living in Italy. Frontiers in oncology. 2014;4:31.
58. Carballo M, Maclean E, Gudumac I. Van Damme P. Hepatitis C and Migration: A Public Health Challenge. J Fam Med. 2016;3(4):1065.
59. Ackermann N, Marosevic D, Hormansdorfer S, et al. Screening for infectious diseases among newly arrived asylum seekers, Bavaria, Germany, 2015. Euro Surveill. 2018;23(10):17–00176.
60. Bil JP, Schrooders PA, Prins M, et al. Integrating hepatitis B, hepatitis C and HIV screening into tuberculosis entry screening for migrants in the Netherlands, 2013 to 2015. Eurosurveillance. 2018;23(11):17–00491.
61. Ravensbergen SJ, Berends M, Stienstra Y, Ott A. High prevalence of MRSA and ESBL among asylum seekers in the Netherlands. PLoS One 2017; 12(4):e0176481.
62. Seedat F, Hargreaves S, Nellums LB, Ouyang J, Brown M, Friedland JS. How effective are approaches to migrant screening for infectious diseases in Europe? A systematic review. Lancet Infect Dis. 2018;18(9):e259–e71.
63. Murcia L, Simon M, Carrilero B, Roig M, Segovia M. Treatment of infected women of childbearing age prevents congenital Trypanosoma cruzi infection by eliminating the Parasitemia detected by PCR. J Infect Dis. 2017;215(9):1452–8.
64. Sicuri E, Munoz J, Pinazo MJ, et al. Economic evaluation of Chagas disease screening of pregnant Latin American women and of their infants in a non endemic area. Acta Trop. 2011;118(2):110–7.
65. Nakken CS, Skovdal M, Nellums LB, Friedland JS, Hargreaves S, Norredam M. Vaccination status and needs of asylum-seeking children in Denmark: a retrospective data analysis. Public Health. 2018;158:110–6.
66. Paxton GA, Rice J, Davie G, Carapetis JR, Skull SA. East African immigrant children in Australia have poor immunisation coverage. J Paediatr Child Health. 2011;47(12):888–92.
67. de Monleon JV, Regnier F, Ajana F, et al. catch-up vaccination of worldwide newcoming (adopted, refugee or migrant) children in France. Arch Pediatr. 2014;21(3):329–34.
68. Jablonka A, Happle C, Wetzke M, et al. Measles, rubella and varicella IgG Seroprevalence in a large refugee cohort in Germany in 2015: a cross-sectional study. Infect Dis Ther. 2017;6(4):487–96.
69. Mipatrini D, Stefanelli P, Severoni S, Rezza G. Vaccinations in migrants and refugees: a challenge for European health systems. A systematic review of current scientific evidence. Pathog Glob Health. 2017;111(2):59–68.
70. Jones G, Haeghebaert S, Merlin B, et al. Measles outbreak in a refugee settlement in Calais, France: January to February 2016. Euro Surveill. 2016;21(11):30167.
71. Lesens O, Baud O, Henquell C, Lhermet Nurse A, Beytout J. Varicella outbreak in Sudanese refugees from Calais. J Travel Med. 2016;23(5):042.
72. Mellou K, Chrisostomou A, Sideroglou T, et al. Hepatitis a among refugees, asylum seekers and migrants living in hosting facilities, Greece, April to 2016. Euro Surveill. 2017;22(4):30448.
73. WHO Regional Office per Europe. WHO-UNHCR-UNICEF Joint Technical Guidance: General Principles of Vaccination of Refugees, Asylum-Seekers and Migrants in the WHO European Region. 3 November 2015. http://www.euro.who.int/en/health-topics/disease-prevention/vaccines-and-immunization/news/news/2015/11/who,-unicef-and-unhcr-call-for-equitable-access-to-vaccines-for-refugees-and-migrants/who-unhcr-unicef-joint-technical-guidance-general-principles-of-vaccination-of-refugees,-asylum-seekers-and-migrants-in-the-who-european-region]. Accessed 24 Aug 2018.
74. European Centre for Disease Prevention and Control. ECDC technical document: infectious diseases of specific relevance to newly-arrived migrants in the EU/EEA. Stockholm; 2015. https://ecdc.europa.eu/sites/portal/files/media/en/publications/Publications/Infectious-diseases-of-specific-relevance-to-newly-arrived-migrants-in-EU-EEA.pdf]. Accessed 24 Aug 2018.
75. Hargreaves S, Nellums LB, Ramsay M, et al. Who is responsible for the vaccination of migrants in Europe. Lancet. 2018;391(10132):1752–4.
76. Giambi C, Del Manso M, Dente MG, et al. Immunization Strategies Targeting Newly Arrived Migrants in Non-EU Countries of the Mediterranean Basin and Black Sea. Int J Environ Res Public Health. 2017;14(5):E459.
77. Ginsburg AS, Klugman KP. Vaccination to reduce antimicrobial resistance. Lancet Glob Health. 2017;5(12):e1176–e7.

78. Kumar S. Reduction in antimicrobial resistance by the way of extensive vaccination. Hum Vaccin Immunother. 2018:1–2.
79. Tagliabue A, Rappuoli R. Changing priorities in Vaccinology: antibiotic resistance moving to the top. Front Immunol. 2018;9:1068.
80. Jansen KU, Knirsch C, Anderson AS. The role of vaccines in preventing bacterial antimicrobial resistance. Nat Med. 2018;24(1):10–9.
81. Atkins KE, Lafferty EI, Deeny SR, Davies NG, Robotham JV, Jit M. Use of mathematical modelling to assess the impact of vaccines on antibiotic resistance. Lancet Infect Dis. 2018;18(6):e204–e13.
82. Wilson ME. Travel and the emergence of infectious-diseases. Emerg Infect Dis. 1995;1(2):39–46.
83. European Centre for Disease Prevention and Control (ECDC). Infectious diseases of specific relevance to newly-arrived migrants in EU/EEA. Stockholm: ECDC; 2015.
84. Soto SM. Human migration and infectious diseases. Clin Microbiol Infect. 2009;15:26–8.
85. Nellums L, Hargreaves S, Thompson H, Friedland JS. Antimicrobial resistance in migrants to Europe. Vienna: European Congress of Clinical Microbiology and Infectious Diseases; 2017.
86. de Smalen AW, Ghorab H, Abd El Ghany M, Hill-Cawthorne GA. Refugees and antimicrobial resistance: a systematic review. Travel Med Infect Dis 2017; 15: 23–28.
87. Nellums LB, Thompson H, Holmes A, et al. Antimicrobial resistance among migrants in Europe: a systematic review and meta-analysis. Lancet Infect Dis. 2018;18(7):796–811.
88. Hargreaves S, Lonnroth K, Nellums LB, et al. Multidrug-resistant tuberculosis and migration to Europe. Clin Microbiol Infect. 2017;23(3):141–6.
89. Trovato A, Reid A, Takarinda KC, et al. Dangerous crossing: demographic and clinical features of rescued sea migrants seen in 2014 at an outpatient clinic at Augusta Harbor, Italy. Confl Health. 2016;10:14.
90. Briody C, Rubenstein L, Roberts L, Penney E, Keenan W, Horbar J. Review of attacks on health care facilities in six conflicts of the past three decades. Confl Health. 2018;12:19.
91. Fouad FM, Sparrow A, Tarakji A, et al. Health workers and the weaponisation of health care in Syria: a preliminary inquiry for the lancet-American University of Beirut Commission on Syria. Lancet. 2017;390(10111):2516–26.
92. Health care in danger. Violent incidents affecting the delivery of health care. January 2012 to December 2013: International Committee of the Red Cross, 2014.
93. Huddleston T, Bilgili O, Joki A-L, Vankova Z. Migrant integration policy index 2015. 2015.
94. United Nations High Commissioner for Refugees (UNHCR). UNHCR Position on the Return of Asylum-Seekers to Greece Under the "Dublin Regulation". Geneva: UNHCR; 2008.
95. United Nations High Commissioner for Refugees (UNHCR). UNHCR Comments on The European Commission Proposal for a Recast Dublin Regulation. Geneva: UNHCR; 2016.
96. Parliamentary Assembly of the Council of Europe. Resolution 2072 (2015). Strasbourg: Council of Europe; 2015.
97. Parliamentary Assembly of the Council of Europe. Resolution 2000 (2014). Strasbourg: Council of Europe; 2014.
98. New York Declaration for Refugees and Migrants. New York: United Nations, 2016.
99. United Nations High Commissioner for Refugees (UNHCR). New York Declaration for Refugees and Migrants. http://www.unhcr.org/new-york-declaration-for-refugees-and-migrants.html. Accessed 13 Mar 2018.
100. Hargreaves S. Europe's migrants face unacceptable humanitarian situation. Lancet Infect Dis. 2016;16(1):27–8.
101. Carballo M, Hargreaves S, Gudumac I, Maclean EC. Evolving migrant crisis in Europe: implications for health systems. Lancet Glob Health. 2017;5(3):e252–e3.
102. Afkhami AA. Can academic medicine Lead the way in the refugee crisis? Acad Med. 2016;91(12):1595–7.
103. UCL-Lancet Commission on Migration and Health. About the Commission. https://www.migrationandhealth.org/about (accessed 12.03.2018).
104. Hanefeld J, Vearey J, Lunt N. Researchers migration M. a global research agenda on migration, mobility, and health. Lancet. 2017;389(10087):2358–9.
105. Bozorgmehr K, Razum O. Effect of restricting access to health care on health expenditures among asylum-seekers and refugees: a quasi-experimental study in Germany, 1994–2013. PLoS One. 2015;10(7):e0131483.
106. Tan TM, Spiegel P, Haskew C, Greenough PG. Does spending on refugees make a difference? A cross-sectional study of the association between refugee program spending and health outcomes in 70 sites in 17 countries. Confl Health. 2016;10:28.
107. Ingleby D, Petrova-Benedict R. Recommendations on access to health services for migrants in an irregular situation: an expert consensus. Brussels: International Organization for Migration (IOM) Regional Office Brussels, Migration Health Division; 2016.
108. World Bank. Migration and development brief, 27 April 2017. 2017.
109. Fromentin V. The long-run and short-run impacts of remittances on financial development in developing countries. 2017.
110. Organisation for Economic Co-operation and Development (OECD). Labour market integration of immigrants and their children: developing, activating and using skills. In: International migration outlook, vol. 2014. Paris: OECD Publishing; 2014.
111. Organisation for Economic Co-operation and Development (OECD). How can migrants' skills be put to use? Migration Policy Debates, 2014. Access 01.10.2017).
112. Macchiavello M. Forced migrants as an under-utilized asset: refugee skills, livelihoods, and achievements in Kampala, Uganda. Working paper no. 95. Geneva: UNHCR; 2003.
113. Commission launches initiative to help refugee scientists and researchers. 2015. http://ec.europa.eu/research/index.cfm?pg=newsalert&year=2015&na=na-051015 (accessed 23.10.2017).
114. Kitching GT, J. Haavik H, Tandstad BJ, Zaman M, Darj E. Exploring the role of ad hoc grassroots organizations providing humanitarian aid on Lesvos. Greece *PLoS Currents*. 2016;8 ecurrents.dis. bd282cd90ade7d4eb63b6bbdb1904d10.
115. Grandi F. World Refugee Day Statement By Filippo Grandi, United Nations High Commissioner for Refugees. 20.06.2017. http://www.unhcr.org/admin/hcspeeches/5948d38e7/world-refugee-day-statement.html (accessed 01.10.2017).

5

Genotyping and distribution of putative virulence factors and antibiotic resistance genes of *Acinetobacter baumannii* strains isolated from raw meat

Marziyeh Tavakol[1], Hassan Momtaz[1*], Parviz Mohajeri[2,3], Leili Shokoohizadeh[4] and Elahe Tajbakhsh[1]

Abstract

Background: *Acinetobacter baumannii* strains with multiple antimicrobial resistance are primarily known as opportunistic nosocomial bacteria but they may also be regarded as emerging bacterial contaminants of food samples of animal origin. Here we aimed to study the molecular characteristics of the *A. baumanni* strains isolated from raw meat samples.

Methods: A total of 22 *A. baumanni* strains were isolated from 126 animal meat samples and were genotyped by ERIC-PCR method and by PCR detection of their virulence and antimicrobial resistance determinants. *A. baumannii* strains with 80% and more similarities were considered as one cluster.

Results: Sixteen different genetic clusters were found amongst the 22 *A. baumanni* strains. Of the 22 strains, 12 (54.54%) had similar genetic cluster. *A. baumannii* strains exhibited the highest percentage of resistance against tetracycline (90.90%), trimethoprim (59.09%), cotrimoxazole (54.54%) and gentamicin (50.00%). *TetA* (81.81%), *tetB* (72.72%), *dfrA1* (63.63%), *aac(3)-IV* (63.63%), *sul1* (63.63%) and *aadA1* (45.45%) were the most commonly detected antibiotic resistance genes. *FimH* (81.81%), *afa/draBC* (63.63%), *csgA* (63.63%), *cnf1* (59.09%), *cnf2* (54.54%) and *iutA* (50.00%) were the most commonly detected virulence factors. *A. baumannii* strains isolated from the chicken meat samples had the highest similarities in the genetic cluster.

Conclusions: *A. baumannii* strains with similar genetic cluster (ERIC-Type) had the same prevalence of antibiotic resistance, antibiotic resistance genes and virulence factors. Genetic cluster of the *A. baumannii* strains is the main factor affected the similarities in the genotypic and phenotypic properties of the *A. baumannii* strains.

Keywords: *Acinetobacter baumannii*, ERIC-PCR, Virulence genes, Antibiotic resistance pattern, Raw meat

Background

Consumption of raw or undercooked meat has been associated with several outbreaks of bacterial foodborne disease all-around the world [1–5]. Bacterial strains isolated from meat are both pathogenic and commensal such as *Staphylococcus aureus*, *Streptococcus* species, *Listeria monocytogenes*, Bacillus spp., Salmonella spp., Campylobacter spp., *Escherichia coli*, *Yersinia enterocolitica*, Acinetobacter spp., Aeromonas spp., Pseudomonas spp. and etc. [2, 3, 6–9]. *Acinetobacter* species are saprophytic, ubiquitous and have emerged as an important nosocomial pathogen due to its ability for survival in the hospital environment on a wide range of dry and moist surfaces [10, 11]. Human infections caused by Acinetobacter species include pneumonia, which is most often related to endotracheal tubes or tracheostomies, endocarditis, meningitis, skin and wound infections, peritonitis in patients receiving peritoneal dialysis, UTI and bacteremia.[10, 11] Acinetobacter spp. and especially *Acinetobacter baumannii* are one of the newly emerged bacteria all-around the world [10, 11]. *A. baumannii* colonizes the respiratory tract, skin, urinary and gastrointestinal systems, and

* Correspondence: hamomtaz@yahoo.com; hamomtaz@iaushk.ac.ir
[1]Department of Microbiology, Shahrekord Branch, Islamic Azad University, PO. Box: 166, Shahrekord, Iran
Full list of author information is available at the end of the article

frequently leads to pneumonia, surgical site infections, catheter-related blood circulatory infections, and urinary tract infections and rarely community acquired pneumonia, meningitis, mediastinitis, osteomyelitis and cholangitis [10, 11].

A. baumannii strains isolated from clinical infections harbored the high prevalence of certain virulence factors including pathogenicity islands (PAI), P fimbriae (*pap* genes), S fimbriae adhesion and F1C (*sfa*), a fimbriae adhesion and Dr. antigen family (*afa/dra*), type 1 fimbriae (*fimH*), fibronectin receptor (*fbn*), serum resistance (*traT*), curli fibers (*csg*), aerobactin (*iutA*), yersiniabactin (*fyuA*), polysaccharide coatings as group II and III capsules (*kpsMT*), cytotoxic necrotizing factors (*cnf*), invasins factors (*IbeA*) and colicin V production (*cvaC*). Moreover, these factors are responsible for adhesion, colonization and invasion of the *A. baumannii* strains into the different target organs [12, 13].

A. baumannii strains are also known to harbor multiple resistance against different types of antibiotics. Documented data revealed that the *A. baumannii* strains isolated from human and animal clinical infections and food stuffs harbored the high prevalence of resistance against different types of antibiotics [14, 15]. The genes that encode resistance against antibiotics and especially *aadA1* (streptomycin), *aac(3)-IV* (gentamicin), *sul1* (sulfonamide), *blaSHV* and *blaCTX-M* (cephalosporins), *cat1* and *cmlA* (chloramphenicol), *tetA* and *tetB* (tetracycline), *dfrA1* (trimethoprim), *qnr* (fluoroquinolones),*imp*, *sim* and *vim* (carbenicillin), and *Oxa-51-like*(oxacillinases) are mainly responsible for occurrence of severe antibiotic resistance [14–16]. In keeping with this, genotyping is one of the best techniques to find the molecular relationship between bacterial strains isolated from different sources. Enterobacterial Repetitive Intergenic Consensus Polymerase Chain Reaction (ERIC-PCR) is one of the best typing methods of DNA fingerprints of bacterial strains. This method has sporadically been used to characterize *A. baumannii* strains isolated from clinical samples [17].

Studies regarding the association of *Acinetobacter* with foodborne illnesses are somewhat limited [10, 11].Therefore, the present investigation was done to study the phenotypic and genotypic characterization of antibiotic resistance and molecular typing of the *A. baumannii* strains isolated from raw meat samples.

Methods

A. baumannii strains

From January 2016 to May 2017, a total of 22 *A. baumannii* strains were isolated from 126 samples of raw chicken, turkey, bovine, ovine and camel meat samples. Meat samples were randomly collected (simple random sampling procedure) from the butchers and shopping center of different parts of the Chaharmahal Va Bakhtiari province, Iran. All isolates were transferred to the Microbiology Research Center of the Islamic Azad University of Shahrekord in cooler with ice-packs.

A. baumanni strains were isolated based on the method described by the Cappuccino and Welsh (2016) [18]. Briefly, the specimens were inoculated initially on blood agar (Merck) and MacConkey agar (Merck) medium and incubated for 24 h at 37 °C. Conventional biochemical methods such as oxidase, citrate, urea urease, malonate consumption, oxidation and fermentation of sugars, motility and indole production were used to identify *A. baumannii*. Additionally, genus Acinetobacter was identified by Gram staining, cell and colony morphology, positive catalase test, negative oxidase test and absence of motility. Speciation of *Acinetobacter* was performed on the basis of glucose oxidation, gelatin liquefaction, beta hemolysis, growth at 37 °C and 42 °C, arginine hydrolysis and susceptibility to chloramphenicol [18]. The isolates were stored in BHI medium containing 15% glycerol at − 20 °C.

PCR confirmation of the *A. baumannii* isolates

Confirmation of *A. baumannii* isolates were done using the PCR method. Presence of the16S–23S ribosomal RNA (*16S–23SrRNA*) gene was analyzed using the PCR method described previously [19]. *A. baumannii* isolates were sub-cultured on TSB media (Merck, Germany) and incubated for 48 h at 37 °C. Genomic DNA was extracted from bacterial colonies using the DNA extraction kit (Cinnagen, Iran) according to manufacturer's instruction. A pair of primers of P-Ab-ITSF (5'-CATTATCAC GGTAATTAGTG-3′) and PAb-ITSB (5'-AGAGCACTG TGCACTTAAG-3′) (208 bp) was used for PCR amplification of the *16S–23SrDNA* gene of the *A. baumanni* according to the method described by Chiang et al., (2011) [19]. Confirmed strains were maintained in slant nutrient agar (Merck, Germany) and stored at − 70 °C on 20% sterile buffered glycerol.

Antibiotic susceptibility testing

Patterns of antimicrobial resistance of the *A. baumanni* strains were studied using the simple disk diffusion technique. The Mueller–Hinton agar (Merck, Germany) medium was used for this purpose. Susceptibility of *A. baumanni*isolates were tested against several types of antibiotics with appropriate disks containing azithromycin (15 μg), erythromycin (15 μg), rifampin (5 μg), nitrofurantoin (300 μg), chloramphenicol (30 μg), imipenem (30 μg), meropenem (10 μg), levofloxacin (5 μg), ciprofloxacin (5 μg), trimethoprim (5 μg), tetracycline (30 μg), ceftazidime (30 μg), cephalotin (30 μg), trimethoprim/sulphamethoxazole(25 μg), tobramycin (10 μg), amikacin (30 μg), gentamicin (10 μg) and streptomycin (10 μg) (produced by PadTan-Teb, Iran), according to the instruction of Clinical and Laboratory Standards Institute [20]. *A. baumanni*

ATCC 19606 was used for quality control organism in antimicrobial susceptibility determination.

Detection of antibiotic resistance genes and virulence factors

Thermo-cycler (Eppendorf Mastercycler 5330, Eppen dorf-Nethel-Hinz GmbH, Hamburg, Germany) was used in all PCR reactions. Table 1 represents the list of primers and PCR conditions used for amplification of virulence factors and antibiotic resistance genes in the *A. baumannii* strains.

Molecular typing of *A. baumannii* isolates using the ERIC-PCR

The primer pair ERIC1: 5′-ATGTAAGCTCCTGG GGATTCAC-3′ and ERIC2: 5′- AAGTAAGTGACTGG GGTGAGCG-3′ were used to amplify intervening fragments of ERIC in the genomic DNA extracted from the bacterial colonies [17]. Amplification reactions were performed in a final volume of 25 μL including 150 μM dNTP mixture, 1.5 U Taq enzyme, 0.5 μM each primer and 1 μL DNA template. The PCR conditions were as follows: initial denaturation (5 min at 94 °C), followed by four cycles of denaturation (1 min at 94 °C), annealing (1 min at 26 °C) and extension (1 min at 72 °C) and 40 cycles of denaturation (30 s at 94 °C), annealing (30 s at 40 ° C) and extension (1 min at 72 °C), followed by the final extension at 72 °C for 10 min [17]. Amplified products of each sample were subjected to electrophoresis in 2% agarose gel containing DNA Safe Stain (CinnaGen, Iran).

Data analysis

Electrophoretic patterns were analyzed either visually or by using the Bionumerics software (Applied Maths, Sint-Martems-Latem, Belgium). The BioNumerics analysis was performed using the Dice coefficient and the unweighted pair group method of averages (UPGMA) with a 1% tolerance limit and 1% optimization. Isolates that clustered with ≥80% similarity were considered to belong to the same ERIC type, respectively.

Statistical analysis

Data were transferred to a Microsoft Excel spreadsheet (version 15; Microsoft Corp., Redmond, WA, USA) for analysis. Using statistical software (version 16; SPSS Inc., Chicago, USA), Chi-square test and Fisher's exact two-tailed test analysis was performed and differences were considered significant at values of $p < 0.05$.

Results

Of 22 tested *A. baumannii* strains, 10 strains were originated from the chicken meat, 4 strains from bovine meat, 3 strains from camel meat, 3 strains from turkey meat and 2 strains from ovine meat.

Figure 1 represent the electrophoretic patterns of the ERIC types of *A. baumannii* strains No 1-17 isolated from raw meat samples. Figure 2 represents the electrophoretic patterns of the ERIC types of *A. baumannii* strains No 18-22 isolated from raw meat samples. Figure 3 shows the results of the molecular typing of the *A. baumannii* strains isolated from different animal origins. *A. baumannii* strains with 80% and more than 80% similarity in the molecular typing were considered as one cluster. In keeping with this, a total of 16 ERIC types were identified. We found that strains no 19 and 22 (originated from chicken meat), 12 and 15 (originated from chicken meat), 6 (originated from bovine meat) and 14 (originated from chicken meat), 1 and 3 (originated from chicken meat), 4 (originated from bovine meat) and 5 (originated from turkey meat) and finally 2 (originated from chicken meat) and 10 (originated from ovine meat) had similar genetic cluster and were related to the 1, 4, 9, 13, 15 and 16 genetic cluster of the *A. baumannii* strains, respectively.

Table 2 represents the antibiotic resistance pattern of the *A. baumannii* strains isolated from different animal origins. *A. baumannii* strains harbored the highest prevalence of resistance against tetracycline (90.90%), trimethoprim (59.09%), co-trimoxazole (54.54%) and gentamicin (50.00%) antibiotics. *A. baumannii* strains of similar molecular cluster (ERIC-type) showed the same pattern of antibiotic resistance (Table 2). *TetA* (81.81%), *tetB* (72.72%), *dfrA1* (63.63%), *aac(3)-IV* (63.63%), *sul1* (63.63%) and *aadA1* (45.45%) were the most commonly detected antibiotic resistance genes. *A. baumannii* strains of the same molecular cluster had the same antibiotic resistance genes (Table 2).

Table 2 also represents the distribution of virulence factors among the *A. baumannii* strains isolated from meat samples of animals. *FimH* (81.81%), *afa/draBC* (63.63%), *csgA* (63.63%), *cnf1* (59.09%), *cnf2* (54.54%) and *iutA* (50.00%) were the most commonly detected virulence factors amongst the *A. baumannii* strains isolated from animal origins. *A. baumannii* strains of same molecular cluster (ERIC-type) had the same virulence factors.

Discussion

Acinetobacter is a nosocomial pathogen. Its ability to infect healthy hosts and its propensity to develop antimicrobial drug resistance is a cause for concern among infectious disease specialty. Although the ubiquitous existence of *A. baumannii* in hospital environment has been considered a routine delusion by several investigations [10, 12–14, 16, 17, 19, 21], different recent reports have undeniably highlighted the presence of the bacterium in different types of animal origins [11, 22, 23]. In recent years, nosocomial infections of *A. baumannii*, as an opportunistic pathogen, are increasing. Treatment of this bacteria especially multi-drug resistant and broad-spectrum beta-lactamases strains is of major concern [11, 22, 23]. These recent works

Table 1 Oligonucleotide primers and PCR conditions used for amplification of the antibiotic resistance genes and virulence factors in the A. baumannii strains of animal origin [19, 34–46]

Target gene	Primer Sequence (5′-3′)	Size of product (bp)	PCR conditions	Volume (50 µl)
draBC	GCTGGGCAGCAAACTGATAACTCTC CATCAAGCTGTTTGTTCGTCCGCCG	750	1 cycle: 95 0C ---------- 4 min. 30 cycle: 95 0C ---------- 50 s 58 0C ---------- 60 s 72 0C ---------- 45 s 1 cycle: 72 0C ---------- 8 min	5 µL PCR buffer 10X 1.5 mM Mgcl2 200 µM dNTP (Fermentas) 0.5 µM of each primers F & R 1.25 U Taq DNA polymerase (Fermentas) 2.5 µL DNA template
cnf1	AAGATGGAGTTTCCTATGCAGGAG CATTCAGAGTCCTGCCCTCATTATT	498		
csgA	ACTCTGACTTGACTATTACC AGATGCAGTCTGGTCAAC	200		
cvaC	CACACACAAACGGGAGCTGTT CTTCCCGCAGCATAGTTCCAT	680		
iutA	GGCTGGACATCATGGGAACTGG CGTCGGGAACGGGTAGAATCG	300		
fyuA	TGATTAACCCCGCGACGGGAA CGCAGTAGGCACGATGTTGTA	880		
cnf2	AATCTAATTAAAGAGAAC CATGCTTTGTATATCTA	543	1 cycle: 94 0C ---------- 6 min. 34 cycle: 95 0C ---------- 50 s 58 0C ---------- 70 s 72 0C ---------- 55 s 1 cycle: 72 0C ---------- 10 min	5 µL PCR buffer 10X 2 mM Mgcl2 150 µM dNTP (Fermentas) 0.75 µM of each primers F & R 1.5 U Taq DNA polymerase (Fermentas) 3 µL DNA template
kpsMT II	GCGCATTTGCTGATACTGTTG CATCCAGACGATAAGCATGAGCA	272		
PAI	GGACATCCTGTTACAGCGCGCA TCGCCACCAATCACAGCCGAAC	930		
papC	GACGGCTGTACTGCAGGGTGTGGCG ATATCCTTTCTGCAGGGATGCAATA	328		
fimH	TGCAGAACGGATAAGCCGTGG GCAGTCACCTGCCCTCCGGTA	508	1 cycle: 95 0C ---------- 4 min. 34 cycle: 94 0C ---------- 60 s 56 0C ---------- 45 s 72 0C ---------- 60 s 1 cycle: 72 0C ---------- 10 min	5 µL PCR buffer 10X 2 mM Mgcl2 200 µM dNTP (Fermentas) 0.5 µM of each primers F & R 1.5 U Taq DNA polymerase (Fermentas) 5 µL DNA template
ibeA	AGGCAGGTGTGCGCCGCGTAC TGGTGCTCCGGCAAACCATGC	170		
PapG II-III	CTGTAATTACGGAAGTGATTTCTG ACTATCCGGCTCCGGATAAACCAT	1070		
sfa/focDE	CTCCGGAGAACTGGGTGCATCTTAC CGGAGGAGTAATTACAAACCTGGCA	410		
traT	GGTGTGGTGCGATGAGCACAG CACGGTTCAGCCATCCCTGAG	290		
aadA1	TATCCAGCTAAGCGCGAACT ATTTGCCGACTACCTTGGTC	447	1 cycle: 94 0C ---------- 6 min. 33 cycle: 95 0C ---------- 70 s 55 0C ---------- 65 s 72 0C ---------- 90 s 1 cycle: 72 0C ---------- 8 min	5 µL PCR buffer 10X 2 mM Mgcl2 150 µM dNTP (Fermentas) 0. 5 µM of each primers F & R 1.5 U Taq DNA polymerase (Fermentas) 2 µL DNA template
aac(3)-IV	CTTCAGGATGGCAAGTTGGT TCATCTCGTTCTCCGCTCAT	286		
sul1	TTCGGCATTCTGAATCTCAC ATGATCTAACCCTCGGTCTC	822		
blaSHV	TCGCCTGTGTATTATCTCCC CGCAGATAAATCACCACAATG	768		
CITM	TGGCCAGAACTGACAGGCAAA	462		

Table 1 Oligonucleotide primers and PCR conditions used for amplification of the antibiotic resistance genes and virulence factors in the A. baumannii strains of animal origin [19, 34–46] *(Continued)*

Target gene	Primer Sequence (5′-3′)	Size of product (bp)	PCR conditions	Volume (50 μl)
	TTTCTCCTGAACGTGGCTGGC			
cat1	AGTTGCTCAATGTACCTATAACC TTGTAATTCATTAAGCATTCTGCC	547		
cmlA	CCGCCACGGTGTTGTTGTTATC CACCTTGCCTGCCCATCATTAG	698		
tet(A)	GGTTCACTCGAACGACGTCA CTGTCCGACAAGTTGCATGA	577		
tet(B)	CCTCAGCTTCTCAACGCGTG GCACCTTGCTGATGACTCTT	634		
dfrA1	CGAGTGCCAAAGGTGAACAGC GAGGCGAAGTCTTGGGTAAAAAC	367		
qnr	GGGTATGGATATTATTGATAAAG CTAATCCGGCAGCACTATTTA	670		
imp	GAATAGAATGGTTAACTCTC CCAAACCACTAGGTTATC	188	1 cycle: 95 0C ----------- 4 min. 30 cycle: 95 0C ----------- 45 s 58 0C ----------- 60s 72 0C ----------- 40 s 1 cycle: 72 0C ----------- 5 min	5 μL PCR buffer 10X 1.5 mM Mgcl2 100 μM dNTP (Fermentas) 1 μM of each primers F & R 1 U Taq DNA polymerase (Fermentas) 2.5 μL DNA template
vim	GTTTGGTCGCATATCGCAAC AATGCGCAGCACCAGGATAG	382		
sim	GTACAAGGGATTCGGCATCG GTACAAGGGATTCGGCATCG	569		
Oxa-23-like	GATCGGATTGGAGAACCAGA ATTTCTGACCGCATTTCCAT	501	1 cycle: 94 0C ----------- 5 min. 32 cycle: 95 0C ----------- 50 s 60 0C ----------- 60 s 72 0C ----------- 70 s 1 cycle: 72 0C ----------- 10 min	5 μL PCR buffer 10X 2.5 mM Mgcl2 200 μM dNTP (Fermentas) 0.5 μM of each primers F & R 1.5 U Taq DNA polymerase (Fermentas) 2 μL DNA template
Oxa-24-like	GGTTAGTTGGCCCCCTTAAA AGTTGAGCGAAAAGGGGATT	246		
Oxa-51-like	TAATGCTTTGATCGGCCTTG TGGATTGCACTTCATCTTGG	353		
Oxa-58-like	AAGTATTGGGGCTTGTGCTG CCCCTCTGCGCTCTACATAC	599		

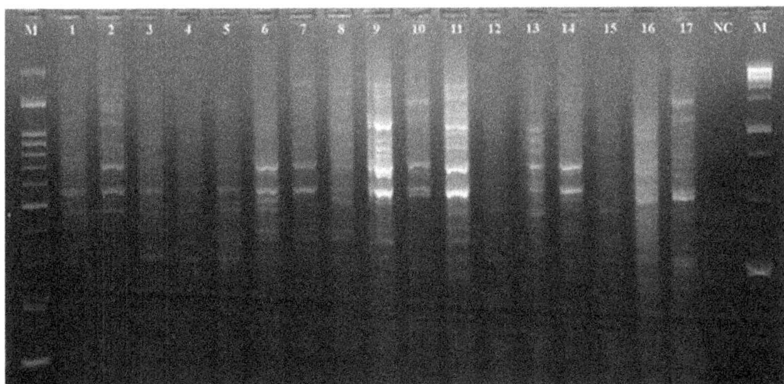

Fig. 1 Electrophoretic patterns of the ERIC types of *A. baumannii* strains No 1–17 isolated from raw meat samples, NC=Negative control, M = DNA Ladder 100 bp, 1Kb

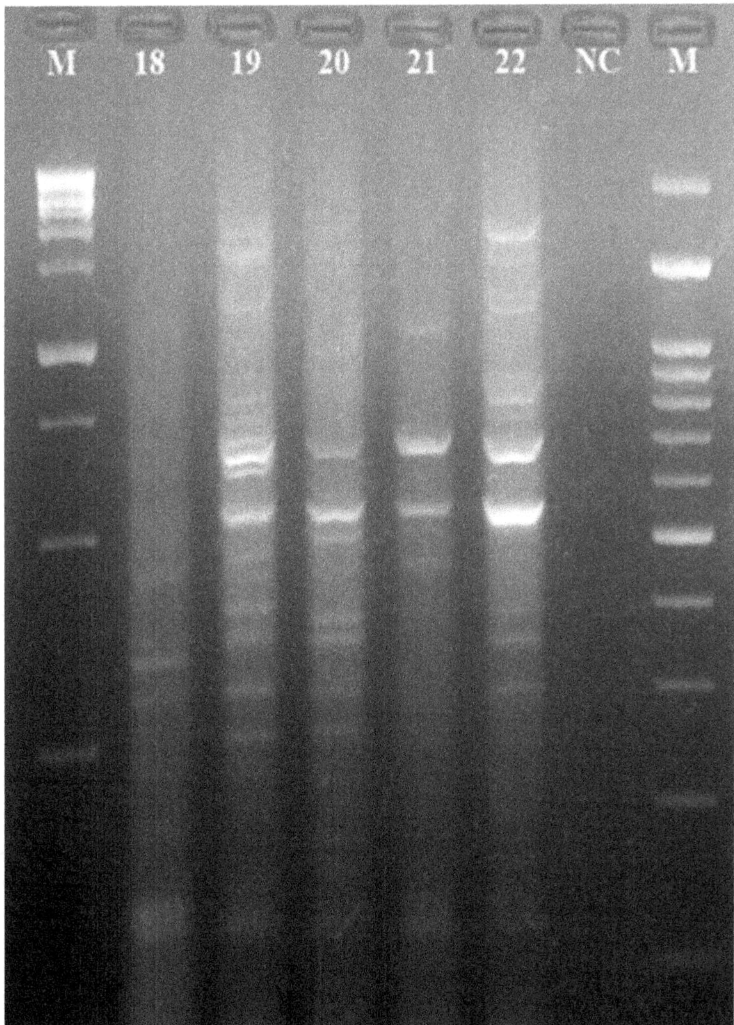

Fig. 2 Electrophoretic patterns of the ERIC types of *A. baumannii* strains No 18–22 isolated from raw meat samples, NC=Negative control, M = DNA Ladder 100 bp, 1Kb

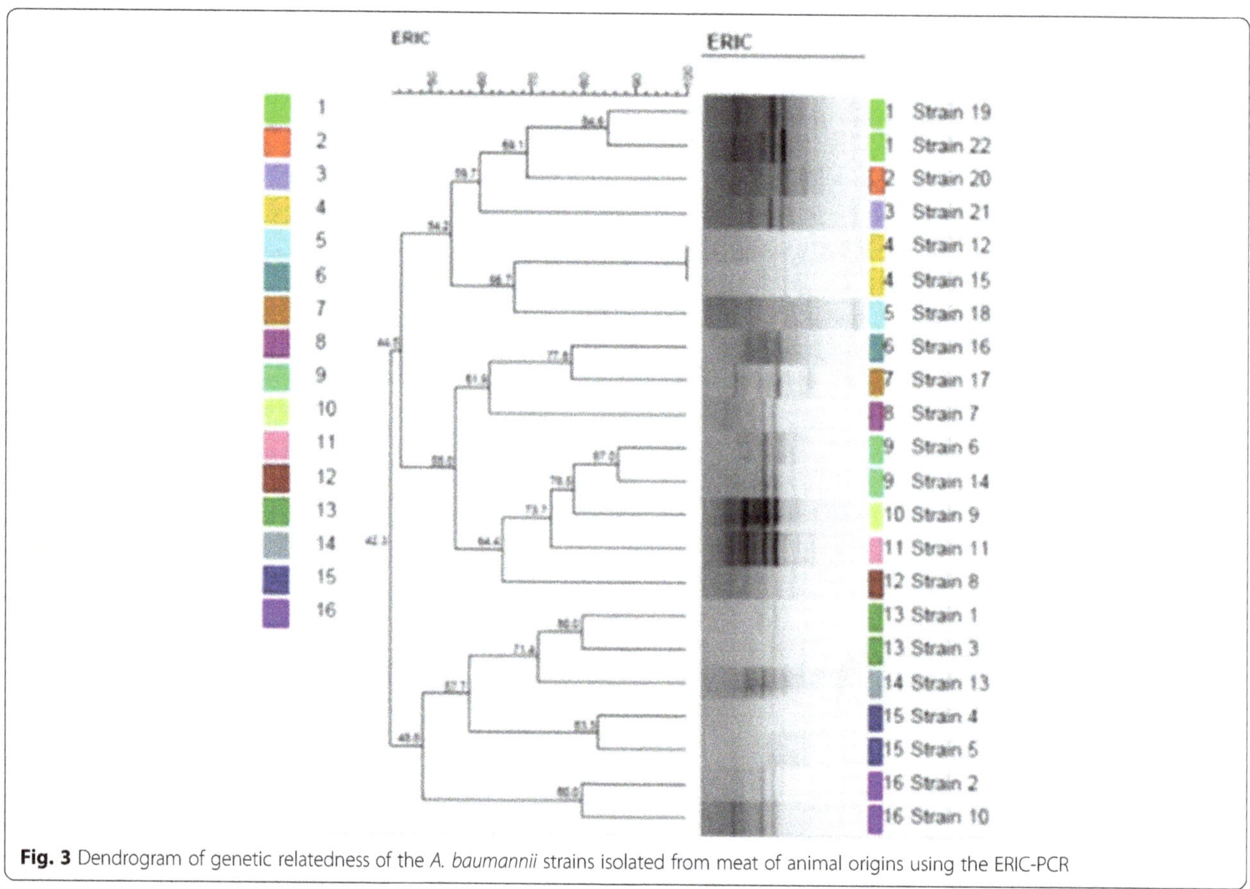

Fig. 3 Dendrogram of genetic relatedness of the *A. baumannii* strains isolated from meat of animal origins using the ERIC-PCR

have mainly been done only on the prevalence rate of *A. baumannii* and in some cases, on antibiotic susceptibility patterns. Reversely, to the best of our knowledge, the study presented here is the first report of the molecular typing, on the distribution of virulence factors and genotypic evaluation of antibiotic resistance of the *A. baumannii* strains isolated from different animal origins. A total of 22 strains of *A. baumannii* were assessed and 16 different genetic cluster were detected. Meat-derived *A. baumannii* strains may originate in the slaughterhouses, butchers and shopping centers especially due to the manipulation of the meat samples.

A. baumannii has previously been recognized as an animal colonizer with diverse distributions in different countries including in Scotland, 1.20% [22] and Senegal, 5.10% [24]. Rafei et al. (2015) [25] reported the high prevalence of *A. baumannii* strains in food samples with animal origins including raw meat, raw milk, and dairy products. The *A. baumannii* strains of the present research were frequently resistant to clinically relevant antibiotics. However, a few isolates displayed low levels of resistance against imipenem, azithromycin, meropenem, rifampin, levofloxacin, ceftazidime and tobramycin. This latter is still among the drugs of choice for the treatment of *A. baumannii* infections in humans and animals in Iran.

A. baumannii strains of the same molecular cluster (ERIC-type) had the same profile of the antibiotic resistance pattern. We also found that all of *A. baumannii* strains originated from chicken meat samples were susceptible to azithromycin and rifampin and resistant against tetracycline. These findings have been supported by several studies conducted on Lebanon [25], Switzerland [26], and France [27].

We found that molecular similarities of 19 and 22, 12 and 15, 6 and 14, 1 and 3, 4 and 5 and finally 2 and 10 *A. baumannii* strains were 84.60%, 100%, 87%, 80%, 83.30% and 80% with each other, respectively. All the other *A. baumannii* strains were classified as differing ERIC types. *A. baumannii* strains recovered from the bovine, camel, turkey and ovine meat samples didn't show any similarity in their molecular typing and there were no similar antibiotic resistance patterns between them. Our findings showed that they also had similar phenotypic pattern of antibiotic resistance. One possible explanation for the similar molecular types of the *A. baumannii* strains recovered from different animal origins is their common source of infection. It may also be due to the close contact between bovine and chicken, bovine and turkey and between chicken and ovine species, facilitating transmission of the *A. baumannii* strains with same molecular type. Unfortunately,

Table 2 Profiles obtained by ERIC-PCR, virulence factors and antimicrobial resistance pattern in *A. baumannii* strains isolated from animal origins

ERIC types[a]	Numbers and source of strains	Antibiotic resistance phenotypes	Antibiotic resistance genes	®
I	19,22 (Chicken meat)	SXT25, TE30, F300	*aadA1, sul1, tetB, sim, oxa-58-like*	*cnf1, csgA, fimH*
II	20 (Chicken meat)	GM10, TE30, TMP5, CIP5, C30, F300	*sul1, tetA, tetB, dfrA1, qnr, cat1, vim*	*ibeA, sfa/focDE, afa/draBC*
III	21 (Chicken meat)	CL30, TE30, TMP5, E15	*tetB, dfrA1, qnr, cmlA, oxa-23-like*	*kpsMTII, PAI, ibeA, traT, afa/draBC, cnf2, csgA, fyuA, fimH*
IV	12,15 (Chicken meat)	S10, GM10, SXT25, TE30, TMP5	*aadA1, aac(3)-IV, sul1, blaSHV, tetA, dfrA1*	*kpsMTII, sfa/focDE, cnf1, iutA*
V	18 (Turkey meat)	TOB10, CL30, CAZ30, TE30, AZM15	*aac(3)-IV, blaSHV, CITM, tetA, tetB*	*cvaC, fimH*
VI	16 (Ovine meat)	GM10, AK30, SXT25, CL30, CAZ30, TE30, TMP5, CIP5, LEV5, MEM10, C30, F300, E15	*aadA1, aac(3)-IV, sul1, blaSHV, CITM, tetA, tetB, dfrA1, cat1, cmlA, sim, oxa-51-like, oxa-23-like*	*kpsMTII, ibeA, papC, papGII, papGIII, traT, afa/draBC, cnf1, cnf2, csgA, iutA, fimH*
VII	17 (Bovine meat)	S10, CAZ30, TE30, TMP5, IPM10, RA5	*aadA1, aac(3)-IV, CITM, dfrA1, imp*	*PAI, papC, papGIII, traT, afa/draBC, cnf1, cnf2, csgA, cvaA, iutA, fyuA, fimH*
VIII	7 (Bovine meat)	F300, RA5	*aadA1, CITM, tetA, tetB, dfrA1, cat1, imp, oxa-51-like, oxa-24-like*	*kpsMTII, PAI, papC, papGIII, traT, afa/draBC, cnf1, cnf2, csgA, iutA, fyuA, fimH*
IX	14 (Chicken meat) 6 (Bovine meat)	GM10, AK30, TOB10, CL30, TE30, CIP5, C30	*aac(3)-IV, sul1, blaSHV, tetA, tetB, dfrA1*	*papGII, papGIII, afa/draBC, cnf1, cnf2, cvaC, fyuA, fimH*
X	9 (Camel meat)	S10, AZM15	*aadA1, tetA*	*PAI, papC, papGII, sfa/focDE, afa/draBC, csgA, cvaC*
XI	11 (Camel meat)	GM10, TOB10, SXT25, TE30, C30, RA5	*aadA1, aac(3)-IV, sul1, tetA, tetB, cmlA*	*ibeA, papGII, sfa/focDE, traT, afa/draBC, cnf2, csgA, cvaC, fimH*
XII	8 (Chicken meat)	S10, AK30, CAZ30, TE30, LEV5, IPM10, C30	*sul1, CITM, tetA, tetB, qnr, cat1, cmlA, vim, oxa-51-like, oxa-23-like, oxa-24-like*	*PAI, ibeA, papGII, sfa/focDE, cnf2, iutA, fimH*
XIII	1,3 (Chicken meat)	SXT25, TE30, TMP5, CIP5, MEM10, E15	*aac(3)-IV, sul1, CITM, tetA, tetB, dfrA1*	*cnf2, csgA, iutA, fimH*
XIV	13 (Turkey meat)	TOB10, TE30, TMP5, CIP5, LEV5, E15	*aadA1, tetA, tetB, dfrA1, oxa-51-like, oxa-24-like*	*ibeA, papC, sfa/focDE, fimH*
XV	5 (Turkey meat) 4 (Bovine meat)	GM10, TOB10, SXT25, TE30, TEP5, E15	*aac(3)-IV, sul1, tetA, tetB*	*afa/draBC, cnf1, cnf2, csgA, cvaC, fimH*
XVI	2 (Camel meat) 10 (Ovine meat)	S10, GM10, TE30, TMP5	*aac(3)-IV, tetA, dfrA1, oxa-58-like*	*sfa/focDE, afa/draBC, cnf1, csgA, cvaC, iutA, fyuA, fimH*

[a]In this table: S10 = Streptomycin, GM10 = Gentamicin, AK30 = Amikacin, TOB10 = Tobramycin, SXT25 = Trimethoprim/sulphamethoxazole, CL30 = Cephalothin, CAZ30 = Ceftazidime, TE30 = Tetracycline, TMP5 = Trimethoprim, CIP5 = Ciprofloxacin, LEV5 = Levofloxacin, IPM10 = Imipenem, MEM10 = Meropenem, C30 = Chloramphenicol, F300 = Nitrofurantoin, AZM15 = Azithromycin, RA5 = Rifampin, E15 = Erythromycin

Iranian ranchers frequently maintain and breed different species of animals and especially bovine, ovine and caprine species in contact to each other. This may cause easy transmission of the *A. baumannii* strains between different species. The high genetic diversity of strains isolated from meat samples has also previously been reported by Lupo et al. (2014) [26] and Carvalheira et al. (2017) [28]. Recent research [21] revealed the similar antibiotic resistance pattern of the *A. baumannii* strains isolated from different types of raw meat samples. They showed that the prevalence of resistance against trimethoprim-sulfamethoxazole, tetracycline, amikacin, tobramycin, ampicillin-sulbactam, meropenem and imipenem were 23.20%, 23.20%, 14.30%, 12.50%, 12.50%, 8.30% and1.20%, respectively which was different to our findings. The prevalence of antibiotic resistant bacteria in meat samples has been attributed, at least partially, to the extensive use of antimicrobials for treatment, prevention and control of diseases and finally for growth stimulate in food-producing animals, since this enhances the antimicrobial selective pressure for strains present. Otherwise, using antibiotics for growth stimulation is allowed in Iran. Low prevalence rate of resistance against carbapenems is due to the fact that these antibiotics are not allowed to treat food-producing animals.

Phenotypic characterization of antibiotic resistance was also confirmed by genotyping analysis of antibiotic resistance. We identified the genes for resistances to aminoglycosides (*aadA1* and *aac(3)-IV*), beta-lactams (bla_{SHV} and bla_{CTM}), chloramphenicol (*cat1* and *cmlA*), tetracyclines (*tetA* and *tetB*), sulfonamides (*sul1* and *dfrA1*), carbenicilins (*imp, sim* and *vim*) and to fluoroquinolones (*qnr*). Furthermore, *A. baumannii* strains harbored their own specific antibiotic resistance genes (Table 2). This part of our study was in agreement with previous researches [21, 29]. Additionally, we found that *A. baumannii* strains of the same molecular cluster (ERIC-type) had the same profile of the antibiotic resistance genes., as follows: strains no 1 and 3 of the same ERIC-type (type XIII) were positive for *CITM,dfrA1, tetA, tetB, aac(3)-IV* and *sul1* which showed their same genetic pattern of antibiotic resistance. Strains no 12 and 15 of the same ERIC-type (type IV) were positive for *tetA, aadA1, aac(3)-IV, blaSHV, dfrA1* and *sul1*. Strains no 19 and 22 of the same ERIC-type (type I) were positive for *tetB, aadA1, sim, oxa-58-like* and *sul1*. Despite of the different animal origin of the *A. baumannii* strains no 6 and 14 of the same ERIC-type (type IX), were positive for *tetA, tetB, aac(3)-IV, sul1, dfrA1* and *blaSHV* antibiotic resistance genes. Additionally, *A. baumannii* strains no 4 and 5 of the same ERIC-type (type XV) had different origins but they harbored *tetA, tetB, sul1* and *aac(3)-IV* antibiotic resistance genes. Finally, *A. baumannii* strains no 2 and 10 of the same ERIC-type (type XVI) were positive for *tetA, aac(3)-IV, dfrA1* and *oxa-58-like* antibiotic resistance. *A. baumannii* strains of other ERIC types had unique pattern of antibiotic resistance.

Virulence of *A. baumannii* is dependent on several other attributes (i.e. “slime”, LPS production and etc.) beside the selected virulence genes listed here [30, 31].

Another notable finding is the high prevalence of certain virulence factors in the *A. baumannii* strains isolated from meat of different animals. The most commonly detected virulence genes amongst these *A. baumannii* strains were *fimH, afa/draBC, csgA, cnf1, cnf2* and *iutA*. Prevalence of non-adhesive virulence factors including *traT* (serum resistance), *cvaC* (colicin V), *ibeA* (invasion), *fyuA* (yersiniabactin) and *PAI* (indicator gene) were low. This finding is in agreement with those of previous researches [30, 31]. Non-adhesive virulence factors play an important role in bacterial survival in special conditions such as in human blood and exposure to serum and poor iron environments contributing to the pathogenesis of extra instestinal diseases. However, presence of these non-adhesive virulence factors may not be essential for pathogenicity of food-borne enteric diseases. The gene *iutA* (aerobactin) has a high prevalence (50.00%) in our strains. Darvishi (2016) [32] reported that the prevalence of *cnf1, csgA, cvaC* and *iutA* virulence factors amongst the *A. baumannii* strains isolated from hospitalized patients were 50%, 70%, 10% and 25%, respectively. Daryanavard and Safaei (2015) [33] reported that the total prevalence of *csga, cnf1, cvaC* and *iutA* virulence genes among the samples of UTIs were 55%, 40%, 10% and 30%, respectively which was similar to our findings. Momtaz et al. (2015) [13] reported that the prevalence of *csga, cnf1, cvaC* and *iutA* virulence genes among the *A. baumannii* strains of clinical infections in Iran were 12.39%, 35.53%, 21.48% and 19%, respectively which was lower than our results.

We also found that the *A. baumannii* strains of the same molecular cluster (ERIC-type) had the same virulence factors. Despite of the different origin of the *A. baumannii* strains no 6 and 14 of the same ERIC-type (type IX), were both positive for *fimH, fyuA, cvaC, cnf1, cnf2, papGII, papGIII,* and *afa/draBC* virulence factors. Furthermore, *A. baumannii* strains no 4 and 5 of the same ERIC-type (molecular type XV) had different origins but they both harbored *fimH, cvaC, csgA, cnf1, afa/draBC* and *cnf2* virulence factors. Finally, *A. baumannii* strains no 2 and 10 of the same ERIC-type (type XVI) were positive for *fimH, fyuA, csgA, afa/draBC, cvaC, iutA, cnf1* and *sfa/focDE* virulence factors. These high similarities in the pattern of virulence factors of the *A. baumannii* strains of same ERIC types recovered from different origins showed that genetic cluster of bacterial strains is closely related to their virulence determinants.

A. baumannii strains isolated from the chicken meat samples had similar molecular type. *A. baumannii* strains isolated from other meat samples did not fall into common molecular types. Two *A. baumannii* strains of bovine origins had similar molecular type with turkey and chicken. A camel and ovine *A. baumannii* strains had also similar molecular type.

Conclusions

In conclusion, we studied the phenotypic and genotypic patterns of antibiotic resistance of the *A. baumannii* strains isolated from meat samples of different animals. High prevalence of resistance against tetracycline, trimethoprim, co-trimoxazole and gentamicin antibiotics and high distribution of *tetA*, *tetB*, *dfrA1*, *aac(3)-IV*, *sul1* and *aadA1* antibiotic resistance genes was established. Besides, *fimH*, *afa/draBC*, *csgA*, *cnf1*, *cnf2* and *iutA* were the most commonly detected virulence factors amongst the *A. baumannii* strains of our study. Twenty-two *A. baumannii* strains were classified into the 16 different genetic clusters according to the results of the ERIC-PCR. We also found that genetic cluster of the strains was closely related to their antibiotic resistance genes and virulence factors. Similarities in the genetic cluster of some strains was also recorded which may represent their similar sources of contamination.

Abbreviations

CLSI: Clinical and Laboratory Standards Institute; ERIC-PCR: Enterobacterial Repetitive Intergenic Consensus-Polymerase Chain Reaction

Acknowledgements

The authors would like to thank Dr. Abbas Farahani for his assistance in sample collection and PCR genetic alignments. This work was financially supported by the Islamic Azad University, Shahrekord Branch, Shahrekord, Iran.

Funding

Hassan Momtaz received Research grants for Research at Islamic Azad University, Shahrekord Branch with grant number 96/1046.

Authors' contributions

MT, HM and LS carried out the molecular genetic studies, participated in the primers sequence alignment and drafted the manuscript. PM and ET carried out the sampling and culture method. HM and MT participated in the design of the study, performed the statistical analysis and writing the manuscript. All authors read and approved the final manuscript.

Consent for publication

Not applicable.

Competing interests

The authors declare that they have no competing interests.

Author details

[1]Department of Microbiology, Shahrekord Branch, Islamic Azad University, P.O. Box: 166, Shahrekord, Iran. [2]Department of Microbiology, School of Medicine, Kermanshah University of Medical Sciences, Kermanshah, Iran. [3]Nosocomial Infection Research Center, Kermanshah University of Medical Sciences, Kermanshah, Iran. [4]Department of Microbiology, School of Medicine, Hamadan University of Medical Sciences, Hamadan, Iran.

References

1. Dehkordi FS, Parsaei P, Saberian S, Moshkelani S, Hajshafiei P, Hoseini SR, et al. Prevalence study of theileria annulata by comparison of four diagnostict techniques in Southwest Iran. Bulgarian J Vet Med. 2012;15(2): 123–30.
2. Momtaz H, Davood Rahimian M, Safarpoor Dehkordi F. Identification and characterization of Yersinia enterocolitica isolated from raw chicken meat based on molecular and biological techniques. J Appl Poult Res. 2013;22(1): 137–45.
3. Momtaz H, Dehkordi FS, Rahimi E, Asgarifar A, Momeni M. Virulence genes and antimicrobial resistance profiles of Staphylococcus aureus isolated from chicken meat in Isfahan province, Iran. J Appl Poult Res. 2013;22(4):913–21.
4. Ghorbani F, Gheisari E, Dehkordi FS. Genotyping of vacA alleles of helicobacter pylori strains recovered from some Iranian food items. Trop J Pharm Res. 2016;15(8):1631–6.
5. Dehkordi FS, Gandomi H, Basti AA, Misaghi A, Rahimi E. Phenotypic and genotypic characterization of antibiotic resistance of methicillin-resistant Staphylococcus aureus isolated from hospital food. Antimicrob Resist Infect Control. 2017;6(1):104.
6. Momtaz H, Safarpoor Dehkordi F, Taktaz T, Rezvani A, Yarali S. Shiga toxin-producing Escherichia coli isolated from bovine mastitic milk: serogroups, virulence factors, and antibiotic resistance properties. Sci World J. 2012;2012.
7. Rahimi E, Sepehri S, Dehkordi FS, Shaygan S, Momtaz H. Prevalence of Yersinia species in traditional and commercial dairy products in Isfahan Province, Iran. Jundishapur J Microbiol. 2014;7(4).
8. Madahi H, Rostami F, Rahimi E, Dehkordi FS. Prevalence of enterotoxigenic Staphylococcus aureus isolated from chicken nugget in Iran. Jundishapur J Microbiol 2014;7(8).
9. Ranjbar R, Masoudimanesh M, Dehkordi FS, Jonaidi-Jafari N, Rahimi E. Shiga (Vero)-toxin producing Escherichia coli isolated from the hospital foods; virulence factors, o-serogroups and antimicrobial resistance properties. Antimicrob Resist Infect Control. 2017;6(1):4.
10. Engür D, Çetinkaya Çakmak B, Kaynak Türkmen M, Telli M, Eyigör M, Güzünler M. A milk pump as a source for spreading Acinetobacter baumannii in a neonatal intensive care unit. Breastfeeding Med. 2014;9(10): 551–4.
11. Gurung M, Nam HM, Tamang MD, Chae MH, Jang GC, Jung SC, et al. Prevalence and antimicrobial susceptibility of Acinetobacter from raw bulk tank milk in Korea. J Dairy Sci. 2013;96(4):1997–2002.
12. Eijkelkamp BA, Stroeher UH, Hassan KA, Paulsen IT, Brown MH. Comparative analysis of surface-exposed virulence factors of Acinetobacter baumannii. BMC Gen. 2014;15(1):1020.
13. Momtaz H, Seifati SM, Tavakol M. Determining the prevalence and detection of the most prevalent virulence genes in Acinetobacter baumannii isolated from hospital infections. Int J Med Lab. 2015;2(2):87–97.
14. Asadollahi P, Akbari M, Soroush S, Taherikalani M, Asadollahi K, Sayehmiri K, et al. Antimicrobial resistance patterns and their encoding genes among Acinetobacter baumannii strains isolated from burned patients. Burns. 2012; 38(8):1198–203.
15. Pourhajibagher M, Hashemi FB, Pourakbari B, Aziemzadeh M, Bahador A. Antimicrobial resistance of Acinetobacter baumannii to imipenem in Iran: a systematic review and meta-analysis. Open Microbiol J. 2016;10:32.
16. Wang H, Wang J, Yu P, Ge P, Jiang Y, Xu R, et al. Identification of antibiotic resistance genes in the multidrug-resistant Acinetobacter baumannii strain, MDR-SHH02, using whole-genome sequencing. Int J Mol Med. 2017;39(2): 364–72.
17. Ying C, Li Y, Wang Y, Zheng B, Yang C. Investigation of the molecular epidemiology of Acinetobacter baumannii isolated from patients and environmental contamination. J Antibiot. 2015;68(9):562.
18. Cappuccino JG, Welsh CT. Microbiology: a laboratory manual. 11rd ed. London: Pearson Education; 2016.
19. Chiang MC, Kuo SC, Chen YC, Lee YT, Chen TL, Fung CP. Polymerase chain reaction assay for the detection of Acinetobacter baumannii in endotracheal aspirates from patients in the intensive care unit. J Microbiol, Immunol Infect. 2011;44(2):106–10.

20. CLSI. Performance standards for antimicrobial susceptibility testing; twenty-fifth informational supplement. CLSI document M100-S25. Wayne: Clinical and Laboratory Standards Institute; 2017.
21. Kiani S, Momtaz H, Serajian AA, Tajbakhsh E. Detection of integrons in Acinetobacter baumannii strains isolated from the nosocomial infections of Ahvaz city and their relation with the resistance pattern. Int J Med Lab. 2016;3(1):50–63.
22. Hamouda A, Findlay J, Al Hassan L, Amyes SG. Epidemiology of Acinetobacter baumannii of animal origin. Int J Antimicrob Agents. 2011; 38(4):314–8.
23. Zordan S, Prenger-Berninghoff E, Weiss R, van der Reijden T, van den Broek P, Baljer G, et al. Multidrug-resistant Acinetobacter baumannii in veterinary clinics, Germany. Emerg Infect Dis. 2011;17(9):1751.
24. Kempf M, Rolain JM, Diatta G, Azza S, Samb B, Mediannikov O, et al. Carbapenem resistance and Acinetobacter baumannii in Senegal: the paradigm of a common phenomenon in natural reservoirs. PLoS One. 2012; 7(6):e39495.
25. Rafei R, Hamze M, Pailhoriès H, Eveillard M, Marsollier L, Joly-Guillou ML, et al. Extra-human epidemiology of Acinetobacter baumannii in Lebanon. Appl Environ Microbiol 2015:AEM-03824.
26. Lupo A, Vogt D, Seiffert SN, Endimiani A, Perreten V. Antibiotic resistance and phylogenetic characterization of Acinetobacter baumannii strains isolated from commercial raw meat in Switzerland. J Food Protect. 2014; 77(11):1976–81.
27. Hauck Y, Soler C, Jault P, Mérens A, Gérome P, Mac Nab C, et al. Diversity of Acinetobacter baumannii in four French military hospitals, as assessed by multiple locus variable number of tandem repeats analysis. PLoS One. 2012; 7(9):e44597.
28. Carvalheira A, Casquete R, Silva J, Teixeira P. Prevalence and antimicrobial susceptibility of Acinetobacter spp. isolated from meat. Int J Food Microbiol. 2017;243:58–63.
29. Farahani Kheltabadi R, Moniri R, Shajari GR, Shirazi N, Hossein M, Musavi SG, et al. Antimicrobial susceptibility patterns and the distribution of resistance genes among Acinetobacter species isolated from patients in shahid Beheshti hospital, Kashan. KAUMS J (FEYZ). 2009;12(4):61–7.
30. Farahami A, Khodarahmi R. Frequency of adhesive virulence factors in Carbapenemase-producing Acinetobacter baumannii isolated from clinical samples. Asian J Biol Sci. 2014;7(4):158–64.
31. Mohajeri P, Sharbati S, Farahani A, Rezaei Z. Evaluate the frequency distribution of nonadhesive virulence factors in carbapenemase-producing Acinetobacter baumannii isolated from clinical samples in Kermanshah. J Nat Sci Biol Med. 2016;7(1):58.
32. Darvishi M. Virulence factors profile and antimicrobial resistance of Acinetobacter baumannii strains isolated from various infections recovered from immunosuppressive patients. Biomed Pharmacol J. 2016;9(3):1057–62.
33. Daryanavard R, Safaei HR. Virulence genes and antimicrobial resistance properties of Acinetobacter baumannii isolated from pediatrics suffered from UTIs. Int J Adv Res Biol Sci. 2015;2(11):272–9.
34. Randall LP, Cooles SW, Osborn MK, Piddock LJ, Woodward MJ. Antibiotic resistance genes, integrons and multiple antibiotic resistance in thirty-five serotypes of Salmonella enterica isolated from humans and animals in the UK. J Antimicrob Chemother. 2004;53(2):208–16.
35. Toro CS, Farfán M, Contreras I, Flores O, Navarro N, Mora GC, et al. Genetic analysis of antibiotic-resistance determinants in multidrug-resistant Shigella strains isolated from Chilean children. Epidemiol Infect. 2005;133(1):81–6.
36. Van TT, Chin J, Chapman T, Tran LT, Coloe PJ. Safety of raw meat and shellfish in Vietnam: an analysis of Escherichia coli isolations for antibiotic resistance and virulence genes. Int J Food Microbiol. 2008;124(3):217–23.
37. Woodford N, Ellington MJ, Coelho JM, Turton JF, Ward ME, Brown S, et al. Multiplex PCR for genes encoding prevalent OXA carbapenemases in Acinetobacter spp. Int J Antimicrob Agents. 2006;27(4):351–3.
38. Mammeri H, Van De Loo M, Poirel L, Martinez-Martinez L, Nordmann P. Emergence of plasmid-mediated quinolone resistance in Escherichia coli in Europe. Antimicrob Agents Chemother. 2005;49(1):71–6.
39. Mendes RE, Kiyota KA, Monteiro J, Castanheira M, Andrade SS, Gales AC, et al. Rapid detection and identification of metallo-β-lactamase-encoding genes by multiplex real-time PCR assay and melt curve analysis. J Clin Microbiol. 2007;45(2):544–7.
40. Marklund BL, Tennent JM, Garcia E, Hamers A, Baga M, Lindberg F, et al. Horizontal gene transfer of the Escherichia coli pap and prs pili operons as a mechanism for the development of tissue-specific adhesive properties. Mol Microbiol. 1992;6(16):2225–42.
41. Le Bouguenec C, Archambaud M, Labigne A. Rapid and specific detection of the pap, afa, and sfa adhesin-encoding operons in uropathogenic Escherichia coli strains by polymerase chain reaction. J Clin Microbiol 1992; 30(5):1189–1193.
42. Johnson JR, Brown JJ, Carlino UB, Russo TA. Colonization with and acquisition of uropathogenic Escherichia coli as revealed by polymerase chain reaction-based detection. J Infect Dis. 1998;177(4):1120–4.
43. Johnson JR, Stell AL. Extended virulence genotypes of Escherichia coli strains from patients with urosepsis in relation to phylogeny and host compromise. J Infect Dis. 2000;181(1):261–72.
44. Huang SH, Wass C, Fu QI, Prasadarao NV, Stins M, Kim KS. Escherichia coli invasion of brain microvascular endothelial cells in vitro and in vivo: molecular cloning and characterization of invasion gene ibe10. Infect Immun. 1995;63(11):4470–5.
45. Yamamoto S, Terai A, Yuri K, Kurazono H, Takeda Y, Yoshida O. Detection of urovirulence factors in Escherichia coli by multiplex polymerase chain reaction. FEMS Immunol Med Microbiol. 1995;12(2):85–90.
46. Schubert S, Rakin A, Karch H, Carniel E, Heesemann J. Prevalence of the "high-Pathogenicity Island" of Yersinia species among Escherichia coliStrains that are pathogenic to humans. Infect Immun. 1998;66(2):480–5.

6

A prospective surveillance study for multidrug-resistant bacteria colonization in hospitalized patients at a Thai University Hospital

Pinyo Rattanaumpawan[1,2], Chatiros Choorat[1,2], Kanchanaporn Takonkitsakul[2], Teerawit Tangkoskul[1,2], Chakrapong Seenama[1,2] and Visanu Thamlikitkul[1,2*]

Abstract

Background: Colonization with multidrug-resistant (MDR) bacteria is a major risk factor for developing subsequent MDR infections.

Methods: We performed a prospective surveillance study in hospitalized patients at Siriraj Hospital. Nasal cavity, throat, inguinal area and rectal swabs were obtained within the first 48-h after admission, on day-5 after hospitalization and then every 7 days until discharge. Target bacteria included extended-spectrum beta-lactamase-producing Enterobacteriaceae (ESBL), carbapenem-resistant-*P.aeruginosa* (CR-PA), carbapenem-resistant-*A.baumannii* (CR-AB) and methicillin-resistant *S.aureus* (MRSA).

Results: From January 2013–December 2014, 487 patients were enrolled. The baseline prevalence of colonization by ESBL, CR-PA, CR-AB and MRSA at any site was 52.2%, 6.8%, 4.7% and 7.2%, respectively. After 3-week of hospitalization, the prevalence of colonization by ESBL, CR-PA, CR-AB and MRSA increased to 71.7%, 47.2%, 18.9% and 18.9%, respectively. Multivariable analysis revealed that diabetes mellitus and recent cephalosporin exposure were the independent risk factors for baseline colonization by ESBL. The independent risk factors for CR-AB and/or CR-PA colonization were cerebrovascular diseases, previous hospitalization, transfer from another hospital/a LTCF and previous nasogastric tube use, whereas those for MRSA colonization were previous fluoroquinolone exposure and previous nasogastric tube use.

Conclusions: The baseline prevalence of colonization by ESBL was relatively high, whereas the baseline prevalence of colonization by CR-PA, CR-AB and MRSA was comparable to previous studies. There was an increasing trend in MDR bacteria colonization after hospitalization.

Background

Antimicrobial resistance (AMR) is considered a major health threat. The consequences of multidrug-resistant (MDR) bacterial infections including high morbidity and mortality and economic loss have been well documented in many studies [1–3]. Colonization by MDR bacteria is considered a potential source of cross-transmission to other patients [4–6]. Moreover, colonization by MDR bacteria was found to be an independent risk factor for developing subsequent MDR bacterial infections in previous studies [5, 7].

The World Health Organization recognized AMR as a global health problem and recommended that Member States should strengthen the knowledge and evidence base through AMR surveillance and research in the global action plan on AMR [8]. Lack of AMR surveillance data contributes to underestimating the magnitude of AMR problem and halting the implementation of AMR control measures.

* Correspondence: visanu.tha@mahidol.ac.th
[1]Division of Infectious Diseases and Tropical Medicine, Bangkok, Thailand
[2]Department of Medicine, Faculty of Medicine Siriraj Hospital, Mahidol University, 2 Wang Lang Rd., Bangkoknoi, Bangkok 10700, Thailand

A surveillance study reported that the prevalence of rectal colonization by ESBL-producing Enterobacteriaceae among newly-hospitalized general medical patients in an Israel teaching hospital was only 8% [9]. After two weeks of hospitalization, the prevalence of colonization increased to 21% [9]. Surprisingly, the prevalence of rectal colonization by extended-spectrum beta-lactamase-producing Enterobacteriaceae in Thai community volunteers was remarkably high (32.0–66.5%) [10, 11].

Similar to ESBL-producing Enterobacteriaceae, the prevalence of *Pseudomonas aeruginosa* (PA) colonization varied across geographic locations. In a United States study, the prevalence of PA rectal colonization among intensive care unit (ICU) patients was 11.6% [12]. However, a recent Spanish study found that the prevalence of rectal colonization by non-drug resistant PA and extensive drug resistant PA in ICU patients was 27.0% and 4.0%, respectively [13].

Based on the data from a recent surveillance study performed in a medical ICU in Korea, active surveillance detected carbapenem-resistant-*Acinetobacter baumannii* (CR-AB) in 15.0% of patients, and approximately one-third of them later developed CR-AB infections [14]. Similar to the Korean study, the prevalence of CR-AB colonization in ICU patients at a US tertiary hospital was 13.5% [15].

Nasal colonization by methicillin-resistant *Staphylococcus aureus* (MRSA) has been widely investigated. The prevalence of MRSA nasal colonization varied from 4.1% in the US national surveillance in-patient data [16] to 9.0% among newly-hospitalized patients in an Israel teaching hospital [9]. Data on MRSA colonization at other sites in the body in addition to the nasal cavity is very limited.

Based on previous scientific evidence, the prevalence of MDR bacteria colonization varied across specific types of MDR bacteria, geographic regions and clinical settings [community, hospital or long-term care facility (LTCF)]. Although many studies have already investigated the prevalence of MDR bacteria colonization, most studies focused only on rectal or stool colonization by MDR gram-negative bacteria and nasal colonization by MRSA. Furthermore, these studies were not longitudinal studies that monitored changes in the prevalence of AMR bacteria colonization after hospitalization.

Given these considerations, we performed a prospective surveillance study for MDR bacteria colonization in hospitalized patients on admission and during hospitalization. The primary objective was to determine the prevalence of colonization by MDR bacteria in newly-hospitalized patients and the prevalence of new acquisition of MDR bacteria during hospitalization. The secondary objective was to identify risk factors for colonization by MDR bacteria and for new acquisition of MDR bacteria. Results from this study helped us determine the magnitude of AMR problem and the natural history of AMR colonization in hospitalized patients. Furthermore, the study could identify the patients at risk for MDR bacteria colonization who may subsequently develop infections due to these bacteria.

Methods

Study design and setting

During a 2-year study period (1 January 2013–31 December 2014), we performed a prospective surveillance study in eight general medical wards at Siriraj Hospital, which is a 2200-bed university hospital located in Bangkok, Thailand. The study protocol was approved by the Siriraj Institutional Review Board.

Study population

The eligible subjects were all adults aged ≥18 years who had been hospitalized in general medical wards for less than 24 h. Subjects who were expected to be discharged or dead within 48 h or those with any contraindications for obtaining clinical specimens (i.e. a neutropenic patient (digital rectal examination or rectal swab culture was contraindicated), or having local infection at the site of surveillance culture) were excluded. Only subjects who agreed to participate and signed informed consent forms were enrolled.

Microbiological surveillance of AMR bacteria

Clinical specimens from four sites including the nasal cavity, throat, skin at the inguinal area and rectum or stool were obtained from each patient within 48 h after hospitalization (time-1). Clinical specimens were subsequently obtained on day 5 ± 1 of hospitalization (time-2) and then every 7 days until the patient left the hospital (time-3, time-4 and so on). All clinical specimens were transferred in Stuart transport medium to the Laboratory of Division of Infectious Diseases, Department of Medicine.

The targeted MDR bacteria were ESBL-producing Enterobacteriaceae, CR-PA, CR-AB and MRSA. MacConkey agar supplemented with ceftriaxone for the isolation of MDR gram-negative bacteria and Mannitol Salt agar for the isolation of staphylococci were used for inoculating the clinical specimens collected from all sites.

Species identification and antimicrobial susceptibility tests were performed according to the performance standards for antimicrobial susceptibility testing recommended by the Clinical and Laboratory Standards Institute 2013 [17]. Species identification was performed using conventional biochemical tests. Identification of ESBL-producing bacteria was confirmed using the combination disc method. MRSA strains were determined using cefoxitin disc (30 mg) screening. Antimicrobial susceptibility testing was performed using the disc diffusion method.

Results of microbiology surveillance were directly reported to the study team and available (per request) for the service team (i.e. a responsible physician, an infectious disease consultant, etc.). However, there was no special infection control intervention for patients with colonization by target MDR-bacteria.

Data collection

Medical records for the enrolled patients were reviewed for demographics, co-morbidities and clinical course. Data on any hospitalization, medication used, intervention and catheter use in the preceding 90 days prior to hospitalization were also obtained. Previous hospitalization included any stay at observation or emergency rooms for periodic monitoring and/or short-term treatment for longer than 24 h within 3 months prior to the index hospitalization.

Statistical analysis

Categorical variables were summarized by frequency and proportion, whereas continuous variables were summarised by mean, median, standard deviation and range as appropriate. The prevalence of colonization by MDR bacteria was reported as percentage with a 95% confidence interval (95% CI). Wilcoxon-type test for trend analysis was performed to identify an increasing trend of colonization over time after hospitalization.

Multivariate logistic analysis was performed to identify the risk factors for colonization by MDR bacteria (at any site) and for new acquisition of MDR bacteria (at any site). A separate model was built for each MDR pathogen including 1) ESBL-producing Enterobacteriaceae; 2) CR-PA and/or CR-AB and 3) MRSA. Primary analysis was performed to compare cases with the specific MDR pathogens to controls without the given pathogen. Additionally, we performed a secondary analysis by comparing cases with the specific MDR pathogen to controls without any colonization.

Any associated variable with a p-value ≤ 0.20 was entered in a forward stepwise manner into the model. Any associated variables with a p-value < 0.20 was entered into the model. The likelihood ratio test was performed to confirm the model fit. For all calculations, a two-tailed p-value of < 0.05 was considered statistically significant. All calculations were performed using STATA version 14.0 (Stata Corp, College Station, TX).

Results

Baseline characteristics of patients

During the study period, 487 patients were enrolled in the study as shown in Fig. 1. The baseline characteristics of patients prior to hospitalization are shown in Table 1. Nearly half (45.4%) of the patients were male, with an average age of 61.7 ± 17.8 years. Previous hospitalization was documented in 43.3% of patients. Additionally, 11.0% and 1.2% of patients had been transferred from another

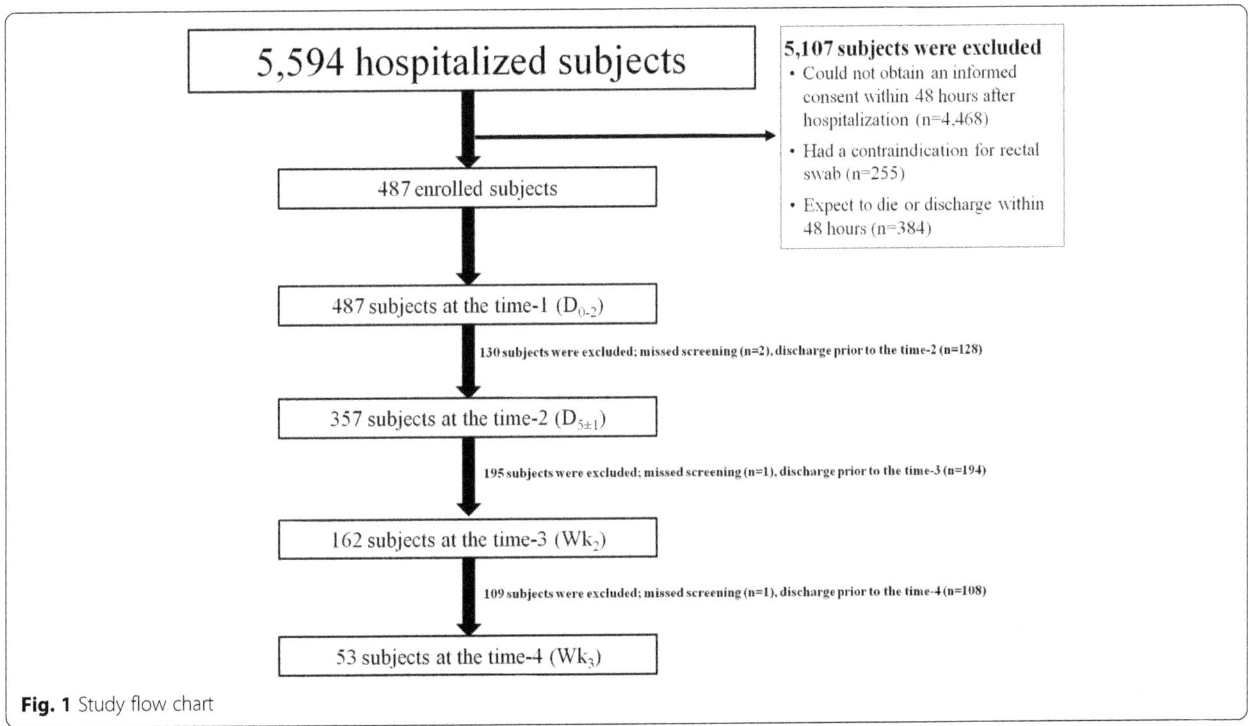

Fig. 1 Study flow chart

Table 1 Baseline characteristics of 487 patients

Baseline characteristics prior to hospitalization	n (%)
Mean age ± SD (years)	61.7 ± 17.8
Male gender	221 (45.4%)
Mean length of hospital stay, days (±SD)	14.5 ± 18.5
Median length of hospital stay, days (range)	10.0 (2.0–303.0)
Previous hospitalization	211 (43.3%)
Transfer status	
From another hospital	56 (11.5%)
From a long-term care facility	6 (1.2%)
Underlying diseases	
Any underlying disease	420 (86.2%)
Hypertension	290 (59.6%)
Diabetes mellitus	184 (37.8%)
Cardiovascular diseases	133 (27.3%)
Cerebrovascular diseases	97 (19.9%)
Chronic liver diseases	88 (18.0%)
Chronic renal diseases	64 (13.1%)
Chronic lung diseases	63 (12.9%)
Malignancy	87 (17.9%)
Solid malignancy	75 (15.4%)
Hematologic malignancy	12 (2.5%)
Hematologic diseases	47 (9.7%)
Prior organ transplantation	7 (1.4%)
Receipt of any immunosuppressive agent within 90 days	75 (15.4%)
HIV infection	16 (3.3%)
Previous antibiotic exposure within 90 days after hospitalization	
Any antibiotic	148 (30.4%)
Penicillins	19 (3.9%)
Cephalosporins	60 (12.3%)
Carbapenems	33 (6.8%)
Beta-lactam/beta-lactamase inhibitors	27 (5.5%)
Fluoroquinolones	46 (9.4%)
Macrolides	19 (3.9%)
Others	42 (8.6%)
Previous use of indwelling catheters within 90 days	
Urinary catheter	73 (15.0%)
Nasogastric tube	45 (9.2%)

hospital or a LTCF, respectively. Majority of patients (94.4%) had at least one underlying disease.

The most common underlying disease was hypertension (59.6%), followed by diabetes mellitus (DM) (37.8%) and cardiovascular disease (27.3%). One-third (30.4%) of patients had previously been exposed to at least one type of antibiotics within the past 3 months. Approximately 15% of patients had a long-term urinary catheter inserted prior to hospitalization. The mean length of stay (LOS) was 14.5 ± 18.5 days, whereas the median LOS was 10 (2–303) days.

Colonization by MDR bacteria in newly-hospitalized patients

The prevalence of colonization by MDR bacteria in newly-hospitalized patients stratified by MDR bacteria species and by colonization site is shown in Table 2. Of the 487 patients evaluated, only 197 were free of colonization (40.5%). The rest (59.5%) were colonized by at least one specific MDR pathogen.

More than half of the patients had ESBL-producing Enterobacteriaceae colonization in at least one body site, primarily in the rectum (47.6%) followed by the inguinal area (16.4%), throat (8.6%) and nasal cavity (2.7%). ESBL-producing *E. coli* (42.3%) were more prevalent than ESBL-producing *K. pneumoniae* (16.6%).

CR-PA was identified in only 4.7% of patients, primarily in the throat (3.7%). Baseline colonization by CR-AB was documented in 12.9% of patients, primarily in the inguinal area (6.6%) followed by the rectum (5.8%), throat (3.3%) and nasal cavity (2.7%).

MRSA was documented in 7.2% of patients, unlike MDR gram-negative bacteria, which primarily colonized in the nasal cavity (4.3%). The risk factors for baseline colonization by each MDR bacteria are reported in the next section.

Colonization by MDR bacteria during hospitalization

Given that some patients were discharged or dead before subsequent clinical specimens were obtained, the number of follow-up specimens decreased over time. Collection of the subsequent specimens was successfully completed in 357 patients (73.3%) at time-2, 162 patients (33.3%) at time-3 and 53 patients (10.9%) at time-4. Overall colonization and colonization by all species of MDR bacteria showed an increasing trend over time as shown in Fig. 2. However, this increasing trend did not reach statistical significance in the test for trend analysis (all p-values > 0.05). The details of colonization by MDR bacteria stratified by MDR bacteria species, colonization site and specimen collection time are shown in Table 3. Due to the small number of new MDR bacteria acquisitions, we did not further investigate the risk factors for new acquisitions of these bacteria.

Risk factors for colonization by ESBL-producing Enterobacteriaceae in hospitalized patients

The risk factors for baseline colonization by ESBL-producing Enterobacteriaceae in 254 patients compared with 233 patients without ESBL-producing Enterobacteriaceae colonization are shown in Table 4. The independent

Table 2 Prevalence of colonization of MDR bacteria in newly-hospitalized patients ($N = 487$) stratified by the specific MDR bacteria and by the specimen collection site

MDR bacteria	All sites, n (%)	Nasal cavity, n (%)	Throat, n (%)	Inguinal area, n (%)	Rectum, n (%)
ESBL-producing Enterobacteriaceae	254 (52.2%)	13 (2.7%)	42 (8.6%)	80 (16.4%)	232 (47.6%)
E. coli	206 (42.3%)	5 (1.0%)	14 (2.9%)	58 (11.9%)	189 (38.8%)
K. pneumoniae	81 (16.6%)	9 (1.8%)	31 (6.4%)	29 (6.0%)	60 (12.3%)
Other Enterobacteriaceae	8 (1.6%)	0	1 (0.2%)	3 (0.6%)	7 (1.4%)
A. baumannii					
Carbapenem-susceptible	88 (18.0%)	13 (2.7%)	43 (8.8%)	34 (7.0%)	32 (6.6%)
Carbapenem-resistant	63 (12.9%)	13 (2.7%)	16 (3.3%)	32 (6.6%)	28 (5.8%)
P. aeruginosa					
Carbapenem-susceptible	33 (6.8%)	10 (2.1%)	11 (2.3%)	18 (3.7%)	12 (2.5%)
Carbapenem-resistant	23 (4.7%)	9 (1.9%)	18 (3.7%)	2 (0.4%)	6 (1.2%)
Staphylococcus aureus					
Methicillin-susceptible	49 (10.0%)	29 (6.0%)	21 (4.3%)	8 (1.6%)	11 (2.3%)
Methicillin-resistant	35 (7.2%)	21 (4.3%)	17 (3.5%)	6 (1.2%)	12 (2.5%)

risk factors from the primary multivariate analysis [Odds Ratio (OR); 95% CI; *p-value*] included underlying DM [1.45;1.00–2.10; $p = 0.05$] and previous exposure to cephalosporin [2.00;1.13–3.54; $p = 0.02$] as shown in Table 7. Secondary analysis identified similar risk factors with a similar OR as shown in the Table 7.

Risk factors for colonization by CR-PA and/or CR-AB in hospitalized patients

Due to the small number of cases with baseline colonization by CR-AB and CR-PA, we combined data on colonization by these two MDR bacteria. A total of 49 patients (10.1%) had at least one clinical specimen that grew CR-PA and/or CR-AB at the baseline. The risk factors for baseline colonization by CR-PA and/or CR-AB in 49 patients compared with 438 patients without this colonization are shown in Table 5. The independent risk factors identified in the primary analysis [OR; 95% CI; *p-value*] included previous hospitalization [2.21;1.07–4.53; $p = 0.03$], transfer from another hospital [2.67;1.19–5.98; $p = 0.02$] or a LTCF [11.51;1.84–71.83; $p = 0.01$], underlying cerebrovascular diseases [2.90;1.37–6.16; $p = 0.005$] and previous nasogastric tube use [2.38;1.002–5.67; $p = 0.05$]. Secondary analysis identified only three independent risk factors, specifically previous hospitalization, underlying cerebrovascular disease and previous nasogastric tube use, with slightly higher ORs. The results for both primary and secondary analyses are shown in Table 7.

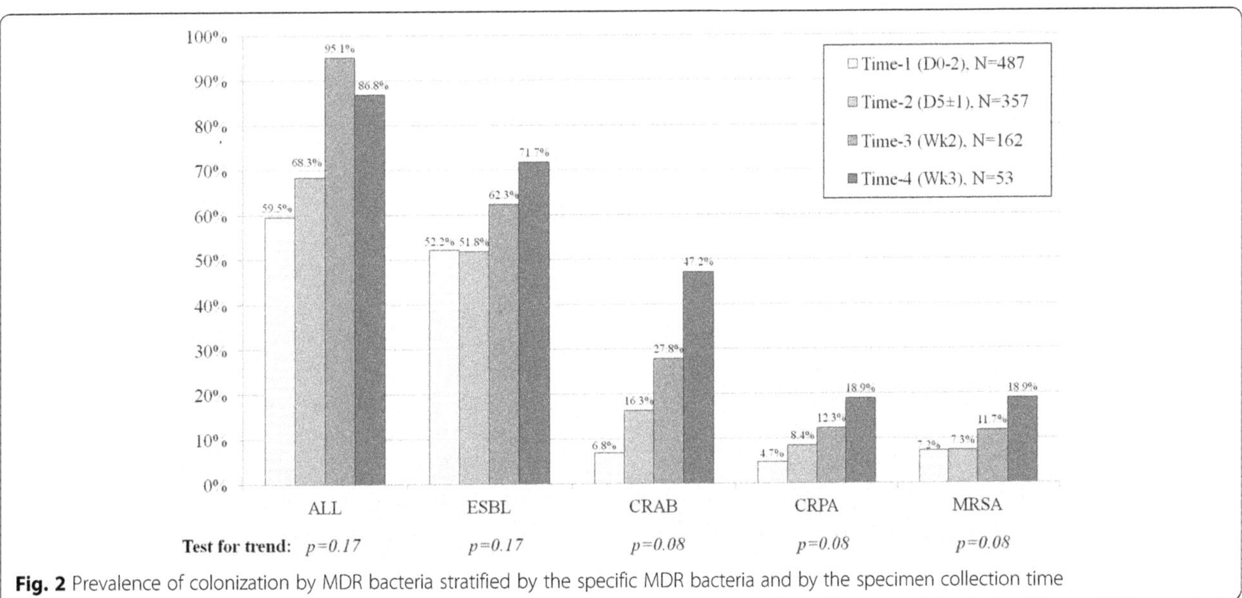

Fig. 2 Prevalence of colonization by MDR bacteria stratified by the specific MDR bacteria and by the specimen collection time

Table 3 Prevalence of colonization on admission and during hospitalization stratified by the specific MDR bacteria, the surveillance culture site and the time of specimen collection

Time	Any site, (%)	Nasal cavity, (%)	Throat, (%)	Inguinal area, (%)	Rectum, (%)
ESBL-producing Enterobacteriaceae					
Time-1 (*N* = 487)	52.2	2.7	9.8	17.5	50.4
Time-2 (*N* = 357)	51.8	3.4	15.1	17.5	46.2
Time-3 (*N* = 162)	62.3	8.3	25.0	21.9	46.2
Time-4 (*N* = 53)	71.7	12.0	28.6	27.1	53.8
ESBL-producing *E. coli*					
Time-1 (*N* = 487)	42.3	1.0	2.9	11.9	38.8
Time-2 (*N* = 357)	41.2	1.3	3.7	10.9	34.3
Time-3 (*N* = 162)	39.5	0.6	3.3	10.3	33.1
Time-4 (*N* = 53)	41.5	2.0	4.1	16.7	32.7
ESBL-producing *Klebsiella* spp.					
Time-1 (*N* = 487)	16.6	1.9	6.4	5.9	12.3
Time-2 (*N* = 357)	19.1	2.2	10.7	5.9	10.4
Time-3 (*N* = 162)	34.6	7.1	19.7	9.7	19.4
Time-4 (*N* = 53)	45.3	1.0	22.5	19.4	19.2
CR-AB					
Time-1 (*N* = 487)	6.8	2.1	2.3	3.7	2.5
Time-2 (*N* = 357)	16.3	4.7	6.7	10.4	8.6
Time-3 (*N* = 162)	27.8	8.3	13.2	15.5	10.0
Time-4 (*N* = 53)	47.2	26.0	24.5	22.9	19.2
CR-PA					
Time-1 (*N* = 487)	4.7	1.6	3.7	0.4	1.2
Time-2 (*N* = 357)	8.4	2.2	5.4	1.8	2.1
Time-3 (*N* = 162)	12.3	5.8	7.2	3.2	3.8
Time-4 (*N* = 53)	18.9	10.0	12.2	2.1	1.9
MRSA					
Time-1 (*N* = 487)	7.2	4.3	3.5	1.2	2.5
Time-2 (*N* = 357)	7.3	3.1	2.2	1.1	2.2
Time-3 (*N* = 162)	11.7	4.9	2.6	3.7	1.2
Time-4 (*N* = 53)	18.9	7.5	5.7	3.7	1.8

Abbreviations: ESBL Extended-Spectrum Beta-Lactamase, *CR-AB* Carbapenem-Resistant *Acinetobacter baumannii*, *CR-PA* Carbapenem-Resistant *Pseudomonas aeruginosa*, *MSSA* Methicillin-Susceptible *Staphylococcus aureus*, *MRSA* Methicillin-Resistant *Staphylococcus aureus*

Risk factors for colonization by MRSA in hospitalized patients

Of the 487 enrolled patients, 35 (7.2%) had at least one clinical specimen that grew MRSA at the baseline. Baseline characteristics for the 35 patients with MRSA colonization and 452 patients without MRSA colonization are shown in Table 6. Independent risk factors for baseline colonization by MRSA [OR; 95% CI; *p-value*] were previous fluoroquinolone exposure [2.76; 1.13–6.74; $p = 0.03$] and previous nasogastric tube use [6.60; 1.13–6.74; $p < 0.001$]. Stronger association between these two factors and baseline colonization by MRSA was documented in secondary analysis as shown in Table 7.

Discussion

The present study revealed a remarkably high prevalence of baseline colonization by ESBL-producing Enterobacteriaceae compared with the prevalence from the Israel study (52.2% vs 8%) [9]. However, our baseline prevalence for faecal colonization by ESBL-producing Enterobacteriaceae (47.6%) was comparable with the prevalence of ESBL colonization among Thai community volunteers (32.0–66.5%) [10, 11].

Two important characteristics, namely DM and previous cephalosporin use, were identified as the independent risk factors for baseline colonization by ESBL-producing Enterobacteriaceae in this study. These findings were

Table 4 Baseline characteristics prior to hospitalization for 254 patients (ESBL-producing Enterobacteriaceae) and 233 controls (no ESBL-producing Enterobacteriaceae)

Baseline characteristics	ESBL+ (*N* = 254)	ESBL- (*N* = 233)	*p*-value
Mean age ± SD (years)	61.4 ± 18.2	61.9 ± 17.4	0.76
Male gender	120 (47.2%)	101 (43.4%)	0.39
Previous hospitalization	115 (45.3%)	96 (41.2%)	0.37
Transfer status			
From another hospital	30 (11.8%)	26 (11.2%)	0.82
From a long-term care facility	4 (1.6%)	2 (0.9%)	0.47
Underlying diseases			
Any underlying disease	225 (88.6%)	195 (83.7%)	0.12
Hypertension	115 (61.0%)	135 (57.9%)	0.49
Diabetes mellitus	106 (41.7%)	78 (33.5%)	0.06
Cardiovascular disease	74 (29.1%)	59 (25.3%)	0.35
Cerebrovascular disease	56 (22.0%)	41 (17.6%)	0.22
Chronic liver disease	43 (16.9%)	45 (19.3%)	0.50
Chronic renal disease	37 (14.6%)	27 (11.6%)	0.33
Chronic lung disease	32 (12.6%)	41 (17.6%)	0.82
Malignancy	46 (18.1%)	41 (17.6%)	0.88
Solid malignancy	42 (16.5%)	33 (14.1%)	0.47
Hematologic malignancy	4 (1.6%)	8 (3.4%)	0.19
Hematologic diseases	26 (10.2%)	21 (9.0%)	0.65
Prior organ transplantation	2 (0.8%)	5 (2.2%)	0.21
Receipt of any immunosuppressive agent	33 (13.0%)	26 (11.2%)	0.54
HIV infection	10 (3.9%)	6 (2.6%)	0.40
Previous antibiotic exposure within 90 days after hospitalization			
Any antibiotic	84 (33.1%)	64 (27.5%)	0.18
Penicillins	12 (4.7%)	7 (3.0%)	0.33
Cephalosporins	40 (15.8%)	20 (8.6%)	0.02
Carbapenems	16 (6.3%)	17 (7.3%)	0.67
Beta-lactam/beta-lactamase inhibitors	10 (3.9%)	17 (7.3%)	0.11
Fluoroquinolones	26 (10.2%)	20 (8.6%)	0.53
Macrolides	11 (4.3%)	8 (3.4%)	0.61
Others	24 (9.5%)	18 (7.7%)	0.50
Previous use of indwelling catheters			
Urinary catheter	40 (15.8%)	33 (14.2%)	0.63
Nasogastric tube	26 (10.2%)	19 (8.2%)	0.43

previously documented in many studies [9, 10]. Underlying DM may be a proxy for recurrent infections, previous antibiotic use and previous hospitalization [10, 18, 19]. Previous exposure to cephalosporin would result in selective pressure against non-ESBL-producing pathogens to become resistant to cephalosporin, leading to colonization in the patients [20].

This study revealed the comparable prevalence of CR-PA colonization (4.7%) compared with the results from the Spanish ICU study (4.0%) [13]. Additionally, the prevalence of CR-AB colonization (12.9%) was similar to the findings from previous studies performed in ICU patients (13.5–15.0%) [14, 15]. Although our study included only hospitalized patients in general medical wards, these patients were sicker than those hospitalized in a general medical ward in developed countries due to resource limitations. These statements could be confirmed due to a very

Table 5 Baseline characteristics prior to hospitalization for 49 patients (with CR-AB and/or CR-PA) and 438 controls (without CR-AB and CR-PA)

Baseline characteristics	CR-AB and/or CR-PA ($n = 49$)	No CR-AB and CR-PA ($n = 438$)	p-value
Mean age ± SD (years)	66.7 ± 18	61.1 ± 17.8	0.04
Male gender	18 (36.7%)	203 (46.4%)	0.20
Previous hospitalization	32 (65.3%)	179 (40.9%)	0.001
Transfer status			
From other hospital	13 (26.5%)	43 (9.8%)	0.001
From a long-term care facility	4 (8.2%)	2 (0.5%)	< 0.001
Underlying diseases			
Any underlying disease	48 (98.0%)	372 (84.9%)	0.01
Hypertension	33 (67.4%)	257 (58.7%)	0.24
Diabetes mellitus	20 (40.8%)	164 (37.4%)	0.64
Cardiovascular disease	16 (32.7%)	117 (26.7%)	0.38
Cerebrovascular disease	23 (46.9%)	74 (16.9%)	< 0.001
Chronic liver disease	9 (18.4%)	79 (18.0%)	0.95
Chronic renal disease	8 (16.3%)	56 (12.8%)	0.49
Chronic lung disease	7 (14.3%)	56 (12.8%)	0.77
Malignancy	7 (14.3%)	80 (18.3%)	0.49
Solid malignancy	7 (14.3%)	68 (15.5%)	0.82
Hematologic malignancy	0	12 (2.7%)	0.24
Hematologic diseases	6 (12.2%)	41 (9.4%)	0.52
Prior organ transplantation	1 (2.0%)	6 (1.4%)	0.71
Receipt of any immunosuppressive agent	6 (12.2%)	- 53 (12.1%)	0.98
HIV infection	1 (2.0%)	15 (3.4%)	0.61
Previous antibiotic exposure within 90 days after hospitalization			
Any antibiotic	26 (53.1%)	122 (27.9%)	< 0.001
Penicillins	1 (2.0%)	18 (4.1%)	0.48
Cephalosporins	10 (20.4%)	50 (11.4%)	0.07
Carbapenems	9 (18.4%)	24 (5.5%)	0.001
Beta-lactam/beta-lactamase inhibitors	7 (14.3%)	20 (4.6%)	0.005
Fluoroquinolones	8 (16.3%)	38 (8.7%)	0.08
Macrolides	4 (8.2%)	15 (3.4%)	0.10
Others	8 (16.3%)	34 (7.8%)	0.04
Previous use of indwelling catheters			
Urinary catheter	19 (38.8%)	54 (12.3%)	< 0.001
Nasogastric tube	16 (32.7%)	29 (6.6%)	< 0.001

high proportion of patients with co-morbidities (> 80%). Furthermore, approximately 40% of our enrolled patients had been previously hospitalized and more than 30% had a previous history of antibiotic exposure. These factors may explain the comparative prevalence of CR-PA and CR-AB colonization.

The independent risk factors for CR-AB and/or CR-PA colonization identified in this study were underlying cerebrovascular disease (CVA), previous hospitalization, transfer from another hospital or a LTCF and previous nasogastric tube use. Previous hospitalization and transfer from another hospital or a LTCF are well known risk factors for colonization by MDR bacteria. Neurologic disease was previously documented as an independent risk factor for PA colonization [12]. Furthermore, underlying CVA may be a proxy of aspiration pneumonia, previous nasogastric tube use, functional disability and previous hospitalization [21].

Table 6 Baseline characteristics prior to hospitalization for 35 patients (with MRSA) and 452 controls (without MRSA)

Baseline characteristics	MRSA (n = 35)	No MRSA (*n* = 452)	*p*-value
Mean age ± SD (years)	66.7 ± 20.1	61.3 ± 17.6	0.09
Male gender	22 (62.9%)	244 (54.0%)	0.31
Previous hospitalization	23 (65.7%)	188 (41.6%)	0.006
Transfer status			
From other hospital	5 (14.3%)	52 (11.3%)	0.59
From a long-term care facility	0	6 (1.3%)	1.00
Underlying diseases			
Any underlying disease	31 (88.6%)	389 (86.1%)	0.68
Hypertension	22 (62.9%)	268 (59.3%)	0.68
Diabetes mellitus	13 (37.1%)	172 (38.1%)	0.92
Cardiovascular disease	12 (34.3%)	121 (26.8%)	0.34
Cerebrovascular disease	15 (42.9%)	82 (18.1%)	< 0.001
Chronic liver disease	5 (14.3%)	83 (18.4%)	0.55
Chronic renal disease	3 (8.6%)	61 (13.4%)	0.60
Chronic lung disease	5 (14.3%)	58 (12.8%)	0.79
Malignancy	6 (17.1%)	81 (17.9%)	0.91
Solid malignancy	5 (14.3%)	70 (15.5%)	0.85
Hematologic malignancy	1 (2.9%)	11 (2.4%)	0.60
Hematologic diseases	3 (8.6%)	44 (9.7%)	1.00
Prior organ transplantation	0	7 (1.6%)	1.00
Receipt of any immunosuppressive agent	4 (11.4%)	55 (12.2%)	1.00
HIV infection	1 (2.9%)	15 (3.3%)	1.00
Previous antibiotic exposure within 90 days after hospitalization			
Any antibiotic	19 (54.3%)	129 (28.5%)	0.001
Penicillins	2 (5.7%)	17 (3.8%)	0.64
Cephalosporins	6 (17.1%)	54 (12.0%)	0.37
Carbapenems	6 (17.1%)	27 (6.0%)	0.01
Beta-lactam/beta-lactamase inhibitor	5 (14.3%)	22 (4.9%)	0.02
Fluoroquinolones	9 (25.7%)	37 (8.2%)	0.001
Macrolides	2 (5.7%)	17 (3.8%)	0.64
Others	5 (14.3%)	37 (8.2%)	0.22
Previous use of indwelling catheters			
Urinary catheter	13 (37.1%)	32 (7.1%)	< 0.001
Nasogastric tube	13 (37.1%)	60 (13.3%)	< 0.001

Our results for the baseline prevalence of MRSA colonization (7.2%) were comparable with results from previous studies [9, 16]. Significant risk factors for MRSA colonization identified in our study included previous fluoroquinolone exposure and previous nasogastric tube use. Previous fluoroquinolone exposure is well documented as an independent risk factor for MRSA colonization in many observational studies [22, 23]. Recent use of nasogastric tube was previously identified to be a significant risk factor for MRSA nasal colonization in end-stage renal disease patients [24].

The present study had several strengths. It was specifically designed to determine the prevalence of MDR bacteria colonization at various sites (nasal cavity, throat, skin at the inguinal area and rectum) and by a variety of important MDR bacteria (ESBL-producing Enterobacteriaceae, CR-PA, CR-AB and MRSA). Additionally, clinical specimens were collected at various time points to capture additional acquisition rates

Table 7 Independent risk factors for baseline colonization by ESBL-producing Enterobacteriaceae, CR-AB and/or CR-PA and MRSA from the primary and secondary analyses

Variables	Adjusted OR [95% CI; *p-value*]	
	Primary Analysis (Case vs non-case)	Secondary Analysis (Case vs No MDR)
1. ESBL-producing *Enterobacteriaceae*	Case ($n = 254$) vs. non-case ($n = 233$)	Case ($n = 254$) vs. no MDR ($n = 197$)
Underlying diabetes mellitus	1.45 [1.00–2.10; $p = 0.05$]	1.49 [1.01–2.20; $p = 0.05$]
Previous cephalosporin exposure	2.00 [1.13–3.54; $p = 0.02$]	2.06 [1.11–3.81; $p = 0.02$]
2. CR-AB and/or CR-PA	Case ($n = 49$) vs. non-case ($n = 438$)	Case ($n = 49$) vs. no MDR ($n = 197$)
Previous hospitalization	2.21 [1.07–4.53; $p = 0.03$]	2.96 [1.40–6.26; $p = 0.004$]
Transfer from another hospital	2.67 [1.19–5.98; $p = 0.02$]	...
Transfer from a LTCF	11.51 [1.84–71.83; $p = 0.01$]	...
Underlying cerebrovascular disease	2.90 [1.37–6.16; $p = 0.005$]	2.68 [1.08–6.64; $p = 0.03$]
Previous nasogastric tube use	2.38 [1.002–5.67; $p = 0.05$]	4.13 [1.27–13.47; $p = 0.02$]
3. MRSA	Case ($n = 35$) vs. non-case ($n = 452$)	Case ($n = 35$) vs. no MDR ($n = 197$)
Previous fluoroquinolone exposure	2.76 [1.13–6.74; $p = 0.03$]	3.85 [1.26–11.80; $p = 0.02$]
Previous use of nasogastric tube	6.60 [1.13–6.74; $p < 0.001$]	12.86 [4.47–36.97; $p < 0.001$]

of colonization by MDR bacteria after hospitalization. Furthermore, we thoroughly collected all clinical characteristics that may be associated with baseline colonization by MDR bacteria.

The present study had some limitations. First, there was a small number of follow-up cultures, with only 53 specimens collected at time-4. Given that sicker patients are more likely to have a longer LOS with more collected clinical specimens, the prevalence of colonization after hospitalization may not represent the true prevalence. Second, the study results may be applicable to only tertiary care university hospitals. As we mentioned before, patients in our study were relatively sicker than those hospitalized at a general medical ward in developed countries.

Conclusion

The prevalence of baseline colonization by ESBL-producing Enterobacteriaceae was relatively high, whereas the prevalence of baseline colonization by CR-PA, CR-AB and MRSA was comparable with the results from previous studies in other geographical locations. There was a slightly increasing trend of MDR bacteria colonization by all important pathogens after hospitalization. However, these observations did not reach statistical significance. Previous antibiotic use and previous nasogastric tube use were the common risk factors for various species of MDR pathogens. The documented risk factors from our study may be used to identify patients who are at a risk for MDR bacterial infection. A study with a larger sample size would be needed to identify the risk factors for acquiring new MDR colonization after hospitalization. Measures to prevent or delay colonization by MDR bacteria in hospitalized patients should be employed.

Abbreviations

AMR: Antimicrobial resistance; CR-AB: Carbapenem-resistant-*A. baumannii*; CR-PA: Carbapenem-resistant-*P. aeruginosa*; CVA: Cerebrovascular disease; DM: Diabetes mellitus; ESBL: Extended-spectrum beta-lactamase-producing; HIV: Human immunodeficiency virus; ICU: Intensive care unit; LTCF: Long-term care facility; MDR: Multidrug-resistant; SD: Standard deviation

Acknowledgements

The authors thank all nurses in eight general medical wards at Siriraj Hospital for their assistance.

Funding

This study was primarily supported by Faculty of Medicine Siriraj Hospital and Health Systems Research Institute (Thailand).

Authors' contributions

PR was responsible for study design, data analysis, data interpretation and writing manuscript. CC and KT were responsible for data collection. TT and CS were responsible for performing all laboratory tests. VT was responsible for study design, data interpretation and writing manuscript. All authors read and approved the final manuscript.

Consent for publication

Not applicable.

Competing interests

The authors declare that they have no competing interests.

References

1. Sheng WH, Chie WC, Chen YC, Hung CC, Wang JT, Chang SC, et al. Impact of nosocomial infections on medical costs, hospital stay, and outcome in hospitalized patients. J Formos Med Assoc. 2005;104:318–26.
2. Schwaber MJ, Carmeli Y. Mortality and delay in effective therapy associated with extended-spectrum beta-lactamase production in Enterobacteriaceae bacteraemia: a systematic review and meta-analysis. J Antimicrob Chemother. 2007;60:913–20.
3. Zimlichman E, Henderson D, Tamir O, Franz C, Song P, Yamin CK, et al. Health care-associated infections: a meta-analysis of costs and financial impact on the US health care system. JAMA Intern Med. 2013;173:2039–46.
4. Hallgren A, Burman LG, Isaksson B, Olsson-Liljeqvist B, Nilsson LE, Saeedi B, et al. Rectal colonization and frequency of enterococcal cross-transmission among prolonged-stay patients in two Swedish intensive care units. Scand J Infect Dis. 2005;37:561–71.
5. Popoola VO, Carroll KC, Ross T, Reich NG, Perl TM, Milstone AM. Impact of colonization pressure and strain type on methicillin-resistant Staphylococcus aureus transmission in children. Clin Infect Dis. 2013;57:1458–60.
6. Mortensen E, Trivedi KK, Rosenberg J, Cody SH, Long J, Jensen BJ, et al. Multidrug-resistant Acinetobacter baumannii infection, colonization, and transmission related to a long-term care facility providing subacute care. Infect Control Hosp Epidemiol. 2014;35:406–11.
7. Reddy P, Malczynski M, Obias A, Reiner S, Jin N, Huang J, et al. Screening for extended-spectrum beta-lactamase-producing Enterobacteriaceae among high-risk patients and rates of subsequent bacteremia. Clin Infect Dis. 2007; 45:846–52.
8. Leung E, Weil DE, Raviglione M, Nakatani H. World Health Organization world health day antimicrobial resistance technical working G the WHO policy package to combat antimicrobial resistance. Bull World Health Organ. 2011;89:390–2.
9. Friedmann R, Raveh D, Zartzer E, Rudensky B, Broide E, Attias D, et al. Prospective evaluation of colonization with extended-spectrum beta-lactamase (ESBL)-producing Enterobacteriaceae among patients at hospital admission and of subsequent colonization with ESBL-producing Enterobacteriaceae among patients during hospitalization. Infect Control Hosp Epidemiol. 2009;30:534–42.
10. Luvsansharav UO, Hirai I, Nakata A, Imura K, Yamauchi K, Niki M, et al. Prevalence of and risk factors associated with faecal carriage of CTX-M beta-lactamase-producing Enterobacteriaceae in rural Thai communities. J Antimicrob Chemother. 2012;67:1769–74.
11. Khamsarn S, Nampoonsak Y, Busamaro S, Tangkoskul T, Seenama C, Rattanaumpawan P, et al. Epidemiology of antibiotic use and antimicrobial resistance in selected communities in Thailand. J Med Assoc Thail. 2016;99:270–5.
12. Harris AD, Jackson SS, Robinson G, Pineles L, Leekha S, Thom KA, et al. Pseudomonas aeruginosa colonization in the intensive care unit: prevalence, risk factors, and clinical outcomes. Infect Control Hosp Epidemiol. 2016;37:544–8.
13. Gomez-Zorrilla S, Camoez M, Tubau F, Periche E, Canizares R, Dominguez MA, et al. Antibiotic pressure is a major risk factor for rectal colonization by multidrug-resistant Pseudomonas aeruginosa in critically ill patients. Antimicrob Agents Chemother. 2014;58:5863–70.
14. An JH, Kim YH, Moon JE, Jeong JH, Kim SH, Kang SJ, et al. Active surveillance for carbapenem-resistant Acinetobacter baumannii in a medical intensive care unit: can it predict and reduce subsequent infections and the use of colistin? Am J Infect Control. 2017; https://doi.org/10.1016/j.ajic.2017.01.016.
15. Latibeaudiere R, Rosa R, Laowansiri P, Arheart K, Namias N, Munoz-Price LS. Surveillance cultures growing carbapenem-resistant Acinetobacter baumannii predict the development of clinical infections: a retrospective cohort study. Clin Infect Dis. 2015;60:415–22.
16. Jarvis WR, Jarvis AA, Chinn RY. National prevalence of methicillin-resistant Staphylococcus aureus in inpatients at United States health care facilities, 2010. Am J Infect Control. 2012;40:194–200.
17. Clinical and Laboratory Standards Institute. Performance standards for antimicrobial susceptibility testing; twentieth informational supplement: M100-S20. Wayne: CLSI; 2013.
18. Pasricha J, Koessler T, Harbarth S, Schrenzel J, Camus V, Cohen G, et al. Carriage of extended-spectrum beta-lactamase-producing enterobacteriacae among internal medicine patients in Switzerland. Antimicrob Resist Infect Control. 2013;2:20.
19. Oguz Mizrakci S, Arda B, Erdem HA, Uyar M, Tunger A, Sipahi OR, et al. Risk factors for gastrointestinal colonization by ESBL-producing Klebsiella pneumoniae and Escherichia coli in anaesthesiology and reanimation intensive care unit. Mikrobiyol Bul. 2013;47:223–9.
20. Dancer SJ. The problem with cephalosporins. J Antimicrob Chemother. 2001;48:463–78.
21. Martino R, Foley N, Bhogal S, Diamant N, Speechley M, Teasell R. Dysphagia after stroke: incidence, diagnosis, and pulmonary complications. Stroke. 2005;36:2756–63.
22. Couderc C, Jolivet S, Thiebaut AC, Ligier C, Remy L, Alvarez AS, et al. Fluoroquinolone use is a risk factor for methicillin-resistant Staphylococcus aureus acquisition in long-term care facilities: a nested case-case-control study. Clin Infect Dis. 2014;59:206–15.
23. Graffunder EM, Venezia RA. Risk factors associated with nosocomial methicillin-resistant Staphylococcus aureus (MRSA) infection including previous use of antimicrobials. J Antimicrob Chemother. 2002;49:999–1005.
24. Wang CY, Wu VC, Wang WJ, Lin YF, Lin YH, Chen YM, et al. Risk factors for nasal carriage of methicillin-resistant Staphylococcus aureus among patients with end-stage renal disease in Taiwan. J Formos Med Assoc. 2012;111:14–8.

7

Phenotypic analysis of antibiotic resistance and genotypic study of the *vacA*, *cagA*, *iceA*, *oipA* and *babA* genotypes of the *Helicobacter pylori* strains isolated from raw milk

Reza Ranjbar[1*], Farid Yadollahi Farsani[2] and Farhad Safarpoor Dehkordi[3]

Abstract

Background: Foods with animal origins and particularly milk play a considerable role in transmission of *Helicobacter pylori*. The current study was performed to assess phenotypic characters of antibiotic resistance and genotyping pattern of *vacA*, *cagA*, *iceA*, *oipA* and *babA2* alleles amongst the *H. pylori* strains isolated from raw milk.

Methods: Six-hundred and thirty raw milk samples were collected and cultured on Wilkins Chalgren anaerobe media. Antibiotic resistance and genotyping patterns were studied using disk diffusion and PCR, respectively.

Results: Sixty-seven out of 630 (10.63%) raw milk samples were positive for *H. pylori*. Ovine raw milk (17.27%) samples had the highest prevalence of *H. pylori*, while camel (5.00%) had the lowest. *H. pylori* strains harbored the highest prevalence of resistance against ampicillin (82.08%), tetracycline (76.11%), amoxicillin (74.62%), metronidazole (65.67%) and erythromycin (53.73%). Prevalence of resistance against more than 10 types of antibiotics was 17.91%. *VacA s1a* (83.58%), *m1a* (80.59%), *s2* (77.61%) and *m2* (68.65%), *cagA* (73.13%) and *babA2* (44.77%) were the most commonly detected genotypes. We found that *S1am1a* (56.71%), *s2m1a* (56.71%), *s1 am2* (43.28%) and *s2 m2* (43.28%) were the most commonly detected genotyping pattern. Frequency of *cagA-*, *oipA-* and *babA2-* genotypes were 26.86%, 62.68% and 55.22%, respectively. We found that S1a/cagA+/iceA1/oipA–/babA2- (28.35%), m1a/cagA+/iceA1/oipA–/babA2- (28.35%) and s2/cagA+/iceA1/oipA–/babA2- (26.86%) were the most commonly detected combined genotyping pattern.

Conclusions: Simultaneous presence of *vacA*, *cagA*, *iceA*, *oipA* and *babA2* genotypes in antibiotic resistant *H. pylori* strains indicates important public health issue regarding the consumption of raw milk. However, additional researches are required to find molecular genetic homology and other epidemiological aspects of *H. pylori* in milk.

Keywords: *Helicobacter pylori*, Raw milk, Antibiotic resistance, Genotyping

* Correspondence: ranjbar@bmsu.ac.ir
[1]Molecular Biology Research Center, Systems Biology and Poisonings Institute, Baqiyatallah University of Medical Sciences, Tehran, Iran
Full list of author information is available at the end of the article

Background

Milk of animals provide a package of key nutrients that are difficult to obtain in diets with limited or no dairy products [1]. Dissimilarly, raw milk is not necessarily safe, as evidenced by higher rates of foodborne illnesses associated with its consumption [2–6]. Likewise, there were so many investigations about the considerable prevalence of some specific foodborne pathogens in raw milk [2–6].

Helicobacter pylori (*H. pylori*) is a microaerophilic and Gram-negative spiral coccoid flagellated bacterium with 2 to 4 μm in length and 0.5 to 1 μm in width. It is known as one of the main causative agents of duodenal ulcer, peptic ulcer disease, gastric adenocarcinoma, type B gastritis and gastric B-cell lymphoma [7–9]. Human stomach is considered as a main reservoir of *H. pylori* strains [7–9]. In keeping with this, foods with animal origins may play an imperative role in transmission of *H. pylori* infections to human [7–9]. Suitable conditions including pH, activated water (AW), moisture and temperature cause *H. pylori* to easily survive in milk [10]. Raw milk [10], pasteurized milk [7–9] and even sterilized food samples [10] have been introduced as possible emerging sources of *H. pylori* infections. Vacuolating Cytotoxin A (*vacA*) and Cytotoxin Associated Gene A (*cagA*) are two important virulence genes with high importance in the pathogenicity of *H. pylori* infections [7–10]. The *vacA* gene is polymorphic, comprising variable signal regions (type *s1* or *s2*) and mid-regions (type *m1* or *m2*). The *s1* type is additionally divided into *s1a*, *s1b* and *s1c* and the *m1* into *m1a* and *m1b* subtypes. The *cagA* gene has been detected in the severe cases of gastrointestinal disorders and peptic ulcers [7–10]. Induced by contact with the epithelium antigen (*iceA*), outer inflammatory protein (*oip*) and blood group antigen-binding adhesin gene (*babA*) are other important pathogenic genotypes of the *H. pylori* strains [7–11]. Genotyping using these virulence markers is considered as one of the best approaches to study the correlations between *H. pylori* isolates from different samples [11].

Antibiotic therapy is one of the best aspects of treatments for *H. pylori* infections. However, therapeutic options have become somewhat restricted because of the presence of severe resistance in some strains of this bacterium [12]. Documented data disclosed that *H. pylori* strains harbored the high prevalence of resistance against different types of antibiotics [12].

Data on the epidemiology and transmission of *H. pylori* is extremely significant in order to prevent its distribution and to identify high-risk populations, especially in areas that have high rates of infections such as Iran [7–10, 13, 14]. Considering the indistinct epidemiological aspects of *H. pylori* in milk and due to the high prevalence of *H. pylori* all-around the world [7–14], the present investigation was performed in order to study the prevalence rate, genotyping patterns and phenotypic evaluation of antibiotic resistance of the *H. pylori* strains isolated from raw milk samples of bovine, ovine, caprine, buffalo and camel.

Methods

Samples

From January to March 2018, total 630 raw milk samples of bovine (*n* = 120), ovine (*n* = 110), caprine (*n* = 130), buffalo (n = 130) and camel (*n* = 140) were arbitrarily collected from the supermarkets of diverse areas of Isfahan province, Iran. All milk samples were collected from traditional dairy farms. Milk samples were kept at refrigerator. Throughout milk collection, the first few squirts were overlooked. The animals which their milk samples collected for this research were clinically healthy, and the milk samples displayed natural physical (color, odor, pH, and density) constancy. Samples (50 ml, in sterile glass bottles) were transported in ice-cooled flasks (at 4 °C) to the laboratory within two hours after collection.

Isolation of helicobacter pylori

Isolation of *H. pylori* bacteria was performed using the culture technique [7–10, 13, 14]. Twenty-five milliliters of milk sample were used for this purpose. Wilkins Chalgren anaerobe broth (Oxoid Ltd., Basingstoke, UK) was used for this purpose. Microaerophilic conditions (5% oxygen, 85% nitrogen and 10% CO_2) was prepared using the MART system (MART system, Lichtenvoorde, The Netherland).

DNA extraction and 16S rRNA-based PCR confirmation

Distinctive colonies of *H. pylori* were additionally approved using the *16S rRNA*-based PCR method. Typical colonies were sub-cultured on Wilkins Chalgren anaerobe broth supplemented with same materials mentioned above [15]. Genomic DNA was then extracted from colonies using a DNA extraction kit (Thermo Fisher Scientific, St. Leon-Rot, Germany). Procedure was performed rendering to the manufacturer's guidelines. Purity (A260/A280) and concentration of extracted DNA were then checked (NanoDrop, Thermo Scientific, Waltham, MA, USA). The truth of the DNA was assessed on a 2% agarose gel stained with ethidium bromide (0.5 μg/mL) (Thermo Fisher Scientific, St. Leon-Rot, Germany). Polymerase Chain Reaction (PCR) was performed using a PCR thermal cycler (Eppendorf Co., Hamburg, Germany) according to reported procedure [15].

Study the antibiotic resistance pattern

There are no accepted standardized methods for testing *H. pylori* antimicrobial susceptibilities and the protocols used in this study were based on recently published guidelines [16] and also those of Performance Standards for Antimicrobial Susceptibility Testing- Clinical and Laboratory Standards Institute - NCCLS, 2007 [17]. Briefly, bacterial suspensions were adjusted to the 0.5 McFarland standard (equivalent to $1–2 \times 10^8$ cfu/ml) and were used to inoculate Muller Hinton agar plates (Merck, Germany). Antimicrobial disks (ampicillin (10 μg), levofloxacin (5 μg), metronidazole (5 μg), clarithromycin (2 μg), amoxicillin (10 μg), streptomycin (10 μg), cefsulodin (30 μg), erythromycin (5 μg), tetracycline (30 μg), trimethoprim (25 μg), furazolidone (1 μg), rifampin (30 μg), and spiramycin (100 μg) (Oxoid, UK)) were applied and the plates were incubated under microaerophilic conditions at 35 °C for 16–18 h. The zones of growth inhibition produced by each antibiotic were measured and interpreted by standard procedure. Reference strains NCTC 13206 (CCUG 38770) and NCTC 13207 (CCUG 38772) were included as quality controls [18].

Genotyping analysis

Frequency of *vacA*, *cagA*, *iceA*, *oipA* and *babA* alleles were assessed using PCR [19–22]. Table 1 characterizes the set of primers and PCR circumstances applied for genotyping of *vacA*, *cagA*, *iceA*, *oipA* and *babA* alleles. Initially, all samples were subjected to pre-tests to found suitable time, temperature and volume of reaction. A programmable DNA thermo-cycler (Eppendorf Mastercycler 5330, Eppendorf-Nethel-Hinz GmbH, Hamburg, Germany) was used in all PCR reactions. PCR grade water and *H. pylori* standard strains (SS1, 26,695, Tx30, J99, 88–23 and 84–183) were used as negative and positive controls, respectively. Ten microliters of PCR product were exposed to electrophoresis in a 2% agarose gel in 1X TBE buffer at 80 V for 30 min, stained with SYBR Green. The UVI doc gel documentation systems (Grade GB004, Jencons PLC, London, UK) was applied for analysis of images.

Statistical analysis

Data were subjected to Microsoft office Excel (version 15; Microsoft Corp., Redmond, WA, USA). Statistical analysis was performed by means of the SPSS 21.0 statistical software (SPSS Inc., Chicago, IL, USA). Chi-square test and Fisher's exact two-tailed test were applied to measure any significant relationship. P value < 0.05 was considered as statistical significant level.

Results

Table 2 represents the prevalence of *H. pylori* in different types of raw milk samples. Sixty-seven out of 630 (10.63%) raw milk samples were positive for *H. pylori* strains. All isolates were also approved by the *16SrRNA* gene PCR amplification. Ovine (17.27%) and caprine (13.84%) raw milk samples had the highest prevalence of *H. pylori* strains, while camel (5.00%) had the lowest. Statistically significant difference was seen between type of samples and prevalence of *H. pylori* strains ($P < 0.05$).

Table 3 represents the antibiotic resistance pattern of *H. pylori* strains isolated from different types of raw milk samples. *H. pylori* strains harbored the highest prevalence of resistance against ampicillin (82.08%), tetracycline (76.11%), amoxicillin (74.62%), metronidazole (65.67%) and erythromycin (53.73%) antibiotic agents. Furthermore, *H. pylori* strains harbored the lowest prevalence of resistance against cefsulodin (13.43%), furazolidone (13.43%), spiramycin (16.41%) and streptomycin (23.88%). Moreover, prevalence of resistance against clarithromycin, levofloxacin, rifampin and trimethoprim antibiotic agents were 47.76%, 38.80%, 32.83% and 34.32%, respectively. Statistically significant difference was seen between type of samples and prevalence of antibiotic resistance ($P < 0.05$). Figure 1 represents the distribution of multi-drug resistant *H. pylori* strains isolated from different types of raw milk samples. We found that all of the *H. pylori* strains isolated from raw milk samples at least had resistance against 3 different types of antibiotics, while prevalence of resistance against more than 3 types of antibiotics (etc) was 94.02%.

Table 4 represents the distribution of genotypes amongst the *H. pylori* strains isolated from different types of raw milk samples. *VacA s1a* (83.58%), *m1a* (80.59%), *s2* (77.61%) and *m2* (68.65%), *cagA* (73.13%) and *babA2* (44.77%) were the most commonly detected genotypes amongst the *H. pylori* strains isolated from different types of raw milk samples. *VacA s1c* (10.44%), *m1b* (28.35%) and *s1b* (32.83%), *iceA2* (19.40%) and *oipA* (37.31%) had the lowest prevalence amongst the *H. pylori* strains isolated from different types of raw milk samples. Statistically significant difference was seen between type of samples and prevalence of genotypes ($P < 0.05$). Additionally, statistically significant difference was seen between the prevalence of *iceA1* and *iceA2* genotypes ($P < 0.05$).

Table 5 represents the genotyping pattern of *H. pylori* strains isolated from different types of raw milk samples. *S1am1a* (56.71%), *s2m1a* (56.71%), *s1 am2* (43.28%) and *s2 m2* (43.28%) were the most commonly detected genotyping pattern of the *vacA* alleles of *H. pylori* strains isolated from different types of raw milk samples. Distribution of *cagA-*, *oipA-* and *babA2-* genotypes were 26.86%, 62.68% and 55.22%, respectively. We found that 10.44% of *H. pylori* strains harbored *iceA1/iceA2* genotyping pattern. *S1cm1b* (1.49%), *s1 cm2* (4.47%), *s1bm1b* (7.46%), *s1cm1a* (7.46%), s1bm2 (11.94%), *s2m1b* (16.41%) and *s1bm1a* (16.41%) had the lowest prevalence

Table 1 Set of primers and PCR circumstances applied for genotyping of *vacA, cagA, iceA, oipA* and *babA* alleles

Genes	Primer Sequence (5'-3')	Size of product (bp)	Volume of PCR reaction (50 μl)	PCR programs
VacA s_1a	F: CTCTCGCTTTAGTAGGAGC R: CTGCTTGAATGCGCCAAAC	213	5 μL PCR buffer 10 x 1.5 mM Mgcl$_2$ 200 μM dNTP (Thermo Fisher Scientific, St. Leon-Rot, Germany) 0.5 μM of each primers F & R 1.25 U Taq DNA polymerase (Thermo Fisher Scientific, St. Leon-Rot, Germany) 2.5 μL DNA template	1 cycle: 95 °C ----------- 1 min. 32 cycle: 95 °C ----------- 45 s 64 °C ----------- 50 s 72 °C ----------- 70 s 1 cycle: 72 °C ----------- 5 min
VacA s_1b	F: AGCGCCATACCGCAAGAG CTGCTTGAATGCGCCAAAC	187		
VacA s_1c	F: CTCTCGCTTTAGTGGGGYT R: CTGCTTGAATGCGCCAAAC	213		
VacA s_2	F: GCTAACACGCCAAATGATCC R: CTGCTTGAATGCGCCAAAC	199		
VacA m_1a	F: GGTCAAAATGCGGTCATGG R: CCATTGGTACCTGTAGAAAC	290		
VacA m_1b	F: GGCCCCAATGCAGTCATGGA R: GCTGTTAGTGCCTAAAGAAGCAT	291		
VacA m_2	F: GGAGCCCCAGGAAACATTG R: CATAACTAGCGCCTTGCA	352		
Cag A	F: GATAACAGCCAAGCTTTTGAGG R: CTGCAAAAGATTGTTTGGCAGA	300	5 μL PCR buffer 10X 2 mM Mgcl$_2$ 150 μM dNTP (Thermo Fisher Scientific, St. Leon-Rot, Germany) 0.75 μM of each primers F & R 1.5 U Taq DNA polymerase (Thermo Fisher Scientific, St. Leon-Rot, Germany) 3 μL DNA template	1 cycle: 94 °C ----------- 1 min. 32 cycle: 95 °C ----------- 60 s 56 °C ----------- 60 s 72 °C ----------- 60 s 1 cycle: 72 °C ----------- 10 min
IceA *IceA1*	F: GTGTTTTTAACCAAAGTATC R: CTATAGCCASTYTCTTTGCA	247	5 μL PCR buffer 10 x 2 mM Mgcl$_2$ 150 μM dNTP (Thermo Fisher Scientific, St. Leon-Rot, Germany) 0.75 μM of each primers F & R 1.5 U Taq DNA polymerase (Thermo Fisher Scientific, St. Leon-Rot, Germany) 3 μL DNA template	1 cycle: 94 °C ----------- 1 min. 32 cycle: 94 °C ----------- 60 s 56 °C ----------- 60 s 72 °C ----------- 60 s 1 cycle: 72 °C ----------- 10 min
IceA2	F: GTTGGGTATATCACAATTTAT R: TTRCCCTATTTTCTAGTAGGT	229/334		
OipA	F: GTTTTTGATGCATGGGATTT R: GTGCATCTCTTATGGCTTT	401	5 μL PCR buffer 10 x 2 mM Mgcl$_2$ 150 μM dNTP (Thermo Fisher Scientific, St. Leon-Rot, Germany) 0.75 μM of each primers F & R 1.5 U Taq DNA polymerase (Thermo Fisher Scientific, St. Leon-Rot, Germany) 3 μL DNA template	1 cycle: 94 °C ----------- 1 min. 32 cycle: 94 °C ----------- 60 s 56 °C ----------- 60 s 72 °C ----------- 60 s 1 cycle: 72 °C ----------- 10 min
BabA	F: CCAAACGAAACAAAAAGCGT R: GCTTGTGTAAAAGCCGTCGT	105–124	5 μL PCR buffer 10 x 2 mM Mgcl$_2$ 150 μM dNTP (Thermo Fisher Scientific, St. Leon-Rot, Germany) 0.75 μM of each primers F & R 1.5 U Taq DNA polymerase (Thermo Fisher Scientific, St. Leon-Rot, Germany) 3 μL DNA template	1 cycle: 94 °C ----------- 1 min. 35 cycle: 94 °C ----------- 60 s 57 °C ----------- 45 s 72 °C ----------- 30 s 1 cycle: 72 °C ----------- 10 min

amongst different genotyping patterns of *H. pylori* strains.

Table 6 represents the combined genotyping pattern of *H. pylori* strains isolated from different types of raw milk samples. We found that s1a/cagA+/iceA1/oipA−/babA2- (28.35%), m1a/cagA+/iceA1/oipA−/babA2- (28.35%), s2/cagA+/iceA1/oipA−/babA2- (26.86%), s1a/cagA+/iceA1/oipA−/babA2+ (25.37%), m1a/cagA+/iceA1/oipA−/babA2+ (25.37%), s2/cagA+/iceA1/oipA−/babA2+ (23.88%), s1a/cagA+/iceA1/oipA+/babA2- (22.38%) and m2/cagA+/iceA1/oipA−/babA2+ (22.38%) were the most commonly detected combined genotyping pattern of *H. pylori* strains isolated from different types of raw milk samples. There were no detected *H. pylori* strains positive for s1b/cagA−/iceA2/oipA+/babA2+, s1c/cagA+/iceA1/oipA+/babA2+, s1c/cagA+/iceA1/oipA+/babA2-, s1c/cagA+/iceA2/oipA+/babA2+, s1c/cagA+/iceA2/oipA+/babA2-, s1c/cagA+/iceA2/oipA−/babA2+, s1c/cagA−/iceA1/oipA+/babA2+, s1c/cagA−/iceA1/oipA+/babA2-, s1c/cagA−/iceA1/oipA−/babA2+, s1c/cagA−/iceA2/oipA+/babA2+, s1c/cagA−/iceA2/oipA+/babA2-, s1c/cagA−/iceA2/oipA−/babA2+, s1c/cagA−/iceA2/oipA−/babA2-, m1b/cagA−/iceA1/oipA

Table 2 Prevalence of *H. pylori* in different types of raw milk samples

Raw milk samples	No samples collected	N (%) of *H. pylori* positive samples	*H. pylori 16SrRNA* PCR confirmation (%)
Bovine	120	9 (7.50)	9 (7.50)
Ovine	110	19 (17.27)	19 (17.27)
Caprine	130	18 (13.84)	18 (13.84)
Buffalo	130	14 (10.76)	14 (10.76)
Camel	140	7 (5.00)	7 (5.00)
Total	630	67 (10.63)	67 (10.63)

+/babA2+ and s1b/cagA−/iceA2/oipA+/babA2+ combined genotyping patterns. Prevalence of s1b/cagA−/iceA1/oipA+/babA2+, s1b/cagA−/iceA1/oipA+/babA2-, s1b/cagA−/iceA2/oipA+/babA2-, s1c/cagA+/iceA1/oipA−/babA2+, s1c/cagA+/iceA2/oipA−/babA2-, s1c/cagA−/iceA1/oipA−/babA2-, s2/cagA−/iceA2/oipA+/babA2+, m1b/cagA−/iceA1/oipA+/babA2-, m1b/cagA−/iceA1/oipA−/babA2+, m1b/cagA−/iceA2/oipA+/babA2- and m2/cagA−/iceA2/oipA+/babA2+ (1.49%) were lower than other detected combined genotyping patterns.

Discussion

H. pylori is a common bacterium with high microbiological and clinical importance and about 50% of the world's population, depending to the geographic location considered, has been estimated to have been infected with this organism. Despite the high incidence of the infection, the reservoir for *H. pylori* and the routes of infection are still indeterminate and various routes of transmission have been recommended [23]. Moreover, epidemiological investigations suggest that transmission of *H. pylori* between individuals happens both via the oral–oral and fecal–oral routes [23]. In keeping with this, fecal–oral transmission has more significant implications than since *H. pylori* may occur in food and water supplies subsequent to fecal contamination [24]. Besides, the isolation of *H. pylori* in drinking water [13, 14], raw vegetables [7, 9], salads [7, 9], meat [25, 26], ready to eat foods [27, 28], sterilized foods [29, 30] and foods with animal origin such as milk [31–35], suggests that these foods may act as vehicles for transmission of *H. pylori* to human population.

The present study was performed to assess the prevalence rate, genotyping patterns and antibiotic resistance properties of *H. pylori* strains isolated from different types of raw milk samples. Totally, 10.63% of raw milk samples were positive for *H. pylori* strains. Prevalence of *H. pylori* strains in raw milk samples of bovine, ovine, caprine, buffalo and camel were 7.50, 17.27, 13.84, 10.76 and 5.00%, respectively. Several studies have been conducted in this field. Talaei et al. (2015) [36] reported that the total prevalence of *H. pylori* strains amongst the cow, sheep, goat and buffalo milk samples were 16.00, 13.79, 4.76, 13.33 and 20.00%, respectively. Quaglia et al. (2008) [35] determined that the prevalence of *H. pylori* strains in sheep, cow and goat milk samples were 33.00%, 50.00% and 25.60%, respectively. Mousavi et al. (2014) [10] described that the prevalence of *H. pylori* strains in bovine, ovine, caprine, buffalo and camel milk samples were 16.66, 35.00, 28.00, 15.00 and 13.30%, respectively. Rahimi and Kheirabadi (2012) [37] noted that the prevalence of *H. pylori* strains in raw bovine, ovine, caprine, buffalo and camel milk samples were 1.41, 12.20, 8.70, 23.40 and 3.60%, respectively. Osman et al. (2015) [38] revealed that the prevalence of *H. pylori* in raw milk samples of different parts of Sudan had a range of 7 to 38%. Similar results have been reported for the high prevalence of *H. pylori* in milk samples from Japan (72.20%) [32], Greece (20.00%) [34], Italy 1.80%) [39] and Iran (16.00%) [40].

Foods presenting intrinsic factors, including water activity higher than 0.97 and pH ranging from 4.9 to 6.0 such as raw milk, theoretically could provide conditions for survival of *H. pylori* [7–9]. Therefore, it is not surprising that the *H. pylori* strains has the high prevalence in raw milk samples of our investigation. High prevalence rate of *H. pylori* in milk samples of our research is may be due to the low levels of hygienic conditions of milking procedure. Furthermore, considering the boost prevalence of *H. pylori* in healthy human carrier, contamination due to poor hygiene management of open package of milk, has more important implications for the transmission of the infection through foods. Milk, that could become contaminated during production or because of low hygiene after the open of package, is considered to be one of the most likely vehicles for infection [31, 32]. Insufficient post-processing hygienic management of the milk, can carry the contamination of the matrix by humans. Despite of the low prevalence of *H. pylori* strains in some kinds of studied milk samples, the infectious dose of *H. pylori* is presumably low [31, 32]. Therefore, it is an important public health threat regarding the consumption of raw milk. The urea-dependent acid resistance of *H. pylori* may account for the long-term survival of *H. pylori* in an acidic environment including raw milk [29]. Higher prevalence of *H. pylori* in raw ovine milk samples is may be due to the more suitable conditions present in ovine milk such as higher fat, protein and water activity and also optimum pH. Furthermore, ovine milk may have a higher qualification for growth and survival of *H. pylori* strains. Moreover, differences in the feed of ovine with bovine, buffalo, camel and even caprine species may affect the prevalence rate of bacteria presented in their milk. Higher prevalence of *H. pylori* in raw ovine milk was also reported by previous investigations [10, 31, 32, 34–43].

Table 3 Antibiotic resistance pattern of *H. pylori* strains isolated from different types of raw milk samples

Type of raw milk samples (N of *H. pylori* strains)	*N* (%) isolates resistant to each antibiotic												
	AM10[a]	Met5	ER5	CLR2	AMX 10	Tet30	Lev5	S10	RIF30	Cef30	TRP25	FZL1	Spi100
Bovine (9)	8 (88.88)	6 (66.66)	4 (44.44)	4 (44.44)	7 (77.77)	7 (77.77)	3 (33.33)	2 (22.22)	3 (33.33)	2 (22.22)	3 (33.33)	2 (22.22)	3 (33.33)
Ovine (19)	18 (94.73)	16 (84.21)	14 (73.68)	13 (68.42)	17 (89.47)	18 (94.73)	12 (63.15)	7 (36.84)	10 (52.63)	4 (21.05)	10 (52.63)	3 (15.78)	3 (15.78)
Caprine (18)	14 (77.77)	12 (66.66)	9 (50)	8 (44.44)	13 (72.22)	13 (72.22)	6 (33.33)	4 (22.22)	5 (27.77)	2 (11.11)	5 (27.77)	3 (16.66)	3 (16.66)
Buffalo (14)	11 (78.57)	8 (57.14)	8 (57.14)	6 (42.85)	10 (71.42)	10 (71.42)	4 (28.57)	2 (14.28)	3 (21.42)	1 (7.14)	4 (28.57)	1 (7.14)	2 (14.28)
Camel (7)	4 (57.14)	2 (28.57)	1 (7.14)	1 (7.14)	3 (42.85)	3 (42.85)	1 (7.14)	1 (7.14)	1 (7.14)	–	1 (7.14)	–	–
Total (67)	55 (82.08)	44 (65.67)	36 (53.73)	32 (47.76)	50 (74.62)	51 (76.11)	26 (38.80)	16 (23.88)	22 (32.83)	9 (13.43)	23 (34.32)	9 (13.43)	11 (16.41)

[a]AM10: ampicillin (10 μg), Met5: metronidazole (5 μg), ER5: erythromycin (5 μg), CLR2: clarithromycin (2 μg), AMX10: amoxicillin (10 μg), Tet30: tetracycline (30 μg), Lev5: levofloxacin (5 μg), S10: streptomycin (10 μg), RIF30: rifampin (30 μg), Cef30: cefsulodin (30 μg), TRP25: trimethoprim (25 μg), FZL1: furazolidone (1 μg) and Spi100: spiramycin (100 μg)

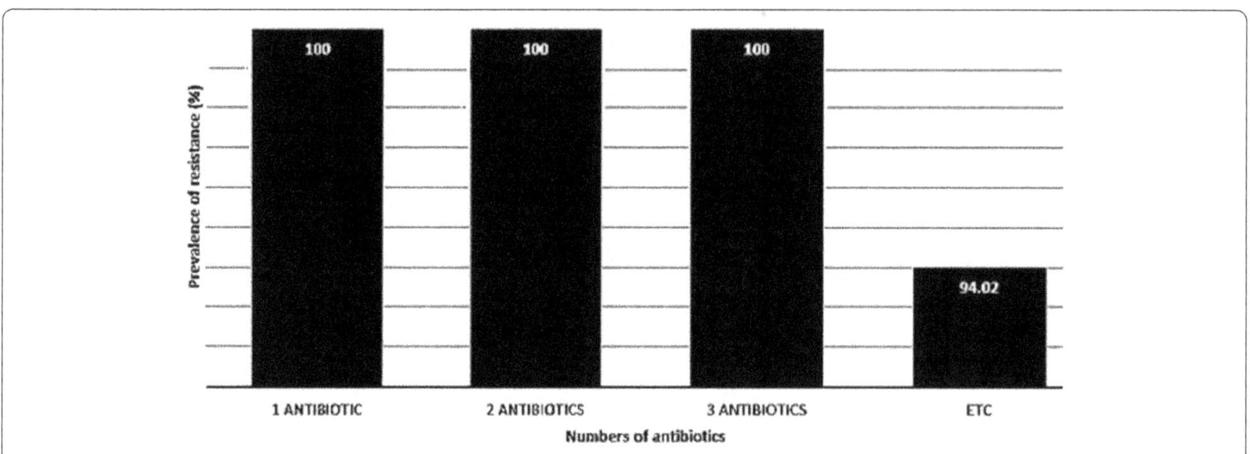

Fig. 1 Distribution of multidrug resistant *H. pylori* strains isolated from different types of raw milk. Multidrug resistant *H. pylori* strains were determined as those who had at least simultaneous resistance against 3 or more than 3 types of antibiotics

Using thorns and thistles in deserts and living away from humans and the polluted environment of cities are the most important probable reasons for the lower prevalence of *H. pylori* in camel milk. Lower prevalence of *H. pylori* in raw camel milk was also reported by previous investigations [10, 37, 44, 45].

We described that *H. pylori* bacteria exhibited the maximum prevalence of resistance against ampicillin, tetracycline, amoxicillin, metronidazole and erythromycin antibiotics. Boost prevalence of resistance against human-based antibiotics such as metronidazole, erythromycin, clarithromycin, levofloxacin, amoxicillin, streptomycin, rifampin, cefsulodin, trimethoprim, furazolidone and spiramycin in *H. pylori* bacteria isolated from raw milk samples characterized their anthropogenic origin. Reversely, boost prevalence of resistance against animal-based antibiotics such as ampicillin and tetracycline in *H. pylori* bacteria isolated from raw milk samples characterized their animal origin. As it displayed, majority of *H. pylori* bacteria exhibited resistance against human-based antibiotics. Extreme, illegal and prohibited prescription of antibiotics in medicine and also veterinary caused momentous surge in antibiotic resistance. Frequent researches have been accomplished, globally. Among plentiful examines performed on the antibiotic resistance of *H. pylori* bacteria, discoveries of Hemmatinezhad et al. (2016) [46] (amoxicillin (94.59%), ampicillin (93.24%), metronidazole (89.18%), tetracycline (72.97%) and erythromycin (58.10%)), Yahaghi et al. (2014) [9] (metronidazole (77.96%), amoxicillin (67.79%), ampicillin (61.01%), and erythromycin (23.72%)) and Mousavi et al. (2014) [10] (ampicillin (84.4%), tetracycline (76.6%), erythromycin (70.5%), metronidazole (70%), and clarithromycin (17.70%)) were similar to our findings. Clinical investigations conducted in Iran, China, India, Nigeria, Taiwan, Senegal, Thailand, Saudi Arabia, Brazil, Egypt, Argentina and Colombia disclosed that *H. pylori* bacteria of human clinical specimens displayed boost prevalence of resistance against aminoglycosides, tetracyclines, penicillins, macrolides and metronidazole [47] which was parallel to our results.

We also found that *vacA s1a, s2, m1a* and *m2, cagA, iceA1, oipA* and *babA2* genotypes, *s1am1a, s2m1a, s1 am2, s2 m2, cagA-, oipA-* and *babA2-* patterns and s1a/cagA+/iceA1/oipA−/babA2-, m1a/cagA+/iceA1/oipA−/babA2-, s2/cagA+/iceA1/oipA−/babA2-, s1a/cagA+/iceA1/oipA−/babA2+, m1a/cagA+/iceA1/oipA−/babA2+, s2/cagA+/iceA1/oipA−/babA2+, s1a/cagA+/iceA1/oipA+/babA2- and m2/cagA+/iceA1/oipA−/babA2+ combined genotyping patterns were the most commonly detected virulence characters of *H. pylori* strains isolated from raw milk samples. High prevalence of *vacA, cagA, iceA1, oipA* and *babA2* genotypes was also reported in the *H. pylori* strains isolated from clinical samples of human and animal species [48–51]. Furthermore, high prevalence of these genotypes has been reported in the *H. pylori* strains isolated from different types of food samples [8–10, 14, 36, 42–45, 52]. Adjacent association of *vacA, cagA, iceA, oipA* and *babA2* genotypes of *H. pylori* bacteria with secretion of interleukin-8 and cytotoxin, adhesion to gastric epithelial cells, occurrence of inflammatory effect, vacuolization, apoptosis procedure in gastric epithelial cells, peptic ulceration, increase acute neutrophilic infiltration, interleukin-10 secretion and inflammation, has been presented previously [48–50]. Since *H. pylori* isolates in our investigation harbored *vacA, cagA, iceA, oipA* and *babA2* genotypes, therefore consumption of raw milk contaminated with virulent strains of *H. pylori* may aggravate duodenal ulceration, gastric mucosal atrophy and gastric cancer. Additionally, some of *H. pylori* isolates were simultaneously positive for more than one detected genotypes which poses their higher pathogenicity. Similar genotyping patterns of *H. pylori* strains

Table 4 Distribution of genotypes amongst the *H. pylori* strains isolated from different types of raw milk samples

Type of raw milk samples (N of *H. pylori* strains)	N (%) isolates harbor each genotype											
	VacA							*CagA*	*IceA*		*OipA*	*BabA2*
	s1a	*s1b*	*s1c*	*s2*	*m1a*	*m1b*	*m2*		*IceA1*	*IceA2*		
Bovine (9)	7 (77.77)	3 (33.33)	1 (11.11)	6 (66.66)	7 (77.77)	3 (33.33)	6 (66.66)	6 (66.66)	4 (44.44)	2 (22.22)	3 (33.33)	4 (44.44)
Ovine (19)	17 (89.47)	8 (42.10)	2 (10.52)	17 (89.47)	17 (89.47)	7 (36.84)	15 (78.94)	16 (84.21)	10 (52.63)	5 (26.31)	9 (50)	10 (52.63)
Caprine (18)	15 (83.33)	6 (33.33)	2 (11.11)	13 (72.22)	14 (77.77)	5 (27.77)	12 (66.66)	13 (72.22)	8 (44.44)	3 (16.66)	7 (38.88)	8 (44.44)
Buffalo (14)	12 (85.71)	4 (28.57)	1 (7.14)	12 (85.71)	12 (85.71)	3 (21.42)	10 (71.42)	11 (78.57)	6 (42.85)	2 (14.28)	5 (35.71)	6 (42.85)
Camel (7)	5 (71.42)	1 (14.28)	1 (14.28)	4 (57.14)	4 (57.14)	1 (14.28)	3 (42.85)	3 (42.85)	3 (42.85)	1 (14.28)	1 (14.28)	2 (28.57)
Total (67)	56 (83.58)	22 (32.83)	7 (10.44)	52 (77.61)	54 (80.59)	19 (28.35)	46 (68.65)	49 (73.13)	31 (46.26)	13 (19.40)	25 (37.31)	30 (44.77)

Table 5 Genotyping pattern of *H. pylori* strains isolated from different types of raw milk samples

Type of raw milk samples (N of *H. pylori* strains)	Genotyping pattern (%)								
	s1am1a	*s1am1b*	*s1 am2*	*s1bm1a*	*s1bm1b*	*s1bm2*	*s1cm1a*	*s1cm1b*	*s1 cm2*
Bovine (9)	5 (55.55)	2 (22.22)	4 (44.44)	2 (22.22)	1 (11.11)	2 (22.22)	1 (11.11)	–	1 (11.11)
Ovine (19)	13 (68.42)	4 (21.05)	11 (57.89)	4 (21.05)	2 (10.52)	3 (15.78)	1 (5.26)	1 (5.26)	1 (5.26)
Caprine (18)	11 (61.11)	3 (16.66)	10 (55.55)	2 (11.11)	1 (5.55)	2 (11.11)	1 (5.55)	–	1 (5.55)
Buffalo (14)	7 (50)	1 (7.14)	3 (21.42)	2 (14.28)	1 (7.14)	1 (7.14)	1 (7.14)	–	–
Camel (7)	2 (28.57)	–	1 (14.28)	1 (14.28)	–	–	1 (14.28)	–	–
Total (67)	38 (56.71)	10 (14.92)	29 (43.28)	11 (16.41)	5 (7.46)	8 (11.94)	5 (7.46)	1 (1.49)	3 (4.47)

Table 5 Genotyping pattern of *H. pylori* strains isolated from different types of raw milk samples *(Continued)*

Type of raw milk samples (N of *H. pylori* strains)	Genotyping pattern (%)									
	s2m1a	*s2m1b*	*s2 m2*	CagA+	CagA-	IceA1/IceA2	OipA+	OipA-	BabA2+	BabA2-
Ovine (19)	15 (78.94)	5 (26.31)	12 (63.15)	16 (84.21)	3 (15.78)	3 (15.78)	9 (47.36)	10 (52.63)	10 (52.63)	9 (47.36)
Caprine (18)	10 (55.55)	3 (16.66)	8 (44.44)	13 (72.22)	5 (27.77)	2 (11.11)	7 (38.88)	11 (61.11)	8 (44.44)	10 (55.55)
Buffalo (14)	7 (50)	1 (7.14)	5 (35.71)	11 (78.57)	3 (21.42)	1 (7.14)	5 (35.71)	9 (64.28)	6 (42.85)	8 (57.14)
Camel (7)	2 (28.57)	-	1 (14.28)	3 (42.85)	4 (57.14)	-	1 (14.28)	6 (85.71)	2 (28.57)	5 (71.42)
Total (67)	38 (56.71)	11 (16.41)	29 (43.28)	49 (73.13)	18 (26.86)	7 (10.44)	25 (37.31)	42 (62.68)	30 (44.77)	37 (55.22)

Table 6 Combined genotyping pattern of *H. pylori* strains isolated from different types of raw milk samples

Combined genotyping patterns	Distribution[a] (%)
s1a/cagA+/iceA1/oipA+/babA2+	13 (19.40)
s1a/cagA+/iceA1/oipA+/babA2-	15 (22.38)
s1a/cagA+/iceA1/oipA−/babA2+	17 (25.37)
s1a/cagA+/iceA1/oipA−/babA2-	19 (28.35)
s1a/cagA+/iceA2/oipA+/babA2+	4 (5.97)
s1a/cagA+/iceA2/oipA+/babA2-	5 (7.46)
s1a/cagA+/iceA2/oipA−/babA2+	6 (8.95)
s1a/cagA+/iceA2/oipA−/babA2-	7 (10.44)
s1a/cagA−/iceA1/oipA+/babA2+	6 (8.95)
s1a/cagA−/iceA1/oipA+/babA2-	8 (11.94)
s1a/cagA−/iceA1/oipA−/babA2+	8 (11.94)
s1a/cagA−/iceA1/oipA−/babA2-	10 (14.92)
s1a/cagA−/iceA2/oipA+/babA2+	2 (2.98)
s1a/cagA−/iceA2/oipA+/babA2-	4 (5.97)
s1a/cagA−/iceA2/oipA−/babA2+	5 (7.46)
s1a/cagA−/iceA2/oipA−/babA2-	5 (7.46)
s1b/cagA+/iceA1/oipA+/babA2+	9 (13.43)
s1b/cagA+/iceA1/oipA+/babA2-	11 (16.41)
s1b/cagA+/iceA1/oipA−/babA2+	12 (17.91)
s1b/cagA+/iceA1/oipA−/babA2-	14 (20.89)
s1b/cagA+/iceA2/oipA+/babA2+	2 (2.98)
s1b/cagA+/iceA2/oipA+/babA2-	3 (4.47)
s1b/cagA+/iceA2/oipA−/babA2+	4 (5.97)
s1b/cagA+/iceA2/oipA−/babA2-	5 (7.46)
s1b/cagA−/iceA1/oipA+/babA2+	1 (1.49)
s1b/cagA−/iceA1/oipA+/babA2-	1 (1.49)
s1b/cagA−/iceA1/oipA−/babA2+	2 (2.98)
s1b/cagA−/iceA1/oipA−/babA2-	2 (2.98)
s1b/cagA−/iceA2/oipA+/babA2+	–
s1b/cagA−/iceA2/oipA+/babA2-	1 (1.49)
s1b/cagA−/iceA2/oipA−/babA2+	2 (2.98)
s1b/cagA−/iceA2/oipA−/babA2-	2 (2.98)
s1c/cagA+/iceA1/oipA+/babA2+	–
s1c/cagA+/iceA1/oipA+/babA2-	–
s1c/cagA+/iceA1/oipA−/babA2+	1 (1.49)
s1c/cagA+/iceA1/oipA−/babA2-	2 (2.98)
s1c/cagA+/iceA2/oipA+/babA2+	–
s1c/cagA+/iceA2/oipA+/babA2-	–
s1c/cagA+/iceA2/oipA−/babA2+	–
s1c/cagA+/iceA2/oipA−/babA2-	1 (1.49)
s1c/cagA−/iceA1/oipA+/babA2+	–
s1c/cagA−/iceA1/oipA+/babA2-	–
s1c/cagA−/iceA1/oipA−/babA2+	–

Table 6 Combined genotyping pattern of *H. pylori* strains isolated from different types of raw milk samples *(Continued)*

Combined genotyping patterns	Distribution[a] (%)
s1c/cagA−/iceA1/oipA−/babA2-	1 (1.49)
s1c/cagA−/iceA2/oipA+/babA2+	–
s1c/cagA−/iceA2/oipA+/babA2-	–
s1c/cagA−/iceA2/oipA−/babA2+	–
s1c/cagA−/iceA2/oipA−/babA2-	–
s2/cagA+/iceA1/oipA+/babA2+	12 (17.91)
s2/cagA+/iceA1/oipA+/babA2-	13 (19.40)
s2/cagA+/iceA1/oipA−/babA2+	16 (23.88)
s2/cagA+/iceA1/oipA−/babA2-	18 (26.86)
s2/cagA+/iceA2/oipA+/babA2+	3 (4.47)
s2/cagA+/iceA2/oipA+/babA2-	4 (5.97)
s2/cagA+/iceA2/oipA−/babA2+	6 (8.95)
s2/cagA+/iceA2/oipA−/babA2-	6 (8.95)
s2/cagA−/iceA1/oipA+/babA2+	5 (7.46)
s2/cagA−/iceA1/oipA+/babA2-	7 (10.44)
s2/cagA−/iceA1/oipA−/babA2+	9 (13.43)
s2/cagA−/iceA1/oipA−/babA2-	10 (14.92)
s2/cagA−/iceA2/oipA+/babA2+	1 (1.49)
s2/cagA−/iceA2/oipA+/babA2-	3 (4.47)
s2/cagA−/iceA2/oipA−/babA2+	4 (5.97)
s2/cagA−/iceA2/oipA−/babA2-	5 (7.46)
m1a/cagA+/iceA1/oipA+/babA2+	12 (17.91)
m1a/cagA+/iceA1/oipA+/babA2-	14 (20.89)
m1a/cagA+/iceA1/oipA−/babA2+	17 (25.37)
m1a/cagA+/iceA1/oipA−/babA2-	19 (28.35)
m1a/cagA+/iceA2/oipA+/babA2+	4 (5.97)
m1a/cagA+/iceA2/oipA+/babA2-	5 (7.46)
m1a/cagA+/iceA2/oipA−/babA2+	6 (8.95)
m1a/cagA+/iceA2/oipA−/babA2-	6 (8.95)
m1a/cagA−/iceA1/oipA+/babA2+	6 (8.95)
m1a/cagA−/iceA1/oipA+/babA2-	7 (10.44)
m1a/cagA−/iceA1/oipA−/babA2+	8 (11.94)
m1a/cagA−/iceA1/oipA−/babA2-	10 (14.92)
m1a/cagA−/iceA2/oipA+/babA2+	2 (2.98)
m1a/cagA−/iceA2/oipA+/babA2-	3 (4.47)
m1a/cagA−/iceA2/oipA−/babA2+	5 (7.46)
m1a/cagA−/iceA2/oipA−/babA2-	5 (7.46)
m1b/cagA+/iceA1/oipA+/babA2+	8 (11.94)
m1b/cagA+/iceA1/oipA+/babA2-	10 (14.92)
m1b/cagA+/iceA1/oipA−/babA2+	10 (14.92)
m1b/cagA+/iceA1/oipA−/babA2-	13 (19.40)
m1b/cagA+/iceA2/oipA+/babA2+	2 (2.98)
m1b/cagA+/iceA2/oipA+/babA2-	3 (4.47)

Table 6 Combined genotyping pattern of *H. pylori* strains isolated from different types of raw milk samples *(Continued)*

Combined genotyping patterns	Distribution[a] (%)
m1b/cagA+/iceA2/oipA–/babA2+	4 (5.97)
m1b/cagA+/iceA2/oipA–/babA2-	4 (5.97)
m1b/cagA–/iceA1/oipA+/babA2+	–
m1b/cagA–/iceA1/oipA+/babA2-	1 (1.49)
m1b/cagA–/iceA1/oipA–/babA2+	1 (1.49)
m1b/cagA–/iceA1/oipA–/babA2-	2 (2.98)
s1b/cagA–/iceA2/oipA+/babA2+	–
m1b/cagA–/iceA2/oipA+/babA2-	1 (1.49)
m1b/cagA–/iceA2/oipA–/babA2+	2 (2.98)
m1b/cagA–/iceA2/oipA–/babA2-	2 (2.98)
m2/cagA+/iceA1/oipA+/babA2+	11 (16.41)
m2/cagA+/iceA1/oipA+/babA2-	13 (19.40)
m2/cagA+/iceA1/oipA–/babA2+	15 (22.38)
m2/cagA+/iceA1/oipA–/babA2-	18 (26.86)
m2/cagA+/iceA2/oipA+/babA2+	2 (2.98)
m2/cagA+/iceA2/oipA+/babA2-	4 (5.97)
m2/cagA+/iceA2/oipA–/babA2+	5 (7.46)
m2/cagA+/iceA2/oipA–/babA2-	6 (8.95)
m2/cagA–/iceA1/oipA+/babA2+	3 (4.47)
m2/cagA–/iceA1/oipA+/babA2-	6 (8.95)
m2/cagA–/iceA1/oipA–/babA2+	8 (11.94)
m2/cagA–/iceA1/oipA–/babA2-	10 (14.92)
m2/cagA–/iceA2/oipA+/babA2+	1 (1.49)
m2/cagA–/iceA2/oipA+/babA2-	3 (4.47)
m2/cagA–/iceA2/oipA–/babA2+	3 (4.47)
m2/cagA–/iceA2/oipA–/babA2-	5 (7.46)

[a]Distribution was achieved based on the total numbers of 67 *H. pylori* isolates

recovered from human clinical samples were also reported previously [53–56].

A possible relationship between virulence factors and antimicrobial resistance has been suggested. A study conducted in 2009 in Ireland reported that the absence of *cagA* may be a risk factor for developing metronidazole resistance [57]. Other studies have found an association between clarithromycin resistance mutations and the less virulent *vacA* genotypes [58]. Another report revealed that *cagE* and *vacA* S1 correlated with clarithromycin and metronidazole resistance [59], while others found that neither *cagA* nor *vacA* was associated with resistance [60, 61]. Therefore, it is important to found any significant relationship between the presence of virulence markers and antibiotic resistance amongst the *H. pylori* strains.

Triple therapy, including two antibiotics, amoxicillin and clarithromycin, and a proton pump inhibitor given for a week has been recommended as the treatment of choice at several consensus conferences [62]. However, this treatment may fail for several reasons, as reported elsewhere [63]. In fact, the main reason for failure was found to be *H pylori* resistance to one of the antibiotics used (that is, clarithromycin). Other treatments have also been proposed, including metronidazole, a drug for which resistance is also a problem although to a lesser extent, as well as tetracycline, fluoroquinolones, and rifamycins for which resistance has become an emerging issue [64]. Results of the present investigation showed that application of furazolidone, streptomycin and cefsulodin may be effective for treatment of the cases of *H. pylori* infections. Reduction in the antibiotic prescription and also prescription of antibiotics according to the results of the disk diffusion can reduce the risk of antibiotic resistance. Using medicinal plants and especially those with high antimicrobial effects is a practical alternative way for treatment of *H. pylori* infection.

Conclusions

To put it in a nutshell, we recognized a great numbers of virulent and resistant *H. pylori* bacteria in raw milk samples of bovine, ovine, caprine, buffalo and camel species. Boost incidence of *H. pylori* bacteria in raw milk characterizes that these samples may be the natural reservoirs of the bacteria and can spread *H. pylori* to human. Moreover, some of the *H. pylori* bacteria of our research harbored *vacA*, *cagA*, *iceA*, *oipA* and *babA2* genotypes together which represents the high pathogenicity. Furthermore, higher prevalence of *iceA1+* strains than *iceA2+*, *oipA-* than *oipA+* and finally *babA2-* than *babA2+* is another important finding of our study. Additionally, presence of 97 diverse combined genotyping patterns with high distribution of s1a/cagA+/iceA1/oipA–/babA2-, m1a/cagA+/iceA1/oipA–/babA2-, s2/cagA+/iceA1/oipA–/babA2-, s1a/cagA+/iceA1/oipA–/babA2+, m1a/cagA+/iceA1/oipA–/babA2+, s2/cagA+/iceA1/oipA–/babA2+, s1a/cagA+/iceA1/oipA+/babA2- and m2/cagA+/iceA1/oipA–/babA2+ is another interesting finding of our research. Similarities in the genotyping pattern of *H. pylori* strains between various milk sources represent their same route of infection. High prevalence of multi-drug resistant *H. pylori* strains shows that raw milk of bovine, ovine, caprine, buffalo and camel species may be reservoir of antibiotic resistant *H. pylori*. Prescription of cefsulodin, furazolidone, spiramycin and streptomycin may be effectual for treatment of cases of *H. pylori* infections due to the consumption of raw milk. Additional researches are essential to recognize the rates of the molecular genetic homology of *H. pylori* bacteria isolated from milk and dairy samples and those of human clinical specimens to confirm the zoonotic aspects of *H. pylori*.

Abbreviations

BabA: Blood group Antigen-Binding Adhesin gene; CagA: Cytotoxin Associated Gene AlceAlnduced by Contact with the Epithelium Antigen; *H. pylori*: Helicobacter pylori; *Oip*: Outer Inflammatory Protein; PCR: Polymerase Chain Reaction; SPSS: Statistical Package for the Social Sciences; VacA: Vacuolating Cytotoxin A

Acknowledgements

The authors would like to thank Prof. Ebrahim Rahimi and Dr. Manouchehr Momeni Shahraki for their assistance in laboratory-based examinations. Authors would also thank from Dr. Mojtaba Masoudimanesh, Dr. Amirthossein Sheikhshahrokh and Dr. Mohammad Hossein Sakhaei Shahreza for their important assistance in the samples collection and statistical analysis. We would also like to thank from the "Clinical Research Development Center of Baqiyatallah hospital" for their kindly cooperation. This study was supported in part by a grant from "Clinical Research Development Center of Baqiyatallah hospital".

Funding

This work was supported by a grant provided from "Clinical Research Development Center of Baqiyatallah hospital" and the Molecular Biology Research Center, Systems Biology and Poisonings Institute, Baqiyatallah University of Medical Sciences, Tehran, Iran (grant no. 97/23).

Authors' contributions

FSD designed the study and carried out the PCR genetic alignment. RR supported the study and carried out the culture-based identification, disk diffusion and statistical analysis. FYF carried out the sample collection and preparation and writing of the manuscript. RR carried out the drafting of the manuscript. All authors read and approved the final manuscript.

Consent for publication

There was no consent for publication.

Competing interests

The authors declare that they have no competing interests.

Author details

[1]Molecular Biology Research Center, Systems Biology and Poisonings Institute, Baqiyatallah University of Medical Sciences, Tehran, Iran. [2]Molecular Biology Research Center, Systems Biology and Poisonings Institute, Baqiyatallah University of Medical Sciences, Tehran, Iran. [3]Young Researchers and Elites Club, Shahrekord Branch, Islamic Azad University, Shahrekord, Iran.

References

1. Thorning TK, Raben A, Tholstrup T, Soedamah-Muthu SS, Givens I, Astrup A. Milk and dairy products: good or bad for human health? An assessment of the totality of scientific evidence. Food Nutr Res. 2016;60:32527.
2. Safarpoor Dehkordi F, Valizadeh Y, Birgani T, Dehkordi K. Prevalence study of Brucella melitensis and Brucella abortus in cow's milk using dot enzyme linked immuno sorbent assay and duplex polymerase chain reaction. J Pure Appl Microbiol. 2014;8:1065–9.
3. Momtaz H, Safarpoor Dehkordi F, Taktaz T, Rezvani A, Yarali S. Shiga toxin-producing Escherichia coli isolated from bovine mastitic milk: serogroups, virulence factors, and antibiotic resistance properties. Sci World J. 2012;2012: 1-9.
4. Rahimi E, Sepehri S, Dehkordi FS, Shaygan S, Momtaz H. Prevalence of Yersinia species in traditional and commercial dairy products in Isfahan Province, Iran. Jundishapur J Microbiol. 2014;7.
5. Ranjbar R, Dehkordi FS, Shahreza MHS, Rahimi E. Prevalence, identification of virulence factors, O-serogroups and antibiotic resistance properties of Shiga-toxin producing Escherichia coli strains isolated from raw milk and traditional dairy products. Antimicrob Resist Infect Control. 2018;7:53.
6. Safarpoor Dehkordi F, Barati S, Momtaz H, Hosseini Ahari SN, Nejat Dehkordi S. Comparison of shedding, and antibiotic resistance properties of listeria monocytogenes isolated from milk, feces, urine, and vaginal secretion of bovine, ovine, caprine, buffalo, and camel species in Iran. Jundishapur J Microbiol. 2013;6:284–94.
7. Atapoor S, Dehkordi FS, Rahimi E. Detection of helicobacter pylori in various types of vegetables and salads. Jundishapur J Microbiol. 2014;7:e10013.
8. Ghorbani F, Gheisari E, Dehkordi FS. Genotyping of vacA alleles of helicobacter pylori strains recovered from some Iranian food items. Trop J Pharm Res. 2016;15:1631–6.
9. Yahaghi E, Khamesipour F, Mashayekhi F, Safarpoor Dehkordi F, Sakhaei MH, Masoudimanesh M, et al. Helicobacter pylori in vegetables and salads: genotyping and antimicrobial resistance properties. Biomed Res Int. 2014;2014:1–11.
10. Mousavi S, Dehkordi FS, Rahimi E. Virulence factors and antibiotic resistance of helicobacter pylori isolated from raw milk and unpasteurized dairy products in Iran. J Venom Anim Toxins Incl Trop Dis. 2014;20:51.
11. Biernat MM, Gościniak G, Iwańczak B. Prevalence of helicobacter pylori cagA, vacA, iceA, babA2 genotypes in polish children and adolescents with gastroduodenal disease. Adv Hyg Experiment Med. 2014;68:1015–21.
12. Alba C, Blanco A, Alarcón T. Antibiotic resistance in helicobacter pylori. Curr Opin Infect Dis. 2017;30:489–97.
13. Ranjbar R, Khamesipour F, Jonaidi-Jafari N, Rahimi E. Helicobacter pylori in bottled mineral water: genotyping and antimicrobial resistance properties. BMC Microbiol. 2016;16:40.
14. Ranjbar R, Khamesipour F, Jonaidi-Jafari N, Rahimi E. Helicobacter pylori isolated from Iranian drinking water: vacA, cagA, iceA, oipA and babA2 genotype status and antimicrobial resistance properties. FEBS Open Bio. 2016;6:433–41.
15. Ho S-A, Hoyle J, Lewis F, Secker A, Cross D, Mapstone N, et al. Direct polymerase chain reaction test for detection of helicobacter pylori in humans and animals. J Clin Microbiol. 1991;29:2543–9.
16. Andrews J. BSAC disc diffusion method for antimicrobial susceptibility testing. 2.1.4 ed. British Society for Antimicrobial Chemotherapy: Birmingham, UK; 2003.
17. NCCLS. Performance Standards for Antimicrobial Susceptibility Testing. Approved Standard M7-A5: Informational Supplement M100- S18. National Committee for Clinical Laboratory Standards: Wayne, PA; 2007.
18. Glupczynski Y, Megraud F, Lopez-Brea M, Andersen L. European multicentre survey of in vitro antimicrobial resistance in helicobacter pylori. Eur J Clin Microbiol Infect Dis. 2001;20:820–3.
19. Yamazaki S, Yamakawa A, Okuda T, Ohtani M, Suto H, Ito Y, et al. Distinct diversity of vacA, cagA, and cagE genes of helicobacter pylori associated with peptic ulcer in Japan. J Clin Microbiol. 2005;43:3906–16.
20. Wang J, Chi DS, Laffan JJ, Li C, Ferguson DA, Litchfield P, et al. Comparison of cytotoxin genotypes of helicobacter pylori in stomach and saliva. Digest Dis Sci. 2002;47:1850–6.
21. Peek JR, Thompson SA, Donahue JP, Tham KT, Atherton JC, Blaser MJ, et al. Adherence to gastric epithelial cells induces expression of a helicobacter pylori gene, iceA, that is associated with clinical outcome. Proc Assoc Am Physicians. 1998;110:531–44.
22. Sheu B, Sheu S, Yang H, Huang A, Wu J-J. Host gastric Lewis expression determines the bacterial density of helicobacter pylori in babA2 genopositive infection. Gut. 2003;52:927–32.
23. Dore MP, Sepulveda AR, El-Zimaity H, Yamaoka Y, Osato MS, Mototsugu K, et al. Isolation of helicobacter pylori from sheep—implications for transmission to humans. Am J Gastroenterol. 2001;96:1396.
24. Bui D, Brown HE, Harris RB, Oren E. Serologic evidence for fecal-oral transmission of helicobacter pylori. Am J Trop Med Hyg. 2016;94:82–8.

25. Mard SA, Khadem Haghighian H, Sebghatulahi V, Ahmadi B. Dietary factors in relation to helicobacter pylori infection. Gastroenterol Res Pract. 2014;2014:1–5.
26. Stevenson TH, Bauer N, Lucia LM, Acuff GR. Attempts to isolate helicobacter from cattle and survival of helicobacter pylori in beef products. J Food Prot. 2000;63:174–8.
27. Poms RE, Tatini SR. Survival of helicobacter pylori in ready-to-eat foods at 4 C. Int J Food Microbiol. 2001;63:281–6.
28. Meng X, Zhang H, Law J, Tsang R, Tsang T. Detection of helicobacter pylori from food sources by a novel multiplex PCR assay. J Food Safety. 2008;28:609–19.
29. Jiang X, Doyle MP. Optimizing enrichment culture conditions for detecting helicobacter pylori in foods. J Food Prot. 2002;65:1949–54.
30. Herrera AG. Helicobacter pylori and food products. Public Health Microbiol. 2004:297–301.
31. Quaglia N, Dambrosio A, Normanno G, Parisi A, Firinu A, Lorusso V, et al. Survival of helicobacter pylori in artificially contaminated ultrahigh temperature and pasteurized milk. Food Microbiol. 2007;24:296–300.
32. Fujimura S, Kawamura T, Kato S, Tateno H, Watanabe A. Detection of helicobacter pylori in cow's milk. Lett Appl Microbiol. 2002;35:504–7.
33. Vale F, Vítor J. Transmission pathway of helicobacter pylori: does food play a role in rural and urban areas? Int J Food Microbiol. 2010;138:1–12.
34. Angelidis AS, Tirodimos I, Bobos M, Kalamaki MS, Papageorgiou DK, Arvanitidou M. Detection of helicobacter pylori in raw bovine milk by fluorescence in situ hybridization (FISH). Int J Food Microbiol. 2011;151:252–6.
35. Quaglia N, Dambrosio A, Normanno G, Parisi A, Patrono R, Ranieri G, et al. High occurrence of helicobacter pylori in raw goat, sheep and cow milk inferred by glmM gene: a risk of food-borne infection? Int J Food Microbiol. 2008;124:43–7.
36. Talaei R, Souod N, Momtaz H, Dabiri H. Milk of livestock as a possible transmission route of helicobacter pylori infection. Gastroenterol Hepatol Bed Bench. 2015;8:S30.
37. Rahimi E, Kheirabadi EK. Detection of helicobacter pylori in bovine, buffalo, camel, ovine, and caprine milk in Iran. Foodborne Pathog Dis. 2012;9:453–6.
38. Osman EY, El-Eragi A, Musa AM, El-Magboul SB. Detection of helicobacter pylori glmM gene in bovine milk using nested polymerase chain reaction. Vet World. 2015;8:913.
39. Bianchini V, Recordati C, Borella L, Gualdi V, Scanziani E, Selvatico E, et al. Helicobacteraceae in bulk tank milk of dairy herds from northern Italy. Biomed Res Int. 2015;2015:1-4.
40. Safaei HG, Rahimi E, Zandi A, Rashidipour A. Helicobacter pylori as a zoonotic infection: the detection of H pylori antigens in the milk and faeces of cows. J Res Med Sci. 2011;16:184.
41. Zamani M, Vahedi A, Maghdouri Z, Shokri-Shirvani J. Role of food in environmental transmission of helicobacter pylori. Caspian J Int Med. 2017;8:146.
42. Talimkhani A, Mashak Z. Prevalence and genotyping of helicobacter pylori isolated from meat, Milk and vegetable in Iran. Jundishapur J Microbiol. 2017;10.
43. Khaji L, Banisharif G, Alavi I. Genotyping of the helicobacter pylori isolates of raw milk and traditional dairy products. Microbiol Res. 2017;8:43–6.
44. Esmaeiligoudarzi D, Tameshkel FS, Ajdarkosh H, Arsalani M, Sohani MH, Behnod V. Prevalence of helicobacter pyloriinIranian milk and dairy products using culture and ureC based-PCR techniques. Biomed Pharmacol J. 2015;8:179–83.
45. Saeidi E, Sheikhshahrokh A. VacA genotype status of helicobacter pylori isolated from foods with animal origin. Biomed Res Int. 2016;2016:1-6.
46. Hemmatinezhad B, Momtaz H, Rahimi E. VacA, cagA, iceA and oipA genotypes status and antimicrobial resistance properties of helicobacter pylori isolated from various types of ready to eat foods. Ann Clin Microbiol Antimicrob. 2016;15:2.
47. Hunt R, Xiao S, Megraud F, Leon-Barua R, Bazzoli F, Van der Merwe S, et al. Helicobacter pylori in developing countries. J Gastrointestin Liver Dis. 2011;20:299–304.
48. Torkan S, Shahreza MHS. VacA, CagA, IceA and OipA genotype status of helicobacter pylori isolated from biopsy samples from Iranian dogs. Trop J Pharmaceu Res. 2016;15:377–84.
49. Dabiri H, Jafari F, Baghaei K, Shokrzadeh L, Abdi S, Pourhoseingholi MA, et al. Prevalence of helicobacter pylori vacA, cagA, cagE, oipA, iceA, babA2 and babB genotypes in Iranian dyspeptic patients. Microb Pathog. 2017;105:226–30.
50. Podzorski RP, Podzorski DS, Wuerth A, Tolia V. Analysis of the vacA, cagA, cagE, iceA, and babA2 genes in helicobacter pylori from sixty-one pediatric patients from the Midwestern United States. Diagn Microbiol Infect Dis. 2003;46:83–8.
51. Momtaz H, Dabiri H, Souod N, Gholami M. Study of helicobacter pylori genotype status in cows, sheep, goats and human beings. BMC Gastroenterol. 2014;14:61.
52. Gilani A, Razavilar V, Rokni N, Rahimi E. VacA and cagA genotypes status and antimicrobial resistance properties of helicobacter pylori strains isolated from meat products in Isfahan province. Iran Iran J Vet Res. 2017;18:97.
53. Pakbaz Z, Shirazi MH, Ranjbar R. Frequency of sabA gene in helicobacter pylori strains isolated from patients in Tehran, Iran. Iran Red Crescent Med J. 2013;15:767.
54. Souod N, Kargar M, Doosti A, Ranjbar R, Sarshar M. Genetic analysis of cagA and vacA genes in helicobacter pylori isolates and their relationship with gastroduodenal diseases in the west of Iran. Iran Red Crescent Med J. 2013;15:371.
55. Farshad S, Alborzi A, Japoni A, Ranjbar R, Asl KH, Badiee P, et al. Antimicrobial susceptibility of helicobacter pylori strains isolated from patients in shiraz, southern Iran. World J Gastroenterol. 2010;16:5746.
56. Ghasemi A, Shirazi M, Ranjbar R, Khorramizadeh M, Daryani N, Hosseini M. The prevalence of cagA and cagE genes in helicobacter pylori strains isolated from different patient groups by polymerase chain reaction. Pak J Biol Sci. 2008;11:2579–83.
57. Taneike I, Nami A, O'Connor A, Fitzgerald N, Murphy P, Qasim A, et al. Analysis of drug resistance and virulence-factor genotype of Irish helicobacter pylori strains: is there any relationship between resistance to metronidazole and cagA status? Aliment Pharmacol Ther. 2009;30:784–90.
58. Boyanova L, Markovska R, Yordanov D, Gergova G, Mitov I. Clarithromycin resistance mutations in helicobacter pylori in association with virulence factors and antibiotic susceptibility of the strains. Microb Drug Resist. 2016;22:227–32.
59. Karabiber H, Selimoglu MA, Otlu B, Yildirim O, Ozer A. Virulence factors and antibiotic resistance in children with helicobacter pylori gastritis. J Pediatr Gastroenterol Nutr. 2014;58:608–12.
60. van Doorn LJ, Glupczynski Y, Kusters JG, Mégraud F, Midolo P, Maggi-Solcà N, et al. Accurate prediction of macrolide resistance in helicobacter pylori by a PCR line probe assay for detection of mutations in the 23S rRNA gene: multicenter validation study. Antimicrob Agents Chemother. 2001;45:1500–4.
61. Godoy AP, Ribeiro ML, Benvengo YH, Vitiello L, Miranda Mde C, Mendonça S, et al. Analysis of antimicrobial susceptibility and virulence factors in helicobacter pylori clinical isolates. BMC Gastroenterol. 2003;3:20.
62. European Helicobacter pylori Study Group. Current European concepts in the management of helicobacter pylori infection. The Maastricht consensus report. Gut. 1997;41:8–13.
63. Mégraud F, Lamouliatte H. The treatment of refractory helicobacter pylori infection. Aliment Pharmacol Ther. 2003;17:1333–43.
64. Mégraud F, Hazell S, Glupczynski Y. Antibiotic susceptibility and resistance. In: Mobley HLT, Mendz GL, Hazell SL, editors. Helicobacter pylori: physiology and genetics. Washington, DC: ASM Press; 2001. p. 511–30.

8

Incidence and outcomes of multidrug-resistant gram-negative bacteria infections in intensive care unit from Nepal- a prospective cohort study

Shraddha Siwakoti[1*], Asish Subedi[2], Abhilasha Sharma[1], Ratna Baral[1], Narayan Raj Bhattarai[1] and Basudha Khanal[1]

Abstract

Background: Infections caused by multi-drug resistant gram-negative bacterial infections are the principle threats to the critically ill patients of intensive care units. Increasing reports of these infections from the Nepalese intensive care unit underline the clinical importance of these pathogens. However, the impact of these infections on the patient's clinical outcome has not yet been clearly evaluated. The objective of our study was to determine the incidence and associated clinical outcome of multi-drug resistant gram-negative bacterial infections in intensive care unit from a tertiary care center of Nepal.

Methods: A prospective cohort study was conducted among adult patients admitted in intensive care unit of B. P Koirala Institute of Health Sciences from July to December 2017. Patients infected with multi-drug resistant gram-negative bacteria, non-multi-drug resistant gram-negative bacteria and those without infection were included. Identification of gram-negative bacteria and their antibiotic susceptibility pattern was performed with standard microbiological methods. Demographic, clinical profiles and outcomes (in-hospital-mortality, intensive care unit and hospital length of stay) were documented.

Results: The incidence rate of multi-drug resistant gram-negative bacteria infections was 47 per 100 admitted patients (64/137) with 128 episodes. *Acinetobacter species* (41%, 52/128) was the commonest followed by *Klebsiella pneumoniae* (28%, 36/128) and *Pseudomonas spp* (21%, 27/128). Patients with multi-drug resistant gram-negative bacteria in comparison to non-multi-drug resistant gram-negative bacteria had high healthcare-associated infections (95%, 61/64 versus 20%, 2/10; $p = < 0.001$). In-hospital-mortality was 38% (24/64), 20% (2/10) and 10% (4/41) in multi-drug resistant, non-multi-drug resistant and uninfected group respectively ($p = 0.007$). After adjustment for independent risk factors, compared to uninfected patients, the odds ratio (CI) for in-hospital-mortality in multi-drug resistant and non-multi-drug resistant group was (4.7[1.4–15.5], $p = 0.01$) and 2.60 [0.38–17.8], $p = 0.32$) respectively. Multi-drug resistant patients also had longer intensive care unit and hospital stay, however, it was statistically insignificant.

Conclusion: The incidence of multi-drug resistant gram-negative bacterial infections was remarkably high in our intensive care unit and showed a significant association with healthcare-associated infections and in-hospital-mortality.

Keywords: ICU, Multidrug-resistant gram-negative bacteria, Healthcare-associated infection, Incidence, Outcome

* Correspondence: shraddha.siwakoti@bpkihs.edu
[1]Department of Microbiology, B. P. Koirala Institute of Health Sciences, Dharan 56700, Nepal
Full list of author information is available at the end of the article

Background

The prevalence of infection is high among patients admitted to intensive care units (ICUs) and it is a major cause of mortality [1, 2]. The extended prevalence of infection in intensive care study reported infection in 51% of patients with gram-negative bacteria (GNB) isolation from 62% of infectious episodes [2]. As a disastrous effect of infection, antimicrobial resistance is an increasing concern in ICUs worldwide [3]. The global scenario shows that gram-positive infections are common in the developed countries ICUs [4]. However, multidrug-resistant gram-negative bacteria (MDR-GNB) infections dominate in the Asia-Pacific region [4, 5] including Nepal [6, 7]. Among MDR-GNB, extended-spectrum beta-lactamases (ESBL) organisms, carbapenemase producing enterobacteriaceae, carbapenem-resistant *Acinetobacter species*, multidrug-resistant *Pseudomonas aeruginosa* are the major culprits. Unfortunately, new antibacterial agents have not been developed in pace with the growth of multidrug-resistant (MDR) organisms [8]. There are now a rising number of reports globally [9] and also from Nepal [6, 7] of MDR-GNB infections in ICUs for which the treatment options are limited. The impact of the MDR-GNB infections can be determined from analyzing clinical outcomes, in-hospital-mortality and the length of ICU or hospital stay [10]. The association of MDR-GNB with a prolonged hospital length of stay (LOS) and mortality remains controversial. Several studies [10, 11] have reported the direct association whereas, others [12, 13] have shown that MDR-GNB infections are not associated with increased hospital LOS and mortality. Previous studies from Nepal have reported a high incidence of MDR-GNB infections from ICU [6, 7], but the impact of these infections on clinical outcome has not been evaluated. Therefore, the objective of our study was to determine the incidence of MDR-GNB infections in the critically ill patients from adult ICU, as well as the clinical outcomes with regard to in-hospital-mortality, ICU and hospital LOS.

Methods

Study design

This prospective cohort study was conducted in seven bedded general adult ICU under the care of the department of Anesthesiology and Critical care unit, B.P Koirala Institute of Health Sciences (BPKIHS), Nepal.

Study population

All consecutive adult patients admitted to the medical ICU from July to December 2017 were eligible for the study. Patients infected with MDR-GNB, non-MDR-GNB and those without infection were included.

Microbiological procedures

Pathogenic bacteria isolated from the clinical specimens from the ICU were further characterized by conventional biochemical tests to identify the specific GNB by using standard microbiologic methods [14]. Antibiotic susceptibility test of GNB strains was done by the Kirby Bauer disc diffusion method on Mueller Hinton agar (MHA) as per the Clinical Laboratory Standard Institute (CLSI) guidelines [15]. Antibiotics of following concentrations were used: ampicillin (10 μg), amikacin (30 μg), gentamycin (10 μg), tobramycin(10 μg), ciprofloxacin (5 μg), levofloxacin (5 μg), chloramphenicol (30 μg), co-trimoxazole (25 μg), ceftazidime (30 μg), cefotaxime (30 μg), cefepime (30 μg), piperacillin (100 μg), carbenicillin (100 μg.), piperacillin-tazobactam (100/10 μg), imipenem (10 μg), tigecycline (30 μg), polymyxin B (300unit), and colistin sulphate (10 μg) from HiMedia Laboratories, India. Disk zone diameters were interpreted according to the CLSI 2017 recommendations. Quality control for culture plates and antibiotic susceptibility was performed using *Escherichia coli* ATCC 25922 and *Pseudomonas aeruginosa* ATCC 27853. All the strains were subjected to various phenotypic methods for the screening and confirmation of the beta lactamases. Strains showing decreased sensitivity to ceftazidime/ cefotaxime were considered as screen positive for ESBL production and were subjected to the following confirmatory phenotypic tests as per the CLSI guidelines [15].

- ESBL- A difference in the zone size of 5 mm between ceftazidime and ceftazidime+ clavulanic acid and cefotaxime and cefotaxime+clavulanic acid discs was considered as confirmed ESBL producer [15].
- Carbapenemase- The screen positive for carbapenemase production was considered for strains showing resistance to carbapenems. A positive modified hodge test (MHT) with appearance of clover leaf at the streaking line was considered as carbapenemase producer as per the CLSI guidelines [15]. A difference in the zone size of 7 mm between Imipenem and Imienem+ EDTA disc in the EDTA disk synergy test was considered as MBL producer [16].

Definitions

Infection-An episode of infection was defined as the isolation of GNB in the presence of compatible signs or symptoms. Healthcare-associated infections (HCAI) and those infections present on admission were included.

Infection occurring > 48 h after admission to the hospital was defined as HCAI.

MDR was defined as non-susceptibility to at least one agent in three or more antimicrobial categories [17].

Diagnostic criteria recommended by CDC was implemented to classify different infections. Pneumonia was considered if purulent tracheobronchial secretion or new pathogenic bacteria isolated from sputum or tracheal aspirate culture with ≥10 [4] colony forming unit/ml and at least two of the following criteria were met: fever (> 38°C); leukocytes > 12,000 or < 4000 cells/ml; new or progressive pulmonary infiltrates on chest X-rays; new onset or worsening cough or dyspnea or tachypnea; or worsening gas exchange.

An episode of blood stream infection (BSI) was defined as one positive blood culture with a recognized pathogen or two positive cultures with same organism drawn on separate occasions with one of the following signs and symptoms: (fever(> 38°C), chills and rigor and hypotension.

An episode of urinary tract infection (UTI) was defined as a positive urine culture of ≥10 [5] colony forming units/ml and with no more than two species of microorganisms, and at least one of following signs or symptoms: fever (> 38°C); dysuria; suprapubic tenderness; costovertebral angle pain or tenderness with no other recognized cause.

An episode of surgical site infection (SSI) was defined as infection which occurred within 30 days after the operation involving skin, subcutaneous tissue or deep soft tissue of the incision and at least one of the following: purulent drainage with or without laboratory confirmation; organisms isolated from an aseptically obtained culture of fluid or tissue; or one of the signs or symptoms of infection: pain or tenderness, localised swelling, redness, or heat.

Based on the presence or absence of infection, patients were categorized into three groups: Uninfected patients- Patients without infection; Non-MDR-GNB patients-Infections attributed to susceptible GNB and MDR-GNB patients- Infections attributed to MDR-GNB.

Patients were included more than once in the analysis for separate episodes of infection.

In cases of polymicrobial infections, the episode was defined as an MDR-GNB case if 1 of the isolates was an MDR-GNB strain.

Previous antibiotic therapy was defined as antibiotic used within 30 days prior to positive culture for GNB.

Empiric antibiotic therapy was considered inappropriate if it did not include at least one antibiotic active against the GNB in vitro. Empirical antibiotic treatment protocols were same for all the groups and the antibiotic was changed after the culture and sensitivity report.

Data collection

Patient demographic characteristics, underlying conditions and reason for hospital admission were recorded in the participant record form at the time of admission. Patient were routinely followed up again each morning and data on clinical or laboratory parameters were collected, including previous antibiotic therapy, clinical manifestations, HCAI, pathogens and antibiotic resistance. The baseline severity of illness were assessed with acute physiology chronic health evaluation II (APACHE II) score [18] and Charlson comorbidity index (CCI) score [19]. Further, the data were collected regarding clinical outcomes that included the ICU stay, hospital stay, discharge and in-hospital-mortality.

Statistical analysis

Data were entered in the MS Excel 2007 and analyzed with STATA version 14 (stata corporation, college station, Tx, USA). Normal distribution of data was tested using histogram, skewness-kurtosis, and shapiro–wilk test. We used kruskal–wallis test for non-parametric data to compare between three groups. Categorical data were analyzed using the chi-square test or fisher's exact test as appropriate. Univariate and multivariate logistic regression analysis was used to compare in-hospital-mortality between the groups. Data are reported as median (IQR), number (percentage), odds ratio (95% confidence interval). Values of $p < 0.05$ was considered statistically significant.

Results

A total of 137 patients were admitted to the ICU during the 6 months study period. There were128 episodes of MDR-GNB infections in 64 patients with an incidence rate of 47 per 100 ICU admissions. There were 41 uninfected and 10 infected cases with 19 episodes of non-MDR-GNB infections (Fig. 1).

Among the GNB infection episodes, incidences of MDR for each of the bacterial strains were reported as 100% (4/4) for *Enterobacter spp*, 100% (2/2) for *Citrobacter spp*, 93% (52/56) for *Acinetobacter spp*, 86% (36/42) for *Klebsiella pneumoniae*, 84% (27/32) for *Pseudomonas spp* and 64%(7/11) for *Escherichia coli*. Polymicrobial infection was present in 28% (18/64) MDR-GNB patients and 10% (1/10) in non-MDR-GNB patients. The detailed results of GNB pattern in the non-MDR-GNB and MDR-GNB group are presented in Table 1.

In the MDR group, bacteria were most frequently isolated from the lower respiratory tract infection (LRTI) (72%, 92/128) followed by BSI (14%, 18/128), UTI and SSI each with (3%, 4/128). Whereas, in the non-MDR group, BSI (53%, 10/19) was the commonest followed by LRTI (42%, 8/19) and UTI (5%, 1/19). MDR-GNB showed variable degree of resistance to different classes of antibiotics as shown in Table 2.

Demographic and clinical characteristics are provided in Table 3.

Patients with MDR-GNB in comparison to non-MDR-GNB were found to have high incidence of previous antibiotic therapy (95%, 61/64 versus 60%, 6/10; p = < 0.001) and HCAI (95%, 61/64 versus 20%, 2/10; $p = < 0.001$).

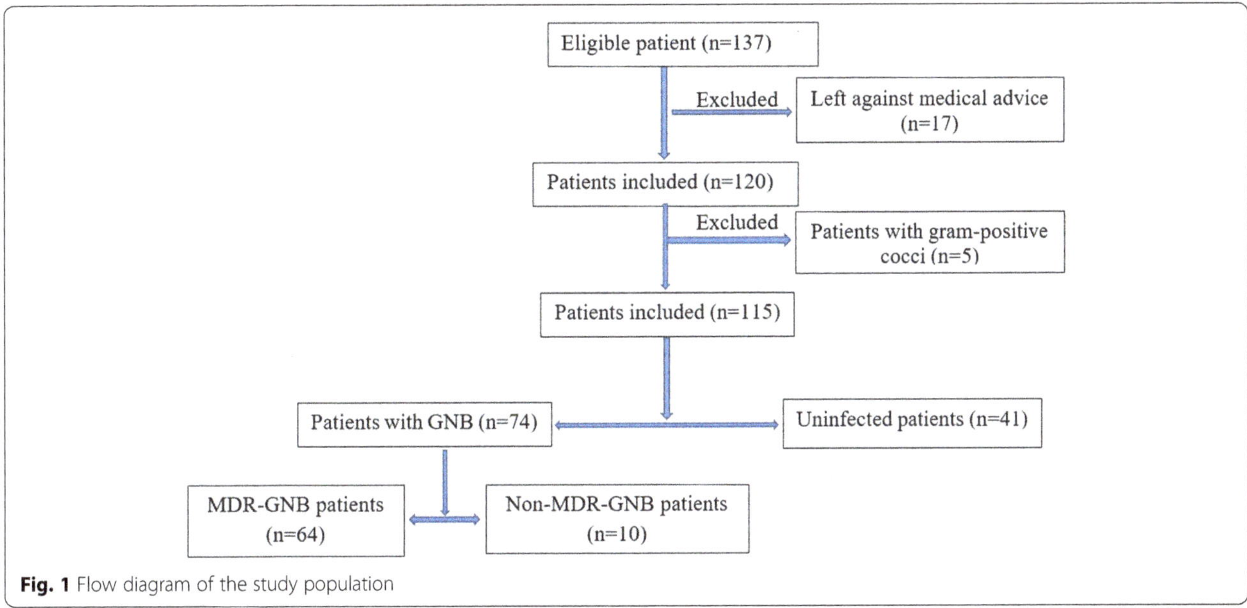

Fig. 1 Flow diagram of the study population

With respect to the clinical outcome, in-hospital-mortality among patients in the MDR group (38%, 24/64) was significantly higher than those in the non-MDR group (20%, 2/10) and uninfected group (10%, 4/41) ($p = 0.007$) as depicted in Table 4. However, no difference was detected when MDR-GNB group was compared to non-MDR-GNB group ($p = 0.47$).

The findings of univariate and multivariate logistic regression for variables associated with in-hospital- mortality are described in Table 5.

After adjustment for independent risk factors, compared to uninfected patients, the odds ratio (CI) for in-hospital-mortality in MDR-GNB group was (4.7[1.4–15.5], $p = 0.01$), while in patients with non-MDR-GNB it was (2.60 [0.38–17.8], $p = 0.32$).

Discussion

The increasing incidence of MDR-GNB infections reported from the different ICU's in Nepal is of great concern [6, 7]. However, most prior work from Nepal has been focused on their incidence and the common mechanism of drug resistance [6, 7]. To our knowledge, this is the first study from Nepal that highlights the association between MDR-GNB infections and various clinical outcomes in ICU admitted patients.

The present study found that MDR-GNB infections was not uncommon in ICU and it accounted for 47 MDR-GNB cases per 100 ICU admission. Despite significant advances in ICU in current years, the incidence of MDR-GNB HCAI remains higher in the ICU compared with other hospital units [20]. In our study, 95% cases of MDR-GNB were associated with HCAI. Similar findings were reported by other recent studies from Nepal which were done by Parajuli et al., Bhandari et al. and khanal et al. which reported 96% [6], 79% [21] and 69% [7] of GNB causing HCAI from ICU were MDR. Rampant antibiotic use, increased prevalence of drug resistance and nonadherence to infection control strategies are the emerging problems in Nepalese ICU's predisposing for the emergence and spread of HCAI [6]. Likewise,

Table 1 Gram-negative bacilli (GNB) infections from ICU ($n = 147$)

Gram negative bacilli isolates	Total GNB	Non-MDR-GNB	MDR-GNB			
			Resistance mechanisms			Total MDR
			ESBL	CP(MBL)	Other	
Acinetobacter spp	56	4(21%)	6	34	12	52(41%)
Pseudomonas spp	32	5(26%)	3	19	5	27(21%)
Klebsiella pneumoniae	42	6(32%)	12	19	5	36(28%)
Escherichia coli	11	4(21%)	6	1	–	7(5.5%)
Enterobacter spp	4	–	2	2	–	4(3%)
Citrobacter spp	2	–	2		–	2(1.5%)
Total	147	19(100%)	31(24%)	75(59%)	22(17%)	128(100%)

Table 2 Antibiotic sensitivity of multidrug-resistant gram negative bacilli ($n = 128$)

Antimicrobial agents	Resistance (%) among bacterial isolates					
	Acinetobacter spp ($n = 52$)	*Pseudomonas spp* ($n = 27$)	*Klebsiella pneumoniae* ($n = 36$)	*Escherichiacoli* ($n = 7$)	*Enterobacter spp* ($n = 4$)	*Citrobacter spp* ($n = 2$)
Levofloxacin	85	88	73	57	100	50
Ciprofloxacin	92	90	82	86	100	100
Amikacin	93	89	76	71	100	50
Gentamycin	93	89	79	71	100	50
Tobramycin	–	87	–	–	–	–
Chloramphenicol	–	–	73	57	100	0
Cotrimoxazole	90	–	73	71	100	50
Ampicillin	–	–	–	100	100	100
Piperacillin	93	90	79		100	100
Piperacillin- Tazobactam	86	82	73	100	100	100
Amoxicillin-clavulanate	–	–	76	100	100	100
Ceftazidime	93	92	92	100	100	100
Cefotaxime	93	92	92	100	100	100
Cefepime	87	90	86	100	100	100
Imipenem	81	82	69	14	100	0
Tigecycline	58	63	57	14	67	0
Polymixin B	0	0	0	0	0	0
Colistin Sulphate	0	0	0	0	0	0

in a study from India, 58% MDR-GNB were isolated from the ICUs specimens from the total received specimens [22]. Another study from India on epidemiology of MDR-GNB isolated from ventilator-associated pneumonia in ICU patients found 88% of total isolates to be GNB, among which 72% were MDR [23]. A systematic review of the burden of MDR HCAI among ICU patients in Southeast Asia showed substantially higher incidence of MDR *Acinetobacter baumannii* (58%) than reported from other parts of globe [24]. These scenario shows high prevalence of MDR-GNB infections in ICUs of Asia including Nepal. The present study showed high frequency of bacterial isolates producing beta-lactamases (MBL 59%, ESBL 24%). Current studies from Nepal also have reported high incidence of ESBL (43% [6], 40% [21], 25% [7]) and MBL (65% [21], 50% [6], 37% [7]) from ICU. Prevalence of ESBL and carbapenemases producing GNB from ICU was 22.7% and 9.6% respectively in a recent study from India [25]. Studies from the west also have shown an increasing trend of ESBL with ICU GNB isolates [20]. Sader and colleagues reported on the prevalence and trends of MDR-GNB occurring in the ICU of the hospitals in the United States and Europe from January 2009 to December 2011 [20]. Over the 3-year study period, rates of ESBL-producing strains of *Escherichia coli* and *Klebsiella spp* from the ICU increased from 11.9 to 17.4% and 27.5–41.8% respectively from 2009 to 2011 [20]. Alike, a SENTRY study also reported that GNB resistance to imipenem increased from 34.5% in 2006 to 59.8% in 2009 across the world [26]. This globally increasing trend of carbapenemase resistance in the ICUs poses a significant concern since it limits the range of therapeutic alternative forcing the clinicians to use agents like colistin which is expensive and associated with significant toxicity [8]. The reports of infections caused by MDR non-fermentative gram-negative bacteria and enterobacteriaceae are increasingly documented from the Nepalese ICU. In this study, 93% of *Acinetobacter spp,* 86% of *Klebsiella pneumoniae,* 84% of *Pseudomonas spp* and 64% of *Escherichia coli* were MDR and a similar result was also reported from Nepal [7]. Excessive use of broad spectrum antibiotics as observed in this study along with inadherence to infection control measures are the main causes for this terrifying rates of MDR infections in our ICU.

In the present study, multivariate analysis showed strong association between MDR-GNB patients and in-hospital-mortality even after adjusting all the confounding factors (Odds ratio: 4.7, *p*-0.01). Ben-David D et al. [11], in a retrospective study on the outcome of carbapenem-resistant *Klebsiella pneumoniae,* (CRKP) BSI, also found mortality to be significantly higher among patients with CRKP compared with those with susceptible *K. pneumoniae* BSI (48% vs.17%). A study by Cosgrove et al. [10] on the impact of the emergence of resistance to third-generation cephalosporins in

Table 3 Baseline and Clinical characteristics of patients

Variables	Uninfected patients; $n = 41$	Patients with MDR-GNB; $n = 64$	Patients with non-MDR-GNB; $n = 10$	*p*-value
Age (years)	43.5(28–56)	53(27–65)	55(40–60)	0.27
Age categories				
< 65	25(61%)	49(76%)	8(80%)	0.18
> 65	16(39%)	15(23%)	2(20%)	
Sex(M/F)	19/23	28/35	4/6	0.95
Reason for admission				
Cardiovascular	9(22%)	16(25%)	6 (60%)	0.89
Respiratory	27(66%)	44 (69%)	3(30%)	
Digestive/Liver	1(2%)	2(3%)	0 (0%)	
Renal	1(2%)	2(3%)	1 (10%)	
Neurological	3(7%)	0 (0%)	0(0%)	
Medical/Surgical admission	35/6	50/14	7/3	0.47
CCI Score	0(0–2)	1(0–3)	1(0–1)	0.77
APACHE Score				
At 24 h	13.5(11–16)	16(12–21)	13(12–15)	0.15
At 48 h	13(11–15)	17(12–20)	13(12–14)	0.08
Duration of ventilation	0(0–7)	10(6–16)	7.5(6–11)	0.22
Previous antibiotic therapy	17(41%)	61(95%)	6(60%)	< 0.001
Aminoglycoside	5(12%)	18(28%)	2(20%)	0.13
Fluoroquinolone	3(7%)	20(31%)	2(20%)	0.009
Macrolide	3(7%)	13(20%)	2(20%)	0.15
Beta-lactam/Beta-lactamase inhibitor	4(10%)	27(42%)	4(40%)	0.001
Cephalosporin	5(12%)	10(16%)	0(0%)	0.49
Carbapenem	1(2%)	22((34%)	0(0%)	< 0.001
Tigecycline	0(0%)	4(6%)	0(0%)	0.29
Clindamycin	0(0%)	6(9%)	0(0%)	0.12
Vancomycin or teicoplanin	0(0%)	23(36%)	1(10%)	< 0.001
Metronidazole	0(0%)	7(11%)	0(0%)	0.06
Duration of prior antibiotics used (days)	0(0–6)	7(6–8)	4(0–5)	< 0.001
Health-care-associated infection		61(95%)	2(20%)	< 0.001

Note: Values are in median (IQR), number, number (%)

Enterobacter spp on patient outcomes also found a significant increase in mortality (Relative risk, 5.02). This may possibly due to that appropriate antibiotic therapy will be started later for MDR-GNB infections in compared to infections caused by antibiotic-sensitive bacteria. In contrary to our findings some of the earlier studies did not find significant associations between MDR-GNB and mortality [12, 13]. However, variation in the clinical virulence of the varieties of GNB prevalent in different geographical areas may be the reasons for these conflicting results. Further, the patients infected by MDR-GNB, compared with those with non-MDR-GNB

Table 4 Clinical outcome of patients

Outcome	Uninfected patients $n = 41$	Patients with MDR-GNB $n = 64$	Patients with non-MDR-GNB $n = 10$	*p*-value
In-hospital-mortality	4(10%)	24 (38%)	2 (20%)	0.007
Discharged	37 (90%)	40 (62%)	8 (80%)	0.007
ICU stay	9(5–12)	13(8–18)	9(7–12)	0.43
Hospital stay	11(8–17)	14(10–21)	9(7–15)	0.93

Note: Values are in median (IQR), number, number (%)

Table 5 Univariate and Multivariate logistic regression for variables associated with hospital mortality

Variables	Univariate analysis		Multivariate analysis	
	Odds ratio (95% CI)	*p* value	Odds ratio (95% CI)	*p* value
MDR GNB[a]	5.46(1.72–17.26)	0.004	4.71(1.42–15.54)	0.01
Non- MDR GNB[a]	2.37(0.36–15.26)	0.36	2.60(0.38–17.83)	0.32
Age	1.00(0.98–1.03)	0.50	1.001(0.96–1.03)	0.95
Male	0.70(0.29–1.66)	0.42	0.59(0.23–1.53)	0.28
CCI Score	1.15(0.84–1.56)	0.36	1.05(0.63–1.72)	0.84
APACHE 24 h	1.07(1.00–1.16)	0.04	1.04(0.91–1.20)	0.48
APACHE 48 h	1.09(1.00–1.17)	0.02	0.38(0.89–1.17)	0.72

Note: [a]In reference to patients without infection

isolates, had a longer average stay in ICU and hospital, however, it did not reached the statistically significant level. As a consequence of prolonged hospitalization, MDR-GNB patients may have the economic impact due to increase in financial burden.

This study had certain limitations, including small sample size and lack of data on inappropriate empiric antibiotic therapy that could possibly influence in-hospital-mortality. Also, genotypic screening for resistance genes could not be performed due to the limited resources.

Conclusion

The present study revealed a high incidence of MDR-GNB infections in ICU. HCAI and in-hospital-mortality were significantly associated with MDR-GNB infection. Likewise, MDR-GNB patients needed prolong ICU and hospital stay, however, it was statistically insignificant. Our study highlights the alarming need of multidisciplinary efforts to address the situation and recommends the implementation of antimicrobial stewardship, continuous surveillance, strict adherence to hand hygiene and contact precautions and regular environmental cleaning to contain the development and spread of antimicrobial resistance among the local isolates.

Abbreviations

APACHE II: Acute physiology and chronic health evaluation II; BPKIHS: B.P Koirala Institute of Health Sciences; BSI: Blood stream infection; CCI: Charlson comorbidity index; CDC: Centers for Disease Control and Prevention (CDC); CLSI: Clinical Laboratory Standard Institute; ECDC: European Centre for Disease Prevention and Control; ESBL: Extended-spectrum beta-lactamases; HCAI: Healthcare-associated infections; ICU: Intensive care unit; IRC: Institutional review committee; LOS: Length of stay; LRTI: Lower respiratory tract infection; MDRGNB: Multi-drug resistant gram-negative bacilli; MHA: Mueller Hinton agar (MHA); MHT: Modified hodge test; SSI: Surgical site infection; UTI: Urinary tract infection; XDR: Extensively drug resistant

Acknowledgements

All staffs of the Department of Microbiology.

Authors' contributions

Conceptualization: SS, AS[1], AS[2], RB, NRB, BK. Investigation and Methodology: SS, RB, AS[2]. Resources: SS, NRB, BK. Supervision: BK, NRB, AS[2]. Statistical analysis: AS[2]. Writing original draft: SS. Writing-review and editing: NRB, AS[1], AS[2], BK. All authors read and approved the final manuscript.

Consent for publication

Informed consent for publication of the findings were taken from patient or from their closest relative.

Competing interests

The authors declare that they have no competing interests.

Author details

[1]Department of Microbiology, B. P. Koirala Institute of Health Sciences, Dharan 56700, Nepal. [2]Department of Anaesthesiology and Critical care, B. P. Koirala Institute of Health Sciences, Dharan, Nepal.

References

1. Vincent JL, Sakr Y, Sprung CL, et al. Sepsis in European intensive care units: results of the SOAP study. Crit Care Med. 2006;34:344–53 PMID: 16424713.
2. Vincent JL, Rello J, Marshall J, et al. International study of the prevalence and outcomes of infection in intensive care units. JAMA. 2009;302:2323–9. https://doi.org/10.1001/jama.2009.1754.
3. Cohen J. Confronting the threat of multidrug-resistant gram-negative bacteria in critically ill patients. J Antimicrob Chemother. 2013;68:490–1. https://doi.org/10.1093/jac/dks460.
4. Chaudhry D, Prajapat B. Intensive care unit bugs in India: How do they differ from the Western world? J Assoc Chest Physicians. 2017;5:10–7. https://doi.org/10.4103/2320-8775.196645.
5. Mendes RE, Mendoza M, Banga Singh KK, et al. Regional resistance surveillance program results for 12 Asia Pacific nations (2011). Antimicrob Agents Chemother. 2013; 5 7(11):5721–5726. doi: https://doi.org/10.1128/AAC.01121-13.
6. Parajuli NP, Acharya SP, Mishra SK, et al. High burden of antimicrobial resistance among gram-negative bacteria causing healthcare associated infections in a critical care unit of Nepal. Antimicrob Resist Infect Control. 2017;6:67. https://doi.org/10.1186/s13756-017-0222-z.
7. Khanal S, Joshi DR, Bhatta DR, et al. -lactamase-producing multidrug-resistant bacterial pathogens from tracheal aspirates of intensive care unit patients at National Institute of neurological and allied sciences. Nepal ISRN Microbiology. 2013; https://doi.org/10.1155/2013/847569.
8. Boucher HW, Talbot GH, Bradley JS, et al. Bad bugs, no drugs: no ESKAPE! An update from the Infectious Diseases Society of America. Clin Infect Dis. 2009;48:1–12.
9. Falagas ME, Bliziotis IA, Kasiakou SK, et al. Outcome of infections due to pan-drug resistant (PDR) gram-negative bacteria. BMC Infect Dis. 2005;5:24. https://doi.org/10.1186/1471-2334-5-24
10. Cosgrove SE. The relationship between antimicrobial resistance and patient outcomes: mortality, length of hospital stay, and health care costs. Clin Infect Dis. 2006;42:82–9. https://doi.org/10.1086/499406.

11. Ben-David D, Kordevani R, Keller N, et al. Outcome of carbapenem resistant Klebsiella pneumoniae bloodstream infections. Clin Microbiol Infect. 2012; 18(1):54–60. https://doi.org/10.1111/j.1469-0691.2011.03478.x.
12. Blot S, Vandewoude K, De Bacquer D, et al. Nosocomial bacteremia caused by antibiotic-resistant gram-negative bacteria in critically ill patients: clinical outcome and length of hospitalization. Clin Infect Dis. 2002;34(12):1600–6. https://doi.org/10.1086/340616.
13. Menashe G, Borer A, Yagupsky P, et al. Clinical significance and impact on mortality of ESBL-producing gram-negative isolates in nosocomial bacteremia. Scand J Infect Dis. 2001;33(3):188–93 PMID: 11303808.
14. Washington CW Jr, Stephen DA, William MJ, et al. Koneman's color atlas and text book of diagnostic microbiology. 6th ed. Philadelphia: Lippincott Williams and Wilkins; 2006.
15. Clinical and Laboratory Standards Institute. Performance standards for antimicrobial susceptibility testing; 27th ed. CLSI supplement. *CLSI Document M100-S27*. Wayne, PA: Clinical and Laboratory Standards Institute; 2017.
16. Yong D, Lee K, Yum JH, et al. Imipenem-EDTA disk method for differentiation of metallo-beta-lactamase-producing clinical isolates of pseudomonas spp. and Acinetobacter spp. J Clin Microbiol. 2002;40(10): 3798–801 PMID: 12354884.
17. Magiorakos AP, Srinivasan A, Carey RB, et al. Multidrug-resistant, extensively drugresistant and pandrug-resistant bacteria: an international expert proposal for interim standard definitions for acquired resistance. Clin Microbiol Infect. 2012;18(3):268–81. https://doi.org/10.1111/j.1469-0691.2011.03570.x.
18. Knaus WA, Draper EA, Wagner DP, et al. APACHE II: a severity of disease classification system. Crit Care Med. 1985;13:818–29 https://doi.org/10.1097/00003246-198510000-00009.
19. Charlson ME, Pompei P, Ales KL, et al. A new method of classifying prognostic comorbidity in longitudinal studies: development and validation. J Chronic Dis. 1987;40:373–83 PMID: 3558716.
20. Sader HS, Farrell DJ, Flamm RK, Jones RN. Antimicrobial susceptibility of gram-negative organisms isolated from patients hospitalized in intensive care units in United States and European hospitals (2009-2011). Diagn Microbiol Infect Dis. 2014;78(4):443–8.
21. Bhandari P, Thapa G, Pokhrel BM, et al. Nosocomial Isolates and Their Drug Resistant Pattern in ICU Patients at National Institute of Neurological and Allied Sciences, Nepal. Int J Microbiol. 2015;2015:572163 https://doi.org/10.1155/2015/572163.
22. Subhedar V, Jain SK. Gram negative super bugs: a new generation of ICU infections, an emerging challenge for health care settings. Am J Microbiol Res. 2016;4:47–50.
23. Gupta R, Malik A, Rizvi M, et al. Epidemiology of multidrug-resistant gram-negative pathogens isolated from ventilator-associated pneumonia in ICU patients. J Glob Antimicrob Resist. 2017;9:47–50. https://doi.org/10.1016/j.jgar.2016.12.016.
24. Teerawattanapong N, Panich P, Kulpokin D, et al. A systematic review of the burden of multidrug-resistant healthcare-associated infections among intensive care unit patients in Southeast Asia: the rise of multidrug-resistant Acinetobacter baumannii. Infect Control Hosp Epidemiol. 2018;39(5):525–33. https://doi.org/10.1017/ice.2018.58.
25. Arora A, Jain C, Saxena S, Kaur R. Profile of drug resistant gram negative bacteria from ICU at a tertiary Care Center of India. Asian J Med Health. 2011;3(3):1–7. https://doi.org/10.9734/AJMAH/2017/31434.
26. Gales AC, Jones RN, Sader HS. Contemporary activity of colistin and polymyxin B against a worldwide collection of gram-negative pathogens: results from the SENTRY antimicrobial surveillance program (2006-09). J Antimicrob Chemother. 2011;66(9):2070–4.

9

Prevalence of different carbapenemase genes among carbapenem-resistant *Acinetobacter baumannii* blood isolates in Taiwan

Teng-Ho Wang[1,2,3], Yi-Shing Leu[4,5], Nai-Yu Wang[6], Chang-Pan Liu[5,6,7,8,9*] and Tsong-Rong Yan[2*]

Abstract

Background: Although the prevalence of the carbapenem-resistant *A. baumannii* (CRAB) has increased in Taiwan, few studies have elucidated the prevalence of different carbapenemase genes in Taiwan. The first objective of this study was to identify the types and prevalence of different carbapenemase genes, and the second objective was to determine the carbapenem antimicrobial susceptibility of carbapenemase producing isolates.

Methods: In total, 269 CRAB blood isolates from four medical centres in Taiwan from 1/1/2009 to 31/12/2013 were analysed. Antimicrobial susceptibilities were determined using the Vitek 2 system. Carbapenemase genes were identified by polymerase chain reaction (PCR) and sequencing. Pulsed-field gel electrophoresis (PFGE) was used to identify the different pulsotypes.

Results: All 269 CRAB isolates had the bla_{OXA-51}-like gene, while 237 (88.1%) had the bla_{OXA-23}-like gene, and 11 (4.09%) had the bla_{OXA-24}-like gene. Twenty-one CRAB isolates (7.81%) contained only the bla_{OXA-51}-like gene. None of the isolates had the bla_{OXA-58}-like gene or the metallo-β-lactamases (MBL)-encoding genes. In 28.69% of isolates with the bla_{OXA-23}-like gene and 90.91% of isolates with the bla_{OXA-24}-like gene, the minimum inhibitory concentrations (MICs) for imipenem were 64 mg/L or more. In 37.55% of isolates with the bla_{OXA-23}-like gene and 100% of isolates with the bla_{OXA-24}-like gene, meropenem MICs were 64 mg/L or more. PFGE analyses indicated that six highly similar genomes which harbored the bla_{OXA-24}-like gene came from three different medical centres.

Conclusion: Our study determined the prevalence of CRAB, the types and prevalence of carbapenemase genes, carbapenem susceptibility among CRAB isolates, and documented that the bla_{OXA-24}-like gene had greater resistance to carbapenem than the bla_{OXA-23}-like gene. We also demonstrated inter-hospital transmission of the highly resistant $bla_{\ OXA-24}$-like gene.

Keywords: *Acinetobacter calcoaceticus-Acinetobacter baumannii* (ACB) complex, Carbapenem-resistant *Acinetobacter baumannii* (CRAB), bla_{OXA-23}-like, bla_{OXA-24}-like, bla_{OXA-51}-like

* Correspondence: joeliu5929@hotmail.com.tw; tryan@ttu.edu.tw
[5]Department of Medicine, MacKay Medical College, New Taipei City, Taiwan
[2]Graduate Institute of Bioengineering, Tatung University, Taipei, Taiwan
Full list of author information is available at the end of the article

Background

Acinetobacter is a Gram-negative bacillus that is common in water and soil. *Acinetobacter* species are recognized as opportunistic pathogens of increasing relevance in healthcare-associated infections, and are particularly likely to cause opportunistic infections in intensive care units (ICUs) [1]. Analysis of healthcare-associated infection data from the Taiwan Nosocomial Infections Surveillance System (TNIS) in 2007–2012 showed that *A. baumannii* complex (AB complex) composed by *A. baumannii, A. nosocomialis* and *A. pittii* was among the top three common causes of infections in ICUs of medical centres and regional hospitals [2].

The *Acinetobacter calcoaceticus-Acinetobacter baumannii* (ACB) complex is composed of *A. calcoaceticus* (genospecies 1), *A. baumannii* (genospecies 2), *A. pittii* (genospecies 3) and *A. nosocomialis* (genospecies 13TU). *A. baumannii* often causes bloodstream infections, and the associated mortality rate is about 43.3% in ICUs [3]. ACB complex species have similar appearances and biochemical reactions, and cannot be distinguished by traditional biochemical reactions or by automatic or semi-automatic identification machines, such as the Vitek 2 system (BioMérieux). Therefore, ACB complex species have often mistakenly been categorized as *A. baumannii.* Precise molecular biological techniques can now be used to identify and accurately distinguish these species. *A. calcoaceticus* is less likely to cause severe disease. However, *A. baumannii, A. nosocomialis,* and *A. pittii* (AB complex) can cause healthcare-associated infections in ICUs. In recent years, the gradual increase of carbapenem-resistant forms of each of these species from hospital isolates has caused great concern. The resistance rate of *Acinetobacter* to carbapenems has exceeded 50% in the United States, South America, India, and China [4]. Data from the TNIS indicated the percentage of carbapenem-resistant Acinetobacter calcoaceticus-Acinetobacter baumannii (CRACB) complex increased from 49.0% in 2007 to 71.2% in 2012 among ICUs in medical centres in Taiwan, and increased from 49.8 to 63% in regional hospitals during the same period [2].

A. baumannii is the most common and important genospecies of *Acinetobacter* and the presence of carbapenemases is the commonest cause of resistance to carbapenems. The carbapenemases in the AB complex include carbapenem-hydrolyzing class D β-lactamases (CHDLs), which consist of OXA-51-like, OXA-23-like, OXA-24-like, and OXA-58-like genes, and class B metallo-β-lactamases, mainly VIM, IMP, and SIM [5]. Our study utilized molecular biological methods to analyze carbapenemase genes in 269 nosocomial carbapenem-resistant *A. baumannii* (CRAB) blood isolates from four medical centres in northern and central Taiwan. The first objective was to identify the types and prevalence of different carbapenemase genes, and the second objective was to determine the carbapenem antimicrobial susceptibility testing of carbapenemase producing isolates.

Methods

Study design

The Inclusion criteria were listed as follows: all the tested strains were isolated from infected patients from 4 tertiary medical centres in Taiwan, randomized to collect up to 100 clones of ACB complex with imipenem or meropenem MICs of at least 8 mg/L in each tertiary medical centres from January of 2009 to December of 2013. The exclusion criteria were that only the first episode was enrolled from patients with ≥2 positive blood cultures, the other blood isolates were excluded. We collected the ACB complex blood isolates using the Vitek 2 system, and further species identification of ACB complex was confirmed by analysis of the RNA polymerase β subunit (*rpo*B) gene. The prevalence of different carbapenemase genes among CRAB was performed by conventional PCR and sequencing. The imipenem and meropenem MICs were tested in all CRAB blood isolates. Additionally, tigecycline, ceftazidime, cefepime, amikacin, ampicillin/sulbactam, piperacillin/tazobactam and colistin MICs were tested for the bla_{OXA-24}-like highly resistant gene only. Antimicrobial susceptibility was tested using the Vitek-2 system and interpreted according to the Clinical and Laboratory Standards Institute (CLSI) guidelines except for the MICs of tigecycline which were interpreted according to the European Committee on Antimicrobial Susceptibility Testing (EUCAST) breakpoints for *Enterobacteriaceae* spp. (MIC > 2 mg/L was defined as resistant). Pulsed-field gel electrophoresis was used to analyse the high resistant *bla_{OXA-24}*-like gene pulsotypes.

Each medical centre was expected to collect 100 ACB complex blood isolates. MacKay Memorial Hospital is a 2200-bed tertiary medical centre in northern Taiwan. Taipei Veterans General Hospital is a 3000-bed tertiary medical centre in northern Taiwan. Tri-Service General Hospital is an 1800-bed tertiary medical centre in northern Taiwan. Changhua Christian Hospital is an 1500-bed tertiary medical centre in central Taiwan. These four medical centres provide both primary and tertiary care, including cancer therapy, intensive care and organ transplantation. They are premier hospitals in Taiwan.

Collection of bacterial isolates

All the tested strains were isolated from infected patients. A total of 357 blood isolates of ACB complex, with imipenem or meropenem MICs of at least 8 mg/L, were collected from January of 2009 to December of 2013 from 4 tertiary medical centres in Taiwan. A total of 357 nonduplicate ACB complex blood isolates were collected from the 4 medical centres. ACB complex blood isolates were stored at −70 °C in tryptic soy broth (BD, MD, USA) supplemented with 20% glycerol (*v*/v). Freezing at − 70 °C in a high percentage of glycerol were employed as cryoprotective agents. All patients were deidentified locally and re-coded. Then the blood isolates were transported to the research laboratory at MacKay Memorial hospital for further study. This study protocol (14MMHIS125) was reviewed and approved by the Institutional Review Boards of the MacKay Memorial Hospital, Taipei, Taiwan.

Species identification

The plates were incubated under aerobic conditions at 36 °C and evaluated for growth after 24 and 48 h. Suspected colonies were further cultivated on blood agar and identified at species level using the automated Vitek MS system (bioMerieux). Antimicrobial susceptibility was tested using Vitek-2 (card AST-N196 and/or N248). All isolates were stored at − 70 °C for analysis of genetic relatedness. Genospecies identification of ACB complex was confirmed by analysis of the RNA polymerase β subunit (*rpo*B) gene according to the protocol by La Scola et al. [6].

Antimicrobial susceptibility testing

Antimicrobial susceptibility was tested using Vitek-2 system. The imipenem and meropenem MICs were tested in all CRAB blood isolates. However, tigecycline, ceftazidime, cefepime, amikacin, ampicillin/sulbactam, piperacillin/tazobactam and colistin MICs were tested for the bla_{OXA-24}-like highly resistant gene only. The MICs of tested antibiotics were interpreted according to the CLSI guidelines, but the MICs of tigecycline were interpreted according to the EUCAST breakpoints for *Enterobacteriaceae* spp. (MIC > 2 mg/L was defined as resistant). *Staphylococcus aureus* ATCC 29213, *Escherichia coli* ATCC25922, *Pseudomonas aeruginosa* ATCC 27853 were measured for quality control. All results were within quality control ranges.

Polymerase chain reaction and sequencing

The ACB complex blood isolates were screened for the following carbapenemase genes by use of conventional PCR and sequencing: bla_{IMP},bla_{VIM}, bla_{NDM}, bla_{SPM}, bla_{GIM}, bla_{SIM}, bla_{KPC}, bla_{GES}, bla_{OXA-23}-like, bla_{OXA-24}-like, bla_{OXA-51}-like, bla_{OXA-58}-like, $bla_{OXA-143}$-like, $bla_{OXA-235}$-like. The sequences of primers are shown in Table 1 [7–12]. Deionized distilled water was used as the negative control. Isolates whose sequences were previously confirmed was used as the positive control. Multiplex PCR were performed. A separate group of 2~ 10 primers (such as bla_{IMP}, bla_{VIM}, bla_{NDM}, bla_{SPM}, bla_{GIM}, bla_{SIM}, bla_{KPC}, bla_{GES}, $bla_{OXA-23-like}$, $bla_{OXA-24-like}$, $bla_{OXA-51-like}$, $bla_{OXA-58-like}$, $bla_{OXA-143-like}$ and $bla_{OXA-235-like}$) were used to test multiplex PCR each time. The PCR condition was one cycle of 95 °C for 10 min, followed by 40 cycles of 94 °C for 1 min, 52 °C for 1 min, 72 °C for 2 min and finally, one cycle of 72 °C for 10 min followed by cooling to 4 °C. A sample of amplified DNA was electrophoresed in an agarose gel and stained with ethidium bromide to assess the purity and size of the more multiplex PCR products. PCR products were visualized by agarose gel electrophoresis stained with ethidium bromide followed by UV light crosslinking. The PCR amplicons were purified for DNA sequencing using a Exo-ProStar™ reagent (GE Healthcare, UK) as per manufacturer instructions and incubated at 37 °C for 30 min, followed by incubation at 80 °C for 15 mins to inactivate the enzymes. The enzyme-treated PCR products were sequenced using the BigDye Terminator v3.1 Cycle Sequencing Kit (Applied Biosystems, Foster City, CA) following instructions provided by the manufacturer. The PCR products were purified using by gel filtration with Sephadex G-50 (GE Healthcare, UK) using spin columns in a MultiScreen™ Filtration System 96 well filter plate (Millipore) to remove unincorporated dye terminators. The final DNA

Table 1 Oligonucleotide primers used in this study

Primer	Sequence (5′-3′)	Reference
OXA-51-like forward	TAA TGC TTT GAT CGG CCT TG	6
OXA-51-like reverse	TGG ATT GCA CTT CAT CTT GG	
OXA-23-like forward	GAT CGG ATT GGA GAA CCA GA	6
OXA-23-like reverse	ATT TCT GAC CGC ATT TCC AT	
OXA-24-like forward	GGT TAG TTG GCC CCC TTA AA	6
OXA-24-like reverse	AGT TGA GCG AAA AGG GGA TT	
OXA-58-like forward	AAG TAT TGG GGC TTG TGC TG	6
OXA-58-like reverse	CCC CTC TGC GCT CTA CAT AC	
OXA-143-F	TGGCACTTTCAGCAGTTCCT	7
OXA-143-R	TAATCTTGAGGGGGCCAACC	
OXA-235-F	TTGTTGCCTT TACTTAGTTGC	8
OXA-235-R	CAAAATTTTAAGACGGAT CG	
Imp-F	GGA ATA GAG TGG CTT AAY TCT C	9
Imp-R	CCA AAC YAC TAS GTT ATC T	
Vim-F	GAT GGT GTT TGG TCG CAT A	9
Vim-R	CGA ATG CGC AGC ACC AG	
Sim-F	TAC AAG GGA TTC GGC ATC G	9
Sim-R	TAA TGG CCT GTT CCC ATG TG	
Gim-F	TCG ACA CAC CTT GGT CTG AA	9
Gim-R	AAC TTC CAA CTT TGC CAT GC	
Spm-F	AAA ATC TGG GTA CGC AAA CG	9
Spm-R	ACA TTA TCC GCT GGA ACA GG	
NDM-F	GGTTTGGCGATCTGGTTTTC	10
NDM-R	CGGAATGGCTCATCACGATC	
KPC-Fm	CGTCTAGTTCTGCTGTCTTG	10
KPC-Rm	CTTGTCATCCTTGTTAGGCG	
GES-C	GTTTTGCAATGTGCTCAACG	11
GES-D	TGCCATAGCAATAGGCGTAG	

sequence reading was performed in an ABI Prism 377 DNA sequencer analyzer (Applied Biosystems, Foster City, CA, USA). Sequence similarity searches were performed with the basic local alignment search tool (BLAST, http://blast.ncbi.nlm.nih.gov/Blast.cgi).

Pulsed-field gel electrophoresis

Eleven isolates with bla_{OXA-24}-like genes among the 357 ACB complex blood isolates were typed by pulsed-field gel electrophoresis following digestion of intact genomic DNA with *Apa*I (New England Biolabs) [13]. The DNA fragments were separated on 1% (*w/v*) SeaKem Gold agarose gels in 0.5% Tris-borate-ethylene diamine tetra-acetic acid buffer using a contour-clamped homogeneous electric field (CHEF) Mapper apparatus (Bio-Rad, Hercules, CA, USA) at a potential of 6 V/cm pulsed from 5 s to 20 s for 19 h at 14 °C [13]. The gels were stained with ethidium bromide and photographed under ultraviolet light. The *Apa*I restriction profiles were initially compared by visual inspection, and isolates were considered closely related if they had differences in fewer than three bands [14]. Computer-assisted analysis using BioNumerics software (Applied Maths, Sint-Martens-Latem, Belgium) was also performed. Cluster analysis was performed by the unweighted pair group method with mathematical averaging. DNA similarity was calculated using the band-based Dice coefficient with a tolerance setting of 1.0% and an optimization setting of 1.0% for the whole profile. Isolates were considered to be in the same cluster if the similarity coefficient was greater than 87% [13].

Results

We collected a total of 357 ACB complex isolates, including 57 from Taipei Veterans General Hospital, and 100 each from the other 3 medical centres. Among these, 334 were CRACB complex truly (93.6%); of which 269 were CRAB isolates (80.5%).

All 269 of the CRAB isolates had the bla_{OXA-51}-like gene, a gene considered intrinsic to *A. baumannii* (Table 2) [15]. The combination of bla_{OXA-23}-like gene and bla_{OXA-51}-like gene had the highest prevalence, (237 isolates, 88.1%). The combination of bla_{OXA-24}-like gene and bla_{OXA-51}-like gene was present in 11 isolates (4.09%), and 21 isolates (7.81%) contained solely the bla_{OXA-51}-like gene without combination with other bla_{OXA}-like genes. None of the isolates had a bla_{OXA-58}-like gene or any of the MBL-encoding genes.

Table 2 Carbapenem resistance among ACB complex blood isolates and distribution of OXA carbapenemase genes in Taiwan

Target allele(s)	No. (%) of isolates
ACB complex by Vitek 2 method	357
CRACB complex by Vitek 2 & AST method	334
CRAB by La Scola's protocol method	269
bla_{OXA-51}-like+bla_{OXA-23}-like	237 (237/269, 88.10%)
bla_{OXA-51}-like+bla_{OXA-24}-like	11 (11/269, 4.09%)
bla_{OXA-51}-like solely	21 (21/269, 7.81%)

Abbreviations here and below: *ACB complex Acinetobacter calcoaceticus-Acinetobacter baumannii* complex, *CRACB complex* carbapenem-resistant *Acinetobacter calcoaceticus-Acinetobacter baumannii* complex, *AST* antimicrobial susceptibility testing, *CRAB* carbapenem-resistant *Acinetobacter baumannii*

Table 3 shows the prevalence of the different carbapenemase genes among CRAB isolates from the four institutions. The highest prevalence in all 4 hospitals was for the combination of bla_{OXA-23}-like gene and bla_{OXA-51}-like gene (75.93–92.77%). The prevalence foe bla_{OXA-51}-like gene solely was 2.17–22.22%, and 0–6.52% for the combination of bla_{OXA-24}-like gene and bla_{OXA-51}-like gene.

Figures 1 and 2 show the distributions of imipenem and meropenem MICs in 269 *A. baumannii* isolates. In isolates with the bla_{OXA-23}-like gene, 28.69% had imipenem MICs of 64 mg/L or more, and 90.91% of isolates with the bla_{OXA-24}-like gene had imipenem MICs of 64 mg/L or more. In isolates with the bla_{OXA-23}-like gene, 37.55% had meropenem MICs of 64 mg/L or more, and all isolates with the bla_{OXA-24}-like gene had meropenem MICs of 64 mg/L or more. Our study showed that the bla_{OXA-24}-like genes were more resistant than bla_{OXA-23}-like genes to carbapenem. Hence we performed PFGE in these bla_{OXA-24}-like highly resistant genes.

PFGE analysis indicated the presence of 11 distinct strains of CRAB among isolates that had both the bla_{OXA-24}-like gene and the bla_{OXA-51}-like gene (Fig. 3). This analysis also indicated the presence of three main PFGE pulsotypes (Fig. 3). Interestingly, six bla_{OXA-24}-like genes of same cluster originated from three different medical centres. It meant that inter-hospital transmission of the highly resistant bla_{OXA-24}-like gene may occur in Taiwan. The MICs values of 11 bla_{OXA-24}-like $_{+}bla_{OXA-51}$-like CRAB isolates against six antimicrobial agents are shown in Table 4. Among the eleven CRAB isolates which harbored both the bla_{OXA-24}-like genes and the bla_{OXA-51}-like genes, the highest sensitivity was for colistin (MICs≦1 mg/L, showed 100% sensitive). Only 9% had MICs≦1 mg/L sensitive for tigecycline, while 64% had MICs = 2 mg/L and intermediate sensitivity, and 27% MICs≧2 mg/L were resistant to tigecycline. Besides, only 9% showed sensitivity to amikacin with MICs = 8 mg/L. All eleven isolates demonstrated total resistance to cefepime (MICs ≧ 64 mg/L), ceftazidime (MICs ≧ 128 mg/L), piperacillin/tazobactam (MICs ≧ 128 mg/L) and ampicillin/sulbactam (MICs ≧ 32 mg/L).

Discussions

Antibiotic over-use has led to an increase in the prevalence of drug-resistant strains of *Acinetobacter*. In the United States, South America, India, and China, more than 50% of *Acinetobacter* species are resistant to carbapenems [4]. At

Table 3 Prevalence of CRAB/ACB complex and OXA carbapenemase genes from four hospitals in Taiwan

2009–2013	MacKay Memorial Hospital	Taipei Veterans General Hospital	Tri-Service General Hospital	Changhua Christian Hospital
CRAB/ACB complex	83/100 = 83%	54/57 = 94.74%	40/100 = 40%	92/100 = 92%
bla_{OXA-23}-like + bla_{OXA-51}-like	77 (77/83 = 92.77%)	41 (41/54 = 75.93%)	35 (35/40 = 87.50%)	84 (84/92 = 91.30%)
bla_{OXA-24}-like + bla_{OXA-51}-like	4 (4/83 = 4.82%)	1 (1/54 = 1.85%)	0 (0/40 = 0.00%)	6 (6/92 = 6.52%)
bla_{OXA-51}-like solely	2 (2/83 = 2.41%)	12 (12/54 = 22.22%)	5 (5/40 = 12.50%)	2 (2/92 = 2.17%)

the same time, carbapenem-resistant *A. baumannii* has become the most common genospecies of the CRACB complex. Our study showed that different hospitals had different CRAB/CRACB complex ratios, but a common feature was that CRAB accounted for most of our CRACB complex blood isolates. Researchers previously reported similar results for three other hospitals in Taiwan and in the US, but different results for Hong Kong, Denmark, and Norway [16–20].

In our study, all CRAB isolates had the bla_{OXA-51}-like gene. The $bla_{OXA-23-like}$ gene was the second commonest carbapenemase gene (88.10%), and its prevalence among CRAB isolates was higher than in previous reports in Taiwan. For example, Kuo et al. reported that the prevalence of the bla_{OXA-23}-like gene was 58% in a hospital in northern Taiwan [21], while Lin et al. reported a 4.2% prevalence in a hospital in northern Taiwan [22]. Chuang et al. reported a prevalence of 7.7% in Taiwan [23]. Our data thus indicate that the prevalence of the $bla_{OXA-23like}$ gene among CRAB isolates is increasing in Taiwan. In agreement with our findings, a report from Italy showed that the bla_{OXA-23}-like enzyme was the most common carbapenemase (81.7%) [24]. Chusri et al. also reported that the prevalence of the bla_{OXA-23}-like gene was 95% in their hospital in Thailand [25]. We think that carbapenem and/or cephalosporin antibiotics overuse could be responsible for the increased prevalence of the bla_{OXA}-23like gene among CRAB isolates. Lack of strict infection control strategy is another cause. We also found that only 4.09% of CRAB isolates had the $bla_{OXA-24-like}$ gene, similar to two other studies in Taiwan (3% and 7.7%) [21, 23]. The findings of Hu et al. report are similar to our study [26]. They found that the prevalence of the bla_{OXA-23}-like gene was 93.5% and the bla_{OXA-24}-like gene was 4.6% in MacKay Memorial Hospital in Taiwan. Our study differed from Hu et al. in that firstly, we investigated the prevalence of different carbapenemase genes among CRAB in multiple tertiary centres (all > 1500 beds) in northern and central Taiwan. Secondly, we compared the MICs to imipenem and meropenem between the *bla*OXA-23-like gene and the *bla*OXA-24-like gene. Lastly, we compared the MICs of the bla_{OXA-24}-like highly resistant gene to ceftazidime, cefepime, amikacin, ampicillin/sulbactam, colistin and piperacillin/tazobactam. Although the bla_{OXA-24}-like gene accounts for only a small percentage of carbapenemase genes, it confers high resistance to carbapenems (Figs. 1 and 2). Since the occurrence of the $bla_{OXA-24-like}$ gene was so rare, we performed PFGE analysis and antimicrobial susceptibility tests for this group. We found that the $bla_{OXA-24-like}$ gene was almost totally resistant to amikacin, cefepime, ceftazidime, piperacillin/tazobactam and ampicillin/sulbactam. In our study, the isolates with $bla_{OXA-24-like}$ gene were 100% sensitive to colistin. The second recommended antibiotic is tigecycline despite the absence of Clinical and Laboratory Standards Institute (CLSI) MICs breakpoints for tigecycline.

Our study showed that the MICs to imipenem and meropenem among CRAB isolates with the bla_{OXA-23}-like gene were much lower than that for those with the bla_{OXA-24}-like

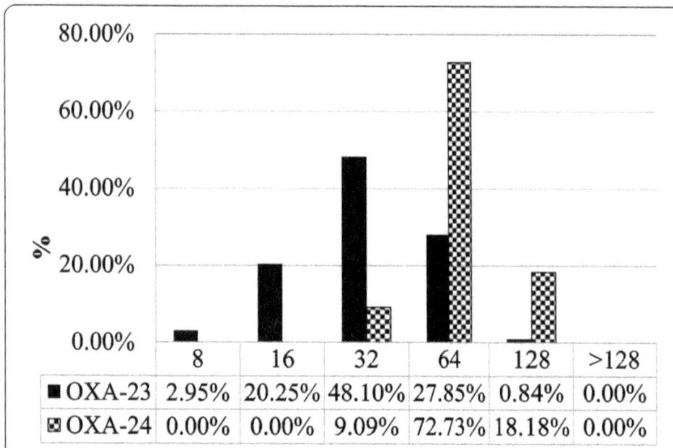

Fig. 1 Distribution of imipenem MICs in 269 CRAB blood isolates with the bla_{OXA-23}-like and bla_{OXA-24}-like genes

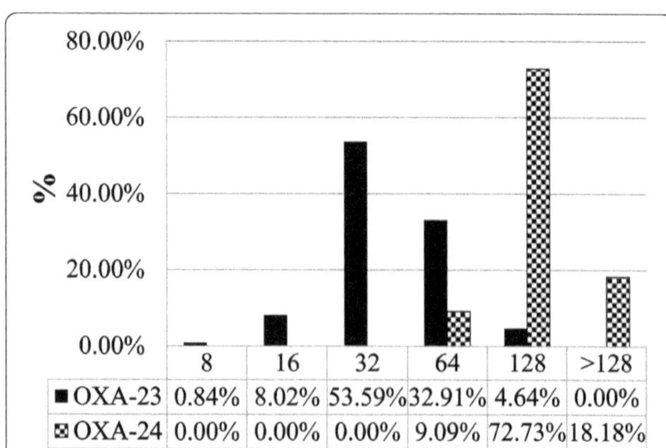

Fig. 2 Distribution of meropenem MICs in 269 CRAB blood isolates with the bla_{OXA-23}-like and bla_{OXA-24}-like genes

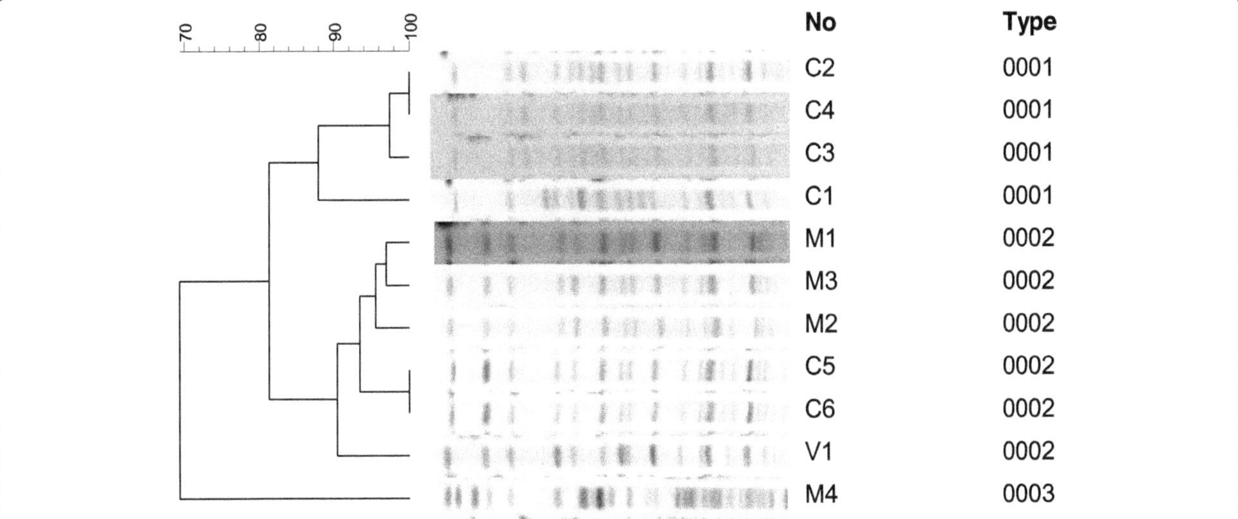

Fig. 3 Pulsed-field gel electrophoresis results of *A. baumannii* isolates that had the bla_{OXA-24}-like and bla_{OXA-51}-like genes. There were 11 distinct genospecies and 3 PFGE dominant types. The scale indicates the percentage of overall genetic similarity. Isolates with the same letter were from the same hospital. M1, M2, M3, C5, C6, and V1 with the same gene cluster came from 3 different hospitals. Letter C: Changhua Christian Hospital. Letter M: MacKay Memorial Hospital. Letter V: Taipei Veterans General Hospital

gene. Thus, the bla_{OXA-24}-like gene appears to confer greater resistance to carbapenem than the bla_{OXA-23}-like gene. We also identified 3 major PFGE types of bla_{OXA-24}-like genes in Taiwan based on ApaI digestion. Six bla_{OXA-24}-like genes of same cluster came from 3 different hospitals (Fig. 3). This suggested that inter-hospital transmission of this resistant gene could occur in Taiwan, and may help to explain the increasing prevalence of more drug-resistant strains of CRAB in Taiwan. There are two reasons that could lead to the facilitated transmission of CRAB strains among hospitals. Firstly, in Taiwan, a patient can gain admission to any tertiary teaching hospital freely, without a doctor's referral. Usually, the same patient had also visited several different tertiary teaching hospitals for different diseases. Secondly, after discharge, many patients carry resistant pathogens from different hospitals in which they were cared for back to the private nursing home or private respiratory care unit where they reside. The resistant strains are easily transmitted in these sites there if no strict infection control strategy. Therefore, we recommend additional infection control interventions for these patients to reduce the spread of resistant strains of CRAB.

What is the prevalence in other countries of the carbapenemase genes found in our study and do they have similar or differing antibiotic susceptibilities? What are the MICs of the bla_{OXA-23}-like gene and the bla_{OXA-24}-like gene to ceftazidime-avibactam, meropenem-vaborbactam or fosfomycin? Future multicenter, multi-country investigations could provide more data on the worldwide prevalence of carbapenemase genes in CRAB isolates and help the treatment of CRAB.

There were some limitations in our study. Firstly, the analysis of antibiotics consumption is not listed in our study. We could not analyse the relationship between the prevalence of the OXA genes and antibiotic drug consumption data in these 4 tertiary teaching hospitals. We were also unable to compare the relationship between the prevalence of the OXA genes and infection control strategy between these 4 tertiary teaching hospitals. Secondly, we did not perform PFGE and antimicrobial

Table 4 The MICs of 11 bla_{OXA-24}-like $_{+}bla_{OXA-51}$-like CRAB isolates for six antimicrobial agents

OXA-24+ OXA-51 (*n* = 11)	CL		TG[a]				AMK		FEP		CAZ	PTZ	AMS		
MICs	≦0.5	1	1	2	4	≧8	8	≧128	64	≧128	≧128	≧128	32	64	128
Percentage	45%	55%	9%	64%	0%	27%	9%	91%	9%	91%	100%	100%	9%	36%	55%
Number of isolates	5	6	1	7	0	3	1	10	1	10	11	11	1	4	6
susceptibility	S	S	S	I	R	R	S	R	R	R	R	R	R	R	R

Abbreviations: *CL* colistin, *TG* tigecycline, *AMK* amikacin, *FEP* cefepime, *CAZ* ceftazidime, *PTZ* piperacillin-tazobactam, *AMS* ampicillin/sulbactam, *R* resistant, *S* sensitive, *I* intermediate

[a]The MICs of tigecycline were interpreted according to the European Committee on Antimicrobial Susceptibility Testing breakpoint for *Enterobacteriaceae* spp. (MIC > 2 mg/L as resistant)

The MICs of the other tested antibiotics were interpreted according to the Clinical and Laboratory Standards Institute (CLSI) guidelines susceptibility tests on all CRAB blood isolates. Thirdly, under or over estimation of imipenem and meropenem non-sensitivity for the *bla*$_{OXA-24}$-like gene is possible due to the small number of *bla*$_{OXA-24}$-like genes (only 11 isolates). Large-scale studies throughout Taiwan are needed to address this limitation.

Conclusions

Our study determined the prevalence of CRAB, the types and prevalence of carbapenemase genes, antibiotic susceptibility among CRAB isolates, and documented that the *bla*$_{OXA-24}$-like gene showed greater resistance to carbapenem than the *bla*$_{OXA-23}$-like gene. We also found evidence of inter-hospital transmission of the highly antimicrobial-resistant *bla*$_{OXA-24}$-like gene in Taiwan. Results of this study are reliable because all isolates were all from blood cultures and not from bacterial colonization. Our findings are helpful in that identification of the type of gene associated with carbapenemase resistance could assist in devising strategies to reduce the transmission of CRAB strains between patients and among hospitals and thus reduce mortality from CRAB infection.

Abbreviations

AB complex: *Acinetobacter calcoaceticus-Acinetobacter baumannii* complex; AB: *Acinetobacter baumannii*; CHDLs: Carbapenem-hydrolyzing class D β-lactamases; CHEF: Contour-clamped homogeneous electric field; CRAB complex: Carbapenem-resistant *Acinetobacter baumannii* complex; CRAB: Carbapenem-resistant *Acinetobacter baumannii*; ICUs: Intensive care units; MBL: Metallo-β-lactamases; MICs: Minimum inhibitory concentrations; PCR: Polymerase chain reaction; PFGE: Pulsed-field gel electrophoresis; TNIS: Taiwan Nosocomial Infections Surveillance System

Acknowledgments

We thank the Microbiology Laboratory personnel who are responsible for collection of bacterial isolates in MacKay Memorial Hospital, Taipei Veterans General Hospital, Tri-Service General Hospital, and Changhua Christian Hospital.

Funding

This study was funded by the grant MMH 103-54, MMH 104-15 and MMH 104-69 from MacKay Memorial Hospital, Taipei, Taiwan.

Authors' contributions

THW: performed data analysis and interpretation, and drafted the manuscript. YSL: analysis of data, critical review of article. NYW: Performed drug susceptibility tests and performed PCR and sequencing. CPL and TRY: Designed protocols and supervised this study. All authors read and approved the final manuscript.

Consent for publication

Not applicable.

Competing interests

The authors declare that they have no competing interests.

Author details

[1]Divison of Infection disease, Department of Internal Medicine, Taipei City Hospital, Zhongxiao Branch, Taipei, Taiwan. [2]Graduate Institute of Bioengineering, Tatung University, Taipei, Taiwan. [3]Division of Infection Control, Taipei City Hospital, Zhongxiao Branch, Taipei, Taiwan. [4]Division of Otolaryngology, MacKay Memorial Hospital, Taipei, Taiwan. [5]Department of Medicine, MacKay Medical College, New Taipei City, Taiwan. [6]Department of Medical Research, MacKay Memorial Hospital, Taipei, Taiwan. [7]Division of Infectious Diseases, Department of Internal Medicine, MacKay Memorial Hospital, Taipei, Taiwan. [8]MacKay College of Medicine, Nursing and Management, Taipei, Taiwan. [9]Infection Control Committee, MacKay Memorial Hospital, Taipei, Taiwan.

References

1. Visca P, Seifert H, Towner KJ. *Acinetobacter* infection--an emerging threat to human health. IUBMB Life. 2011;63:1048–54.
2. Centers for Disease Control (Taiwan). Annual Report of Nosocomial Infections Surveillance System in Taiwan 2007 and 2014. Available at: https://www.cdc.gov.tw/english/info.aspx?treeid=00ED75D6C887BB27&nowtreeid=F0131176AA46D5DB&tid=1A8C498AF5F8AF5D. Accessed 1 Jan 2018.
3. Wisplinghoff H, Bischoff T, Tallent SM, Seifert H, Wenzel RP, Edmond MB. Nosocomial bloodstream infections in US hospitals: analysis of 24,179 cases from a prospective nationwide surveillance study. Clin Infect Dis. 2004;39:309–17.
4. Kim UJ, Kim HK, An JH, Cho SK, Park KH, Jang HC. Update on the epidemiology, treatment, and outcomes of carbapenem-resistant *Acinetobacter* infections. Chonnam Med J. 2014;50:37–44.
5. Poirel L, Nordmann P. Carbapenem resistance in *Acinetobacter baumannii*: mechanisms and epidemiology. Clin Microbiol Infect. 2006;12:826–36.
6. La Scola B, Gundi VA, Khamis A, Raoult D. Sequencing of the *rpoB* gene and flanking spacers for molecular identification of *Acinetobacter* species. J Clin Microbiol. 2006;44:827–32.
7. Woodford N, Ellington MJ, Coelho JM, Turton JF, Ward ME, Brown S, et al. Multiplex PCR for genes encoding prevalent OXA carbapenemases in *Acinetobacter* spp. Int J Antimicrob Agents. 2006;27:351–3.
8. Higgins PG, Lehmann M, Seifert H. Inclusion of OXA-143 primers in a multiplex polymerase chain reaction (PCR) for genes encoding prevalent OXA carbapenemases in *Acinetobacter* spp. Int J Antimicrob Agents. 2010;35:305–14.
9. Higgins PG, Pérez-Llarena FJ, Zander E, Fernández A, Bou G, Seifert H. OXA-235, a novel class D β-lactamase involved in resistance to carbapenems in *Acinetobacter baumannii*. Antimicrob Agents Chemother. 2013;57:2121–6.
10. Ellington MJ, Kistler J, Livermore DM, Woodford N. Multiplex PCR for rapid detection of genes encoding acquired metallo-beta-lactamases. J Antimicrob Chemother. 2007;59:321–2.
11. Poirel L, Walsh TR, Cuvillier V, Nordmann P. Multiplex PCR for detection of acquired carbapenemase genes. Diagn Microbiol Infect Dis. 2011;70:119–23.
12. Queenan AM, Bush K. Carbapenemases: the versatile beta-lactamases. Clin Microbiol Rev. 2007;20:440–58.
13. Seifert H, Dolzani L, Bressan R, van der Reijden T, van Strijen B, Stefanik D, et al. Standardization and interlaboratory reproducibility assessment of pulsed-field gel electrophoresis-generated fingerprints of *Acinetobacter baumannii*. J Clin Microbiol. 2005;43:4328–35.
14. Tenover FC, Arbeit RD, Goering RV, Mickelsen PA, Murray BE, Persing DH, et al. Interpreting chromosomal DNA restriction patterns produced by pulsed-field gel electrophoresis: criteria for bacterial strain typing. J Clin Microbiol. 1995;33:2233–9.
15. Turton JF, Woodford N, Glover J, Yarde S, Kaufmann ME, Pitt TL. Identification of *Acinetobacter baumannii* by detection of the bla$_{OXA-51}$-like carbapenemase gene intrinsic to this species. J Clin Microbiol. 2006;44:2974–6.
16. Lee YC, Huang YT, Tan CK, Kuo YW, Liao CH, Lee PI, et al. *Acinetobacter baumannii* and *Acinetobacter* genospecies 13TU and 3 bacteraemia: comparison of clinical features, prognostic factors and outcomes. J Antimicrob Chemother. 2011;66:1839–46.
17. Lee HY, Chen CL, Wu SR, Huang CW, Chiu CH. Risk factors and outcome analysis of *Acinetobacter baumannii* complex bacteremia in critical patients. Crit Care Med. 2014;42:1081–8.
18. Chuang YC, Sheng WH, Li SY, Lin YC, Wang JT, Chen YC, et al. Influence of genospecies of *Acinetobacter baumannii* complex on clinical outcomes of patients with *Acinetobacter* bacteremia. Clin Infect Dis. 2011;52:352–60.

19. Fitzpatrick MA, Ozer E, Bolon MK, Hauser AR. Influence of ACB complex genospecies on clinical outcomes in a U.S. hospital with high rates of multidrug resistance. J Inf Secur. 2015;70:144–52.
20. Wisplinghoff H, Paulus T, Lugenheim M, Stefanik D, Higgins PG, Edmond MB, et al. Nosocomial bloodstream infections due to *Acinetobacter baumannii*, *Acinetobacter pittii* and *Acinetobacter nosocomialis* in the United States. J Inf Secur. 2012;64:282–90.
21. Kuo HY, Yang CM, Lin MF, Cheng WL, Tien N, Liou ML. Distribution of bla_{OXA}-carrying imipenem-resistant *Acinetobacter* spp. in 3 hospitals in Taiwan. Diagn Microbiol Infect Dis. 2010;66:195–9.
22. Lin YC, Hsia KC, Chen YC, Sheng WH, Chang SC, Liao MH, et al. Genetic basis of multidrug resistance in *Acinetobacter* clinical isolates in Taiwan. Antimicrob Agents Chemother. 2010;54:2078–84.
23. Chuang YC, Sheng WH, Lauderdale TL, Li SY, Wang JT, Chen YC, et al. Molecular epidemiology, antimicrobial susceptibility and carbapenemase resistance determinants among *Acinetobacter baumannii* clinical isolates in Taiwan. J Microbiol Immunol Infect. 2014;47:324–32.
24. Principe L, Piazza A, Giani T, Bracco S, Caltagirone MS, Arena F, et al. Epidemic diffusion of OXA-23 producing *Acinetobacter baumannii* isolates in Italy: results of the first cross-sectional countrywide survey. J Clin Microbiol. 2014;52:3004–10.
25. Chusri S, Chongsuvivatwong V, Rivera JI, Silpapojakul K, Singkhamanan K, McNeil E, et al. Molecular epidemiology and spatiotemporal analysis of hospital-acquired *Acinetobacter baumannii* infection in a tertiary care hospital in southern Thailand. J Hosp Infect. 2017;95:53–8.
26. Hu YF, Hou CJ, Kuo CF, Wang NY, Wu AY, Leung CH, et al. Emergence of carbapenem-resistant *Acinetobacter baumannii* ST787 in clinical isolates from blood in a tertiary teaching hospital in northern Taiwan. J Microbiol Immunol Infect. 2017;50:640–5.

10

Predictive factors for multidrug-resistant gram-negative bacteria among hospitalised patients with complicated urinary tract infections

Aina Gomila[1,2,3*], Evelyn Shaw[1,2,3], Jordi Carratalà[1,2,3,4], Leonard Leibovici[5], Cristian Tebé[3], Irith Wiegand[6], Laura Vallejo-Torres[7], Joan M. Vigo[8], Stephen Morris[7], Margaret Stoddart[9], Sally Grier[9], Christiane Vank[6], Nienke Cuperus[10], Leonard Van den Heuvel[10], Noa Eliakim-Raz[5], Cuong Vuong[6], Alasdair MacGowan[9], Ibironke Addy[6] and Miquel Pujol[1,2,3] on behalf of COMBACTE-MAGNET WP5- RESCUING Study

Abstract

Background: Patients with complicated urinary tract infections (cUTIs) frequently receive broad-spectrum antibiotics. We aimed to determine the prevalence and predictive factors of multidrug-resistant gram-negative bacteria in patients with cUTI.

Methods: This is a multicenter, retrospective cohort study in south and eastern Europe, Turkey and Israel including consecutive patients with cUTIs hospitalised between January 2013 and December 2014. Multidrug-resistance was defined as non-susceptibility to at least one agent in three or more antimicrobial categories. A mixed-effects logistic regression model was used to determine predictive factors of multidrug-resistant gram-negative bacteria cUTI.

Results: From 948 patients and 1074 microbiological isolates, *Escherichia coli* was the most frequent microorganism (559/1074), showing a 14.5% multidrug-resistance rate. *Klebsiella pneumoniae* was second (168/1074) and exhibited the highest multidrug-resistance rate (54.2%), followed by *Pseudomonas aeruginosa* (97/1074) with a 38.1% multidrug-resistance rate. Predictors of multidrug-resistant gram-negative bacteria were male gender (odds ratio [OR], 1.66; 95% confidence interval [CI], 1.20–2.29), acquisition of cUTI in a medical care facility (OR, 2.59; 95%CI, 1.80–3.71), presence of indwelling urinary catheter (OR, 1.44; 95%CI, 0.99–2.10), having had urinary tract infection within the previous year (OR, 1.89; 95%CI, 1.28–2.79) and antibiotic treatment within the previous 30 days (OR, 1.68; 95%CI, 1.13–2.50).

Conclusions: The current high rate of multidrug-resistant gram-negative bacteria infections among hospitalised patients with cUTIs in the studied area is alarming. Our predictive model could be useful to avoid inappropriate antibiotic treatment and implement antibiotic stewardship policies that enhance the use of carbapenem-sparing regimens in patients at low risk of multidrug-resistance.

Keywords: Multidrug-resistance, Complicated urinary tract infection, Gram-negative bacteria, Predictive model of multidrug-resistance gram-negative bacteria

* Correspondence: agomilagrange@gmail.com
[1]Department of Infectious Diseases, Hospital Universitari de Bellvitge, Institut Català de la Salut (ICS-HUB), Feixa Llarga s/n, L'Hospitalet de Llobregat, 08907 Barcelona, Spain
[2]Spanish Network for Research in Infectious Diseases (REIPI RD12/0015), Instituto de Salud Carlos III, Madrid, Spain
Full list of author information is available at the end of the article

Background

Urinary tract infections (UTIs) are one of the most common bacterial infections [1]. Complicated urinary tract infections (cUTIs), occurring in individuals with functional or structural urinary tract abnormalities, are a leading cause of hospital admissions, hospital-acquired infections, and antibiotic use [2].

The prevalence of cUTIs is difficult to assess accurately. Data from the most recent point prevalence survey of healthcare-associated infections (HAIs) in European acute care hospitals showed that UTI was the third most common cause, accounting for 19% of estimated 3.2 million overall cases of HAIs [3]. This figure, although huge, clearly underestimates the overall cUTI incidence in Europe because it did not include patients developing cUTIs in the community and in long-term care facilities (LTCFs). In LTCFs, cUTIs occur in more than one million patients annually [4]. Aging, comorbidities, and an increasing number of invasive urologic procedures for both diagnosis and treatment have been related to this high prevalence of cUTIs in the European population.

Antibiotic resistance has become a major healthcare problem in Europe and worldwide [5, 6]. Currently, multidrug-resistant (MDR) gram-negative bacteria (GNB) pose a threat in hospitals and nursing homes [7]. According to the recent Annual Report of the European Antimicrobial Resistance Surveillance Network (EARS-Net) [8], MDR rates showed large variations across Europe, being higher in southern and south-eastern Europe than in northern Europe. Patients with suspected cUTIs are frequently treated empirically with broad-spectrum antibiotics. Developing a model that helps select patients at high risk for MDR could be useful when choosing empirical antibiotic regimens and in antibiotic stewardship policies.

Considering the lack of contemporary data on hospitalised patients with cUTIs, we aimed to determine the prevalence of MDR among hospitalised patients with cUTIs in countries with high MDR-GNB prevalence and develop a predictive model to determine the risk of MDR-GNB infections, which would be useful to select more targeted antibiotic regimens avoiding the frequent treatment with broad-spectrum antibiotics.

Methods

Study design

The COMBACTE-MAGNET, WP5 RESCUING Study was a multicenter, retrospective, observational cohort study including hospitalised patients with cUTI from January 2013 to December 2014. Data was collected from patients who were diagnosed with cUTI as the primary cause of hospitalisation and from patients who were hospitalised for other reasons but who developed cUTIs during their hospitalization [9]. This study conformed to the STROBE guidelines for reporting observational studies [10].

Setting and patients

The study was conducted in Bulgaria (2 hospitals), Greece (2 hospitals), Hungary (3 hospitals), Israel (3 hospitals), Italy (3 hospitals), Romania (2 hospitals), Spain (3 hospitals) and Turkey (2 hospitals). Patients were identified by searching for the appropriate International Classification of Diseases (ICD)-9 Clinical Modification (CM) or ICD-10 CM Codes [11, 12] at discharge from hospital (diagnoses are detailed in Additional file 1). All patients who met the criteria for cUTI were selected for data collection. In order to avoid selection bias, each hospital included 50 to 60 consecutive patients with cUTI until achieving the total estimated sample size of 1000 patients.

Complicated urinary tract infection inclusion criteria followed the Food and Drug Administration (FDA) guidance on cUTI [13], and consisted on:

- Patients with UTI and at least one of the following underlying conditions: a) indwelling urinary catheter; b) urinary retention (at least 100 mL of residual urine after voiding); c) neurogenic bladder; d) obstructive uropathy (e.g., nephrolithiasis, fibrosis); e) renal impairment caused by intrinsic renal disease (estimated glomerular filtration rate < 60 mL/min); f) renal transplantation; g) urinary tract modifications, such as an ileal loop or pouch; or h) pyelonephritis.
- And at least one of the following signs or symptoms: a) chills or rigors associated with fever or hypothermia (temperature > 38 °C or < 36 °C); b) flank pain (pyelonephritis) or pelvic pain (cUTI); c) dysuria, urinary frequency, or urinary urgency; or d) costovertebral angle tenderness on physical examination.
- And urine culture with $\geq 10^5$ colony-forming units/mL of uropathogen (no more than two species) or;
- At least one blood culture growing possible uropathogens (no more than two species) with no other evident site of infection.

The exclusion criteria were as follows: a) patients aged < 18 years, b) diagnosis of prostatitis according to FDA guidance, c) polymicrobial infections including *Candida* spp., d) polymicrobial infections including more than two bacterial species, or e) cUTI with *Candida* spp. as sole uropathogen, d) patients with uncomplicated cystitis.

If a patient had more than one episode of cUTI during the same hospitalisation, only the first episode was included.

Data collection and validation

Data on demographic characteristics, comorbidities, place of acquisition of infection, signs and symptoms of infection, laboratory and microbiology, imaging tests, management of infection including antibiotic therapy and interventional procedures, details of discharge and outcome of infection, including death if applicable, were reviewed by professionals who received web-database training sessions. For data collection, an access-controlled web-based electronic case report form was used. At each site, a screening log was kept of the patients with infections detected according to the ICD codes, detailing the excluded patients and the reasons for exclusion. To confirm data quality, study sites were monitored and audited by a contract research organization (CRO) from Utrecht, Netherlands.

Definitions

Acquisition of cUTI in a medical care facility was considered if it was:

- Hospital-acquired: if it started ≥48 h after hospital admission.
- Healthcare-associated: if it was detected at hospital admission or within the first 48 h of hospitalization, with the patient fulfilling any of the following criteria: 1) receiving intravenous therapy, wound care, or specialized nursing care at home in the previous 30 days; 2) admission in the hospital or haemodialysis ward or receiving intravenous chemotherapy in the previous 30 days; 3) hospitalization for ≥2 days in the previous 90 days; 4) residence in a long-term care facility; 5) underwent invasive urinary procedure within the previous 30 days; or 6) having a long-term indwelling urinary catheter.

We used the following categories for cUTIs:

- UTI related to indwelling urinary catheterization, including long-term, short-term, or intermittent catheterization
- Pyelonephritis with no other urinary tract modification, defined as sepsis, flank pain or costovertebral angle tenderness
- UTI related to anatomical urinary tract modification, including any urinary diversion procedure, nephrostomy or stents, or renal transplants
- UTI related to obstructive uropathy, including any obstruction intrinsic or extrinsic to the urinary tract, such as lithiasis, tumor, ureteral herniation, or prostate hyperplasia
- UTI related to other events that do not fall under any other category

Multidrug resistance was defined according to an international expert proposal by Magiorakos et al. [14], as non-susceptibility to at least one agent in three or more antimicrobial categories (extended-spectrum penicillins, carbapenems, cephalosporins, aminoglycosides, and fluoroquinolones). Extensively drug-resistance (XDR) was defined as non-susceptibility to at least one agent in all but two or fewer antimicrobial categories (i.e., bacterial isolates remaining susceptible to only one or two categories) tested for a determined microorganism.

Outcomes

The primary outcome was the presence of MDR, as previously defined.

Secondary outcomes included the following:

- Estimation of the MDR prevalence in each country and participating hospital
- Definition of the most prevalent microbiology according to source of infection
- Assessment of the resistance rate of the main GNB to the different antimicrobial classes

Statistical methods

The chi-square or Fisher's exact test was used to compare categorical data, and Student's t-test or the Mann-Whitney U test to compare continuous data, as appropriate. The quantile-quantile normality plot and Kolmogorov-Smirnov test were used to assess whether a continuous variable was normally distributed.

Predictive model of MDR in patients with cUTI

Countries and hospitals presented a non-homogeneous MDR baseline risk. To account for such variations, a mixed-effects logistic regression model to predict the risk of MDR in patients with cUTIs, including all different epidemiological and clinical variables, was built using hospitals as clusters. First, a stepwise selection method based on the Akaike Information Criterion was performed to identify variables that explained the bulk of MDR infections. Adequacy of the final model was assessed by collinearity, influential observations, and residuals. To evaluate discrimination properties, the Hosmer-Lemeshow goodness-of-fit test was used. Moreover, the bootstrapping resampling method was used to improve the robustness of estimated standard errors. Results were given as odds ratios (OR) and 95% confidence intervals (95% CI). All tests were two-tailed, and a p-value of < 0.05 was considered statistically significant.

All data were analyzed using R software (2017). R Foundation for Statistical Computing, Vienna, Austria.

Results

Patients' epidemiological characteristics and univariate analysis of MDR-GNB

Fifty-two cases were excluded due to lack of information on the presence of MDR, leaving a final sample of 948 patients. Among them, 1074 bacterial isolates were obtained.

The patients' clinical characteristics are shown in Table 1. Females comprised 56%, the mean age was 65.8 ± 18.2 years, 34.4% were admitted due to conditions other than cUTIs, 17.4% came from LTCFs, and 46% were functionally dependent. Factors associated with MDR by univariate

Table 1 Patients' epidemiological characteristics and univariate analysis of multidrug-resistance in gram-negative bacteria

	Entire Cohort ($n = 948$)	Susceptible ($n = 691$)	MDR ($n = 257$)	*p*-Value
Male gender, n (%)	420 (44.3)	270 (39.1)	150 (58.4)	< 0.001
Mean age (SD), years	65.8 (18.2)	65.6 (18.6)	66.5 (16.8)	0.526
Elective admission, n (%)	141 (14.9)	97 (14)	44 (17.1)	0.236
Admission reason: conditions other than cUTI, n (%)	326 (34.4)	214 (31)	112 (43.6)	< 0.001
Place of residency: long-term care facility, n (%)	165 (17.4)	98 (14.2)	67 (26.1)	< 0.001
Underlying disease, n (%)				
Acute myocardial infarction	79 (8.3)	56 (8.1)	23 (8.9)	0.676
Congestive heart failure	182 (19.2)	134 (19.4)	48 (18.7%)	0.804
Peripheral vascular disease	70 (7.4)	55 (8)	15 (5.8)	0.267
Cerebrovascular disease	182 (19.2)	122 (17.7)	60 (23.3)	0.048
Dementia	130 (13.7)	93 (13.5)	37 (14.4)	0.709
Chronic pulmonary disease	135 (14.2)	91 (13.2)	44 (17.1)	0.122
Connective tissue disease	21 (2.2)	15 (2.2)	6 (2.3)	0.879
Peptic ulcer	46 (4.9)	34 (4.9)	12 (4.7)	0.873
Diabetes mellitus	250 (26.4)	186 (26.9)	64 (24.9)	0.531
Chronic kidney disease	263 (27.7)	191 (27.6)	72 (28)	0.909
Hemiplegia	86 (9.1)	58 (8.4)	28 (10.9)	0.233
Leukaemia	9 (0.9)	6 (0.9)	3 (1.2)	0.673
Lymphoma	13 (1.4)	11 (1.6)	2 (0.8)	0.338
Chronic liver disease	50 (5.3)	35 (5.1)	15 (5.8)	0.637
Solid tumour	114 (12.3)	75 (11.1)	39 (15.4)	0.075
Metastatic tumour	47 (5)	35 (5.1)	12 (4.7)	0.803
Valvulopathy	88 (9.3)	69 (10)	19 (7.4)	0.221
HIV infection	10 (1.1)	8 (1.2)	2 (0.8)	0.611
Charlson index ≥ 3, n (%)	418 (44.1)	299 (43.3)	119 (46.3)	0.403
Organ transplant, n (%)	65 (6.9)	45 (6.5)	20 (7.8)	0.492
Immunosuppression, n (%)	94 (9.9)	64 (9.3)	30 (11.7)	0.270
Steroids, n (%)	68 (7.2)	46 (6.7)	22 (8.6)	0.313
Functional capacity: dependent, n (%)	436 (46.1)	298 (43.3%)	138 (53.9)	0.003
Prior UTI (within the previous year), n (%)	247 (26.1)	167 (24.2)	80 (31.2)	0.027
Prior antibiotics (within the previous 30 days), n (%)	190 (20.1)	120 (17.4)	70 (27.6)	0.001
Prior quinolone	64 (6.8)	38 (5.5)	26 (10.2)	0.010
Prior Penicillin	55 (5.8)	35 (5.1)	20 (7.9)	0.103
Prior cephalosporin	42 (4.4)	27 (3.9)	15 (5.9)	0.188
Prior Carbapenem	22 (2.3)	10 (1.4)	12 (4.7)	0.003
Prior other antibiotics	51 (5.4)	31 (4.5)	20 (7.9)	0.042
Acquisition in a medical care facility, n (%)	410 (43.2)	244 (35.3)	166 (64.6)	< 0.001
Source of cUTI, n (%)				
Indwelling urinary catheterisation	308 (32.5)	189 (27.4)	119 (46.3)	< 0.001
Pyelonephritis with normal tract anatomy	196 (20.7)	164 (23.7)	32 (12.5)	< 0.001
Obstructive uropathy	152 (16)	114 (16.5)	38 (14.8)	0.523
Urinary tract diversion	84 (8.9)	64 (9.3)	20 (7.8)	0.476

Table 1 Patients' epidemiological characteristics and univariate analysis of multidrug-resistance in gram-negative bacteria *(Continued)*

	Entire Cohort ($n = 948$)	Susceptible ($n = 691$)	MDR ($n = 257$)	*p*-Value
Other	208 (21.9)	160 (23.2)	48 (18.7)	0.139
Shock/severe sepsis, n (%)	140 (15.9)	104 (16.2)	36 (14.9)	0.635

MDR multidrug resistance, *SD* standard deviation, *cUTI* complicated urinary tract infection, *HIV* human immunodeficiency virus, *UTI* urinary tract infection

analysis were male gender, admission due to reasons other than cUTIs, residing in LTCF, dependent functional capacity, UTI within the previous year, antibiotic treatment within the previous 30 days, acquisition of cUTI in a medical care facility, and presence of an indwelling urinary catheter.

Most frequent bacterial aetiology and patterns of antimicrobial resistance

Of all bacterial isolates ($n = 1074$), the most frequent was *Escherichia coli*, isolated in 52% of samples, followed by *Klebsiella pneumoniae* in 15.6%, *Pseudomonas aeruginosa* in 9%, *Proteus mirabilis* in 7.3%, and *Enterococcus* spp. in 3.2%. Only these 5 bacteria were evaluated due to their clinical significance. *Escherichia coli* was mainly related to pyelonephritis with normal urinary tract (76.5%), while *K. pneumoniae* was more frequently associated with urinary tract diversion (22.6%). *Pseudomonas aeruginosa, P. mirabilis* and *Enterococcus* spp. were significantly related to the presence of an indwelling urinary catheter (18.8%, 25.6% and 5.8% respectively) (Table 2).

Significant differences in MDR rate occurred between the different participating hospitals, ranging from < 20% in some countries such as Hungary and Spain to almost 60% in other countries such as Bulgaria and Greece (Fig. 1a). The MDR rates by hospital varied in accordance with the country's trend (Fig. 1b).

The antimicrobial resistance patterns according to the most frequent GNB are shown in Table 3. *Escherichia coli* had a fluoroquinolone resistance rate of 39.5%, a third-generation cephalosporin (3GC) resistance rate of 24.2% and a MDR rate of 14.5%. *Klebsiella pneumoniae* exhibited the highest MDR rate (54.2%), followed by *P. aeruginosa* (38.5%) and *P. mirabilis* (24.1%). By antibiotic class, fluoroquinolones had the highest resistance rates (39.5% in *E. coli*, 56.5% in *K. pneumoniae*, 42.1% in *P. aeruginosa*, and 55.7% in *P. mirabilis*), followed by 3GC and aminoglycosides (Table 3). Resistance to carbapenems was 32.6% in *P. aeruginosa*, 19.6% in *K. pneumoniae* and 2.3% in *E. coli*.

Predictive model of MDR-GNB in patients with cUTIs

Identified predictive factors for MDR risk are reported in Table 4. The resulting equation and an illustrative example for calculating MDR-GNB risk are described in Additional file 1. The proposed model had good discrimination for MDR prediction, with a 0.80 statistic (area under the receiver operating characteristic curve) (Fig. 2). Calibration was also excellent, with a good observed/expected ratio of MDR risk by deciles of predicted risk (Fig. 3a) and by hospital (Fig. 3b).

The factors that best predicted the bulk of MDR presence were male gender (odds ratio [OR], 1.66; 95% confidence interval [CI], 1.20–2.29), acquisition of cUTI in a medical care facility (OR, 2.59; 95% CI, 1.80–3.71), presence of an indwelling urinary catheter (OR, 1.44; 95% CI, 0.99–2.10), having a UTI within the previous year (OR, 1.89; 95% CI, 1.28–2.79), and antibiotic treatment within the previous 30 days (OR, 1.68; 95% CI, 1.13–2.50) (Table 4).

Table 2 Most frequent bacterial aetiology of complicated urinary tract infections according to source of infection (sources = 948, isolations = 1074)

Source ($n = 948$)	*E. coli* $n = 559$ (52%)	*K. pneumoniae* $n = 168$ (15.6%)	*P. aeruginosa* $n = 97$ (9%)	*P. mirabilis* $n = 79$ (7.3%)	*Enterococcus* spp. $n = 34$ (3.2%)
Indwelling urinary catheterisation ($n = 308$), n (%)	124 (40.3%)	63 (20.4%)	58 (18.8%)	40 (25.6%)	18 (5.8%)
Pyelonephritis with normal tract anatomy ($n = 196$), n (%)	150 (76.5%)	25 (12.7%)	4 (2.0%)	13 (6.6%)	0 (0.0)
Obstructive uropathy ($n = 152$), n (%)	98 (64.4%)	26 (17.1%)	12 (7.9%)	11 (7.2%)	5 (3.3%)
Urinary tract diversion ($n = 84$), n (%)	48 (57.1%)	19 (22.6%)	10 (11.9%)	2 (2.4%)	4 (4.8%)
Others ($n = 208$), n (%)	139 (66.8%)	35 (16.8%)	13 (6.2%)	13 (6.2%)	7 (3.4%)

E. coli, Escherichia coli; *K. pneumoniae, Klebsiella pneumoniae*; *P. aeruginosa, Pseudomonas aeruginosa*; *P. mirabilis, Proteus mirabilis*; *Enterococcus* spp., Enterococcus species. First column include all sources of infection ($n = 948$), and first raw include the five more frequent bacteria taking as denominator the total number of isolations ($n = 1074$). All other isolates up to the total number are not included in the table. Denominators in central boxes are the total number of each row (sources)

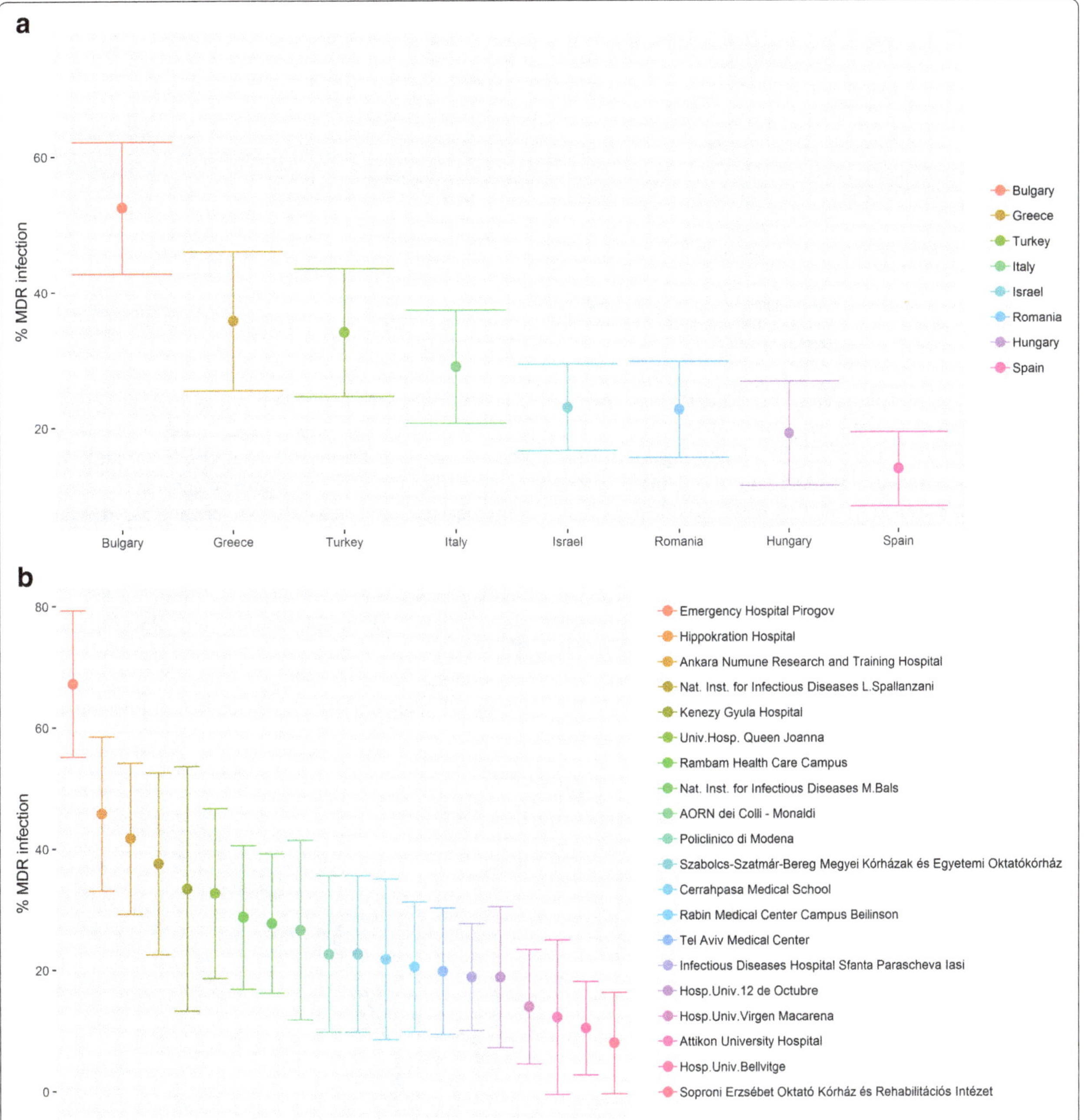

Fig. 1 Cumulative multidrug-resistant gram-negative bacteria incidence with 95% confidence interval by country (**a**) and by hospital (**b**). Figure 1 shows the cumulative incidence with 95% confidence interval of multidrug-resistant (MDR) gram-negative bacteria in complicated urinary tract infection observed in each participating country (**a**) and in each participating hospital (**b**). Hosp. Univ. 12 de Octubre: Hospital Universitario 12 de Octubre, Hosp. Univ. Virgen Macarena: Hospital Universitario Virgen de la Macarena, Hosp. Univ. Bellvitge: Hospital Universitari de Bellvitge

Discussion

This large, multicenter, retrospective cohort study of hospitalised patients with cUTIs provides a comprehensive update about antibiotic resistance in countries with high MDR incidence. In this cohort, *K. pneumoniae* had the highest MDR rate among all the GNB analysed, and fluoroquinolones had the highest resistance rates. We developed a model to predict the risk of cUTIs caused by MDR organisms, in order to avoid inappropriate treatment and help establish antibiotic stewardship policies.

In our cohort, *E. coli* continues to be the most frequent cause of cUTI, as previously observed [15, 16]. Although it was associated with low MDR levels, it showed a fluoroquinolone resistance rate of almost 40% and a 3GC resistance rate of 24%. Previous studies already described an increased resistance rate of *E. coli* to fluoroquinolones and

Table 3 Patterns of antimicrobial resistance to main antibiotic groups by the four most frequent gram-negative bacteria

	AMG-R n (%)	FQ-R n (%)	3GC-R n (%)	P/T-R n (%)	CARB-R n (%)	MDR n (%)	XDR n (%)
E. coli (*n* = 559)	108 (19.3)	221 (39.5)	135 (24.2)	57 (10.2)	13 (2.3)	81 (14.5)	2 (0.4)
K. pneumoniae (*n* = 168)	77 (45.8)	95 (56.5)	98 (58.3)	64 (38.1)	33 (19.6)	91 (54.2)	23 (13.7)
P. aeruginosa (*n* = 97)	36 (37.9)	40 (42.1)	47 (49.5)	30 (31.6)	31 (32.6)	36 (38.5)	16 (16.8)
P. mirabilis (*n* = 79)	29 (36.7)	44 (55.7)	20 (25.4)	9 (11.4)	4 (5.0)	19 (24.1)	1 (1.3)

AMG-R aminoglycoside-resistant, *FQ-R* fluoroquinolone-resistant, *3GC-R* third-generation cephalosporin-resistant, *P/T-R* piperacillin/tazobactam-resistant, *CARB-R* carbapenem-resistant, *MDR* multidrug-resistant, *XDR* extensively drug-resistant, *E. coli, Escherichia coli; K. pneumoniae, Klebsiella pneumoniae; P. aeruginosa, Pseudomonas aeruginosa; P. mirabilis, Proteus mirabilis*

trimethoprim-sulfamethoxazole, precluding their use as empiric treatment in mild and severe infections [16, 17]. Similar to our results, the Study for Monitoring Antimicrobial Resistance Trends (SMART) in the United States showed a 35% resistance rate of *E. coli* to ciprofloxacin [18]. This high fluoroquinolone resistance rate contrasts with the 20% reported by the EARS-Net in 2016 [8]. However, the rate was obtained by including northern European countries that had low antimicrobial resistance rates. On the contrary, the south-eastern countries showed rates similar to those observed in our study. Besides, the EARS-Net included only invasive isolates, a sample profile quite different to ours. MDR rates similar to our results were also observed in the Asia-Pacific region [19].

In our cohort, *K. pneumoniae* was the second most frequent microorganism, showing a remarkably carbapenem-resistance rate of almost 20% and having ileal loop or urinary diversion as the most frequent source of infection.

Table 4 Predictive model of multidrug-resistant gram-negative bacteria in patients with complicated urinary tract infection: a mixed-effects logistic regression model

Factors	OR	95% CI	*p*-Value
(Intercept)	0.1	0.06–0.16	< 0.001
Gender (male)	1.66	1.20–2.29	0.002
Acquisition in a medical facility	2.59	1.80–3.71	< 0.001
Indwelling urinary catheter	1.44	0.99–2.10	0.06
UTI within the previous year	1.89	1.28–2.79	0.001
Antibiotics within the previous 30 days	1.68	1.13–2.50	0.011

OR odds ratio, *CI* confidence interval, *UTI* urinary tract infection
Potential predictors included in the predictive model were age, sex, source of infection, place of residency, functional capacity score, personal history of myocardial infarction, congestive heart failure, peripheral vascular disease, cerebrovascular disease, dementia, chronic pulmonary disease, ulcer disease, diabetes mellitus, chronic kidney disease, hemiplaegia, solid tumor, liver disease, metastatic tumor, Charlson score, infection acquisition site, presence of indwelling urinary catheter, urinary retention, organ transplant, kidney organ transplant, immunosuppressive therapy, active chemotherapy, corticosteroid therapy, UTI within the previous year, previous 30-day antibiotic treatment (including previous treatment with quinolones, penicillins, cephalosporins, carbapenems, and other antibiotics), infection severity, neurogenic bladder, obstructive uropathy, other urinary tract modification, and chronic renal impairment

The countries with the highest rate of carbapenem-resistant *K. pneumoniae* were Greece and Turkey, while those with the lowest were Spain and Hungary. This study did not analyse the type of resistance mechanisms present in Enterobacteriaceae; nevertheless, phenotypic resistance to carbapenems commonly results from acquiring carbapenemases that affect even the latest generations of penicillins and cephalosporins, in addition to other antibiotic families such as aminoglycosides and fluoroquinolones. The European survey of carbapenemase-producing Enterobacteriaceae (EuSCAPE), performed in 2013–2014 in Europe, Turkey, and Israel, showed that *K. pneumoniae* and

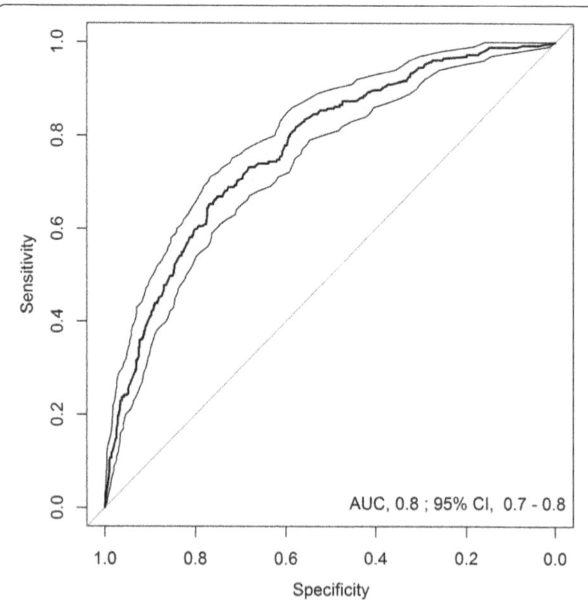

Fig. 2 Receiver operating characteristic curve of the predictive model of multidrug-resistance in gram-negative bacteria. Figure 2 shows the evaluation of the discriminative power of the mixed-effects logistic regression predictive model for multidrug-resistant gram-negative bacteria among patients with complicated urinary tract infection by the receiver operating characteristic curve using observed multidrug-resistance incidence as the gold standard. AUC, area under the curve; CI, confidence interval

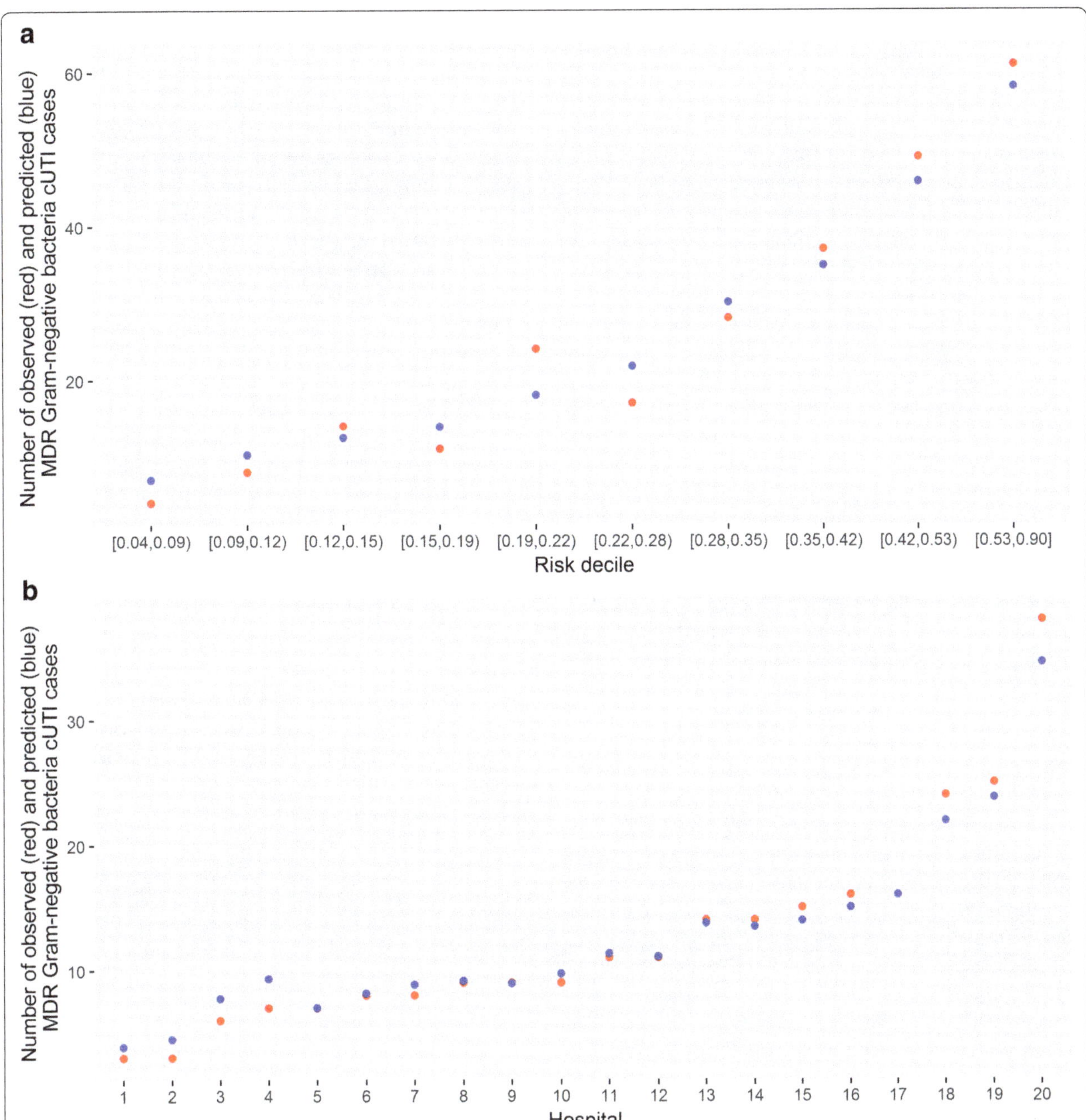

Fig. 3 Observed versus predicted multidrug-resistant gram-negative bacteria risk, stratified by deciles of predicted risk (**a**) and by hospital (**b**). **a** shows the observed to expected events by probability deciles and (**b**) shows the observed to expected events by hospital. Events are defined as multidrug-resistant (MDR) gram-negative bacteria complicated urinary tract infections. Hospitals included in (**b**) are: 1. Soproni Erzsébet Oktató Kórház és Rehabilitációs Intézet, 2. Hospital Universitari de Bellvitge, 3. Attikon University Hospital, 4. Hospital Universitario Virgen de la Macarena, 5. Hospital Universitario 12 de Octubre, 6. Infectious Diseases Hospital Sfanta Parascheva Iasi, 7. Tel Aviv Medical Center, 8. Rabin Medical Center Campus Beilinson, 9. Cerrahpasa Medical School, 10. Szabolcs-Szatmár-Bereg Megyei Kórházak és Egyetemi Oktatókórház, 11. Policlinico di Modena, 12. AORN dei Colli – Monaldi, 13. National Institute for Infectious Diseases Matei Bals, 14. Rambam Health Care Campus, 15. University Hospital Queen Joanna, 16. Kenezy Gyula Hospital, 17. National Institute for Infectious Diseases Lazzaro Spallanzani, 18. Ankara Numune Research and Training Hospital, 19. Hippokration Hospital, 20. Emergency Hospital Pirogov

E. coli produced carbapenemases, mainly KPC-type and OXA-48-like, in the countries represented in our study [20]. However, 29% of *K. pneumoniae* isolates had unidentified mechanisms of carbapenem resistance, and almost 10% of *K. pneumoniae* isolates were resistant to all antibiotics tested, consistent with our findings.

P. aeruginosa isolates showed a carbapenem-resistance rate that reached 32%. In this case, the presence of a urinary catheter was the most frequently associated factor. Countries with the greatest rates of carbapenem-resistant *P. aeruginosa* included Italy and Turkey, while those with the lowest rates were Israel and Hungary. The mechanisms of MDR in *P. aeruginosa* have been related to the production of cephalosporinases, combined with mutations that decrease carbapenem permeability of the bacterial cell wall [21–23]. The selective antibiotic pressure caused by broad-spectrum antibiotics favours the emergence of MDR strains, and once it is produced, its reversion is very slow [24].

We have developed and internally validated a clinical predictive model for hospitalised patients with suspected cUTIs that helps determine the risk of MDR-GNB infections, considering the country's baseline risk. This model may be useful in reducing inappropriate empirical antibiotic treatment that leads to poor clinical outcomes in these patients [25]. It may also help implement antibiotic stewardship programs that enhance the use of carbapenem-sparing antibiotic regimens in patients at low risk for MDR [24, 26]. The severity of infection based on physician's clinical judgement and severity scores needs to be assessed, since non-severe cUTI will probably benefit more from receiving treatment based on susceptibility testing [27]. Importantly, however, more severe cases with potentially serious consequences of treatment failure could benefit from applying our model.

The most reliable factor that predicted MDR was the acquisition of cUTIs in medical care facilities, mostly LTCFs. Most patients admitted to LTCFs are old, have comorbidities, and are functionally dependent. These patients frequently receive repeated courses of antibiotics for various reasons, including cUTIs. Thus, LTCFs have been identified as important reservoirs of MDR-GNB [28]. Besides patients having had a UTI within the previous year and having received antibiotics within the previous month, other predictive factors for MDR identified by our model have been also described by other authors [29, 30]. All of them reflect high cumulative exposure to antibiotics and, consequently, selection of MDR endogenous flora.

Male UTI is usually considered complicated due to the more complex urinary tract anatomy. This implies longer antibiotic treatments and frequent relapse of infection, resulting in repeated antibiotic exposure and higher risk of MDR [31].

The presence of a urinary catheter has been associated with a higher risk of UTI [32, 33] and infections caused by microorganisms with higher intrinsic resistance, such as *P. aeruginosa* and *Enterococcus* spp. [1]. Our study reaffirmed this observation since *P. aeruginosa* was significantly associated with urinary catheter use. The catheter inhibits the defence mechanisms of the urinary tract epithelium against bacteria and facilitates the rapid invasion of the bladder by microorganisms colonizing the device. The urinary catheter also promotes the development of bacterial biofilm, where antibiotics do not achieve significant concentrations [34].

The main limitation of this study is that the model has been validated in a group of hospitals from south and eastern Europe, Turkey and Israel and the results may not be generalizable to other populations. Therefore, further external validation is necessary to confirm our results. Also, the retrospective design and approach for identifying cases could have led to underestimate non-severe cases occurring in patients admitted due to other reason than cUTI and who developed cUTI during the hospitalisation. On the other hand, difficult to treat MDR-GNB cUTIs could have been more easily identified. The main strength of the study is its large-scale, multicenter, and multinational design including 948 patients and the case-validation system. Furthermore, the effect of possible differences in MDR baseline risk by each hospital on the main outcome was considered to create the predictive model.

Conclusions

The current high rate of MDR-GNB infections among hospitalised patients with cUTIs is alarming in south and eastern Europe, Turkey and Israel. A high MDR rate has been observed among *K. pneumoniae* and *P. aeruginosa* isolates. Our study developed a predictive model that could be useful in determining the risk for MDR-GNB cUTI, with the purpose of targeting patients at high risk with broad-spectrum antibiotics and guiding the implementation of antibiotic stewardship policies that enhance the use of carbapenem-sparing antibiotic regimens in patients at low risk for MDR-GNB.

Abbreviations

95%CI: 95% confidence interval; CRO: Contract research organization; cUTIs: Complicated urinary tract infections; EARS-Net: European Antimicrobial Resistance Surveillance Network; EuSCAPE: European survey of carbapenemase-producing Enterobacteriaceae; FDA: Food and Drug Administration; GNB: Gram-negative bacteria; HAIs: Healthcare-associated infections; ICD-9 (– 10) CM: International Classification of Diseases-9 (– 10) Clinical Modification; KPC: *Klebsiella pneumoniae* carbapenemase; LTCFs: Long-term care facilities; MDR: Multidrug-resistance; OR: Odds ratio; OXA: Oxacillinase; SMART: Study for Monitoring Antimicrobial Resistance Trends; STROBE: Strengthening the Reporting of Observational studies in Epidemiology; UTIs: Urinary tract infections; XDR: Extensively drug-resistance

Acknowledgements

COMBACTE-MAGNET, RESCUING Study Group members: Tanya Babitch, Dora Tancheva, Rossitza Vatcheva-Dobrevska, Sotirios Tsiodras, Emmanuel Roilides, Istvan Várkonyi, Judit Bodnár, Aniko Farkas, Yael Zak-Doron, Yehuda Carmeli, Emanuele Durante Mangoni, Cristina Mussini, Nicola Petrosillo, Andrei Vata, Adriana Hristea, Julia Origüen, Jesus Rodriguez-Baño, Arzu Yetkin, and Nese Saltoglu.

Funding

This research project received support from the Innovative Medicines Initiative Joint Undertaking under grant agreement n° 115523 | 115620 | 115737 resources of which are composed of financial contribution from the European Union Seventh Framework Programme (FP7/2007–2013) and EFPIA companies in kind contribution. The research leading to these results was conducted as part of the COMBACTE-MAGNET consortium. For further information please refer to www.COMBACTE.com.

Authors' contributions

AG, LL and MP conceived and designed the study. AG, JC and MP were major contributors in writing the manuscript. ES, LL, IW, CV, CV, IA participated in the design of the study and coordination and helped to draft the manuscript. CT performed the statistical analysis of data. All authors read and approved the final manuscript.

Consent for publication

No applicable.

Competing interests

Authors IA, CV, IW, and CV belong to EFPIA (European Federation of Pharmaceutical Industries and Association) member companies in the IMI JU and costs related to their part in the research were carried by the respective company as in kind contribution under the IMI JU scheme. Other authors declare no potential conflicts.

Author details

[1]Department of Infectious Diseases, Hospital Universitari de Bellvitge, Institut Català de la Salut (ICS-HUB), Feixa Llarga s/n, L'Hospitalet de Llobregat, 08907 Barcelona, Spain. [2]Spanish Network for Research in Infectious Diseases (REIPI RD12/0015), Instituto de Salud Carlos III, Madrid, Spain. [3]Institut d'Investigació Biomèdica de Bellvitge (IDIBELL), Feixa Llarga s/n, L'Hospitalet de Llobregat, 08907 Barcelona, Spain. [4]University of Barcelona, Barcelona, Spain. [5]Department of Medicine E, Beilinson Hospital, Rabin Medical Center, Petah Tikva; Sackler Faculty of Medicine, Tel Aviv University, Tel Aviv, Israel. [6]AiCuris Anti-infective Cures GmbH, Wuppertal, Germany. [7]UCL Department of Applied Health Research, University College London, London, UK. [8]Informatics Unit, Fundació Institut Català de Farmacologia, Barcelona, Spain. [9]Department of Medical Microbiology, Southmead Hospital, North Bristol NHS Trust, Bristol, UK. [10]Julius Center for Health Sciences and Primary Care, University Medical Center Utrecht, Utrecht, Netherlands.

References

1. Flores-Mireles AL, Walker JN, Caparon M, Hultgren SJ. Urinary tract infections: epidemiology, mechanisms of infection and treatment options. Nat Rev Microbiol. 2015;13(5):269–84.
2. Tandogdu Z, Wagenlehner FME. Global epidemiology of urinary tract infections. Curr Opin Infect Dis. 2016;29(1):73–9.
3. European Centre for Disease Prevention and Control. Point prevalence survey of healthcare-associated infections and antimicrobial use in European acute care hospitals 2011–2012. Available at: https://ecdc.europa.eu/sites/portal/files/media/en/publications/Publications/healthcare-associated-infections-antimicrobial-use-PPS.pdf. Accessed 8 May, 2018.
4. European Centre for Disease Prevention and Control (ECDC). Point prevalence survey of healthcare-associated infections and antimicrobial use in European long-term care facilities. April–May 2013. Stockholm; 2014. Available at: https://ecdc.europa.eu/sites/portal/files/media/en/publications/Publications/healthcare-associated-infections-point-prevalence-survey-long-term-care-facilities-2013.pdf. Accessed 8 May, 2018.
5. Levy SB, Marshall B. Antibacterial resistance worldwide: causes, challenges and responses. Nat Med. 2004;10(12s):S122–9.
6. Centers for Disease Control and Prevention (CDC). Antibiotic resistance threats in the United States, 2013. Available at: http://www.cdc.gov/drugresistance/threat-report-2013/index.html. Accessed 8 May, 2018.
7. Mody L, Krein SL, Saint S, Min LC, Montoya A, Lansing B, et al. A targeted infection prevention intervention in nursing home residents with indwelling devices: a randomized clinical trial. JAMA Intern Med. 2015;175(5):714–23.
8. Surveillance Report. Surveillance of antimicrobial resistance in Europe 2016. Available at: https://ecdc.europa.eu/sites/portal/files/documents/AMR-surveillance-Europe-2016.pdf. Accessed 8, May, 2018.
9. Shaw E, Addy I, Stoddart M, Vank C, Grier S, Wiegand I, et al. Retrospective observational study to assess the clinical management and outcomes of hospitalised patients with complicated urinary tract infection in countries with high prevalence of multidrug resistant gram-negative bacteria (RESCUING). BMJ Open. 2016;6(7):e011500.
10. von Elm E, Altman DG, Egger M, Pocock SJ, Gøtzsche PC, Vandenbroucke JP, et al. Strengthening the reporting of observational studies in epidemiology (STROBE) statement: guidelines for reporting observational studies. BMJ. 2007;335(7624):806–8.
11. International Classification of Diseases, Ninth Revision, Clinical Modification, ICD-9-CM. Available at: https://www.cdc.gov/nchs/icd/icd9cm.htm. Accessed 14 Mar 2018.
12. International Classification of Diseases, Tenth Revision, Clinical Modification, ICD-10-CM. Available at: https://www.cdc.gov/nchs/icd/icd10cm.htm. Accessed 14 Mar 2018.
13. Complicated Urinary Tract Infections: Developing Drugs for Treatment. Guidance for Industry. U.S. Department of Health and Human Services, Food and Drug Administration Center for Drug Evaluation and Research (CDER), 2015. http://www.fda.gov/downloads/Drugs/Guidances/ucm070981.pdf. Accessed 8 May 2018.
14. Magiorakos AP, Srinivasan A, Carey RB, Carmeli Y, Falagas ME, Giske CG, et al. Multidrug-resistant, extensively drug-resistant and pandrug-resistant bacteria: an international expert proposal for interim standard definitions for acquired resistance. Clin Microbiol Infect. 2012;18(3):268–81.
15. Nicolle LE, AMMI Canada Guidelines Committee* ACG. Complicated urinary tract infection in adults. Can J Infect Dis Med Microbiol. 2005;16:349–60.
16. Bader MS, Loeb M, Brooks AA. An update on the management of urinary tract infections in the era of antimicrobial resistance. Postgrad Med. 2017;129(2):242–58.
17. Bader MS, Hawboldt J, Brooks A. Management of complicated urinary tract infections in the era of antimicrobial resistance. Postgrad Med. 2010;122(6):7–15.
18. Bouchillon SK, Badal RE, Hoban DJ, Hawser SP. Antimicrobial susceptibility of inpatient urinary tract isolates of gram-negative bacilli in the United States: results from the study for monitoring antimicrobial resistance trends (SMART) program: 2009–2011. Clin Ther. 2013;35(6):872–7.
19. Hsueh P, Hoban DJ, Carmeli Y, Chen S, Desikan S, Alejandria M, et al. Consensus review of the epidemiology and appropriate antimicrobial therapy of complicated urinary tract infections in Asia-Pacific region. J Inf Secur. 2011;63(2):114–23.
20. Grundmann H, Glasner C, Albiger B, Aanensen DM, Tomlinson CT, Andrasević AT, et al. Occurrence of carbapenemase-producing Klebsiella pneumoniae and Escherichia coli in the European survey of carbapenemase-producing Enterobacteriaceae (EuSCAPE): a prospective, multinational study. Lancet Infect Dis. 2017;17(2):153–63.
21. Bonomo RA, Burd EM, Conly J, Limbago BM, Poirel L, Segre JA, et al. Carbapenemase-Producing Organisms: A Global Scourge. Clin Infect Dis. 2018;66(8):1290–7.
22. Vasoo S, Barreto JN, Tosh PK. Emerging Issues in Gram-Negative Bacterial Resistance: An Update for the Practicing Clinician. Mayo Clin Proc. 2015; 90(3):395–403.
23. Exner M, Bhattacharya S, Christiansen B, Gebel J, Goroncy-Bermes P, Hartemann P, et al. Antibiotic resistance: What is so special about multidrug-resistant Gram-negative bacteria? GMS Hyg Infect Control. 2017;12:Doc05.
24. Palacios-Baena ZR, Gutiérrez-Gutiérrez B, Calbo E, Almirante B, Viale P, Oliver A, et al. Empiric therapy with Carbapenem-sparing regimens for bloodstream infections due to extended-Spectrum β-lactamase-producing Enterobacteriaceae: results from the INCREMENT cohort. Clin Infect Dis. 2017;65(10):1615–23.
25. Zilberberg MD, Nathanson BH, Sulham K, Fan W, Shorr AF. Carbapenem resistance, inappropriate empiric treatment and outcomes among patients hospitalized with Enterobacteriaceae urinary tract infection, pneumonia and sepsis. BMC Infect Dis. 2017;17(1):279.
26. Ostrowsky B, Banerjee R, Bonomo RA, Cosgrove SE, Davidson L, Doron S, et al. Infectious Diseases Physicians: Leading the Way in Antimicrobial Stewardship. Clin Infect Dis. 2018;66(7):995–1003.

27. Eliakim-Raz N, Babitch T, Shaw E, Addy I, Wiegand I, Vank C, et al. Risk factors for treatment failure and mortality among hospitalised patients with complicated urinary tract infection: a multicentre retrospective cohort study, RESCUING Study Group. Clin Infect Dis. 2018; https://doi.org/10.1093/cid/ciy418.
28. Magiorakos AP, Burns K, Rodríguez-Baño J, Borg M, Daikos G, Dumpis U, et al. Infection prevention and control measures and tools for the prevention of entry of carbapenem-resistant Enterobacteriaceae into healthcare settings: guidance from the European Centre for Disease Prevention and Control. Antimicrob Resist Infect Control. 2017;6:113.
29. Vazquez-Guillamet MC, Vazquez R, Micek ST, Kollef-Marin H. Predicting resistance to piperacillin-Tazobactam, Cefepime and Meropenem in septic patients with bloodstream infection due to gram-negative Bacteria. Clin Infect Dis. 2017;65(10):1607–14.
30. Bischoff S, Walter T, Gerigk M, Ebert M, Vogelmann R. Empiric antibiotic therapy in urinary tract infection in patients with risk factors for antibiotic resistance in a German emergency department. BMC Infect Dis. 2018;18(1):56.
31. Karlowsky JA, Lagacé-Wiens PRS, Simner PJ, DeCorby MR, Adam HJ, Walkty A, et al. Antimicrobial resistance in urinary tract pathogens in Canada from 2007 to 2009: CANWARD surveillance study. Antimicrob Agents Chemother. 2011;55(7):3169–75.
32. Hooton TM, Bradley SF, Cardenas DD, Colgan R, Geerlings SE, Rice JC, et al. Diagnosis, prevention, and treatment of catheter-associated urinary tract infection in adults: 2009 international clinical practice guidelines from the Infectious Diseases Society of America. Clin Infect Dis. 2010;50(5):625–63.
33. Pallett A, Hand K. Complicated urinary tract infections: Practical solutions for the treatment of multiresistant gram-negative bacteria. J Antimicrob Chemother. 2010;65 Suppl 3:iii25–33.
34. Tenke P, Kovacs B, Bjerklund Johansen TE, Matsumoto T, Tambyah PA, Naber KG. European and Asian guidelines on management and prevention of catheter-associated urinary tract infections. Int J Antimicrob Agents. 2008;31:68–78.

11

Enumerating the economic cost of antimicrobial resistance per antibiotic consumed to inform the evaluation of interventions affecting their use

Poojan Shrestha[1,2], Ben S. Cooper[2,3], Joanna Coast[4], Raymond Oppong[5], Nga Do Thi Thuy[6,7], Tuangrat Phodha[8], Olivier Celhay[3], Philippe J. Guerin[1,2], Heiman Wertheim[6,9] and Yoel Lubell[2,3*]

Abstract

Background: Antimicrobial resistance (AMR) poses a colossal threat to global health and incurs high economic costs to society. Economic evaluations of antimicrobials and interventions such as diagnostics and vaccines that affect their consumption rarely include the costs of AMR, resulting in sub-optimal policy recommendations. We estimate the economic cost of AMR per antibiotic consumed, stratified by drug class and national income level.

Methods: The model is comprised of three components: correlation coefficients between human antibiotic consumption and subsequent resistance; the economic costs of AMR for five key pathogens; and consumption data for antibiotic classes driving resistance in these organisms. These were used to calculate the economic cost of AMR per antibiotic consumed for different drug classes, using data from Thailand and the United States (US) to represent low/middle and high-income countries.

Results: The correlation coefficients between consumption of antibiotics that drive resistance in *S. aureus*, *E. coli*, *K. pneumoniae*, *A. baumanii*, and *P. aeruginosa* and resistance rates were 0.37, 0.27, 0.35, 0.45, and 0.52, respectively. The total economic cost of AMR due to resistance in these five pathogens was \$0.5 billion and \$2.9 billion in Thailand and the US, respectively. The cost of AMR associated with the consumption of one standard unit (SU) of antibiotics ranged from \$0.1 for macrolides to \$0.7 for quinolones, cephalosporins and broad-spectrum penicillins in the Thai context. In the US context, the cost of AMR per SU of antibiotic consumed ranged from \$0.1 for carbapenems to \$0.6 for quinolones, cephalosporins and broad spectrum penicillins.

Conclusion: The economic costs of AMR per antibiotic consumed were considerable, often exceeding their purchase cost. Differences between Thailand and the US were apparent, corresponding with variation in the overall burden of AMR and relative prevalence of different pathogens. Notwithstanding their limitations, use of these estimates in economic evaluations can make better-informed policy recommendations regarding interventions that affect antimicrobial consumption and those aimed specifically at reducing the burden of AMR.

Keywords: Antimicrobial resistance, Antibiotic resistance, Cost of resistance, Economic cost, Economic evaluations

* Correspondence: yoel@tropmedres.ac
[2]Centre for Tropical Medicine and Global Health, Nuffield Department of Medicine, University of Oxford, Oxford, UK
[3]Mahidol Oxford Tropical Medicine Research Unit Faculty of Tropical Medicine, Mahidol University, 420/6 Rajvithi Road, Bangkok 10400, Thailand
Full list of author information is available at the end of the article

Background

Human antimicrobial consumption, whether or not clinically warranted, is associated with propagation of antimicrobial resistance (AMR) [1, 2]. This and other key drivers of AMR are listed in Fig. 1, notably widespread antibiotic use prophylactically and as growth promoters in agriculture [3].

Treatment of resistant infections is associated with higher costs for second line drugs, additional investigations, and longer hospitalisation [4]. Other indirect costs associated with AMR include productivity losses due to excess morbidity and premature mortality. These costs can be conceptualised as a negative externality to antimicrobial consumption accrued by all members of society, which are not reflected in the market price of antimicrobials [5, 6].

In addition to curative use in infectious diseases, antimicrobials are widely used presumptively, in mass treatment programmes (anti-helminths, antimalarials), and as prophylactics in surgical procedures and alongside immunocompromising treatments [2, 7]. Many other healthcare interventions such as vaccinations, diagnostics, and treatments for infectious diseases affect antimicrobial consumption, and consequently increase or decrease the risks of AMR. Economic evaluations of such interventions, however, have failed to internalise the potential costs of AMR into the analyses, leaving policymakers to intuitively consider these alongside more tangible costs and benefits in the evaluation [4, 8]. This can result in uninformed decision making, as the cost of AMR is likely to be under- or over-estimated by policymakers, if it is considered at all [4, 8, 9].

In 1996 Coast et al. argued that the omission of the cost of AMR in economic evaluation is partly explained by the challenges to its quantification [4], with extensive uncertainties surrounding resistance mechanisms, paucity and poor quality of relevant data, and other methodological challenges [5, 10]. The (mis)perception that the impact of AMR will only be felt in future years might also deter analysts from including them in the evaluation, assuming policymakers operate with a myopic view of health gains and costs. As confirmed in a recent review, very few attempts have since been made to quantify the externality of AMR [11].

Policymakers and key stakeholders, however, appear increasingly concerned with AMR, with unprecedented funding being allocated to interventions to mitigate its impact. In late 2016 the UN General Assembly held a special meeting on the topic, passing a unanimous resolution from Member States committing to adopt such measures [12]. Without enumerating the cost of AMR per antimicrobial consumed, it will be difficult to determine

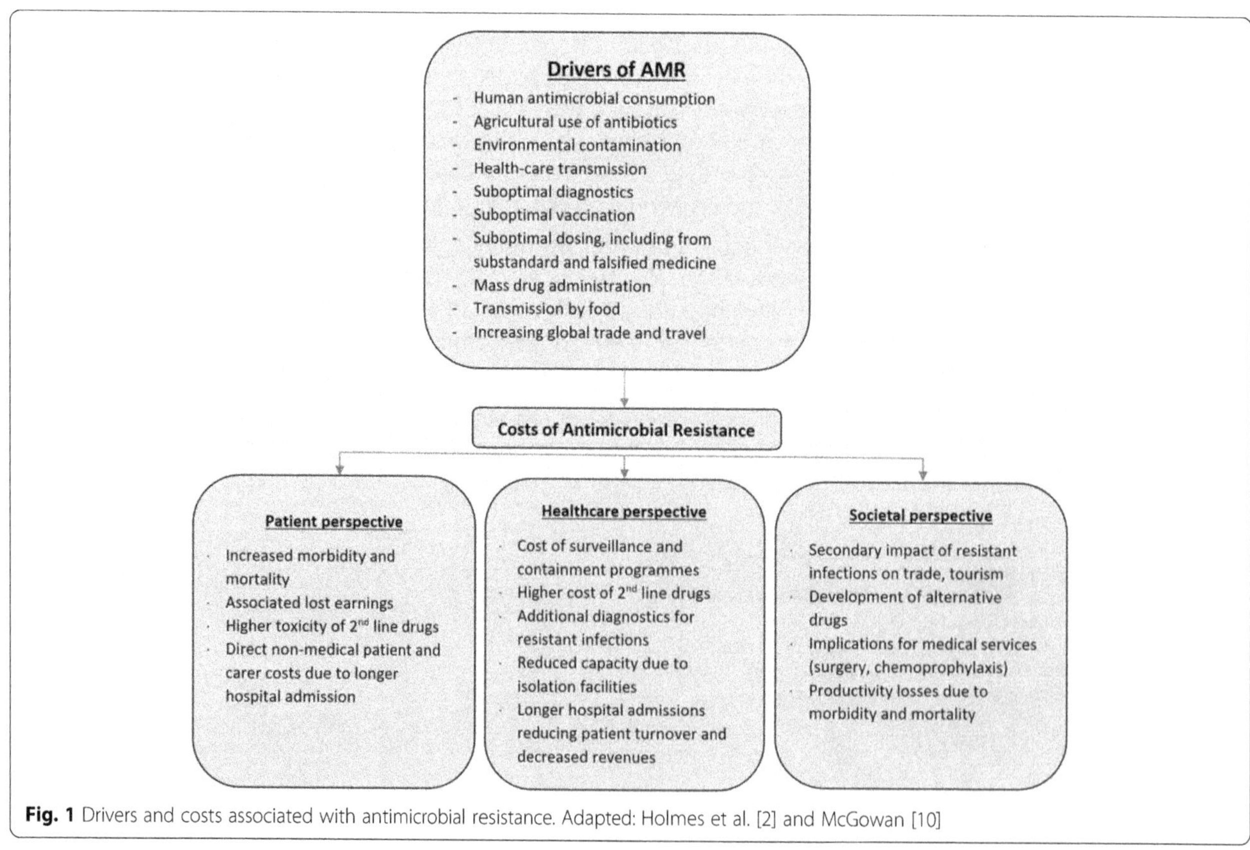

Fig. 1 Drivers and costs associated with antimicrobial resistance. Adapted: Holmes et al. [2] and McGowan [10]

the allocative efficiency of these investments, and particularly so in low/middle income countries (LMICs) with more tangible causes of ill-health to invest in.

Therefore, despite the challenges, there is a clear need for costing the negative externality of AMR that can be affixed to the consumption of antimicrobials. The rare occasions where this has been done indicate the importance of such efforts. In a German hospital setting, for example, the use of a single defined daily dose of a second or third generation cephalosporin was associated with €5 and €15 respectively in costs of AMR [6]. The current analysis produced a menu of economic costs of AMR per antibiotic consumed for a variety drug classes, stratified into LMICs and high-income country settings. The output can be applied in future economic evaluations of interventions that involve or affect antibiotic consumption.

Methods

Economic costs of resistance

The economic cost of AMR is narrowly defined as the incremental cost of treating patients with resistant infections as compared with sensitive ones, and the indirect productivity losses due to excess mortality attributable to resistant infections. We therefore make a fundamental conservative assumption that resistant infections replace, rather than add to the burden of sensitive infections, even though there are strong indications that for Methicillin resistant *Staphylococcus aureus* (MRSA), for instance, the burden is additive to that of Methicillin sensitive *Staphylococcus aureus* (MSSA) [13]. We estimate these direct and indirect costs for the following key pathogens:

1. *Staphylococcus aureus* (*S. aureus*) resistant to Oxacillin
2. *Escherichia coli* (*E. coli*) resistant to 3rd generation cephalosporin
3. *Klebsiella pneumoniae (K. pneumonia)* resistant to 3rd generation cephalosporin
4. *Acinetobacter baumanii (A. baumanii)* resistant to carbapenems
5. *Pseudomonas aeruginosa (P. aeruginosa)* resistant to carbapenems

We focus our analysis on Thailand and the United States as representatives of low/middle and high-income country settings, respectively.

Total economic loss

This is captured through the addition of the direct and indirect economic effects of AMR. The direct economic cost refers to the direct medical cost attributable to the treatment of a resistant infection as compared with the costs of treating a susceptible strain of the pathogen, and the indirect cost refers to the cost to society due to productivity losses attributable to premature excess deaths due to resistance.

Direct cost to the provider

We use the product of the number of resistant infections due to each of the above organisms, and the direct incremental medical cost attributable to resistance in the respective infections (Table 1). The number of infections and deaths per infection for the US was obtained from the Centers for Disease Control and Prevention (CDC) [14]. The unit cost per infection was obtained from a study reporting the incremental cost of resistant bacterial infections based on the Medical Expenditure Panel Survey, with data available for 14 million bacterial infections of which 1.2 million were estimated to be antibiotic resistant [15]. These costs were inflation adjusted to 2016 US$ using the US consumer price index [16].

Estimates for the number of resistant infections and deaths in Thailand were available from two studies deriving their estimates from hospital records. The first report, published in 2012, estimated the number of AMR deaths at 38,000 [17], but we opted for the more conservative estimates in a 2016 study reporting approximately 19,000 AMR attributable deaths annually [18]. We obtained the unit cost per infection from the first of these studies, which included only the costs for antibiotics. We used an estimated excess length of stay (LoS) of 5 days for all gram negative bacteria based on the excess LoS for resistant *E. coli* infections [19] while for MRSA we assumed no excess LoS as compared with MSSA [20]. We then applied a cost of $38 per bed-day in a secondary hospital in Thailand to any excess LoS [21, 22]. Costs were adjusted to 2016 US$ by converting to US$ at the year they were reported, and inflation adjusted using the World Bank Gross Domestic Product (GDP) deflator for Thailand.

Indirect cost

Mortality figures were converted into productivity losses taking the human capital approach, by multiplying them by an assumed ten productive life years lost per death, based on a study of survival post intensive care unit (ICU) admission in Thailand, which reported similar results for high income settings [22], with a sensitivity analysis of 5–20 productive years lost per death. The number of years lost was then multiplied by GDP per capita to generate the productivity losses per death. A 3% discount rate along with a 1% annual productive growth rate was applied to these values.

Resistance modulating factor (RMf)

As illustrated in Fig. 1, human antimicrobial consumption is one of a host of factors driving AMR, and

Table 1 Incidence and mortality of resistant infections per 100,000, and the excess direct cost per resistant infection

	Mortality per 100,000		Infections per 100,000		Direct medical costs per infection	
	Thailand [18]	US [14]	Thailand	US	Thailand (US$) [17]	US (US$) [15]
S.aureus	4.1	3.5	29.5	25.2	1551	1415
E. coli	0.9	0.2	13.3	3.3	956	1415
K. pneumoniae	0.4	0.5	6.5	7.8	956	1415
A. baumanii	22.4	0.2	326.9	2.3	1749	1415
P.aeruginosa	0.4	0.1	6.1	2.1	1601	1415
TOTAL	28.2	4.6	382.3	40.7		

different drug classes are implicated in propagating resistance in different pathogens. The Resistance Modulating factor (RMf) approximates the proportional contribution of human antimicrobial consumption towards the total cost of AMR. Correlation coefficients were calculated to study the strength of the relationship between consumption of antibiotic classes assumed to be implicated in driving resistance in each pathogen, and the rates of resistance observed to their first line treatments. It was assumed that drug classes that were implicated in driving resistance in each pathogen (Table 2) did so equally [23, 24]. Data points for consumption (from 2008 to 2014) and resistance (from 2008 to 2015) were obtained from 44 countries and included total consumption in both hospital and community settings [25].

The ecological association between the consumption of antibiotics implicated in driving resistance and the level of resistance was measured using Pearson's correlation coefficient, ρ_p for each pathogen p, considering the correlation between average resistance rates from 2008 to 2015 and the average of antibiotic consumption between 2008 and 2014. This is given by

$$\frac{\mathrm{cov}(\mathrm{R_p}, \mathrm{Q_p})}{\sigma_{R_p}\sigma_{Q_p}} \quad (1)$$

where R_p is the log transformed average annual measure of resistance for pathogen p (defined as the proportion of non-susceptible isolates), and Q_p is the log-transformed mean consumption of implicated antibiotics. The denominators represent corresponding standard deviations. The lower and upper bounds of the 95% coefficient confidence intervals (CI) were used in the sensitivity analysis.

Model for the economic cost of AMR per antibiotic consumed

Putting together the costs of AMR, the RMf, and the consumption of antibiotics that drive resistance in each pathogen, we established the cost of AMR attributable to the use of a Standard Unit (SU) and a full course of eight antibiotic drug classes. One SU is a measure of volume based on the smallest identifiable dose given to a patient, dependent on the pharmaceutical form (a pill, capsule, tablet or ampoule) [26]. The cost of AMR per SU is thus calculated as.

$$cAMR_d = \sum \frac{\rho_p * (DC_p + IC_p)}{Q} \quad (2)$$

where $cAMR$ is the cost of AMR per standard unit of antibiotic d consumed, DC the direct cost of treatment and IC the indirect costs for each pathogen p, and Q is the annual consumption of antibiotics assumed to be implicated in driving resistance in the pathogen p. For each drug d the costs on the right of the equation are summed up for all pathogens in which it is implicated in driving resistance, as shown in Eq. 2.

The resulting economic costs per SU of antibiotic consumed in each pathogen were then aggregated to calculate the cumulative economic cost per antibiotic consumed for each drug class in each country, including only the infections in which the particular drug class was assumed to

Table 2 Drug classes implicated in increasing the risk of resistance in each organism

Organism (Resistance)	Drug classes implicated for propagating the respective resistance						
S.aureus (Oxacillin)	Quinolones	Cephalosporins		BSP[a]	NSP[a]		Macrolides
E. coli (3GC[a])	Quinolones	Cephalosporins	Glycopeptides	BSP	Aminoglycoside		Macrolides
K. pneumoniae (3GC)	Quinolones	Cephalosporins	Glycopeptides	BSP	Aminoglycoside	Carbapenem	Macrolides
A. baumanii (Carbapenem)	Quinolones	Cephalosporins	Glycopeptides	BSP	Aminoglycoside	Carbapenem	
P. aeruginosa (Carbapenem)	Quinolones	Cephalosporins	Glycopeptides	BSP	Aminoglycoside	Carbapenem	

[a]*BSP* Broad Spectrum Penicillin, *NSP* Narrow spectrum penicillin, *3GC* 3rd Generation Cephalosporin

propagate resistance. For example, as quinolones are assumed to drive resistance in all 5 pathogens the cost of resistance per SU of quinolones would be the sum of the cost of resistance shown in Eq. 2 for all 5 pathogens.

Model outputs are also presented in terms of the cost of AMR per full course of treatment. While in reality there will be much variation in the number of SUs per course depending on the indication, patient age and other factors, we use a pre-specified number of SU per adult full course of antibiotics according to the British National formulary (BNF) [27]. The number of SU per full course ranged from 3 SU for a full course of macrolide antibiotics to 28 SU per full course of quinolones. The number of SUs per course for all classes is presented in Additional file 1: Table S1.

Sensitivity analysis

The lower and the upper bound costs of AMR are calculated using the confidence intervals of the RMf and a range of 5–20 productive life years assigned to each excess death to calculate the indirect cost.

Data entry, verification, and analysis were done in Microsoft Excel 2016. Calculation of the correlation coefficients was done in R version 3.2.2 (R Foundation for Statistical Computing, Vienna, Austria). A web interface for the model where readers can vary parameter estimates and test model assumptions was developed using R-Shiny (RStudio, Boston, US) [28].

Results

The resistance modulating factor

As shown in Table 3, a positive relationship was confirmed between consumption of antibiotics assumed to be implicated in resistance, and the average resistance rates in all pathogens, with correlation coefficients ranging from 0.27 in *E. coli* ($p = 0.07$) to 0.52 in *P. aerginosa* ($p = 0.0006$).

Direct and indirect costs of AMR

The total economic cost of AMR due to drug resistance in the five pathogens was $0.5 billion and $2.8 billion in Thailand and the United States, respectively. This is disaggregated into direct and the indirect costs for each of the organisms in the two countries in Tables 4 and 5, respectively. As an illustration, the direct and indirect annual cost of AMR in Thailand due to MRSA was estimated at $29 million and $151 million, respectively. After adjusting for the relative contribution of human consumption using the RMf, the direct and indirect economic loss was estimated to be $11 million and $56 million.

Economic cost of AMR per antibiotic consumed

With the total economic cost of AMR for each pathogen multiplied by its RMf in the numerator, and the consumption data for the relevant drug classes in the denominator, the economic cost of AMR of one SU of antibiotic for each pathogen was calculated (Table 6). Thus any antibiotic implicated in driving resistance in *S. aureus* (Table 2) would have an economic cost of AMR of $0.07 per SU in the Thai setting, and if a full course of the same drug consisted of 10 units this would imply a cost of $0.69 per full course.

As most antibiotics are assumed to drive resistance in more than one infection, the costs need to be aggregated for all relevant pathogens to obtain the cumulative cost of AMR attributable to the consumption of one SU of that antibiotic. For a broad spectrum penicillin that is assumed to drive resistance in all pathogens, the estimated cost of AMR would be $6.95 per course of 10 SU in Thailand. The costs in Table 6 were therefore aggregated for each drug class where it was assumed to drive resistance in each of the organisms. Table 7 presents the cumulative economic cost per SU and per full course by drug class.

Sensitivity analysis

The lower and the upper bound costs of AMR were calculated using the confidence intervals of the RMf (Table 3) and a range of 5–20 productive life years assigned to each excess death for the indirect cost of AMR. Table 8 shows the resulting range of economic costs for a SU and a full course of antibiotic consumed in Thailand and US. Hence, in Thailand, the best case scenario would see a cost of AMR of $2.93 per course of co-amoxiclav and the worst would be $32.16.

Discussion

Evidence-based policy draws on economic evaluation to allocate resources most efficiently [29], but this is entirely

Table 3 Pearson's correlation coefficient showing ecological associations between average consumption (2008–14) and corresponding resistance (2008–15)

Organism / resistance	Correlation coefficient (95% CI, *p*-values)
S. aureus resistant to oxacillin	0.37 (0.08–0.61, $p = 0.016$)
E. coli resistant to 3rd generation cephalosporin	0.27 (– 0.03–0.53, $p = 0.07$)
K. pneumoniae resistant to 3rd generation cephalosporin	0.35 (0.06–0.59, $p = 0.019$)
A. baumanii resistant to carbapenem	0.45 (0.15–0.68, $p = 0.005$)
P. aeruginosa resistant to carbapenem	0.52 (0.25–0.72, $p = 0.0006$)

Table 4 Direct cost to the providers due to human antibiotic consumption in each resistant infection

	Thailand					United States				
	S. aureus	*E. coli*	*K. pneumoniae*	*A. baumanii*	*P. aeruginosa*	*S. aureus*	*E. coli*	*K. pneumoniae*	*A. baumanii*	*P. aeruginosa*
Total infections	18,725	11,116	15,239	36,553	6118	80,461	10,400	24,900	7300	6700
Cost per infection	1551	956	956	1749	1601	1415	1415	1415	1415	1415
Direct cost (million US$)	29.0	10.6	14.6	63.9	9.8	113.8	14.7	35.2	10.3	9.5
RMf	0.37	0.27	0.35	0.45	0.52	0.37	0.27	0.35	0.45	0.52
Direct cost due to human consumption (million US$)	10.7	2.9	5.1	28.8	5.1	42.1	4.0	12.3	4.6	4.9

dependent on the inclusion of all pertinent costs and benefits associated with interventions under consideration. This is, to our knowledge, a first attempt at estimating the costs of AMR per antibiotic consumed by drug class and across national income brackets. We chose simple and transparent methods and restricted our assessment to the current burden of AMR, rather than more uncertain future projections, and to tangible factors including only direct medical costs and productivity losses due to AMR attributable deaths. Even within this restrictive framework there is much uncertainty surrounding interactions between antibiotic consumption, development of resistance, and its economic implications, but our underlying assumptions and parameter estimates were conservative.

The cost per SU of antibiotic differed between the US and Thailand for several reasons. First, the burden of AMR is considerably higher in Thailand, with a total of 28 AMR associated deaths per 100,000 as compared with 4.6 per 100,000 in the US (Table 1). Furthermore, the two countries had different epidemiological profiles, such as a higher burden of *Acinetobacter* associated mortality in Thailand as compared with the dominance of MRSA in the US. There were also notable differences in the cost data between the two countries; as the unit costs per infection for Thailand were only available from hospital settings, they tended to be higher than those in the US, which included both hospital and community settings. Other factors contributing to this difference are the higher GDP per capita and lower per capita consumption of antibiotics in the US.

The costs of AMR for drug classes also varied widely, driven primarily by the degree to which they were assumed to propagate resistance in the selected infections; NSPs were assumed to drive resistance only in *S. aureus*, while cephalosporins were implicated in resistance in all pathogens. The costs per full course of antibiotics were mostly determined by the number of SU per course, which for glycopeptides is high - a full course of vancomycin being 56 SU (four daily over 14 days) as compared with three daily units for a course of azithromycin (Additional file 1: Table S1).

Very few attempts have been made to quantify the cost of AMR per antibiotic consumed and internalise them in evaluations of interventions that involve or affect the use of antimicrobials. A recent study by Oppong et al. was one of the first attempts to do so in an evaluation focusing on antibiotic treatment of respiratory infections, demonstrating the decisive impact this had on outcomes [30]. Their estimate for the cost of AMR, however, assumed that resistance is driven exclusively by human antimicrobial consumption and that consumption of all drug classes contribute to resistance in all pathogens equally. It also ignored the considerable differences in the burden of resistance across countries, as apparent in the much higher burden of AMR in Thailand compared with that in the US. An earlier study evaluating the cost-effectiveness of malaria rapid tests used a similarly

Table 5 Productivity losses due to excess deaths attributable to resistant infection (Indirect Cost)

	Thailand					United States				
	S. aureus	*E. coli*	*K. pneumoniae*	*A. baumanii*	*P. aeruginosa*	*S. aureus*	*E. coli*	*K. pneumoniae*	*A. baumanii*	*P. aeruginosa*
Excess deaths	2799	597	288	15,168	270	11,285	690	1620	500	440
GDP/capita (US$)[a]	5907					57,466				
Indirect Cost (million US$)	150.5	32.1	15.5	815.3	14.5	5901.4	360.8	847.2	261.5	230.1
RMf	0.37	0.27	0.35	0.45	0.52	0.37	0.27	0.35	0.45	0.52
Indirect cost due to human consumption (million US$)	55.7	8.7	5.4	366.9	7.6	2183.5	97.4	296.5	117.7	119.7

[a] Data from World Bank

Table 6 Cost per Standard Unit (SU) and full course antibiotic consumed per resistant organism

	Thailand					United States				
	S. aureus	*E. coli*	*K. pneumoniae*	*A. baumanii*	*P. aeruginosa*	*S. aureus*	*E. coli*	*K. pneumoniae*	*A. baumanii*	*P. aeruginosa*
Direct Cost (million US$)	11	3	5	29	5	42	4	12	5	5
Indirect Cost (million US$)	56	9	5	367	8	2184	97	297	118	120
Total economic loss (million US$)	66	12	11	396	13	2226	101	309	122	125
Antibiotics consumed (million SU)	965	774	778	683	683	4797	3867	4646	3888	3888
Direct cost per SU	0.01	0.00	0.01	0.04	0.01	0.01	0.00	0.00	0.00	0.00
Indirect Cost per SU	0.06	0.01	0.01	0.54	0.01	0.46	0.03	0.06	0.03	0.03
Cost per SU	0.07	0.01	0.01	0.58	0.02	0.46	0.03	0.07	0.03	0.03
Cost per full course[a]	0.69	0.15	0.14	5.80	0.19	4.64	0.26	0.66	0.31	0.32

[a] Assuming a full course comprises of 10 standard units

crude estimate for the cost of antimalarial resistance, also showing the large impact this had in swaying results and conclusions [31]. Elbasha, building on previous work by Phelps [32] estimated the deadweight loss of resistance due to overtreatment and found a higher cost of AMR of $35 (2003) per course of amoxicillin in the US context [33].

Several studies have explored the correlation between antimicrobial consumption and resistance [34–36]. The correlation coefficients in the current study are smaller than prior estimates. For example, the coefficient for resistance in *E. coli* in this analysis was 0.27 (Table 4) in comparison to 0.74 from Goossens et al. [34]. This could be explained by the latter using 14 European countries in contrast to 44 countries from different regions in our study, and more abundant data for European countries that enabled correlating between the consumption and resistance of specific drugs, rather than drug classes as done here. The smaller coefficients imply a conservative assessment of the cost of AMR attributable to human antibiotic consumption.

Kaier et al. derived measures of association between antibiotic consumption and resistance from a time-series analysis using a multivariate regression model with different drug classes [37]. This would be a better approach for calculating the RMf, rather than the ecological associations used here. We were restricted, however, by having only 10 years of consumption data and even sparser and more heterogeneous resistance data.

There were many assumptions and limitations in the analysis (see Additional file 1: Table S2). One key limitation was the inclusion of a limited number of organisms, while consumption of the same antibiotics could drive resistance in other organisms with additional costs. The Thai estimates also focused only on the burden of AMR within hospital settings, excluding the possible excess burden in primary care and the community. These and other listed limitations result in a conservative estimate of the economic costs of AMR in our model.

Taking the human capital approach to productivity losses implies much higher estimates than would have been derived using friction costs; given the context of this analysis, trying to capture the full societal costs of AMR, this was deemed appropriate. This is essentially equivalent to the widespread use of GDP/capita as a proxy for the ceiling ratio in cost-effectiveness analyses to classify interventions as cost-effective.

The direct medical costs assigned to resistant infections were derived very differently in each country; the US estimates were taken from a recent study providing a national estimate of the incremental healthcare cost of treating millions of patients with antibiotic sensitive and resistant infections [15]. The Thai estimates used rudimentary costing methods, largely relying on expert

Table 7 Cumulative cost per SU and per antibiotic course by drug class (US$)

		Quinolones	Cephalosporin	Glycopeptides	BSP[a]	NSP[a]	Carbapenem	Aminoglycoside	Macrolide
Thailand	per SU	0.7	0.7	0.6	0.7	0.1	0.6	0.6	0.1
	per course	19.5	9.7	35.1	10.4	2.8	12.8	12.5	0.3
US	per SU	0.62	0.6	0.2	0.6	0.5	0.1	0.2	0.6
	per course	17.4	8.7	8.7	9.3	18.6	2.7	3.1	1.7

[a] *BSP* Broad spectrum penicillin, *NSP* Narrow spectrum penicillin

Table 8 Range of economic costs per full course of antibiotics using outputs from the sensitivity analysis (US$)

	Thailand		United States	
Antibiotic (Drug class)	Cost per SU	Cost per full course	Cost per SU	Cost per full course
Levofloxacin (Quinolone)	0.2–2.1	5.5–60.0	0.1–1.8	2.1–51.2
Ceftriaxone (Cephalosporin)	0.2–2.1	2.7–30.0	0.1–1.8	1.0–25.6
Vancomycin (Glycopeptide)	0.2–2.0	10.4–109.4	0.0–0.5	1.1–25.5
Co-amoxiclav (BSP)	0.2–2.1	2.9–32.2	0.1–1.8	1.1–27.4
Phenoxymethylpenicillin (NSP)	0.0–0.2	0.4–7.6	0.1–1.4	2.2–54.9
Meropenem (Carbapenem)	0.2–1.9	3.9–40.1	0.0–0.4	0.4–7.6
Amikacin (Aminoglycoside)	0.2–2.0	3.7–39.1	0.0–0.5	0.4–9.1
Azithromycin (Macrolide)	0.0–0.3	0.0–0.8	0.1–1.7	0.2–5.0

opinion to estimate the cost of antibiotics required to treat resistant infections.

The selection of drug classes implicated in propagation of resistance in the respective organisms were based on limited available evidence [24]. This might explain some apparent anomalies, like the relatively low costs for NSPs, which were assumed to drive resistance only in *S. aureus*. Another reason for this anomaly relates to the entire framework of the analysis, whereby the cost of AMR is approximated from its current (or recent) estimated burden, rather than projections of what will happen if resistance to last line drugs, such as carbapenem, were to spread, for which there are alarming early indications. Such an approach is arguably more relevant than focusing on the present burden of AMR, but it requires many more strong and contestable assumptions.

The data on consumption and resistance levels used to derive the RMf were limited to 10 years and a causal relationship was assumed. For many pathogens and types of infections, however, this is not realistic as increasing resistance could alter consumption patterns as patients and physicians adapt their behaviour in order to provide the best possible treatment in a changing environment of resistance and therefore counteract the assumed dose-response relationship.

These rudimentary estimates for the economic cost of AMR per antibiotic consumed could be improved upon in several ways in future work as better data become available. In addition to addressing the above limitations, the link between human antibiotic consumption and resistance can be disaggregated into hospital vs. community use. The model can be further extended to other organisms including parasites and viruses and their varying distribution in different health sectors and geographical locations (global/regional/country/hospital/community).

Conclusions

The estimates of the economic costs of AMR per antibiotic consumed in this analysis were high. Incorporation of such estimates in economic evaluation of interventions that affect the use of antibiotics will better portray their true costs and benefits, and could act as a catalyst for more efficient deployment of interventions to mitigate the burden of AMR. We highlight the limitations of the analysis to emphasise the need for further development of the methods, and point to the notable differences in the costs of AMR per antibiotic consumed between the two countries and within the different drug classes to encourage their adaptation to other settings as relevant data become available.

Abbreviations

AMR: Antimicrobial resistance; BNF: British National formulary; CDC: Center for disease control and prevention; CI: Confidence interval; GDP: Gross Domestic product; ICU: Intensive care unit; LMICs: Low/middle income countries; LoS: Length of stay; MRSA: Methicillin resistant *Staphylococcus aureus*; MSSA: Methicillin sensitive *Staphylococcus aureus*; RMf: Resistance modulating factor; SU: Standard unit; US: United States

Acknowledgements

We thank Ms. Nistha Shrestha for her contribution in the data compiling process. We also thank Professor Lisa White, Dr. Pan-Ngum Wirichada and other members of the Mathematical and Economic Modelling group at the Mahidol Oxford Tropical Medicine Research Unit for their helpful feedback for a presentation of this analysis.

Authors' contribution

YL and PS conceptualised and designed the study. PS, YL and BC analysed and interpreted the data. PS and YL drafted the manuscript. JC, RO, OC, NDTT, TP, PG and HW revised the manuscript for intellectual content. OC designed the web-interface. All authors read and approved the final manuscript.

Funding

This work was supported by the Wellcome Trust Major Overseas Programme in SE Asia [grant number 106698/Z/14/Z]. The initial analysis formed the basis of the dissertation project funded by the MSc in International Health and Tropical Medicine programme at the University of Oxford, undertaken by PS. PS was funded by the Weidenfeld – Hoffmann Trust for the MSc.

Consent for publication
Not applicable.

Competing interests
The authors declare that they have no competing interests.

Author details
[1]Infectious Diseases Data Observatory, University of Oxford, Oxford, UK. [2]Centre for Tropical Medicine and Global Health, Nuffield Department of Medicine, University of Oxford, Oxford, UK. [3]Mahidol Oxford Tropical Medicine Research Unit Faculty of Tropical Medicine, Mahidol University, 420/6 Rajvithi Road, Bangkok 10400, Thailand. [4]School of Social and Community Medicine, University of Bristol, Bristol, UK. [5]Health Economics Unit, School of Health and Population Sciences, University of Birmingham, Birmingham, UK. [6]Oxford University Clinical Research Unit-Ha Noi, Ha Noi, Vietnam. [7]National Hospital for Tropical Diseases, Hanoi, Vietnam. [8]Faculty of Pharmacy, Mahidol University, Bangkok, Thailand. [9]Department of Medical Microbiology, Radboud Center of Infectious Diseases, Radboudumc, Nijmegen, Netherlands.

References
1. Davies J, Davies D. Origins and evolution of antibiotic resistance. Microbiol Mol Biol Rev. 2010;74:417–33.
2. Holmes AH, Moore LSP, Sundsfjord A, Steinbakk M, Regmi S, Karkey A, et al. Understanding the mechanisms and drivers of antimicrobial resistance. Lancet. 2015;387:176–87.
3. Landers TF, Cohen B, Wittum TE, Larson EL. A review of antibiotic use in food animals: perspective, policy, and potential. Public Health Rep. 2012;127:4–22.
4. Coast J, Smith RD, Millar MR. Superbugs: should antimicrobial resistance be included as a cost in economic evaluation? Health Econ. 1996;5:217–26.
5. Coast J, Smith RD, Millar MR. An economic perspective on policy to reduce antimicrobial resistance. Soc Sci Med. 1998;46:29–38.
6. Kaier K, Frank U. Measuring the externality of antibacterial use from promoting antimicrobial resistance. PharmacoEconomics. 2010;28:1123–8.
7. Do NTT, Ta NTD, Tran NTH, Than HM, Vu BTN, Hoang LB, et al. Point-of-care C-reactive protein testing to reduce inappropriate use of antibiotics for non-severe acute respiratory infections in Vietnamese primary health care: a randomised controlled trial. Lancet Glob Heal. 2016;4:e633–41.
8. Coast J, Smith R, Karcher AM, Wilton P, Millar M. Superbugs II: How should economic evaluation be conducted for interventions which aim to contain antimicrobial resistance? Health Econ. 2002;11:637–47.
9. Gandra S, Barter DM, Laxminarayan R. Economic burden of antibiotic resistance: how much do we really know? Clin Microbiol Infect. 2014;20:973–9.
10. McGowan JE. Economic impact of antimicrobial resistance. Emerg Infect Dis. 2001;7:286–92.
11. Leal JR, Conly J, Henderson EA, Manns BJ. How externalities impact an evaluation of strategies to prevent antimicrobial resistance in health care organizations. Antimicrob Resist Infect Control. 2017;6:53.
12. Friedrich MJ. UN leaders commit to fight antimicrobial resistance. JAMA. 2016;316:1956.
13. Mostofsky E, Lipsitch M, Regev-yochay G. Is methicillin-resistant Staphylococcus aureus replacing methicillin-susceptible S. Aureus? J Antimicrob Chemother. 2011;66:2199–214.
14. Centers for Disease Control and Prevention. Antibiotic resistance threats in the United States, 2013; 2013. p. 114.
15. Thorpe KE, Joski P, Johnston KJ. Antibiotic-Resistant Infection Treatment Costs Have Doubled Since 2002, Now Exceeding $2 Billion Annually. Health Aff. 2018;37:662–9.
16. US Department of Labor Bureau of Labor Statistics. Inflation calculator. CPI Inflation Calculator. https://data.bls.gov/cgi-bin/cpicalc.pl. Accessed 15 Aug 2017.
17. Pumart P, Phodha T, Thamlikitkul V, Riewpaiboon A, Prakongsai P, Limwattananon S. Health and economic impacts of antimicrobial resistance in Thailand. J Health Serv Res Policy. 2012;6:352–60.
18. Lim C, Takahashi E, Hongsuwan M, Wuthiekanun V, Thamlikitkul V, Hinjoy S, et al. Epidemiology and burden of multidrug-resistant bacterial infection in a developing country. eLife. 2016;5:e18082.
19. de Kraker MEA, Wolkewitz M, Davey PG, Koller W, Berger J, Nagler J, et al. Burden of antimicrobial resistance in European hospitals: excess mortality and length of hospital stay associated with bloodstream infections due to Escherichia coli resistant to third-generation cephalosporins. J Antimicrob Chemother. 2011;66:398–407.
20. de Kraker MEA, Wolkewitz M, Davey PG, Grundmann H. Clinical impact of antimicrobial resistance in European hospitals: excess mortality and length of hospital stay related to methicillin-resistant Staphylococcus aureus bloodstream infections. Antimicrob Agents Chemother. 2011;55:1598–605.
21. Riewpaiboon A. Standard cost lists for health economic evaluation in Thailand. J Med Assoc Thail. 2014;97(SUPPL. 5):S127–34.
22. Luangasanatip N, Hongsuwan M, Lubell Y, Limmathurotsakul D, Teparrukkul P, Chaowarat S, et al. Long-term survival after intensive care unit discharge in Thailand: a retrospective study. Crit Care. 2013;17:R219.
23. MacAdam H, Zaoutis TE, Gasink LB, Bilker WB, Lautenbach E. Investigating the association between antibiotic use and antibiotic resistance : impact of different methods of categorising prior antibiotic use. Int J Antimicrob Agents. 2006;28:325–32.
24. Tacconelli E. Antimicrobial use: risk driver of multidrug resistant microorganisms in healthcare settings. Curr Opin Infect Dis. 2009;22:352–8.
25. The Center for Disease Dynamics Economics and Policy. ResistanceMap beta. http://resistancemap.cddep.org. Accessed 22 Jun 2016.
26. Van Boeckel TP, Gandra S, Ashok A, Caudron Q, Grenfell BT, Levin SA, et al. Global antibiotic consumption 2000 to 2010 : an analysis of national pharmaceutical sales data. Lancet Infect Dis. 2014;14:742–50.
27. NICE National Institute for Health and Care Excellence. British National Formulary. https://bnf.nice.org.uk/drug/. Accessed 3 Aug 2016.
28. AMR Costing App. https://moru.shinyapps.io/amrcost/. Accessed 9 Feb 2018.
29. Chisholm D, Evans DB. Economic evaluation in health: saving money or improving care? J Med Econ. 2007;10:325–37.
30. Oppong R, Smith RD, Little P, Verheij T, Butler CC, Goossens H, et al. Cost effectiveness of amoxicillin for lower respiratory tract infections in primary care: an economic evaluation accounting for the cost of antimicrobial resistance. Br J Gen Pract. 2016;66:e633–9.
31. Lubell Y, Reyburn H, Mbakilwa H, Mwangi R, Chonya S, Whitty CJM, et al. The impact of response to the results of diagnostic tests for malaria: cost-benefit analysis. BMJ. 2008;336:202–5.
32. Phelps CE. Bug / drug resistance sometimes less is more. Med Care. 1989;27:194–203.
33. Elbasha EH. Deadweight loss of bacterial resistance due to overtreatment. Health Econ. 2003;12:125–38.
34. Goossens H, Ferech M, Vander Stichele R, Elseviers M. Outpatient antibiotic use in Europe and association with resistance: a cross-national database study. Lancet. 2005;365:579–87.
35. Albrich WC, Monnet DL, Harbarth S. Antibiotic selection pressure and resistance in Streptococcus pneumoniae and Streptococcus pyogenes. Emerg Infect Dis. 2004;10:514–7.
36. Van De Sande-Bruinsma N, Grundmann H, Verloo D, Tiemersma E, Monen J, Goossens H, et al. Antimicrobial drug use and resistance in Europe. Emerg Infect Dis. 2008;14:1722–30.
37. Kaier K, Hagist C, Frank U, Conrad A, Meyer E. Two time-series analyses of the impact of antibiotic consumption and alcohol-based hand disinfection on the incidences of nosocomial methicillin-resistant Staphylococcus aureus infection and Clostridium difficile infection. Infect Control Hosp Epidemiol. 2009;30:346–53.

12

Antibiotic resistance, virulence factors and genotyping of Uropathogenic *Escherichia coli* strains

Maryam Raeispour and Reza Ranjbar*

Abstract

Background: The way of treating different types of infectious diseases is really important. Using genotyping method, we can determine the genetic relatedness between the organisms with different resistance profile from different sources. The aim of this study was to determine antibiotic resistance and genotyping of uropathogenic *Escherichia coli* (UPEC) strains using pulsed field gel electrophoresis (PFGE).

Method: *Escherichia coli* (*E. coli*) strains were recovered from the patients with urinary tract infections (UTI) whom admitted in several major hospitals in Tehran. Antibiotic susceptibility testing was done according to CLSI guideline. The present of some virulence factor have been detected using PCR assay. Genotyping of the strains was performed by PFGE and all PFGE profiles were subjected to data processing.

Result: In total, 60 *E. coli* strains were subjected to the study. Most of *E. coli* isolates were resistant to cefepime (100%) and cephalothin (74%) and susceptible to imipenem (100%), vancomycin (100%) and doxycycline (100%). Among the UPEC isolates the prevalence of fimbriae type I (*fimH*), hemolysin (*hlyA*) and aerobactin (*aer*) genes were 89%, 60% and 90%, respectively. The PFGE differentiated *E. coli* strains into 33 different genetic clusters. Majority (30%) of them including PFGE type 11 generated 15 bands, while PFGE type 2 was the lowest (2%) prevalent group with 9 bands.

Conclusion: The result showed that the antibiotic resistance is escalating rapidly. UPEC strains causing infections are more likely to harbor certain virulence genes. Our finding also showed *E. coli* strains isolated under the study were belonged to the diverse clones.

Keywords: *Escherichia coli*, PFGE, UTIs, Virulence genes

Background

One of the most common bacterial infections is urinary tract infection (UTI) that accounts for a considerable amount of morbidity and high medical costs and also can lead to significant mortality. While UTI affects men and women it's most common among women except at early infancy. Approximately 90% of all UTIs in young women are caused by *E. coli* which is a gram-negative, rod-shaped bacterium and a member of the normal intestinal microorganism. Virulence factors are important in severe UTIs [1, 2]. Some of the virulence genes of UPEC strains are aerobactin (*aer*), P fimbriae (*pap*), hemolysin (*hly*), type 1 fimbriae, afimbrial adhesin I (*afa* I), cytotoxic necrotizing factor 1 (*cnf* 1), S fimbriae (*sfa*), adhesins and fimbriae. The other virulence genes that have a role in pathogenecity of organism are: *kpsMT, ompT, usp, iroN, iha, set 1, astA*, group II capsule synthesis; *sfa*/*foc*, S and *F1C*fimbriae; *iutA, traT*, serum resistance; and *fimH* [3–5].

In the past recent years, the spectrum and frequency of antimicrobial-resistant UTIs have raised [6, 7]. The resistant patterns of bacteria have been varied by geographical location and by time so periodically testing of antibiotic resistant is really important. *E. coli* strains are the leading causes of serious bacterial infections in health society and very different antibiotic patterns have been reported based on the source [8, 9]. Mobile genetic elements including transposons, plasmids and integrons contribute to lateral transfer of resistance genes in

* Correspondence: ranjbarre@gmail.com
Molecular Biology Research Center, Systems Biology and Poisonings Institute, Baqiyatallah University of Medical Sciences, Tehran, Iran

bacteria. *E. coli* can be intrinsically resistant to some special antibiotics and have gens which are responsible for resistance to some of antibiotics such as aminoglycosides, flouroquinolones and β-lactamas [10, 11].

Several studies on various pathotypes of Iranian *E. coli* isolates have done in which a high level of virulence and antibiotic resistance genes have been reported [1, 12–14].

For identification of bacterial infection sources, it is influential to establish relationships between different isolates of bacteria. It helps to determine the contamination sources, gaining insights into the distribution of pathogens, understanding how much pathogens changed over time, to choose the best treatment of diseases, and reducing the risks of antibiotic resistances [15]. Many different typing methods have been established that have been very useful in describing the epidemiology of infectious diseases. The earlier methods were based on phenotypic typing while modern methods have been based on genome components of bacteria [16, 17]. DNA-based approaches have become potentially powerful methods in microbial typing. These techniques consist of analysis of plasmid profiles [18], RFLP (Restriction Fragment Length Polymorphism) [19], Ribotyping [20, 21], MLST (Multi Locus Sequence Typing) [22], VNTR (Variable Number Tandem Repeat) [23, 24], RAPD (Randomly Amplification of Polymorphic DNA) [25, 26], AP-PCR (Arbitrary Pprimed PCR) [27], Rep-PCR (Repetitive extragenic palindromic) [28], ERIC-PCR (Enterobacterial Repetitive Intergenic Consensus) [29, 30], Microarray [5, 31] and PFGE (Pulsed-Field Gel electrophoresis) [32, 33].

The characteristic of typing methods such as discriminatory power, ease of performance, reproducibility, ease of interpretation, and the cost is really important to gain appropriate results. A broad range of methods used to type *E. coli* but PFGE is a commonly used technique for generating DNA fingerprints [28, 34]. PFGE is nominated as the gold standard technique for typing foodborne bacteria [35, 36]. We aimed the current study to determine antibiotic resistance and genotyping of uropathogenic *E. coli* strains isolated from the patients with urinary tract infections in Tehran.

Method

The uropathogenic *E. coli* isolates were collected from several major hospitals in Tehran during May to November 2016. The bacterial isolates were identified as *E. coli* by standard microbiological and biochemical method. The growth of a single colony with counts> 10^5 colony forming unit/ml were considered as positive urine cultures. All *E. coli* isolates were inoculated on MacConkey agar then incubated for 24 h at 37 °C. The typical purple colonies were then streaked on Eosin Methylene Blue (EMB) agar plates and were incubated for 20 h at 37 °C. Those colonies with metallic green morphology were subjected to biochemical tests, including hydrogen sulfide, citrate, urease and indol [13].

Antimicrobial susceptibility testing

Antimicrobial susceptibility was tested by the Kirby-Bauer disk diffusion method. Antimicrobial agents tested were amikacin (30 μg), cephalexin (10 μg), ciprofloxacin (5 μg), cefalothin (30 μg), cefexime (5 μg), cefpodoxime (10 μg), cephazolin (30 μg), cefepime (30 μg), doxycycline (10 μg), nitrofurantoin (30 μg), gentamycine (10 μg), nalidixic acid (30 μg), norfloxacin (5 μg), cotrimoxazole (30 μg), tetracycline (30 μg), imipenem (10 μg), and vancomycin (30 μg). These antibiotics belong to β-lactamas, glycopeptides, aminoglycosides, quinolones and tetracycline classes [10]. The resistance to above mentioned antibiotics was determined according to the breakpoint proposed by CLSI [37]. For quality-control *E. coli* ATCC®25,922™ was used.

Detection of virulence factor

Genomic DNA of UPEC isolates were extracted using DNA extraction kit (AccuPrep® Genomic DNA Extraction Kit, Bioneer, South Korea), after preparation cultured cells with PBS buffer. Binding buffer (GC) was mixed with the samples and incubated for 10 min at 60 ° C then washing buffers were added and samples were spined according to the manufacturer's instructions. Then elution buffer was added to the genomic DNA and stored at − 20 °C.

All UTI isolates were screened for carriage of *fimH*, *hlyA* and *aer* virulence factors. PCR assays were used to reveal the prevalence of these virulence genes using specific primers. The amplification reaction were carried out in a final volume of 25 μl containing 200 μM of deoxynucleotide triphosphates (dNTPs), 2.5 μl of 10X PCR buffer, 0.7 mg/μl $MgCl_2$, 0.6 units of Taq polymerase, 10 pmol of each primer, and 2 μl of sample DNA. The PCR products were analyzed with gel electrophoresis on 2% agarose, followed by staining with EtBr solution after 1 h under 80v and visualized using an ultraviolet (UV) transilluminator. Primer sequences and PCR machine conditions are shown in Table 1.

Pulsed field gel electrophoresis procedure

All the PFGE steps were accomplished following the CDC-standardized procedure used by all PulsedNet laboratories with some changes [38]. Colonies from an overnight culture were suspended in TE buffer (5 mmol/liter Tris-HCL [pH 8.0] 1 M, 10 mmol/liter EDTA 0.5 M) at a wavelength of 600 nm (OD = 0.8–1.2). Then proteinase K, 20 mg/ml added to suspension and mixed with sodium dodecyl sulphate and 1% melted SeaKem Gold agarose and pipette into plug moulds and left at 4 ° C. After solidation, each plug was transferred to a falcon

Table 1 Primers and cycling conditions for the PCR assays

Gene	Primer sequence	Size (bp)	Cycling condition	Reference
hlyA	F: AACAAGGATAAGCACTGTTCTGGCT R: ACCATATAAGCGGTCATTCCCGTCA	1177	1 cycle of 95 °C for 5 min;30 cycles of 94 °C for 1 min, 64 °C for 1 min, 72 °C for 1 min; 72 °C for 8 min final extension	[58]
FimH	F:GAGAAGAGGTTTGATTTAACTTATTG R: AGAGCCGCTGTAGAACTGAGG	559	1 cycle of 95 °C for 5 min;30 cycles of 94 °C for 1 min, 60 °C for 1 min, 72 °C for 1 min; 72 °C for 8 min final extension	[60]
aer	F: GCTGGGCAGCAAACTGATAACTCTC R: CATCAAGCTGTTTGTTCGTCCGCCG	602	1 cycle of 95 °C for 5 min;30 cycles of 94 °C for 1 min, 62 °C for 1 min, 72 °C for 1 min; 72 °C for 8 min final extension	[58]

containing 5 ml cell lysis buffers (2.5 ml Tris-HCL [pH 8.0] 1 M, 5 ml EDTA 0.5 M, 5 ml Sarcosyl 10%) and proteinase K and then incubate overnight at 52 °C. The plugs were washed three times for 30 min in sterile distilled water and twice for 30 min in TE buffer at 52 °C on an orbital shaker. 2 mm of *E. coli* colonies plugs were digested overnight with 50 U of *Xba*I restriction enzyme. And *Salmonella* Braenderup H2812 was used as size standard which after digestion with *Xba*I generates fragments ranging from 20.5 to 1135 kb and cover the fragment ranges generated by *E. coli* strains [39].

After restriction digestion the plugs were placed in refrigerator for 30 min. PFGE was performed with the CHEF DR-III (Bio-Rad Laboratories) system using a 1% Ultra pure agarose gel in 2 l 0.5 TBE (Tris-base, EDTA, boric acid). The electrophoresis condition were set as follows: initial switch time, 2.2 s, final switch time, 54.2 s, run time 20 h, include angle 120°, gradient, 6 V/cm, temperature, 14 °C. The gel was stained for 30 min with EthBr, 0.5 mg/ml and then the fingerprinting profile was observed by Uvitec system by illuminated UV wave to the gel.. The PFGE profiles were compared using In silico stimulation of molecular experiment with a dice similarity coefficient and UPGMA analysis to create the dendrogram. To analyze genetic relatedness, cut off line at 85% was considered [38–41].

Results

Bacterial isolates and antibiotic susceptibility testing

Over 6-month period, a total of 60 *E. coli* strains were isolated and subjected to this study. Distribution of the isolates based on patient's gender and location in Tehran is shown in Table 2. As it is represented in Fig. 3, these 60 isolates identified to be multidrug resistant (MDR). The different prevalence of each antibiotic resistance was as follows: cefepime (100%), cefalothin (74%), cefpodexime (67%), nalidixic acid (63%), cotrimoxazole (54%), cefixime (50%), cephazolin (50%), tetracycline (50%), norfloxacin (43%), ciprofloxacin (34%), cephalexin (30%), gentamycin (19%), nitrofurantoin (10%), amikacin (8%), doxycycline (0%), imipenem (0%), and vancomycin (0%). (Table. 2).

PCR assay

The PCR amplified successfully *aer, fimH* and *hlyA* genes with 602 bp, 559 bp and 1177 bp amplicons respectively. The PCR results of some representative isolates are shown in Fig. 1. Among 60 UPEC isolates, *aer* was the most prevalent virulence gene ($n = 54$, 90%) followed by *fimH* ($n = 53$, 89%) and *hlyA* ($n = 36$, 60%). All of the isolates carried at least one virulence gene.

Pulsed field gel electrophoresis

After observing PFGE profiles fingerprinting (Fig. 2), clustering analysis performed and 33 PFGE pulsotypes were detected for *E. coli* isolates as seen in the dandrogram (Fig. 3). Eighteen clusters including (pulsotypes 2,3,9,11,16,17 and 21) were consist of only one strain, 9 clusters including (pulsotypes 7,14,29 and 31) consist of 2 strains, 2 clusters including (pulsotypes13and 26) consist of 3 strains, 2 clusters including (pulsotypes1 and 19) consist of 4 strains, and 2 clusters including (pulsotypes 12 and 22) consist of 5 strains. Distribution of the pulsutypes is shown in Table 2.

Discussion

E. coli is considered as the cause of 80–90% of UTIs that today is one of the most common bacterial infections [42]. Because of unreasonable use of antibiotics, the bacterial resistance has been raised. In this study, we reported a high value of multidrug resistance among the uropathogenic *E. coli* strains. Resistance to cefepime was very high (100%) and after that the strains were resistant to cefalothin (74%) and cefpodoxime (67%). Also high sensitivity to imipenem, vancomycin and doxycycline (100%), amikacin (92%) and nitrofurantoin (90%) have been observed. High levels of susceptibility to imipenem, amikacin, nitrofurantoin and also high levels of resistance to tetracycline and ampicilline have been reported in other studies in Iran [6, 13].

Our results in some cases are consistent with those reported by Niranjan and Malini. They evaluated antibiotic resistance of 119 *E. coli* isolated from UTI patients. The isolates were resistant to ampicillin (88.4%), amoxicillin (74.4%), norfloxacin (74.2%), ceftiriaxone (71.4%) and sensitive to amikacin (82.6%), nitrofurantoin (82.1%) and imipenem (98.9%) [43].

No resistance to vancomycin, imipenem and doxycycline was observed among the studied isolates. In previous studies a high sensitivity to imipenem has been also

Table 2 Date of isolation, age, sex and location of patients admitted to the hospital; isolates divided in different pulsotype

Pulsotype	Isolation(NO.)	Sex	Age(year)	Patient location	Date of isolation
1	13u	F	27	North	30/05/2016
	8u	F	79	North	18/05/2016
	84u	F	52	Northeast	26/05/2016
	94u	F	20	Northeast	18/07/2016
2	30u	F	41	West	22/11/2016
3	4u	F	24	Center	25/11/2016
4	6u	F	63	West	10/10/2016
5	21u	M	55	West	06/08/2016
	23u	M	62	West	23/08/2016
6	7u	F	26	North	11/07/2016
7	28u	F	52	Center	14/09/2016
	9u	F	87	Center	23/10/2016
8	59u	F	34	East	18/05/2016
	73u	F	56	East	13/10/2016
9	72u	F	78	North	18/09/2016
10	100u	F	74	East	06/08/2016
	19u	M	71	Northeast	10/08/2016
11	71u	M	68	Center	18/05/2016
12	10u	M	47	Northwest	03/06/2016
	5u	M	56	Northwest	01/07/2016
	82u	F	48	Northwest	29/06/2016
	24u	F	39	North	03/07/2016
	31u	F	72	North	03/07/2016
13	12u	F	68	North	05/09/2016
	32u	M	70	West	12/09/2016
	11u	F	29	West	03/09/2016
14	62u	M	82	East	28/10/2016
	81u	M	74	Northeast	20/10/2016
15	58u	M	68	North	16/11/2016
	60u	F	50	North	11/11/2016
16	70u	F	73	Center	11/07/2016
17	79u	F	59	Northwest	18/07/2016
18	83u	F	54	Northwest	26/05/2016
19	20u	M	71	Northwest	18/09/2016
	89u	M	67	North	30/07/2016
	92u	F	49	Center	22/08/2016
	97u	F	59	Center	10/08/2016
20	14u	M	64	Northeast	06/08/2016
21	80u	F	40	East	11/10/2016
22	16u	F	24	Northeast	28/10/2016
	18u	M	66	Northeast	18/10/2016
	74u	F	27	Northeast	23/09/2016
	76u	F	46	West	22/10/2016
	25u	F	38	West	18/10/2016

Table 2 Date of isolation, age, sex and location of patients admitted to the hospital; isolates divided in different pulsotype *(Continued)*

Pulsotype	Isolation(NO.)	Sex	Age(year)	Patient location	Date of isolation
23	86u	M	53	West	24/05/2016
	87u	F	36	North	26/05/2016
	93u	M	83	North	26/05/2016
24	15u	F	27	Center	25/08/2016
25	99u	F	70	Center	14/08/2016
26	17u	F	36	West	25/09/2016
	26u	M	68	West	23/09/2016
27	78u	F	24	Center	11/10/2016
28	2u	F	77	Northeast	25/05/2016
	3u	M	68	Northeast	17/08/2016
29	35u	F	74	Center	15/07/2016
30	88u	F	31	Center	11/07/2016
31	61u	F	26	North	24/06/2016
	98u	F	47	North	13/06/2016
32	77u	F	33	Center	11/10/2016
33	85u	F	33	West	30/05/2016

reported [43–46]. These antibiotics seems to be a good choice for the treatment of UTI caused by *E. coli* but it should be considered that unlimited use of these antibiotics can gradually lead to increasing antibiotic resistant. Shakya, did a research on antibiotic resistance of *E. coli* strains isolated from Indian children. The results showed that the strains have been resistant to nalidixic acid (45%), tetracycline (37%), ampicillin (37%), trimethoprim/sulfamethoxazole (29%), amoxicillin/clavulanic acid (29%), imipenem (0.0%) [45].

Susceptibility to amikacin in our study was high as it was in studies carried out in other parts of the world [43, 46, 47]. However, the resistance to tetracycline in our study was 50% while in another study it was reported to be 26% [48].

In the present study, it has been shown that resistant to gentamicin (19%) and nitrofurantoein (10%) was low among *E. coli* isolates and it was partially similar to the study reported by Adib and his colleagues. They showed that 54.16% of the isolates were resistant to nalidixic acid, 36.45% to gentamycin, 71% to cefazolin, 29.18% to ciprofloxacin, 14.58% to cefepime, 6.25% to nitrofurantoin, and 0.0% to imipenem [44]. However in other studies the resistance against gentamycin for *E.coli* isolates in Iran was about 93% and 62% [12, 14]. Villar et al. reported 99% and 98 susceptibility to imipenem and amikacin respectively for their uropathogenic *E. coli* strains that is consistent with our results [46].

In this study, we have shown the presence of *aer*, *fimH* and *hylA* genes in UPEC isolates (Fig. 3). Almost all of the isolates harbored *aer* gene, which is responsible for obtaining iron. The frequency of *aer* gene in our study is higher than recent studies [49, 50].One of the secreted toxine factors in *E. coli* strains is *hlyA*, which implicated in tissue damage and dysfunction of local immune responses. This study showed a higher prevalence of *hlyA* among UPEC strains in contrast to other studies [49, 50]. Of note, *FimH* is highly conserved and extremely common among *E. coli* isolates. *FimH* mediates UPEC adherence to the urothelium cells, and helps the

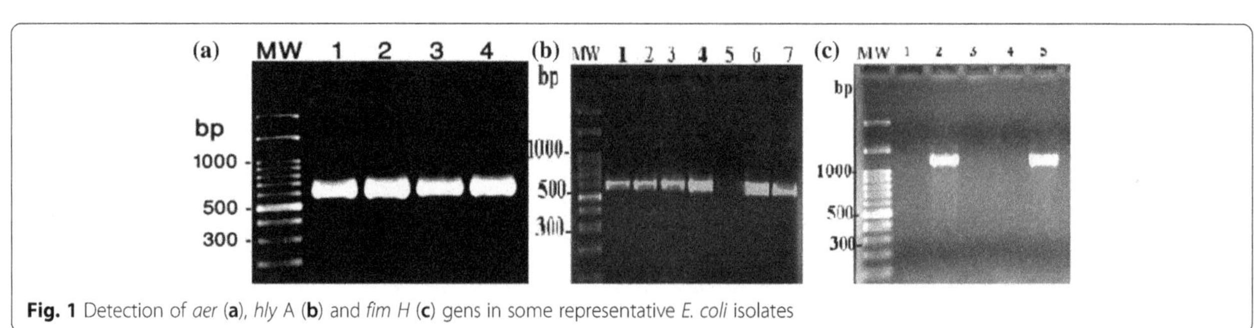

Fig. 1 Detection of *aer* (**a**), *hly* A (**b**) and *fim H* (**c**) gens in some representative *E. coli* isolates

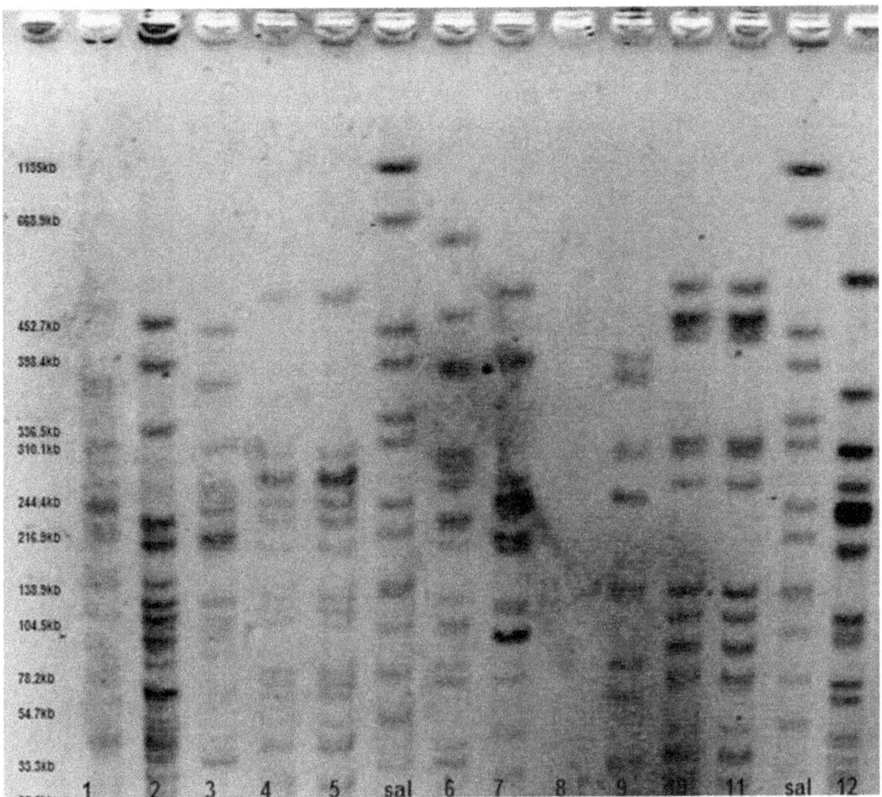

Fig. 2 Representative PFEG profiles of some *E. coli* strains; *Salmonella* Braenderup used as molecular size standard (1135–28.8 kb)

formation of intracellular bacterial biofilms [51]. The distribution of *fimH* gene in our strains is in agreement with other published data [1, 49, 52].

Information about the source of the infections and relatedness between bacterial agents is helpful for preventing measures and choosing the best treatment [35]. In recent studies PFGE, as a gold standard method, has been used for DNA fingerprinting and epidemiologic studies successfully. PFGE is a high discriminatory and reproducible typing method that is used in CDC laboratories [34, 53]. This study provides more information on the distribution of urinary isolates of *E. coli* strains. We applied PFGE technique for separating fragments of DNA chromosome digested using XbaI restriction enzyme. This enzyme has been proved to be more powerful and it is the most common used restriction enzyme for UPEC outbreaks [54–56], and was successfully used in this study to discriminate between the isolates from the UTI patients in some major hospital in Tehran. By using XbaI enzyme the analyzed isolates generated an exclusive profile with the number of DNA bands between 9 and15 and the bands from 33.3kbp to 1135kpb, while other studies have shown different number of bands and different molecular weights. Anvarinejad et al. reported 9 to 16 DNA bands with molecular size of 2 to 660kbp in molecular typing of *E. coli* isolates from patients with cyctitis and pyelonephritis [57]. Dong et al. reported 15–20 distinct bands in genotyping of Shiga toxin produced by *E. coli* isolates [41]. Ejrnaes et al. reported 15–20 bands with 50kbp to 1200kbp molecular sizes by typing UPEC strains [8].

In the current study, based on drown dendrogram 33 clusters with 85% similarity were found among 60 isolates. The strains with 12 and 15 bands had the highest percentage of 30% and 25% respectively, and the lowest percentage was for the strains with the 9 (2%). The pattern No. 10 with 12 bands and No. 12 with 15 bands were repeated more than other patterns in the present study (Fig. 2). By considering the distinct pulsotypes obtained in this study it seems that there is genetic heterogeneity of *E. coli* in the region. Of note, between 60 MDR isolates collected from 6 different locations in Tehran 84% of isolates belonged to the Center had specific types and 16% of isolates of North and Northwest had similar PFGE patterns, while in Northeast only 30% of isolates had specific patterns and other types were also found in other locations during 6 month of study. There was no defined pattern between the time of collection and PFGE profiles of *E. coli* isolates. Patrick and Padman investigated the efficacy of PFGE in a study of

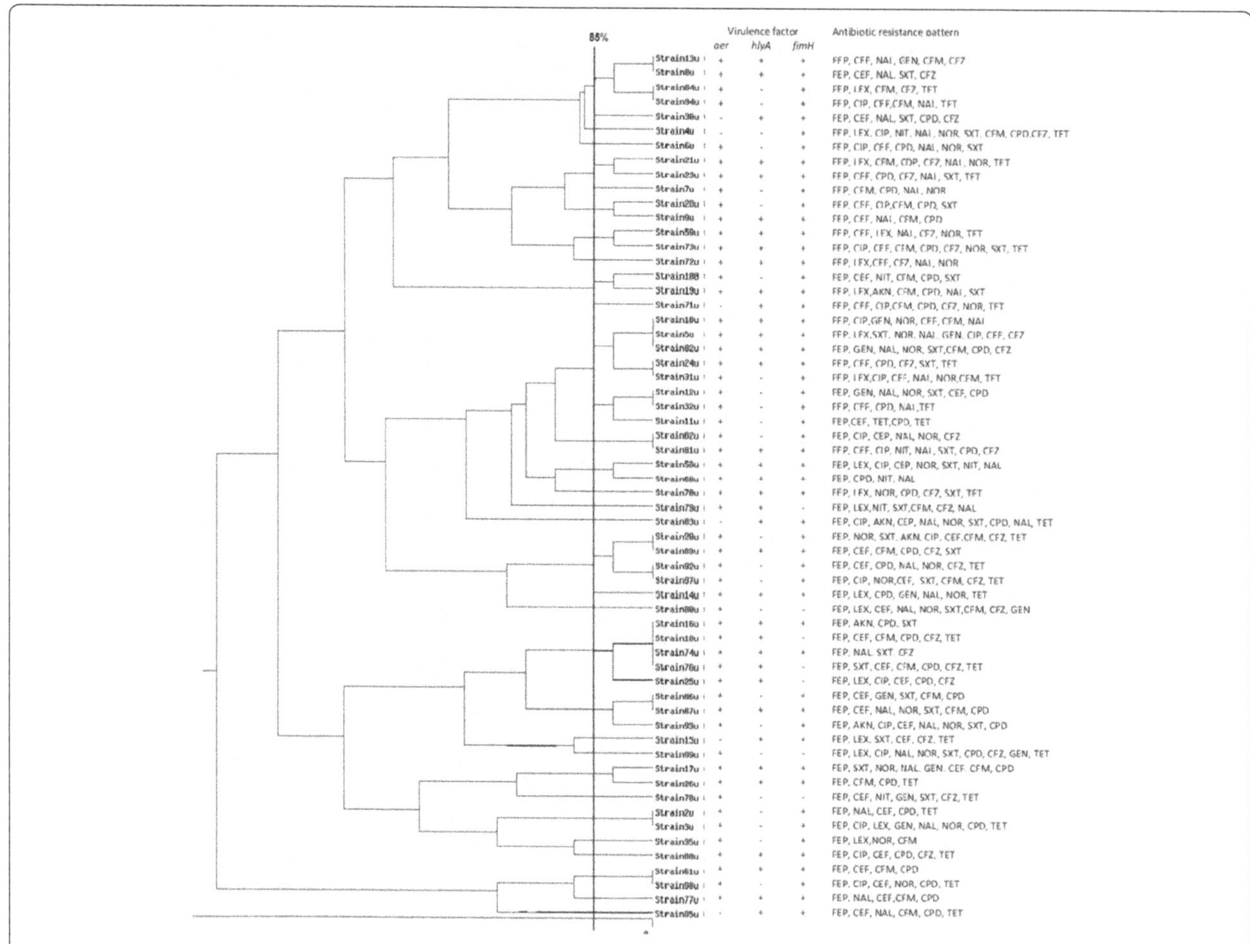

Fig. 3 Dendrogram of 60 *E. coli* isolates based on PFGE patterns after digestion with enzyme *Xba*I associated with present of virulence factors (*fimH*, *hlyA* and *aer*) and antibiotic resistance pattern; AKN, amikacin; *LEX*, cephalexin; *CIP*, ciprofloxacin; *CEF*, cefexime; *CDP*, cefpodexim; *CFZ*, cephazolin; *FEP*, cefepime; *NIT*, nitrofurantoin; *GEN*, gentamycin; *NAL*, nalidixic acid; *NOR*, norfloxacin; *SXT*, cotrimoxazole; *TET*, tetracyclin

extended spectrum beta lactamase (ESBL) enzymes produced by pathogen (*Escherichia coli* and *klebsiella* pneumonia) [53]. Miyuki and his colleagues used PFGE-CHEF for epidemiological study of *E. coli* O157: H7 isolates collected from 1997 to 2000 in Northern Ireland and compared the results to phage typing analysis. They reported that PFGE-CHEF typing proved to have a greater ability to distinguish *E. coli* O157 isolates, while phage typing has been shown to be less efficient [58]. Jones et al. used PFGE for determining the presence of *E. coli* O_{157} and *Salmonella* isolates in an outbreak and concluded that 20% of clusters were attributed to the same source [59]. Xiaoli et al. in China did a study about the genotypic characteristic of multidrug-resistance UTIs *E. coli* by PFGE. Forty PFGE types were observed for 51 MDR *E. coli* isolates at the cut off value of 85% [40].

Considering the high diversity of genetic relatedness between our MDR isolates there was not special pattern for antibiotic resistant. However, we found that isolates belonging to pulsotype 3 were resistant to 65% of antibiotics, while isolates in pulsotype 29 were resistant to 23% of antibiotics.

Conclusion

The present study demonstrates that considering the high number of *E. coli* types in the previous studies our conclusions are not surprising. The PFGE applied in the study was shown to be more powerful. PFGE is an appropriate choice for identifying the sources, clonal relatedness and spread of *E. coli* isolates in the hospitals. The result showed that the antibiotic resistance among uropathogenic *E. coli* under study is escalating rapidly. The PFGE types 3, 18, 25 that consist of 5% of isolates were more associated with antimicrobial resistant. Despite some exception such as PFGE type 1 and 22, most of the isolates in the same type followed similar virulence factors pattern. The information obtained from the similarity of the pulsotypes among isolates can help physicians to understand antibiotic resistant patterns of the different isolates from different sources and have a correct choice in prescribing antibiotic medicine.

Acknowledgements
We would like to thank from the "Clinical Research Development Center of Baqiyatallah hospital" for their kindly cooperation. This study was supported financially by "Clinical Research Development Center of Baqiyatallah hospital".

Authors' contribution
MR performed laboratory works, analyzed the data and drafted the paper. RR designed the study, interpreted the data and revised the manuscript. All authors read and approved the final manuscript.

Consent for publication
Not applicable.

Competing interests
The authors declare that they have no competing interests.

References

1. Momtaz H, et al. Uropathogenic *Escherichia coli* in Iran: serogroup distributions, virulence factors and antimicrobial resistance properties. Ann Clin Microbiol Antimicrob. 2013;12(1):8.
2. Johnson JR. Virulence factors in *Escherichia coli* urinary tract infection. Clin Microbiol Rev. 1991;4(1):80–128.
3. Soto S, et al. Prevalence of the set-1B and astA genes encoding enterotoxins in uropathogenic *Escherichia coli* clinical isolates. Microb Pathog. 2009;47(6):305–7.
4. Bauer RJ, et al. Molecular epidemiology of 3 putative virulence genes for *Escherichia coli* urinary tract infection–usp, iha, and iroN*E. coli*. J Infect Dis. 2002;185(10):1521–4.
5. Jahandeh N, et al. Uropathogenic *Escherichia coli* virulence genes: invaluable approaches for designing DNA microarray probes. Central European journal of urology. 2015;68(4):452.
6. Farshad, S., et al., Microbial susceptibility, virulence factors, and plasmid profiles of uropathogenic *Escherichia coli* strains isolated from children in Jahrom, Iran. Archives of Iranian Medicine (AIM), 2012. 15(5).
7. Tajbakhsh E, et al. Prevalence of class 1 and 2 integrons in multi-drug resistant *Escherichia coli* isolated from aquaculture water in Chaharmahal Va Bakhtiari province, Iran. Ann Clin Microbiol Antimicrob. 2015;14(1):37.
8. Ejrnaes K, et al. Pulsed-field gel electrophoresis typing of *Escherichia coli* strains from samples collected before and after Pivmecillinam or placebo treatment of uncomplicated community-acquired urinary tract infection in women. J Clin Microbiol. 2006;44(5):1776–81.
9. Anderson KL, Whitlock JE, Harwood VJ. Persistence and differential survival of fecal indicator bacteria in subtropical waters and sediments. Appl Environ Microbiol. 2005;71(6):3041–8.
10. Davies J, Davies D. Origins and evolution of antibiotic resistance. Microbiology and Molecular Biology Reviews : MMBR. 2010;74(3):417–33.
11. Blair JMA, et al. Molecular mechanisms of antibiotic resistance. Nat Rev Microbiol. 2014;13:42.
12. Ranjbar R, et al. Shiga (Vero)-toxin producing *Escherichia coli* isolated from the hospital foods; virulence factors, o-serogroups and antimicrobial resistance properties. Antimicrobial Resistance & Infection Control. 2017;6(1):4.
13. Heidary M, Momtaz H, Madani M. Characterization of Diarrheagenic antimicrobial resistant *Escherichia coli* isolated from pediatric patients in Tehran. Iran Iranian Red Crescent Medical Journal. 2014;16(4):e12329.
14. Momtaz H, et al. Serogroups, virulence genes and antibiotic resistance in Shiga toxin-producing *Escherichia coli* isolated from diarrheic and non-diarrheic pediatric patients in Iran. Gut Pathogens. 2013;5(1):39.
15. Singh A, et al. Application of molecular techniques to the study of hospital infection. Clin Microbiol Rev. 2006;19(3):512–30.
16. Rivas, L., et al., Typing and Subtyping Methods for Pathogenic *Escherichia coli*, in Detection and Typing Strategies for Pathogenic *Escherichia coli*. 2015, Springer. p. 67–99.
17. Ranjbar R, et al. Typing methods used in the molecular epidemiology of microbial pathogens: a how-to guide. The new microbiologica. 2014;37(1):1–15.
18. Ranjbar R, et al. Isolation of clinical strains of Pseudomonas aeruginosa harboring different plasmids. Pakistan journal of biological sciences: PJBS. 2007;10(17):3020–2.
19. Arjomandzadegan M, et al. Prevalence of mutations at codon 463 of katg gene in MDR and XDR clinical isolates of *mycobacterium tuberculosis* in Belarus and application of the method in rapid diagnosis. Acta Microbiol Immunol Hung. 2011;58(1):51–63.
20. Ranjbar R, et al. Increased isolation and characterization of *Shigella sonnei* obtained from hospitalized children in Tehran, Iran. Journal of health, population, and nutrition. 2008;26(4):426.
21. Ranjbar R, et al. Characterization of endemic *Shigella boydii* strains isolated in Iran by serotyping, antimicrobial resistance, plasmid profile, ribotyping and pulsed-field gel electrophoresis. BMC research notes. 2008;1(1):74.
22. Ranjbar R, Elhaghi P, Shokoohizadeh L. Multilocus Sequence Typing of the Clinical Isolates of *Salmonella Enterica* Serovar *Typhimurium* in Tehran Hospitals. Iranian Journal of Medical Sciences. 2017:**41**(2).
23. Ranjbar R, Memariani M, Memariani H. Diversity of variable number tandem repeat loci in *Shigella* species isolated from pediatric patients. International journal of molecular and cellular medicine. 2015;4(3):174.
24. Ranjbar R, et al. Distribution of virulence genes and genotyping of CTX-M-15-producing *Klebsiella pneumoniae* isolated from patients with community-acquired urinary tract infection (CA-UTI). Microb Pathog. 2016;100:244–9.
25. Pourshafie M, et al. Dissemination of a single *Vibrio cholerae* clone in cholera outbreaks during 2005 in Iran. J Med Microbiol. 2007;56(12):1615–9.
26. Sadeghifard, N., R. Ranjbar, and J. Zaeimi, Antimicrobial susceptibility, plasmid profiles, and RAPD-PCR typing of *Acinetobacter* bacteria. 2011.
27. Ranjbar R, et al. Molecular characterisation of epidemic isolates of *Vibrio cholerae* O1 recovered from an outbreak occurred in different parts of Iran in 2005. Clinical Microbiology & Infection. 2009;15(4):S371.
28. Ranjbar R, et al. Genomic fingerprints of *Escherichia coli* strains isolated from surface water in Alborz province, Iran. BMC research notes. 2017;10(1):295.
29. Ranjbar R, Ghazi FM. Antibiotic sensitivity patterns and molecular typing of *Shigella sonnei* strains using ERIC-PCR. Iran J Public Health. 2013;42(10):1151.
30. Hosseini MJ, Kaffashian AR. An outbreak of shigellosis due to *Shigella flexneri serotype* 3a in a prison in Iran. Archives of Iranian medicine. 2010;13(5):413.
31. Khakabimamaghani S, et al. GelClust: a software tool for gel electrophoresis images analysis and dendrogram generation. Comput Methods Prog Biomed. 2013;111(2):512–8.
32. Pooideh M, et al. Molecular Epidemiology of *Mycobacterium tuberculosis* Isolates in 100 Patients With Tuberculosis Using Pulsed Field Gel Electrophoresis. Jundishapur journal of microbiology. 2015;8(7).
33. Ranjbar R, et al. Genetic relatedness among isolates of *Shigella sonnei* carrying class 2 integrons in Tehran, Iran, 2002–2003. BMC Infect Dis. 2007;7(1):62.
34. Askarian Nameghi S. Genotyping *Escherichia coli* isolates by pulsed-field gel electrophoresis. Institutionen för livsvetenskaper. 2007.
35. Sabat A, et al. Overview of molecular typing methods for outbreak detection and epidemiological surveillance. Euro Surveill. 2013;18(4):20380.
36. Van Belkum A, et al. European Society of Clinical Microbiology and Infectious Diseases (ESCMID) Study Group on Epidemiological Markers (ESGEM). 2007. Guidelines for the validation and application of typing methods for use in bacterial epidemiology. Clin Microbiol Infect. 2007; 13(146):1469–0691.2007.
37. Performance Standards for Antimicrobial Susceptibility Testing. 27th ed. CLSI supplement M100. Clinical and Laboratory Standards Institute, Wayne, PA, USA, 2017.
38. Ribot EM, et al. Standardization of pulsed-field gel electrophoresis protocols for the subtyping of *Escherichia coli* O157: H7, *Salmonella*, and *Shigella* for PulseNet. Foodbourne Pathogens & Disease. 2006;3(1):59–67.
39. Control, C.f.D. and Prevention, Standard operating procedure for PulseNet PFGE of *Escherichia coli* O157: H7, *Escherichia coli* non-O157 (STEC), *Salmonella* serotypes, *Shigella sonnei* and *Shigella flexneri*. Centers for Disease Control and Prevention, Atlanta, 2013.
40. Cao X, et al. Genotypic characteristics of multidrug-resistant *Escherichia coli* isolates associated with urinary tract infections. APMIS. 2014;122(11): 1088–95.
41. Dong H-J, et al. Prevalence, virulence potential, and pulsed-field gel electrophoresis profiling of Shiga toxin-producing *Escherichia coli* strains from cattle. Gut pathogens. 2017;9(1):22.
42. Ejrnæs K. Bacterial characteristics of importance for recurrent urinary tract infections caused by *Escherichia coli*. Dan Med Bull. 2011;58(4):B4187.

43. Niranjan V, Malini A. Antimicrobial resistance pattern in *Escherichia coli* causing urinary tract infection among inpatients. Indian J Med Res. 2014;139(6):945.
44. Adib N, et al. Antibiotic resistance profile and virulence genes of uropathogenic *Escherichia coli* isolates in relation to phylogeny. Trop Biomed. 2014;31(1):17–25.
45. Shakya P, et al. Antibiotic resistance among *Escherichia coli* isolates from stool samples of children aged 3 to 14 years from Ujjain, India. BMC Infect Dis. 2013;13(1):477.
46. Villar HE, et al. Frequency and antibiotic susceptibility patterns of urinary pathogens in male outpatients in Argentina. The Journal of Infection in Developing Countries. 2014;8(06):699–704.
47. Jakovljević E, et al. A one-year prospective study on the antibiotic resistance of *E. coli* strains isolated in urinary specimens of children hospitalized at the university pediatric medical Center in Novi sad, Serbia. Infection. 2013;41(6): 1111–9.
48. Melo DB, et al. Antimicrobial resistance and genetic diversity of *Escherichia coli* isolated from humans and foods. Braz J Microbiol. 2015;46(4):1165–70.
49. Tarchouna M, et al. Distribution of uropathogenic virulence genes in *Escherichia coli* isolated from patients with urinary tract infection. Int J Infect Dis. 2013;17(6):e450–3.
50. Jalali HR, et al. Genotyping of virulence factors of Uropathogenic *Escherichia coli* by PCR. Novelty in Biomedicine. 2015;3(4):177–81.
51. Wiles TJ, Kulesus RR, Mulvey MA. Origins and virulence mechanisms of uropathogenic *Escherichia coli*. Exp Mol Pathol. 2008;85(1):11–9.
52. Usein CR, et al. Prevalence of virulence genes in *Escherichia coli* strains isolated from Romanian adult urinary tract infection cases. J Cell Mol Med. 2001;5(3):303–10.
53. Akpaka PE, Jayaratne P. Usefulness of pulsed field gel electrophoresis assay in the molecular epidemiological study of extended spectrum beta lactamase producers. Gel electrophoresis-advanced techniques. 2012:193–202.
54. Watabe M, et al. Epidemiological study of *E. coli* O157: H7 isolated in Northern Ireland using pulsed-field gel electrophoresis (PFGE). The Ulster medical journal. 2008;**77**(3):168.
55. Maluta RP, et al. Frequencies of virulence genes and pulse field gel electrophoresis fingerprints in *Escherichia coli* isolates from canine pyometra. Vet J. 2014;202(2):393–5.
56. Basim E, Basim H. Pulsed-field gel electrophoresis (PFGE) technique and its use in molecular biology. Turk J Biol. 2001;25(4):405–18.
57. Anvarinejad M, et al. Genotypic analysis of *E. coli* strains isolated from patients with cystitis and pyelonephritis. Iranian Red Crescent Medical Journal. 2012;14(7):408.
58. Yamamoto S, et al. Detection of urovirulence factors in *Escherichia coli* by multiplex polymerase chain reaction. FEMS Immunol Med Microbiol. 1995;12(2):85–90.
59. Jones TF, et al. Characteristics of clusters of *Salmonella* and *Escherichia coli* O157 detected by pulsed-field gel electrophoresis that predict identification of outbreaks. Foodborne Pathog Dis. 2016;13(12):674–8.
60. Struve C, Krogfelt KA. In vivo detection of *Escherichia coli* type 1 fimbrial expression and phase variation during experimental urinary tract infection. Microbiology. 1999;145(10):2683–90.

13

Resistance pattern and maternal knowledge, attitude and practices of suspected Diarrheagenic *Escherichia coli* among children under 5 years of age in Addis Ababa, Ethiopia

Yeshwondm Mamuye GebreSilasie[1], Kassu Desta Tullu[2] and Addisu Gize Yeshanew[1*]

Abstract

Background: Diarrheal illness remains one of the leading causes of morbidity and mortality among children under 5 years of age worldwide, especially in developing countries. Diarrheagenic *Escherichia coli* (DEC) is the major cause of gastroenteritis in children in the developing world and is associated with high resistance levels to antibiotics. The aims of this study were to isolate and determine susceptibility patterns of DEC among children under 5 years of age with acute diarrhea and to assess maternal knowledge, attitude and practice towards childhood diarrhea.

Methods: A cross sectional study was conducted from August–December 2015 at 3 selected health institutions. Stool samples were cultured and isolated *E. coli* species were run for antimicrobial susceptibility testing using disk diffusion method. In addition, children's caretakers were interviewed using structured questionnaires including a Knowledge, Attitude and Practice (KAPs) survey. Bivariate and multivariate logistic regression analysis was used to quantify the effect of different risk factors on bacterial related diarrhea.

Results: A total of 253 children, 115 males and 138 females with acute diarrhea were enrolled. *E. coli* was identified in a total of sixty-one children (24.1%), followed by *Shigella* (9.1%) and *Salmonella* (3.95%). Additionally, eighty-six children (34.0%) had parasites identified in stool samples. *E. coli* isolates showed 83.6% resistance to ampicillin and augmentin followed by, trimethoprim-sulfamethoxazole (62.3%). Multiple resistances were observed in 72.1% of isolates; however, more than 90% of the strains were sensitive to ciprofloxacin and ceftriaxone. Caretakers identified the following as causes of infection: contaminated food and water (83.4%), microorganisms (55.3%), inadequate breast milk (54.1%), teething (45.1%), house flies (43.1%) and evil eye (15.8%). No hand washing before meals and low levels of knowledge had a significant association with *E. coli* infection ($p < 0.05$).

Conclusion: In children with suspected diarrheagenic *E. coli,* we observed a high frequency of multidrug resistant *E. coli*. Furthermore, study subjects with low awareness about source, cause and symptoms of the disease were more likely to acquire suspected diarrheagenic *E. coli* infections. Thus, there is a need for more education in addition to continuous surveillance of the prevalence and antibiotic susceptibility pattern of diarrheal bacterial isolates in hospitals and in the community.

Keywords: Resistance patterns, Suspected diarrheagenic *E. coli*, KAPs

* Correspondence: konjoaddisu@gmail.com; addisu.gize@sphmmc.edu.et
[1]Department of Microbiology, St. Paul's Hospital Millennium Medical College, P.O.Box 1271, Addis Ababa, Ethiopia
Full list of author information is available at the end of the article

Background

Diarrhea is the third most common cause of deaths among children in sub-Saharan Africa and one of the main causes of hospital admissions in rural areas [1]. It is still considered one of the foremost causes of death in children, accounting for approximately 2 million deaths each year worldwide [2, 3]. In developing countries like Ethiopia, diarrheal diseases are major causes of infant and child mortality and morbidity [4].

Syndromes of diarrhea can be caused by bacterial, viral and parasitic infections of either single or multiple etiologic agents [5]. Suspected Diarrheagenic *Escherichia coli* (DEC) are considered to be the most common of the many recognized enteropathogenic organisms, particularly in developing countries and in diarrhea-associated deaths in children under five [6].

Moreover, the emergence of antimicrobial-drug resistance, including resistance to the new and potent antimicrobial agents, is a major public health concern especially in resource-limited countries, like Ethiopia, where bacterial infections are still among the major causes of death, especially for children, it is of particular concern [7, 8].

Anti-diarrheal, anti-amoebic and anti-bacterial medications have little role in the management of diarrhea, on the basis of WHO guidelines [9]. However, timely management of the children with fluids resuscitation has substantially declined the mortality and morbidity from acute infectious diarrhea [3]. In Ethiopia, evidence is lacking regarding maternal care-taking and environmental risk factors that contribute to acute diarrhea and the case management of diarrhea. Thus, in view of increasing diarrheal disease and emergence of antimicrobial resistance internationally, there is a need identify misconceptions or misunderstandings about transmission of diarrheal illness in the community in addition to determining resistance patterns of isolated bacterial pathogens involved in diarrheal illness. A Knowledge, Attitude and Practices (KAP) survey is a quantitative method that provides access to quantitative and qualitative information used in multiple studies to understand gaps in knowledge. Therefore, this study provides important input on the emergence of antimicrobial resistance and maternal KAPs to design appropriate control measures for Ethiopian children. This study also will improve awareness to clinicians and local communities in terms of potential targets for intervention strategies.

Methods

Study area and population

The study was conducted at outpatient pediatric departments of selected health institutions (Selam health center, Addis Ketema health center, and St. Paul's Hospital Millennium Medical College) in Addis Ababa, Ethiopia from August–December 2015. Addis Ababa is the capital and largest city of Ethiopia. Addis Ababa had an estimated population of 3,384,569 according to the 2007 population census, with annual growth rate of 3.8%. These numbers were initially underestimated, as such; there are no accurate demographic data on Addis Ababa. However, more than 10% of the Ethiopian population can be attributed to children under five years of age.

Sample size and sampling procedures

The sample size for the study was calculated using the formula ($n = (z\alpha/2)2$ p (1-p)/ d2) for estimating a single population proportion at 95% confidence interval (CI) ($Z\alpha/2 = 1.96$), 5% margin of error. Therefore, based on previous prevalence of *E. coli*, 20.8% study in other health facilities, the total sample size is 253 [10]. This sample size was also applied for caretakers to investigate their KAP. To get those study subjects, we utilized a randomly sampling techniques in which patients from the 3 selected heatlh institutes were our sampling frame (the population from which the samples were chosen). Specifically, we reviewed the daily data about patient flow from the selected health institutions to get the total of $n = 253$ subjects or to achieve our total sample size. Consequently, if an average daily patient flow to the pediatric department was = 30, then our sampling fraction become (253/30 = 8.4) that means almost 8. Then we selected random number from between 1 and 8, for example if that number is 3, the 1st selected study individual will be 3, then the 2nd will be (3 + 8 = 11), then the 3rd will be (11 + 8 = 19, then the 4th one will be (19 + 8 = 27)...., will continue the pattern of sequence by jumping 8 individuals until the selected participants will become total of 253 study subjects (3,11,19,27,35,43,51,59,67,75,83, etc., will be selected individual for the study until the sum of all selected individuals equaled 253 subjects).

Data collection

Stool sample collection

We followed the same study protocol as previously published work for resistance patterns of *Shigella* and *Salmonella spp* among under 5 children with acute diarrhea [11]. Trained nurses used a pretested questionnaire to first interview the mother or primary caretaker. The mother or primary caretaker was then given a clean plastic stool container and oriented about sample collection. Once collected, protozoa parasites were identified through direct microscopy using a saline wet mount at each study sites by experienced laboratory technicians/technologists. Part of the stool was kept in Cary-Blair transport media, and transported in an icebox to the microbiology department of St. Paul's Hospital Millennium Medical College (SPHMMC) for further microbiological investigations.

Culture identification and antimicrobial drug susceptibility test methods

Enteric pathogen underwent overnight incubation with Selenite-F Broth enrichment media for further multiplication. This was then subsequently sub-cultured onto MacConkey agar (MAC), Salmonella-Shigella agar (SSA) and Deoxycholate citrate agar (DCA), and then incubated aerobically at 37 °C for 24 h. After overnight incubation, colonies that exhibited characteristics of *Salmonella* and *Shigella* species were identified by conventional biochemical methods [12]. Because of many enteric bacteria can also grow in the enrichment broth, further detection techniques were performed to ensure specific isolation of *E. coli* colonies. Suspicious colonies were transferred to Triple Sugar Iron (TSI) agar, tryptone broth, arabinose broth, and urea broth and incubated for 20 h at 35 °C. Then H_2S-positive, urease-positive, arabinose non-fermenting and indole-negative strains were rejected. Both *E. coli* and *Shigella* are anaerogenic (i.e. produce little or no gas) and non-motile, therefore to differentiate *E. coli* from *Shigella*, slow lactose fermenters were examined for lysine decarboxylase, mucate, and acetate reactions. *Shigella sonnei* was characterized based on a negative indole reaction and slow or non-fermentation of lactose [12, 13].

Shortly, colonies were first examined for lactose fermentation on MacConkey agar. The oxidase and indole tests were performed from a companion blood agar plate. *E. coli* strains were identified as lactose fermenting, betaglucuronidase and indole positive, and oxidase negative. Once suspected diarrheagenic *E. coli* and other enteric bacteria were isolated, drug susceptibility testing was performed using disc diffusion method. Susceptibility testing for all isolates was done and interpreted on the basis of CLSI guidelines [12]. Quality control was performed to check the quality of the medium, the potency of the antibiotic, and assay setup errors. Each new lot was quality controlled before use by testing the *E. coli* ATCC 25922 standard strains as we describe it previously [11–14].

Maternal knowledge, attitude and practices

A structured questionnaire was designed to collect information regarding socio-demographics and KAP of the study participants about diarrhea. The questionnaire was first developed in English and translated into Amharic (the local language), and then pre-tested in non-selected health institutions via pilot study for assessing content validity, appropriateness, and question comprehensibility. Then, the questionnaire was revised when necessary. A total of three nurses, one from each selected study area were selected to collect data. Training was given to the data collectors for two days on how to conduct the interview, content of the questionnaire, data quality, and ways to approach respondents. The first author checked the questionnaires for completeness every day. Incomplete questionnaires were returned to data collectors for correction by revisiting the caretakers. Five percent of the interviewed caretakers were randomly selected and re-interviewed by the first author. The KAP survey contains a total of 33 items. Thirteen items were knowledge related questions. Each correct response was assigned score 1 and wrong response was assigned 0 (zero). Thus for 13 items, the maximum attainable score was 13 and minimum was 0. Nine rating-scale items were for measuring the attitude of caretaker towards childhood diarrhea. The positive items were scored as 1 = strongly disagree, 2 = disagree, 3 = neutral, 4 = agree, and 5 = strongly agree. Scoring was reversed for negative items. Eleven items were for measuring the practice of the mother.

Operational definition

Suspected diarrheagenic *E. coli* (DEC) in this study was defined as a strain of *E. coli* spp. isolated from children under five years with acute diarrhea and considered as pathogenic.

Diarrhea was defined as at least three loose stools in 24 h including at least one of nausea, vomiting, abdominal cramps or fever symptoms.

The level of Knowledge, Attitude and Practices was classified according to the following: a poor knowledge corresponded to a score below 50%, and good knowledge referred to a score ≥ 50%. A score ≥ 50% was a "positive level" and a score of < 50% was classified as "negative level" of attitude of caretakers toward childhood diarrhea. A score < 50% was "poor" and a score ≥ 50% was considered as "good" level of practice.

Data analysis

Data were double entered, cross-checked using Epi-data version 3.3, and analyzed using SPSS version 20. Enteric bacteria prevalence was determined by dividing the number of individuals infected with enteric bacteria by the total number of individuals examined for bacterial infection. Frequency distribution tables were used to quantify enteric bacterial and parasitic infection, in addition to knowledge of respondents related to sign symptoms, causes, transmission, prevention and control measures of diarrhea. Logistic regression was used to examine the association between independent predictors and dependent enteric bacterial infection. Bivariate and multivariate logistic regression analysis was used to quantify the effect of different risk factors including KAP on bacterial related diarrhea. Values were considered statistically significant at $p < 0.05$.

Ethical considerations

The study obtained ethical clearance from the Department Research and Ethical Review Committee (DRERC) of Addis Ababa University School of Allied Health Sciences, Department of Medical Laboratory sciences and each of the selected health institutes. Written informed consent was obtained from voluntary participants and parents or primary caretakers for children during data collection. Individuals who were found positive for bacteria and parasite were treated as per the national guidelines.

Results

Socio-demographic characteristics of children and prevalence of diarrhea

As mentioned, this is a part of work from the previous published study [11]. A total of 253 primary caretakers were interviewed and provided stool samples from children for enteric bacterial and parasite identification. The mean age of the patients was 2.61 years with standard deviation (SD) of 1.26 years. In regards to caretakers, most of respondents (87%) were females ($n = 220$). For all respondents, 66.0% were between 26 and 40 years, ranging from 16 to 52 years with a median of 29 years; 86.2% were married ($n = 218$), and 64.9% had completed a primary education ($n = 164$). The majority of caretakers (53.4%) were house wives ($n = 135$); and the income for 47% of caretaker's ($n = 119$) was less than 500 ETB (18 USD) per month. 5.5% of the caretakers had completed secondary or a higher level of education (Table 1).

Enteric bacteria were isolated from 94 (37.2%) of the children tested. The predominant isolated organisms were suspected diarrheagenic *E. coli* spp. ($n = 64$ or 24.1%), followed by *Salmonella* species ($n = 23$ or 9.1%) and *Shigella* species ($n = 10$ or 3.95%). 34% of samples ($n = 86$) were positive for parasites; the most frequently identified protozoan parasites were *E. histolytica/dispar* ($n = 45$ or 17.8%), followed by *G. lambia* ($n = 26$ or 10.3%), *H. nana* ($n = 9$ or 3.6%), *A. lumbricoides* ($n = 5$ or 2.0%) and *S. stercolaris* ($n = 1$ or 0.4%).

Antimicrobial sensitivity results of isolates

The antimicrobial susceptibility testing was done for all suspected diarrheagenic *E. coli* isolates using disk diffusion method. Zones of inhibition were measured by using caliper meter and interpreted as sensitive (S), intermediate (I), and resistance(R) respectively on the basis of CLSI guide lines [14].

Suspected diarrheagenic *E. coli* (DEC) were isolated from 24.1% of stool samples. Among patients who had suspected diarrheagenic *E. coli* infections, the resistance rates were high for ampicillin (83.6%), augmentin (83.6%), trimethoprim-sulfamethoxazole (62.3%), and medium for chloramphenicol (21.3%), nalidixic acid (19.7%), and gentamicin (11.5%). Low levels of resistance were observed against ciprofloxacin (4.9%) and ceftriaxone (3.3%) (Table 2).

Antimicrobial resistance to one or more antibiotics was very high among the suspected diarrheagenic *E. coli* species isolated in the study (83.6%). Multiple resistances (resistance for two or more commonly used antibiotics) were observed in 85.2% of the DEC species isolated. One of the isolated strains of suspected diarrheagenic *E. coli* was resistant for seven antibiotics. Furthermore, susceptibility to all eight antibiotics tested was observed for 3 (4.9%) of the isolates.

Knowledge, attitude and practice (KAP) towards diarrhea

Out of 253 respondents, 83.4% ($n = 211$) had heard of diarrhea, and 70.8% ($n = 179$) of them mentioned diarrhea as one of the major health problems of the community. 97.9% of caretakers ($n = 247$) used pipe water as the primary source of water in home. However, two patients used stagnant water sources and both were positive for enteric pathogens. On bivariate analysis, low income, < 500 ETB (OR = 3.77, 95% CI = 1.454–9.77, *P*-value = 0.006), 500–1000 ETB (OR = 6.47, 95% CI = 1.922–21.775, *P*-value = 0.003) and absence of hand washing before and after meal (OR = 0.12, 95% CI = 0.02–0.062, *P*-value = 0.03) were important independent predictors of suspected diarrheagenic *E. coli* infections. However, multivariate logistic analysis revealed that only poor hand washing practice had a statistically significant association with detection of suspected diarrheagenic *E. coli* infection. Children from households that wash their hands before and after meals are 81% less likely to have DEC infection compared to children from households who don't wash their hands (AOR = 0.19, 95% CI = 0.144–0.775, *P*-value = 0.004) (Table 3).

From a total of 253 respondents, 158 (62.5%) of them stated diarrhea as a common childhood illness in their area. 225 (88.9%) respondents associated the sources of children's diarrheal infection with poor personal and environmental hygiene (Table 4).

The majority of respondents, 92.5% ($n = 234$) and 78.3% ($n = 198$) mentioned frequent diarrhea and abdominal pain as important and noticeable symptoms of childhood diarrhea, respectively. However, a few (3.6%) participants were not aware of the signs and symptoms.

Regarding their practice, the majority of the caretakers went to health centers, and no one sought out traditional healers. 91.7% ($n = 232$) participants went to health centers, 7.5% ($n = 19$) went to hospitals, and 0.8% ($n = 2$) went to private clinics for medical treatment. Any fluid intake, defined as taking of any fluid drinks in addition to oral rehydration solutions, was noted as a control mechanism in 89.3% ($n = 226$) of respondents. Consequently, more than 90% of the caretakers used oral rehydration solution (ORS) as a treatment option (Table 5).

56.1% ($n = 142$) and 9.1% ($n = 23$) of caretakers used raw milk and raw meat, respectively. However, there was no statistically significant association detected

Table 1 Distributions of socio-demographic characteristics of children and caretakers at the selected public health institutions in Addis Ababa, Ethiopia, 2015

Study Subjects	Variable	Category	Frequency, $n = 253$	Percent
	Sex	Male	115	45.5
		Female	138	54.5
Children		< 1 yrs	32	12.6
	Age	1-2 yrs	72	28.5
		2-3 yrs	64	25.3
		> 3 yrs	84	33.6
	Sex	Male	33	13.0
		Female	220	87.0
	Age	≤25 yrs	78	30.0
		26-40 yrs	167	66.0
		≥41 yrs	8	3.2
Caretakers	Marital Status	Single	15	6.0
		Married	218	86.2
		Divorced	12	4.7
		Other	8	3.1
	Educational Status	Illiterate	42	16.6
		Primary	164	64.9
		Secondary	33	13.0
		Higher education	14	5.5
	Occupation	Government	25	9.9
		Merchant	63	24.9
		Housewife	135	53.4
		Others	30	11.8
	Monthly Income	< 500 ETB	119	47.0
		501–1000 ETB	41	16.2
		1001–1500 ETB	12	4.8
		> 1500 ETB	5	2.0
		Others	76	30.0

ETB Ethiopian Birr

between users and non-users with culture positivity. Of all respondents, 97.2% ($n = 246$) endorsed proper latrine usage. In general, children from caretakers with a low knowledge score were three times more likely to be exposed to *E. coli* infection than children from caretakers with a good knowledge score.

Discussion

The overall isolation prevalence rate of suspected diarrheagenic *E. coli* in diarrheic stool samples was found to be 24.1%. This result was consistent with studies done in Ethio-Swedish Children's Hospital, Addis Ababa Ethiopia, and Tanzania, where 20.8% and 22.9% rates of *E. coli* isolates have been reported respectively [10, 15]. However, our rates were lower compared to a 46.88% and 60.0% prevalence of suspected diarrheagenic *E. coli* from studies done in North West Italy and Nigeria, respectively [16, 17]. In contrast, our participants had higher rates of suspected diarrheagenic *E. coli* when compared to a study in the US of both inpatients (4.7%) and emergency room (10.0%) subjects [18]. Put together, the differences noted in the various populations might be due to age, socio-economic factors, and the nature of the public water supply.

83.6% of suspected diarrheagenic *E. coli* isolates were resistant to ampicillin (83.6%) and augmentin (83.6%). This in to contrast to other studies in other parts of Ethiopia, where ampicillin resistance was 93.70% [19]. This might be due to the difference in study design, place, age and period. The high prevalence of resistance to these drugs could be explained by the longtime use of this antibiotic to treat enteric bacterial infection, thereby ensuring selection pressure and maintenance of this resistance. Studies done in Peru, Iran, Nigeria, and Tanzania also show that diarrheagenic *E. coli* exhibited high levels of antimicrobial drug resistance [20–23].

In this study, multidrug resistance to two or more antibiotics (85.2%) was more commonly observed than resistance to a single drug (3.3%). Despite the high proportion of antimicrobial resistance observed among suspected diarrheagenic *E. coli* isolates, these organisms remain highly susceptible to ciprofloxacin and ceftriaxone, which are now the drugs of choice in many areas. This finding is in agreement with other studies done in Nigeria and Tanzania [18, 21–24].

Table 2 Antimicrobial susceptibility patterns of *E. coli* isolates among children under five years of age at the selected public health institutions in Addis Ababa, Ethiopia, 2015

Enteropathogen (n)	Interpretation	Antibiotics							
		Amp	Aug	SXT	C	CIP	Gen	Na	CRO
Suspected Diarrheagenic *E. coli* (61)	S (%)	11.5	9.8	36.1	72.1	93.4	63.9	73.8	96.7
	I (%)	4.9	6.6	1.6	6.6	1.6	24.6	6.6	0
	R (%)	83.6	83.6	62.3	21.3	4.9	11.5	19.7	3.3

[*] *S* sensitive, *I* intermediate, and *R* resistant, *Amp* Ampicillin, *Aug* Augmentin, *SXT* trimethoprim-sulfamethoxazole, *C* Chloramphenicol, *NA* Nalidixic Acid, *CIP* Ciprofloxacin, *Gen* Gentamicin, *CRO* Ceftriaxone, *n* number

Table 3 Associations of risk factor with culture positivity of *E. coli* at the selected public health institutions in Addis Ababa, Ethiopia, 2015

Variables	Suspected Diarrheagenic *E. coli*					*P*-Value
	Negative, N (%)	Positive, N (%)	COR (CI)	*P*-Value	AOR (CI)	
Marital Status						
Never Married	12(75.0)	4(25.0)	1	0.93		
Ever Married	180(75.9)	57(24.1)	0.95(0.29–3.1)			
Educational status						
Illiterate	29(69.0)	13(31.0)	1.28(0.17–9.9)	0.33		
Primary school	126(76.8)	38(23.2)	0.73(0.09–5.8)	0.51		
Secondary school	26(78.8)	7(21.2)	1.06(0.15–7.8)	0.40		
Higher education	11(78.6)	3(21.4)	1			
Occupation						
Government	19(76.0)	6(24.0)	1			
Merchant	49(77.8)	14(22.2)	0.19((0.2–1.9)	0.30		
Housewife	101(74.8)	34(25.2)	0.38(0.4–3.5)	0.41		
Others	23(76.7)	7(23.3)	3.12(0.3–30.7)	0.33		
Monthly Income						
< 500	98(72.1)	38(27.9)	3.8(1.5–9.8)	0.006*	0.12(−0.05-001)	0.060
501–1000	37(69.8)	16(30.2)	6.5(1.9–21.8)	0.003*	0.22(0.64-1.3.)	0.056
1001–1500	27(84.4)	5(15.6)	1.3(0.12–12.2)	0.61	1.13(0.22–5.74)	0.880
> 1501	30(93.8)	2(6.2)	1			
Family previous diarrhea						
Yes	22(71.0)	9(29.0)	1.47(0.53–1.4)	0.64		
No	170(76.6)	52(23.4)	1			
Attending day care						
Yes	73(79.3)	19(20.7)	1			
No	119(73.9)	42(26.1)	1.3(0.7–2.4)	0.35		
Feeding practice						
Exclusive breast milk	35(89.7)	4(10.3)	1			
Breast milk & solid food	58(72.5)	22(27.5)	3.5(1.07–11.0)	0.07		
Solid food only	95(73.6)	34(26.4)	3.5(1.1–11.2)	0.08		
Formula Milk	4(80.0)	1(20)	2.6(0.23–34.4)	0.28		
Proper usage of latrine						
Yes	187(76.0)	59(24.0)	1			
No	5(71.4	2(28.6)	0.7(0.05–11.6)	0.83		
Raw meat usage						
Yes	111(78.2)	2(8.7)	0.26(0.06–1.2)	0.08		
No	81(73.0)	59(25.7)	1			
Hand washing before & after meal						
Yes	190(77.2)	56(22.8)	1			0.004*
No	2(28.6)	5(71.4)	0.12(0.02–0.6)	0.03*		0.2(0.2-8)
Sources of water						
Pipe	188(76.1)	59(23.9)	1			
Other	4(66.7)	2(33.3)	1.6(0.29–8.9)	0.60		

Table 3 Associations of risk factor with culture positivity of *E. coli* at the selected public health institutions in Addis Ababa, Ethiopia, 2015 *(Continued)*

Variables	Suspected Diarrheagenic *E. coli*					*P*-Value
	Negative, N (%)	Positive, N (%)	COR (CI)	*P*-Value	AOR (CI)	
Knowledge						
Good	168(79.2)	44(20.6)	1			
Poor	24(58.5)	17(41.5)	2.65(1.3–5.4)	0.008*	2.70(1.33-5.5)	
Attitude						
Positive	173 (77.6)	50(22.4)	1			
Negative	19 (63.3)	11(36.7)	1.8(0.88–4.11)	0.163		
Practice						
Good	181(76.1)	57(23.9)	1			
Poor	11(73.3)	4(26.7)	1.4(0.4–4.7)	0.582		

*Statistically significant, *CI* 95% confidence interval, *COR* crude odds ratio, *AOR* adjusted odds ratio
Adjusted OR (adjusted odds ratio from multivariable logistic regression model) = when the effect of one factor on E. coli prevalence is evaluated the analysis was adjusted for other remaining factors listed in the table

A few of the caretakers had completed a higher level of education, and their children had a lower frequency of suspected diarrheagenic *E. coli* isolation. This is similar to a study showing a 54% risk reduction for severe disease among mothers with 7 or more years of education [25–27].

The features of acute diarrhea vary from place to place depending on local meteorology, geography, and socioeconomic variables [16]. However, common presenting features of suspected diarrheagenic *E. coli* include diarrhea that was watery or bloody, with or without mucus, fever, vomiting and abdominal pains. Similarly, in our cohort, the most useful signs and symptoms for the diagnosis of *E. coli* were the complaints of watery diarrhea, as reported in other studies [19].

Drinking of unsafe water and contaminated foods are often considered to increase exposure to enteropathogens and have been associated with increased rates of acute diarrhea [3]. This finding is contrary to a study in India that shows teething (64.3%), evil eye (46%), contact with another case (36.6%), worm infestation (22.6%), dirty water (15.3%), and dirty environment (6%) as causes [27].

Of all, 93.7% of the caretakers agreed that personal hygiene is an effective means to prevent childhood diarrhea and 88.5% mentioned breast milk. Moreover, during episodes of diarrheal illnesses, 92.5% ($n = 234$) of the mothers preferred breast milk. This attitude and practice is consistent with findings in Gondar, Ethiopia, that showed breast-feeding is protective factor [28]. This is also supported by other findings; breast-feeding especially if it is the only source of nutrition, has been shown to protect children against the development of diarrhea in Africa, as elsewhere in the developing world [3].

The majority of the caretakers went to health centers and no one consulted traditional healers. This is in agreement with studies done in other country [26]. 89% of mothers ($n = 226$) preferred fluids in contrast with other studies in Nepal where 15.7% preferred fluids [29]. Oral rehydration therapy was used as a treatment solutions for majority (90.9%) of caretakers, in contrast to other findings in India, where only 13(4.3%) preferred ORS [27]. This difference might be due to the educational status of the participant, as it is shown in the current study only 42 (16.6%) of the study subjects were illiterate as compared to 70% the previous study.

Conclusion

We detected a high frequency of multi drug resistance suspected diarrheagenic *E. coli* in isolated bacteria in children under 5 with acute diarrheal illness. The majority of the participants' caregivers had a good level of awareness when asked about the potential causes of diarrhea (e.g. which is mostly due to poor sanitation). Additionally, there was a statistically significant association detected between low levels of knowledge and suspected diarrheagenic *E. coli* culture positivity. This indicated that those respondents, who have low awareness about source, cause and symptoms of the disease were more likely to acquire suspected diarrheagenic *E. coli* infections. Thus, there is a need for further education in the community about how diarrhea illnesses are transmitted. Additionally, while our data suggest ciprofloxacin or ceftriaxone are good choices for empiric therapy of suspected diarrheagenic *E. coli*, antimicrobial resistance patterns can evolve. Hence, there is a still need for continuous surveillance of the prevalence and antibiotic susceptibility pattern of diarrheal bacterial isolates in hospitals and in the community.

Table 4 Distributions of respondents according to knowledge and attitude towards the symptom and cause of childhood diarrhea at the selected public health institutions in Addis Ababa, Ethiopia, 2015

Cause, Symptoms and prevention of diarrhea	Variable	Frequency (%)
Cause of childhood diarrhea mentioned	Poor personal hygiene	225 (88.9)
	Contaminated food/water	211 (83.4)
	Microorganisms	140 (55.3)
	Inadequate breast milk	137 (54.1)
	Teething	116 (45.8)
	Evil eye	40 (15.8)
	House flies	109 (48.1)
	Do not know	6 (2.4)
Sign/symptoms of childhood diarrhea	3–4 times loose stool per day	234 (92.5)
	Abdominal pain	198 (78.3)
	Fever	165 (65.2)
	Vomiting	140 (55.3)
	Tenesmus	134 (53.1)
	Do not known	9 (3.6)
Cause to worsens childhood diarrhea	Contact with infected people	228 (90.1)
	High fluid intake	122 (48.2)
	Formula milk	120 (47.4)
Preventive methods	Oral rehydration solutions	240 (94.9)
	Personal hygiene	237 (93.7)
	Breast milk	224 (88.1)
	Clean water intake	162 (64.0)
	Anti-diarrheal treatment	123 (48.6)
	Antibiotics	53 (20.9)
	Traditional medicine	22 (8.7)
	Do not know	12 (4.7)

Note: Percentages do not add up to 100 because of multiple responses

Table 5 Practices of respondents towards childhood diarrhea prevention and control at the selected public health institutions in Addis Ababa, Ethiopia, 2015

Variables	Frequency (%)
Exclusive breast feeding	234 (92.5)
Oral rehydration solutions	230 (90.9)
Any fluid intake in addition to ORS	226 (89.3)
Anti-diarrheal treatment	31 (12.3)
Antibiotics treatment	13 (5.1)
Traditional medicines	1 (0.4)
Do not use	2 (0.8)

Note: Percentages do not add up to 100 because of multiple responses

Combined efforts should be also implemented to reduce childhood death rates by improving the knowledge, attitude, and practices level aimed at improving environmental (i.e. water sources) and personal hygiene (i.e. hand washing). Therefore, intensive health education is a public health priority that, together with more judicious use of antimicrobials, could preserve antimicrobial efficacy and substantially reduce diarrheal illness.

Abbreviations

CI: Confidence Interval; CLSI: Clinical Laboratory Standard Institutes; DCA: Deoxycholate citrate agar; DEC: Diarrheagenic *Escherichia coli*; DRERC: Department Research and Ethical Review Committee; *E. coli*: *Escherichia coli*; ETB: Ethiopian Birr; KAPs: Knowledge, attitude, and practices; MAC: MacConkey agar; SPHMMC: St. Paul's Hospital Millennium Medical College; SSA: *Salmonella Shigella* agar; WHO: World Health Organization.

Acknowledgements

The authors would like to thank School of Medical Laboratory Technology, Addis Ababa University and staff members of St. Paul's Hospital Millennium Medical College administration and laboratory staff facilitating the overall the research work. We would also like to extend our profound gratitude to the study subjects without their consent and the provision of the demanded information this research work would not have been real. Last but not least we would like to acknowledge Amy Vercler, Admin Assistant of the SPHMMC and Oludare A. Odumade, MD/PhD, Global Health Pediatric Researcher / Intermediate Care Program Hospitalist, Division of Medical Critical Care / Boston Children's Hospital / Harvard Medical School, United States, who enriched language edition this manuscripts.

Funding

This study was funded by Addis Ababa University, Ethiopia. Funder has role in the study design and data collection but has no any role in writing the manuscript.

Authors' contribution

YM Principal investigator of the study, study design, data collection, laboratory work, and data analysis; AG & KD Study design and data analysis and supervision of the work; AG drafting the manuscript and revising it critically for important intellectual content. All authors contributed to the write up. All authors commented and approved the final manuscript.

Consent for publication

Written informed consent was taken from study participants for publication explaining: the objective and benefit of the finding of the study and their personal identifiers was not attached.

Competing interests

The authors declare that they have no competing interests.

Author details

[1]Department of Microbiology, St. Paul's Hospital Millennium Medical College, P.O.Box 1271, Addis Ababa, Ethiopia. [2]Department of Microbiology, School of Medical Laboratory Sciences, College of Health Science, Addis Ababa University, Addis Ababa, Ethiopia.

References

1. Ina´ c MM, Euse´ b VM, Joaquim R, et al. Etiology of diarrhea in children younger than 5 years of age admitted in a rural hospital of southern Mozambique. Am J Trop Med Hyg. 2007;76(3):522–7.
2. Kosek M, Bern C, Guerrant R. The global burden of diarrheal disease, as estimated from studies published between 1992 and 2000. Bulle World Health Organ. 2003;81:197–204.
3. Bryce J, Boschi-pinto C, Shibuya K, Black RE. WHO Child Health Epidemiology Reference Group WHO estimates of the causes of death in children. Lancet. 2005;365:1147–52.
4. Tiruneh M. Serodiversity and antimicrobial resistance pattern of *Shigella* isolates at Gondar University teaching hospital, Northwest Ethiopia. Jpn J Infect Dis. 2009;62:93–7.
5. O'Ryan M, Prado V, Pickering LK. A millennium update on pediatric diarrheal illness in the developing world. Semin Pediatr Infect Dis. 2005;16:125–36.
6. Viswanathan VK, Hodges K, Hecht G. enteric infection meets intestinal function. Rev Microbiol. 2009;7:110–9.
7. World Health Organization (WHO). Global strategy for containment of antimicrobial resistance. WHO Geneva, 2001; http://www.who.int/drugresistance/en. (Accessed 22 Apr 2012).
8. Isenbarger DW, Hoge CW, Srijan A, Pitarangsi C, Vithayasai N, Bodhidatta L, et al. Comparative antibiotic resistance of diarrheal pathogens from Vietnam and Thailand, 1996-1999. Emerg Infect Dis. 2002;8:175–80.
9. Vu Nguyen T, Van Le P, Huy Le C, Weintraub A. Antibiotic resistance in Diarrheagenic Escherichia coli and Shigella strains isolated from children in Hanoi, Vietnam. Antimicrob Agents Chemother. 2005;49(2):816–9.
10. Asrat D. Screening for enteropathogenic Escherichia coli (EPEC) in paediatric patients with diarrhoea and controls using pooled antisera. Ethiop Med J. 2001;39(1):23–8.
11. Mamuye Y, Metaferia G, Birhanu A, Desta K, Fantaw S. Isolation and antibiotic susceptibility patterns of Shigella and Salmonella among under 5 children with acute Diarrhoea. Clinical Microbiology. 2015;4:1.
12. Chees Brough M. District laboratory practice in tropical countries. ECBS edition .Cambridge University Press, 2002; (2):97–182.
13. Feng, P., Weagant, S. D., and Jinneman, K. (2015). Bacteriological Analytical Manual Chapter 4a Diarrheagenic Escherichia coli. Available at: http://www.fda.gov/Food/FoodScienceResearch/LaboratoryMethods/ucm070080.htm.
14. Clinical and Laboratory Standards Institute (CLSI). Performance Standards for Antimicrobial Disk Susceptibility Tests; Approved Standard—Ninth Edition. USA: Pennsylvania: CLSI. Pennsylvania 19087–1898; 2010.
15. Moyo SJ, Maselle SY, Matee MI, Langeland N, Mylvaganam H. Identification of diarrheagenic *Escherichia coli* isolated from infants and children in dares salaam, Tanzania. BMC Infect Dis. 2007;7:92.
16. Amisano G, Fornasero S, Migliaretti G, Caramello S, Tarasco V. &Savino F. Diarrheagenic Escherichia coli in acute gastroenteritis in infants in north-West Italy. New Microbiol. 2011;34:45–51.
17. Akinjogunla OJ, Eghafona NO, Ekoi OH. Diarrheagenic *Escherichia coli* (DEC): prevalence among in and ambulatory patients and susceptibility to antimicrobial chemotherapeutic agents. J Bacteriol Res. 2009;1(3):34–8.
18. Cohen MB, Nataro JP, Bernstein DI, Hawkins J, Roberts N, Staat MA. Prevalence of diarrheagenic Escherichia coli in acute childhood enteritis: a prospective controlled study. J Pediatr. 2005;146(1):54–61.
19. Agumas LG, Belachew GG, Tekle EL, Mekonnen A. Multiple drug resistance patterns of fecal isolates of enteric bacterial species in Tigray, Northern Ethiopia: A 10-year retrospective analysis. J Pharm Res. 2011;10(4):3259–63.
20. Nataro JP, Kaper JB. Diarrheagenic *Escherichia coli*. Clin Microbiol Rev. 1998; 11:142–201.
21. Ochoa TJ, Ruiz J, Molina M, Del Valle LJ, Vargas M, Gil AI. High frequency of antimicrobial drug resistance of Diarrheagenic *Escherichia coli* in infants in Peru. Am. J. Trop. Med. Hyg. 2009;81(2):296–301.
22. Vila J, Vargas M, Casals C, Urassa H, Mshinda H, Schellemberg D, et al. antimicrobial resistance of Diarrheagenic Escherichia coli isolated from children under the age of 5 years from Ifakara, Tanzania. Antimicrobial Agents Chemother. 1999;43(12):3022–4.
23. Jafari F, Hamidian M, Rezadehbashi M, Doyle M, Salmanzadeh-ahrab S, Derakhshan F, et al. Prevalence and antimicrobial resistance of diarrheagenic Escherichia coli and Shigella species associated with acute diarrhea in Tehran, Iran. Can J Infect Dis Med Microbiol. 2009;20(3):56–62.
24. Okeke IN, Aboderin OA, Byarugaba DK, Ojo KK, Opintan JA. growing problem of multidrug- resistant enteric pathogens in Africa. Emerg Infect. 2007;13(11):1640–6.
25. Carattoli A. Resistance plasmid families in Entrobacteriaceae. Antimicrobial Agents and Chemoter. 2009;53(6):2227–38.
26. Labay EM, Bhuiyan SU, Hongkrailert N. Risk factors relating to the diarrheal disease occurrence among under 5 children at Samut Sakhon Province. Thailand J Pub Heal and Dev. 2007;5(3):63–74.
27. Kapoor P, Raiput VJ. Knowledge, attitude and practice in diarrhea. Indian Pediatr. 1993;33:319–20.
28. Rishi PM, Amsalu F, Lawrence HM, Sisay Y, Bradley RS. Risk factors and case Management of Acute Diarrhea in North Gondar zone, Ethiopia. J Health Popul Nutr. 2010;28(3):253–63.
29. Rehan HS, Gautam K, Gurung K. Mothers needs to know more regarding management of childhood acute diarrhea. *Indian*. J Prev Soc Med. 2003;34(1 & 2):41–5.

14

Hospital acquired vancomycin resistant enterococci in surgical intensive care patients – a prospective longitudinal study

Stefanie Kampmeier[1*†], Annelene Kossow[1†], Larissa Monika Clausen[1], Dennis Knaack[2], Christian Ertmer[3], Antje Gottschalk[3], Hendrik Freise[3] and Alexander Mellmann[1]

Abstract

Background: Vancomycin resistant enterococci (VRE) occur with enhanced frequency in hospitalised patients. This study elucidates the prevalence of VRE on admission among surgical intensive care unit (SICU) patients, whether these patients are at special risk for VRE acquisition and which risk factors support this process.

Methods: Patients admitted to SICUs of the University Hospital Münster were examined during August–October 2017. VRE screening was performed within 48 h after admission and directly prior to discharge of patients. In parallel risk factors were recorded to estimate their effect on VRE acquisition during SICU stay.

Results: In total, 374 patients (68% male) with a median age of 66 years were admitted to one of the SICUs during the investigation period. Of all, 336 patients (89.8%) were screened on admission and 268 (71.7%) on discharge. Nine patients were admitted with previously known VRE colonisation. Twelve (3.6%) further patients were VRE positive on admission. During ICU stay, eight (3.0%) additional patients turned out to be VRE colonised. Risk factors found to be significantly associated with VRE acquisition were median length of stay on the ICU (14 vs. 3 days; $p = 0.01$), long-term dialysis (12.5% vs. 2.0% of patients; $p = 0.05$), and antibiotic treatment with flucloxacillin (28.6% vs. 7.2% of patients; $p = 0.01$) or piperacillin/tazobactam (57.1% vs. 26.6% of patients; $p = 0.01$).

Conclusions: SICU patients are not at special risk for VRE acquisition. Previous stay on a SICU should therefore not be considered as specific risk factor for VRE colonisation.

Keywords: Vancomycin resistant enterococci, Hospital-acquisition, Risk factors, Surgical intensive care patients

Background

Enterococci are an emerging pathogen in hospitalised patients [1]. These pathogens ubiquitously occur in the hospital environment and show a high tenacity on inanimate surfaces [2–4]. As a result, enterococcal infections emerge with a rising frequency. Additionally, enterococci have the ability of acquiring resistances to multiple antimicrobial agents and the capacity to transfer resistances to other pathogens via mobile genetic elements [5–7]. For this reason the prevalence of vancomycin resistant enterococci (VRE) has increased intensively [1]. Vancomycin resistance is associated with enhanced mortality, e.g. among patients with enterococcal blood stream infections [8]. Within hospital settings prevention of VRE transmission is therefore a major objective.

Infection control strategies to control VRE vary, depending on local guidelines. Usually bundle strategies are applied to prevent transmission of VRE between two patients [9]. These include contact precautions, intensified disinfection strategies, the usage of personal protective equipment and active surveillance [10, 11]. In this context, screening strategies are controversially discussed [12]. Both, generalised screening and a risk-adaptive screening, are possible approaches. Regarding the latter, the question arises, which patient groups should be included. Acquisition of VRE in critical ill patients has been associated with prolonged duration of hospital stay, previous hospitalisations, antibiotic

* Correspondence: Stefanie.Kampmeier@ukmuenster.de
†Stefanie Kampmeier and Annelene Kossow contributed equally to this work.
1Institute of Hygiene, University Hospital Münster, Robert-Koch-Strasse 41, 48149 Münster, Germany
Full list of author information is available at the end of the article

treatment, long-term dialysis and immunosuppression [13–15]. Surgical intensive care patients host a variety of these risk factors, although not explicitly mentioned as risk clientele. Whether surgical intensive care patients per se are at a special risk to acquire VRE and should therefore be included in a risk adapted screening upon subsequent admission to a hospital has not yet been investigated. The present work addresses these questions and investigates risk factors making a VRE acquisition more probable.

Methods

Clinical setting and infection control measures

The 1500-bed University Hospital Münster comprises four interdisciplinary SICUs, hosting abdominal-, trauma-, neuro-, vascular- and thoracic-surgery patients. In total, capacity of all ICUs is 43 beds at its maximum distributed over 26 patient rooms.

Routinely, screening for multidrug-resistant organisms includes an admission-screening for methicillin-resistant *Staphylococcus aureus* (MRSA) and multidrug-resistant Gram-negative bacteria according to the national German guidelines is established [16, 17]. After coincidental detection of VRE in screening swabs and clinical samples of SICU patients, a prospective investigation was initiated, concentrating on VRE acquisition during a stay on a SICU.

Extended hygiene measures in case of VRE detection include contact isolation in a separate room; cohorting of multiple VRE patients is possible. Sanitary facilities are strictly separated and staff is instructed to wear personal protective equipment in case of entering a patient room, consisting of gloves, and gowns. Surface cleaning disinfection was performed once a day.

Detection of risk factors for VRE acquisition

During the 2-month study period (August – October 2017), risk factors for VRE acquisition were prospectively recorded during the entire in-patient stay. These risk factors included demographic data (age, gender), the duration of stay on the respective SICU, underlying diseases (haemato-oncological, immunosuppressive diseases [e.g. autoimmune-disease, malignancies, HIV-infection, immunomodulatory drug treatment], hepatic insufficiency, liver transplantation, renal insufficiency, long-term dialysis) and medication (systemic glucocorticoid and antibiotic treatment) attributed to VRE acquisition and previous contacts to the healthcare system (admission from a foreign or domestic hospital, admission from an (in-house) ICU) [13–15, 18]. Patients with a pre-existing VRE status were not included in the analysis, in order to detect risk factors of VRE acquisition on the SICU ward.

VRE screening, culture, antibiotic resistances, PCR testing methods

VRE screening was performed upon patients' admission on the SICU as well as upon discharge of patients from the SICU in order to detect VRE acquisition during SICU stay. Hospital-acquired VRE was defined as acquisition > 48 h after hospitalisation on the SICU. All VRE not acquired during SICU stay were defined as pre-existing VRE. Swabs were obtained rectally (5 cm *ab ano*) (Transwab® m40 compliant, mwe, Corsham, Wiltshire, UK) and subsequently streaked onto chromogenic selective agar (VRESelect™, Biorad, Hercules, California, USA). Suspected colonies were confirmed via MALDI-TOF-MS (Bruker Corporation, Bremen, Germany). Susceptibility testing was performed in accordance with the current European Committee on Antimicrobial Susceptibility Testing (EUCAST) standards for clinical breakpoints (version 7.0) using the VITEK® 2 system (BioMérieux, Nürtingen, Germany). Vancomycin resistance was confirmed by the detection of *vanA*, *vanB*, *vanC1* and *vanC2/3* using the GenoType Enterococcus system (Hain Lifescience, Nehren, Germany). Additionally, subsequent whole genome sequence-based typing confirmed presence of *van*--genes in these isolates.

Whole genome sequence-based typing

In order to elucidate the clonal relationship of VRE -strains, isolates were compared genetically via whole genome sequencing (WGS) using the Illumina MiSeq platform (Illumina Inc., San Diego, USA) and laboratory procedures as described previously [19]. Coding regions were compared in a gene-by-gene approach (core genome multilocus sequence typing, cgMLST) using the SeqSphere+ software version 4.1 (Ridom GmbH, Münster, Germany) [20]. To visualize the clonal relationship a minimum-spanning tree was generated using the same software. Genotypes that differed in ≤3 cgMLST targets were rated as closely related and highly suspected for a hospital-acquired transmission. For backwards compatibility with classical molecular typing, i. e. MLST, the MLST sequence types (ST) were extracted from the WGS data in silico.

Statistical analysis

All data are expressed as absolute numbers or percentage, if not stated otherwise. Independent risk factors were determined in a two-step analysis. First, a univariate analysis was performed, selecting potential risk factors. Chi-Square test was used for categorical and the two-sided student's t-test for comparison of numerical data. Second, a logistic regression was performed to ascertain the independency of risk factors. Statistical significance was declared at $p \leq 0.05$.

Results

Screening adherence, acquired VRE, genotypes

Table 1 shows the detailed results of screening data. Of 374 admitted patients, 336 were screened on admission and 268 on discharge respectively, not considering patients with a confirmed VRE status prior to admission or discharge. In total eight hospital-acquired VRE could be detected. Of all pre-existing VRE (on admission), six presented a *vanA*, 14 a *vanB* and one both genotypes. Of all hospital-acquired VRE, one hosted a *vanA* and seven a *vanB* genotype.

Antimicrobial resistance expressions

In total, 29 VRE isolates of 26 patients (one patient was readmitted twice and one patient once) were tested for antimicrobial resistance expressions. Table 2 gives a detailed overview of tested substances.

Whole genome sequence-based typing and VRE transmission

Of all 29 isolates 25 were subjected to whole genome sequencing. In patients with repetitive VRE detections and the same antimicrobial resistance expression, only the first isolate was undertaken the sequencing procedure. One isolate was not sequenced. Analysing the MLST ST of all sequenced isolates, ST117 was most prevalent (64.0%) followed by ST80 (24.0%) and ST721 (11.0%) (see also Table 2). A genetical comparison with the help of the cgMLST scheme, based on 1423 genes present in all isolates, revealed six clusters, comprising two, three, five and six isolates respectively (Fig. 1). Two of these clusters contain genotypes of pre-existing isolates and isolates detected in both screenings. Six out of eight VRE isolates (204, 283, 291, 314, 361, 372) detected in patients on discharge, who were previously tested negative for VRE on admission, are genetically closely related to isolates detected in other patients, suggesting a transmission of one VRE clone on ward in these cases (see also Fig. 2). The other two isolates (300, 302) detected on discharge are genetically unrelated to other isolates, which can be attributed to selection of VRE e.g. via antibiotic application in these patients or a false-negative screening result on admission.

Analysis of risk factors in SICU patients

Risk factors were compared between the group of hospital-acquired VRE-patients and all patients being not VRE-colonised or infected hospital-acquired. Patients with a pre-existing VRE status were not included in the analysis, in order to detect risk factors of VRE acquisition on the SICU ward. Risk factors to have a significant influence on VRE acquisition in this patient clientele were found to be long-term dialysis ($p = 0.05$), the median duration of stay ($p = 0.01$), and an antibiotic treatment with flucloxacillin (duration of treatment for 5.3 days [$p = 0.01$]) or piperacillin/tazobactam (duration of treatment for 4.6 days [$p = 0.01$]), while an antibiotic treatment per se did not show a significant risk profile. Further results of the risk factor analyses can be found in Table 3. The multivariate analysis found the duration of stay and flucloxacillin treatment to be statistically significant as shown in Table 4.

Discussion

Control of VRE is an emerging topic, patients and healthcare workers have to cope with. An important aspect for prevention of transmission is the early recognition of VRE via screening strategies. Here, the question was addressed, whether SICU patients acquire VRE during their stay and which factors put them at special risk for acquisition. VRE acquisition rate (3.0%) on the SICU was lower than the initial prevalence (3.6%) on admission of all patients. Additionally, no hospital-acquired infection but only colonisations occurred. Distribution of detected *van*-genotypes and MLST ST (*vanB*-genotype and ST117 were most prevalent) are thereby in accordance with national results and trends published for German healthcare institutions recently [21]. In contrast to another retrospective study investigating hospital-acquired VRE, where the acquisition rate was 28.6%, on different wards including surgical and internal ICUs and lacking a generalised VRE screening, acquisition of VRE in our investigation was comparably low [22]. Further investigations on haemato-oncological patients revealed one third of these patients to develop hospital-acquired VRE [18]. SICU patients should per se not be considered as a specific risk clientele for VRE acquisition in comparison with these patients.

Table 1 Screening data of SICU-admitted patients ($n = 374$) during August to October 2017

	Screening result				
	Positive			Negative	Total
	vanA genotype	*vanB* genotype	*vanA* and *vanB* genotype		
Pre-existing VRE	6 (66.7%)	3 (33.3%)	0 (0%)	/	9
Screening on admission	0 (0%)	11 (3.3%)	1 (0.3%)	324 (96.4%)	336
Screening on discharge	1 (0.4%)	7 (2.6%)	0 (0%)	260 (97.0%)	268

Table 2 Collection dates, *van*-genotypes, MLST sequence types and antimicrobial resistance expression of VRE strains detected in SICU patients. Each row represents a single patient

Isolate no.	Collection date	Positive result	MLST ST	*Van* - genotype	AMP	SAM	AX	AMC	PRL	TPZ	IPM	CIP	LEV	VAN	TEC	QD	TGC	LNZ	CN-HLR	S-HLR
001 123	15/08/2017 01/09/2017	On admission Pre-existing	ST80 ST80	*vanB* *vanB*	r	r	r	r	r	r	r	r	r	r	s	s	s	r	–	–
021 119 143	07/07/2017 31/08/2017 04/09/2017	Pre-existing Pre-existing Pre-existing	ST721 ST721 ST721	*vanA* *vanA* *vanA*	r	r	r	r	r	r	r	r	r	r	r	s	s	s	+	–
025	02/07/2017	Pre-existing	ST117	*vanB*	r	r	r	r	r	r	r	r	r	r	s	s	s	s	–	–
076	25/08/2017	On admission	ST117	*vanB*	r	r	r	r	r	r	r	r	r	r	s	s	s	s	–	+
085	02/08/2017	Pre-existing	ST721	*vanA*	r	r	r	r	r	r	r	r	r	r	r	s	s	s	+	+
126	05/09/2017	On admission	ST117	*vanB*	r	r	r	r	r	r	r	r	r	r	s	s	s	s	–	–
189	12/09/2017	On admission	ST80	*vanB*	r	r	r	r	r	r	r	r	r	r	s	s	s	s	–	+
204	26/09/2017	On discharge	ST80	*vanB*	r	r	r	r	r	r	r	r	r	r	s	s	s	s	–	+
235	20/09/2017	On admission	ST117	*vanB*	r	r	r	r	r	r	r	r	r	r	s	s	s	s	–	–
248	27/03/2017	Pre-existing	ST721	*vanA*	r	r	r	r	r	r	r	r	r	r	r	s	s	s	+	–
251	22/09/2017	On admission	NS	*vanA + B*	r	r	r	r	r	r	r	r	r	r	r	r	s	s	+	+
256	22/09/2017	On admission	ST117	*vanB*	r	r	r	r	r	r	r	r	r	r	s	s	s	s	–	–
283	02/10/2017	On discharge	ST117	*vanB*	r	r	r	r	r	r	r	r	r	r	s	s	s	s	–	–
291	05/10/2017	On discharge	ST80	*vanB*	r	r	r	r	r	r	r	r	r	r	s	s	s	s	–	–
300	04/10/2017	On discharge	ST80	*vanA*	r	r	r	r	r	r	r	r	r	r	r	r	s	s	–	+
302	25/10/2017	On discharge	ST117	*vanB*	r	r	r	r	r	r	r	r	r	r	s	s	s	s	–	–
314	13/10/2017	On discharge	ST117	*vanB*	r	r	r	r	r	r	r	r	r	r	s	s	s	s	–	–
330	06/10/2017	On admission	ST117	*vanB*	r	r	r	r	r	r	r	r	r	r	s	s	s	s	–	+
335	04/10/2017	Pre-existing	ST80	*vanB*	r	r	r	r	r	r	r	r	r	r	s	s	s	s	–	–
338	09/10/2017	On admission	ST117	*vanB*	r	r	r	r	r	r	r	r	r	r	s	s	s	s	–	–
348	11/10/2017	On admission	ST117	*vanB*	r	r	r	r	r	r	r	r	r	r	s	r	s	s	–	+
351	11/10/2017	On admission	ST117	*vanB*	r	r	r	r	r	r	r	r	r	r	s	s	s	s	–	–
352	02/04/2013	Pre-existing	ST117	*vanA*	r	r	r	r	r	r	r	r	r	r	r	r	s	s	+	+
361	22/10/2017	On discharge	ST117	*vanB*	r	r	r	r	r	r	r	r	r	r	s	s	s	s	–	–
366	13/10/2017	On admission	ST117	*vanB*	r	r	r	r	r	r	r	r	r	r	s	s	s	s	–	–
372	30/10/2017	On discharge	ST117	*vanB*	r	r	r	r	r	r	r	r	r	r	s	s	s	s	–	–

MLST Multilocus sequence typing; *AMP* Ampicillin, *SAM* Ampicillin/sulbactam, *AX* Amoxicillin, *AMC* Amoxicillin/clavulanic acid, *PRL* Piperacillin, *TPZ* Piperacillin/tazobactam, *IPM* Imipenem, *CIP* Ciprofloxacin, *LEV* Levofloxacin, *VAN* Vancomycin, *TEC* Teicoplanin, *QD* Quinopristin/dalfopristin, *TGC* Tigecyclin, *LNZ* Linezolid, *CN-HLR* Gentamicin-high level resistance, *S-HLR* Streptomycin-high level resistance; *r* Resistant, *s* Susceptible, + – positive, – - negative, *NS* not sequenced

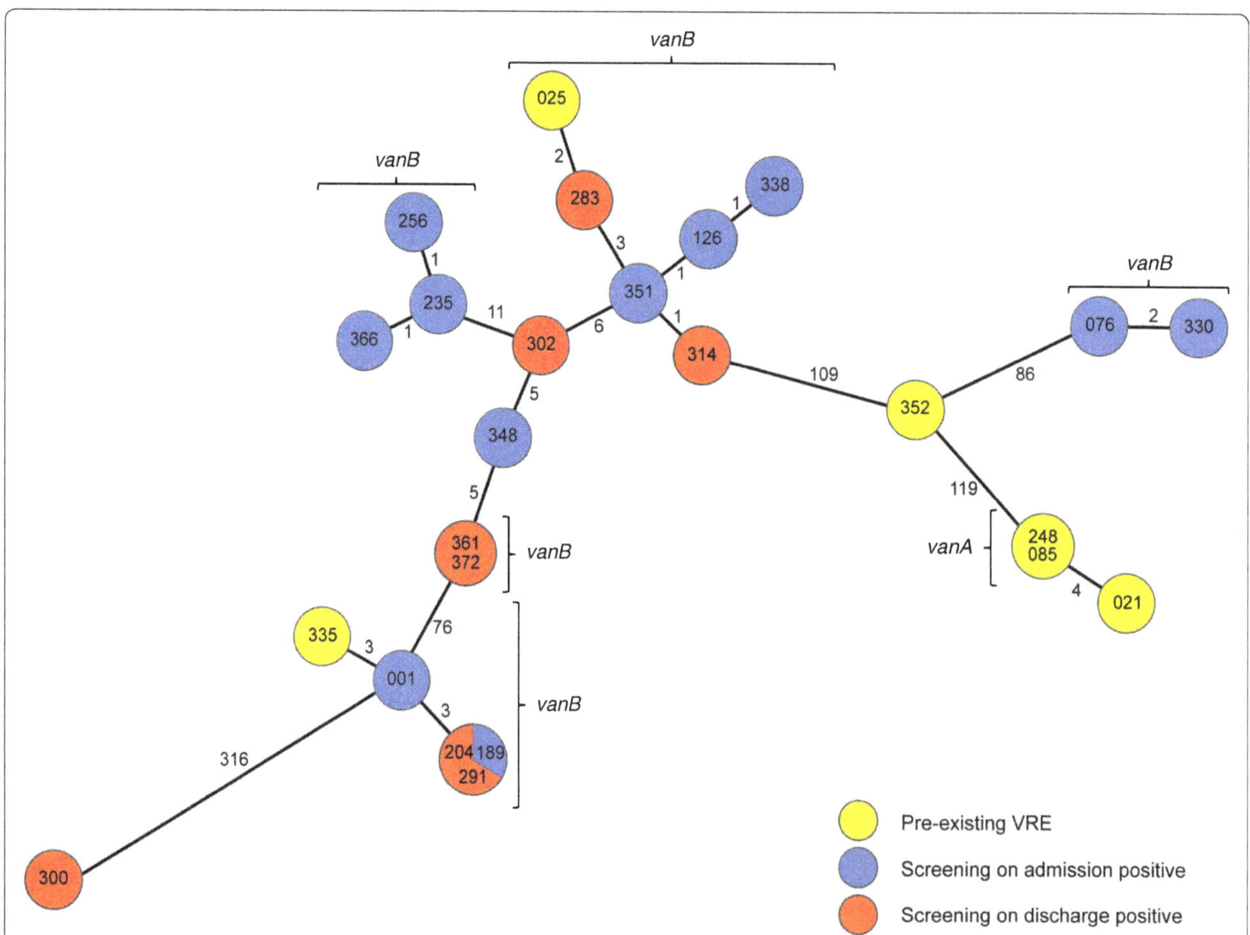

Fig. 1 Minimum spanning tree of VRE isolates illustrating their genotypic relationship. Minimum spanning tree of 25 VRE strains isolated from intensive care unit patients with VRE anamnesis (*yellow*) and detected during screening on admission (*blue*) and on discharge (*red*) during August and October 2017 based on 1423 cgMLST target genes [20], pairwise ignoring missing values. Genotypes are numbered chronologically in order of patients' admission on ICU. Each dot represents one genotype. Size of dots correlates with the number of identical genotypes. Numbers near to the connecting lines show the number of alleles differing between two genotypes. Whole Genome Sequencing revealed six clusters of VRE, one *vanA*-cluster and five *vanB*-clusters

Nevertheless, since hospital-acquired VRE colonisations occurred in our patients, risk factors supporting a VRE acquisition in this group of patients were assessed. Here, the median duration of stay, long-term dialysis and the antibiotic treatment with flucloxacillin or piperacillin/tazobactam were found to be the predominant risk factors. These data correspond with previously investigated risk factors and certainly cannot be considered independently but presuppose each other [23, 24], as also verified by the multivariate analysis. Other risk factors that were found to play an important role in VRE acquisition in other patient clientele could not be verified for our SICU patients. Here, the attributed risk of VRE acquisition after cephalosporin treatment needs to be mentioned. Due to perioperative antibiotic prophylaxis standards, especially referring to cardiac surgery patients, approximately 60% of all admitted patients received cefuroxime; however, this did not lead to an increased VRE acquisition rate. This is noteworthy, since cephalosporine use promotes selection of enterococci and thereby VRE due to intrinsic resistance mechanisms. Nevertheless, previous studies could confirm, that cephalosporine use per se during hospitalization does not result in an enhanced VRE carriage [14]. Interestingly, since the duration of application of flucloxacillin and piperacillin/tazobactam did not vary significantly among the hospital-acquired VRE and the non VRE group, the present results suggest that few antibiotic applications can be sufficient to potentially select VRE. The impact of relatively low numbers of antibiotic administrations on selection of certain pathogens corroborates similar findings for the selection of *Clostridium difficile* [25].

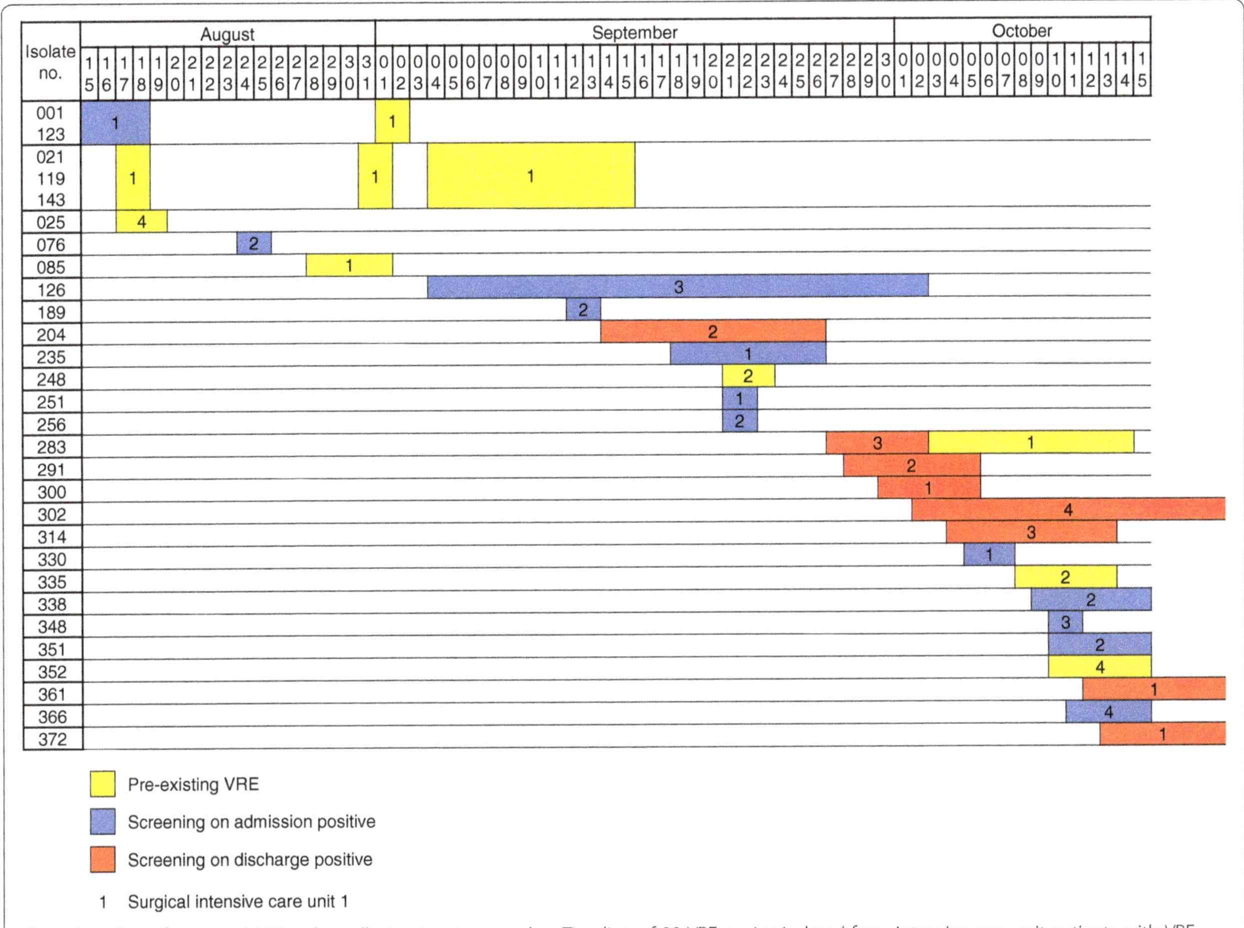

Fig. 2 Timeline of detected VRE isolates illustrating time overlap. Timeline of 29 VRE strains isolated from intensive care unit patients with VRE anamnesis (*yellow*) and detected during screening on admission (*blue*) and on discharge (*red*) during August and October 2017. Each row represents one patient. Numbers within coloured boxes indicate the surgical intensive care unit the patient was admitted to. Isolates 302, 361 and 372, detected in screening on discharge, were identified after end the of study period, but included, as the patients, strains were isolated from, were admitted during the observation period

Previous contacts to VRE confirmed patients are often mentioned as a major risk factor in VRE acquisition [26]. Considering the present core genome analysis of isolates, transmission of VRE on ward could not explicitly be excluded in some cases. This may be due to the transmission of this pathogen on inanimate surfaces in advance to the final diagnosis of the VRE status. Hence in case of a confirmed VRE status, adequate basic and, if necessary, intensified hygienic measures consisting of bundle strategies including contact precautions, usage of personal protective equipment, appropriate disinfection strategies, screening of contact patients and antibiotic stewardship should be implemented to avoid transmissions as good as possible.

Our study has limitations. First, the study period was relatively short. Additional risk factors might have been revealed in case of a longer study period. Moreover, distribution of detected MLST ST in found VRE could have been different. Second, we evaluated risk factors promoting VRE carriage, e.g. flucloxacillin and piperacillin/tazobactam application, but did not investigate the pathophysiological background. Future (prospective) studies are needed to reveal underlying mechanisms. Nevertheless, our findings are in accordance with results published previously [27]. Environmental sampling was not performed during the present study, which could have uncovered the role of inanimate surfaces in VRE transmission, especially in cases of clonality of isolates. Another limitation is the problem of screening sensitivity. Here, only one rectal swab was applied on admission and on discharge respectively, which can lead underestimation of VRE prevalence. However, since screening was performed the same way on admission and on discharge, acquisition rate of VRE during SICU stay can still be assessed precisely.

Table 3 Characteristics and risk factors of admitted surgical intensive care patients with and without hospital-acquired VRE

Characteristic	All admitted patients (n = 374)	Patients with acquired VRE (*n* = 8)	Patients without acquired/ pre-existing VRE (*n* = 345)	*p*-value
Demographic data				
Median age (years)	66 (range: 14–91)	71.5 (range: 50–78)	65 (range: 14–91)	0.43
Male gender	254 (67.9%)	4 (50.0%)	241 (69.9%)	0.23
Median duration of stay (days)	3 (range: 1–45)	14 (range: 7–30)	3 (range: 1–45)	*0.01*
Underlying disease/treatment				
Haemato-oncological disease	62 (16.6%)	1 (12.5%)	58 (16.8%)	0.74
Immunosuppressive disease	71 (19.0%)	1 (12.5%)	66 (19.1%)	0.63
Hepatic insufficiency	17 (4.5%)	0 (0%)	15 (4.3%)	0.55
Liver transplantation	8 (2.1%)	0 (0%)	8 (2.3%)	0.66
Renal insufficiency	51 (13.6%)	2 (25.0%)	41 (11.9%)	0.26
Long-term dialysis	10 (2.7%)	1 (12.5%)	7 (2.0%)	*0.05*
Systemic glucocorticoid treatment	36 (9.6%)	1 (12.5%)	32 (9.2%)	0.76
Antibiotic treatment	218 (58.3%)	7 (87.5%)	207 (60.0%)	0.11
Ampicillin	7 (3.2%)	0 (0%)	4 (1.9%)	0.76
Amoxicillin	14 (6.4%)	0 (0%)	13 (6.3%)	0.58
Flucloxacillin	20 (9.2%)	2 (28.6%)	15 (7.2%)	*0.01*
Piperacillin/tazobactam	62 (28.4%)	4 (57.1%)	55 (26.6%)	*0.01*
Cefuroxime	130 (59.6%)	1 (14.2%)	127 (61.4%)	0.16
Ceftriaxone	7 (3.2%)	0 (0%)	3 (1.4%)	0.79
Meropenem	41 (18.8%)	2 (28.6%)	36 (17.4%)	0.19
Clindamycin	7 (3.2%)	0 (0%)	7 (3.4%)	0.68
Daptomycin	8 (3.7%)	0 (0%)	5 (2.4%)	0.73
Linezolid	3 (1.4%)	0 (0%)	3 (1.4%)	0.79
Rifampicin	13 (6.0%)	0 (0%)	10 (4.8%)	0.63
Erythromycin	7 (3.2%)	0 (0%)	6 (2.9%)	0.71
Vancomycin	19 (8.7%)	0 (0%)	16 (7.7%)	0.53
Fosfomycin	7 (3.2%)	0 (0%)	6 (2.9%)	0.71
Trimethoprim/Sulfamethoxazole	6 (2.8%)	0 (0%)	6 (2.9%)	0.71
Metronidazole	8 (3.7%)	0 (0%)	7 (3.4%)	0.68
Previous contact to healthcare system				
Admission from a foreign hospital	1 (0.3%)	0 (0%)	1 (0.3%)	0.88
Admission from a domestic hospital	188 (50.2%)	5 (62.5%)	173 (50.0%)	0.49
Admission from an intensive care unit	90 (24.1%)	4 (50.0%)	76 (22.0%)	0.06

Statistical significance was declared at $p \leq 0.05$ (see italicized entries)

Table 4 Multivariate analysis: risk factors associated with VRE acquisition

Risk factors ($p \leq 0.05$)	Odds Ratio	95% CI
Duration of stay	0.90	0.84–0.96
Long-term-dialysis	0.08	0.01–1.10
Flucloxacillin treatment	0.09	0.01–0.60
Piperacillin/tazobactam treatment	0.24	0.05–1.13

Conclusion

Compared to patient clienteles previously investigated [23, 28–30], SICU patients per se are not at higher risk of VRE acquisition if hygiene measures are applied as recommended. If a risk adapted screening policy is applied as practised in other national institutions [22], stay on a SICU should not be considered as a risk factor for screening upon admission to a healthcare facility.

Abbreviations

SICU: Surgical intensive care unit; VRE: Vancomycin resistant enterococci

Authors' contributions
SK and AK: Conception and design of the study, acquisition, analysis and interpretation of data, drafting article. LMC and DK: Acquisition, analysis and interpretation of data, revising article critically. CE, AG and HF: Interpretation of data, revising article critically. AM: Conception and design of the study, interpretation of data, revising article critically. All authors have seen and approved the final version of the manuscript.

Consent for publication
Not applicable.

Competing interests
The authors declare that they have no competing interests.

Author details
[1]Institute of Hygiene, University Hospital Münster, Robert-Koch-Strasse 41, 48149 Münster, Germany. [2]Institute of Medical Microbiology, University Hospital Münster, Münster, Germany. [3]Department of Anaesthesiology, Intensive Care and Pain Medicine, University Hospital Münster, Münster, Germany.

References
1. European Center for Disease Prevention and Control. Data from the ECDC Surveillance Atlas - Antimicrobial resistance. https://ecdc.europa.eu/en/antimicrobial-resistance/surveillance-and-disease-data/data-ecdc. Accessed 05 Nov 2017.
2. Kramer A, Schwebke I, Kampf G. How long do nosocomial pathogens persist on inanimate surfaces? A systematic review. BMC Infect Dis. 2006;6:130.
3. Sample ML, Gravel D, Oxley C, Toye B, Garber G, Ramotar K. An outbreak of vancomycin-resistant enterococci in a hematology-oncology unit: control by patient cohorting and terminal cleaning of the environment. Infect Control Hosp Epidemiol. 2002;23:468–70.
4. McDermott H, Skally M, O'Rourke J, Humphreys H, Fitzgerald-Hughes D. Vancomycin-resistant enterococci (VRE) in the intensive care unit in a nonoutbreak setting: identification of potential reservoirs and epidemiological associations between patient and environmental VRE. Infect Control Hosp Epidemiol. 2018;39:40–5.
5. Pinholt M, Gumpert H, Bayliss S, Nielsen JB, Vorobieva V, Pedersen M, et al. Genomic analysis of 495 vancomycin-resistant enterococcus faecium reveals broad dissemination of a vanA plasmid in more than 19 clones from Copenhagen, Denmark. J Antimicrob Chemother. 2017;72:40–7.
6. Bender JK, Kalmbach A, Fleige C, Klare I, Fuchs S, Werner G. Population structure and acquisition of the *vanB* resistance determinant in German clinical isolates of *Enterococcus faecium* ST192. Sci Rep. 2016;6:21847.
7. Gawryszewska I, Zabicka D, Hryniewicz W, Sadowy E. Linezolid-resistant enterococci in polish hospitals: species, clonality and determinants of linezolid resistance. Eur J Clin Microbiol Infect Dis. 2017;36:1279–86.
8. DiazGranados CA, Zimmer SM, Klein M, Jernigan JA. Comparison of mortality associated with vancomycin-resistant and vancomycin-susceptible enterococcal bloodstream infections: a meta-analysis. Clin Infect Dis. 2005;41:327–33.
9. Reyes K, Bardossy AC, Zervos M. Vancomycin-Resistant Enterococci. Epidemiology, Infection Prevention, and Control Infect Dis Clin North Am. 2016;30:953–65.
10. Derde LP, Cooper BS, Goossens H, Malhotra-Kumar S, Willems RJ, Gniadkowski M, et al. Interventions to reduce colonisation and transmission of antimicrobial-resistant bacteria in intensive care units: an interrupted time series study and cluster randomised trial. Lancet Infect Dis. 2014;14:31–9.
11. Price CS, Paule S, Noskin GA, Peterson LR. Active surveillance reduces the incidence of vancomycin-resistant enterococcal bacteremia. Clin Infect Dis. 2003;37:921–8.
12. Faron ML, Ledeboer NA, Buchan BW. Resistance mechanisms, epidemiology, and approaches to screening for vancomycin-resistant enterococcus in the health care setting. J Clin Microbiol. 2016;54:2436–47.
13. Zacharioudakis IM, Zervou FN, Ziakas PD, Rice LB, Mylonakis E. Vancomycin-resistant enterococci colonization among dialysis patients: a meta-analysis of prevalence, risk factors, and significance. Am J Kidney Dis. 2015;65:88–97.
14. Papadimitriou-Olivgeris M, Drougka E, Fligou F, Kolonitsiou F, Liakopoulos A, Dodou V, et al. Risk factors for enterococcal infection and colonization by vancomycin-resistant enterococci in critically ill patients. Infection. 2014;42:1013–22.
15. Ford CD, Lopansri BK, Haydoura S, Snow G, Dascomb KK, Asch J, et al. Frequency, risk factors, and outcomes of vancomycin-resistant enterococcus colonization and infection in patients with newly diagnosed acute leukemia: different patterns in patients with acute myelogenous and acute lymphoblastic leukemia. Infect Control Hosp Epidemiol. 2015;36:47–53.
16. Robert Koch Institut. Empfehlungen zur Prävention und Kontrolle von Methicillin-resistenten *Staphylococcus aureus*-Stämmen (MRSA) in medizinischen und pflegerischen Einrichtungen. Epi Bull. 2014;57:696–732.
17. Robert Koch Institut. Hygienemaßnahmen bei Infektionen oder Besiedlung mit multiresistenten gramnegativen Stäbchen. Epi Bull. 2012;55:1311–54.
18. Ford CD, Lopansri BK, Gazdik MA, Webb B, Snow GL, Hoda D, et al. Room contamination, patient colonization pressure, and the risk of vancomycin-resistant enterococcus colonization on a unit dedicated to the treatment of hematologic malignancies and hematopoietic stem cell transplantation. Am J Infect Control. 2016;44:1110–5.
19. Mellmann A, Bletz S, Boking T, Kipp F, Becker K, Schultes A, et al. Real-time genome sequencing of resistant Bacteria provides precision infection control in an institutional setting. J Clin Microbiol. 2016;54:2874–81.
20. de Been M, Pinholt M, Top J, Bletz S, Mellmann A, van Schaik W, et al. Core genome multilocus sequence typing scheme for high- resolution typing of *Enterococcus faecium*. J Clin Microbiol. 2015;53:3788–97.
21. Robert Koch Institut. Eigenschaften, Häufigkeit und Verbreitung von Vancomycin-resistenten Enterokokken (VRE) in Deutschland - Update 2015/2016. Epi Bull. 2017;46:519–27.
22. Remschmidt C, Behnke M, Kola A, Pena Diaz LA, Rohde AM, Gastmeier P, et al. The effect of antibiotic use on prevalence of nosocomial vancomycin-resistant enterococci- an ecologic study. Antimicrob Resist Infect Control. 2017;6:95.
23. D'Agata EM, Green WK, Schulman G, Li H, Tang YW, Schaffner W. Vancomycin-resistant enterococci among chronic hemodialysis patients: a prospective study of acquisition. Clin Infect Dis. 2001;32:23–9.
24. Pan SC, Wang JT, Chen YC, Chang YY, Chen ML, Chang SC. Incidence of and risk factors for infection or colonization of vancomycin-resistant enterococci in patients in the intensive care unit. PLoS One. 2012;7:e47297.
25. Hensgens MP, Goorhuis A, Dekkers OM, Kuijper EJ. Time interval of increased risk for Clostridium difficile infection after exposure to antibiotics. J Antimicrob Chemother. 2012;67:742–8.
26. Tacconelli E, Cataldo MA. Vancomycin-resistant enterococci (VRE): transmission and control. Int J Antimicrob Agents. 2008;31:99–106.
27. Karki S, Land G, Aitchison S, Kennon J, Johnson PD, Ballard SA, et al. Long-term carriage of vancomycin-resistant enterococci in patients discharged from hospitals: a 12-year retrospective cohort study. J Clin Microbiol. 2013;51:3374–9.
28. Vydra J, Shanley RM, George I, Ustun C, Smith AR, Weisdorf DJ, et al. Enterococcal bacteremia is associated with increased risk of mortality in recipients of allogeneic hematopoietic stem cell transplantation. Clin Infect Dis. 2012;55:764–70.
29. Flokas ME, Karageorgos SA, Detsis M, Alevizakos M, Mylonakis E. Vancomycin-resistant enterococci colonisation, risk factors and risk for infection among hospitalised paediatric patients: a systematic review and meta-analysis. Int J Antimicrob Agents. 2017;49:565–72.
30. Ziakas PD, Pliakos EE, Zervou FN, Knoll BM, Rice LB, Mylonakis E. MRSA and VRE colonization in solid organ transplantation: a meta-analysis of published studies. Am J Transplant. 2014;14:1887–94.

15

Send more data: a systematic review of mathematical models of antimicrobial resistance

Anna Camilla Birkegård[1*], Tariq Halasa[2], Nils Toft[2], Anders Folkesson[3] and Kaare Græsbøll[1]

Abstract

Background: Antimicrobial resistance is a global health problem that demands all possible means to control it. Mathematical modelling is a valuable tool for understanding the mechanisms of AMR development and spread, and can help us to investigate and propose novel control strategies. However, it is of vital importance that mathematical models have a broad utility, which can be assured if good modelling practice is followed.

Objective: The objective of this study was to provide a comprehensive systematic review of published models of AMR development and spread. Furthermore, the study aimed to identify gaps in the knowledge required to develop useful models.

Methods: The review comprised a comprehensive literature search with 38 selected studies. Information was extracted from the selected papers using an adaptation of previously published frameworks, and was evaluated using the TRACE good modelling practice guidelines.

Results: None of the selected papers fulfilled the TRACE guidelines. We recommend that future mathematical models should: a) model the biological processes mechanistically, b) incorporate uncertainty and variability in the system using stochastic modelling, c) include a sensitivity analysis and model external and internal validation.

Conclusion: Many mathematical models of AMR development and spread exist. There is still a lack of knowledge about antimicrobial resistance, which restricts the development of useful mathematical models.

Background

The discovery of antimicrobials in medicine in the 1920s was regarded as a miracle. Since then, millions of lives have been saved as a result of this treatment. However, history has shown that the introduction of any kind of antimicrobial compound into human or veterinary medicine is swiftly followed by emerging resistance to that compound [1]. Antimicrobial resistance (AMR) is threatening our ability to treat common infectious diseases, resulting in prolonged illness, disability and death [2]. Multidrug and even pan-resistant organisms are now a worldwide problem. Despite the difficulty in estimating the actual costs of AMR, the true economic burden is substantial [3]. The estimated economic consequences of AMR in Europe in 2007 were at least €1.5 billion, while they were estimated to be $55 billion in the US in 2000 (cited from Gandra et al., 2014 [3]). It is therefore of utmost importance to limit the emergence and spread of AMR.

AMR is spreading globally - not just in the human population, but also in animal populations and the environment. Furthermore, there is consistent evidence that an exchange of bacteria resistant to antimicrobials and AMR determinants exists between these different compartments [4]. AMR determinants have been shown to survive in environments such as sludge and wastewater treatment systems [5, 6], thus allowing for the transmission of infectious bacteria and accelerating the problem of AMR.

Mathematical models have become important decision support tools in medicine and public health [7]. They have helped in improving our understanding of the development, emergence and spread of AMR [7, 8]. In addition, they can identify gaps in our knowledge, and

* Correspondence: acbir@dtu.dk
[1]Department of Applied Mathematics and Computer Science, Technical University of Denmark, Asmussens Allé Building 303B, 2800 Kgs. Lyngby, Denmark
Full list of author information is available at the end of the article

direct research towards missing information for important parameters and processes in the modelled system. However, in 2006, Opatowski et al. [7] published a review on mathematical models on AMR and concluded that there was still a need for major improvements of AMR models such as regarding implementing important features of pathogen including resistance mechanisms and inter-species cooperation. Continual evaluation of published mathematical models is therefore necessary for us to recognise the progress in AMR modelling. Gaps in our knowledge can be identified, and this can be used to set the agenda and form suitable hypotheses for future research in the fight against AMR.

Grimm et al. [9] updated the TRACE paradigm that was established in 2010 with the aim of developing guidelines to produce useful models. The TRACE paradigm includes eight elements that, when followed, ensure that models are clearly communicated when published. These elements are: 1) Problem formulation (clear formulation of the objective and a description of the context of the model); 2) Model description (written description of model elements to allow readers to understand and replicate the model); 3) Data evaluation (an assessment of the quality of data used to parameterise the model); 4) Conceptual model evaluation (a list and explanation of the most important conceptual design decisions); 5) Implementation verification (internal validation of the model, testing for programming errors and assessing model performance); 6) Model output verification (external validation, testing whether the model output matches the observations); 7) Model analysis (mainly sensitivity analysis); 8) Model output corroboration (a comparison of model output with data that were not used to create the model). For a full description of the TRACE elements, see Grimm et al. [9].

Since the comprehensive systematic review of mathematical models between 1993 and 2006 was conducted by Temime et al. [10], a number of additional reviews have been published [7, 8, 11]. However, these reviews either focused on models linking antibiotic use to AMR [11] or modelling AMR in populations (humans and bacteria) and hospitals [7], and did not include exclusively within-host models [8]. These systematic reviews did not examine models of AMR in relation to animal populations and the environment. However, a comprehensive review of mathematical models of AMR should consider models of all relevant populations and ecosystems in order to target the AMR problem from a One-Health perspective. In this way, researchers from different fields could benefit from experiences and advances in the other fields.

The objective of this review was to assess the usefulness of mathematical and simulation models of AMR development and/or spread in individuals and/or populations of humans, animals and bacteria, as well as in the environment. We also aimed to identify gaps in the knowledge needed to provide useful models of AMR. The assessment was achieved using a systematic review. The published models were then summarised and compared using an adapted version of previously developed frameworks [7, 8]. Furthermore, the strengths and weaknesses of the models were discussed using the TRACE paradigm [9] .

Methods

This is a systematic review following the PRISMA guidelines [12] without the use of an existing review protocol.

Selection of papers and search criteria

The search was performed in PubMed and Web of Science on 6th February 2017. We used the following search terms:

In PubMed three searches were performed:

1) (((((((antimicrobial) OR antibiotic) OR antibacterial) AND "last 10 years"[PDat])) AND resistan*) AND model[Title]) AND "last 10 years"[PDat] AND English[lang]).
2) (((((((antimicrobial) OR antibiotic) OR antibacterial) AND "last 10 years"[PDat])) AND resistan*) AND model[Title]) AND "last 10 years"[PDat] AND English[lang]).

In Web of Science three searches were performed:

1) TS = (resistan*) AND (TS = (antibacterial) OR TS = (antimicrobial) OR TS = (antibiotic)) AND TITLE: (model*) ENGLISH, ARTICLE, REVEIW, 2006–2017 & TS = (resistan*)
2) (TS = (antibacterial) OR TS = (antimicrobial) OR TS = (antibiotic)) AND TITLE: (population dynamic*) ENGLISH, ARTICLE, REVIEW, 2006–2017
3) TS = (resistan*) AND (TS = (antibacterial) OR TS = (antimicrobial) OR TS = (antibiotic)) AND TITLE: (simulat*) ENGLISH, ARTICLE, REVIEW, 2006–2017

We checked for duplicates between the two databases, and excluded papers based on titles. More papers were excluded after the abstracts of all papers were screened. Finally, following full screening of the papers, some were deemed not to fulfil the inclusion criteria and were therefore excluded (Fig. 1). The screening of abstracts and full papers was carried out by three of the authors, with each person reading 2/3 of the abstracts and 2/3 of the full papers.

Papers were included if they: 1) presented not previous published mathematical models that represented the development and/or spread of AMR; 2) modelled AMR in bacteria, humans, animal or the environment, and 3)

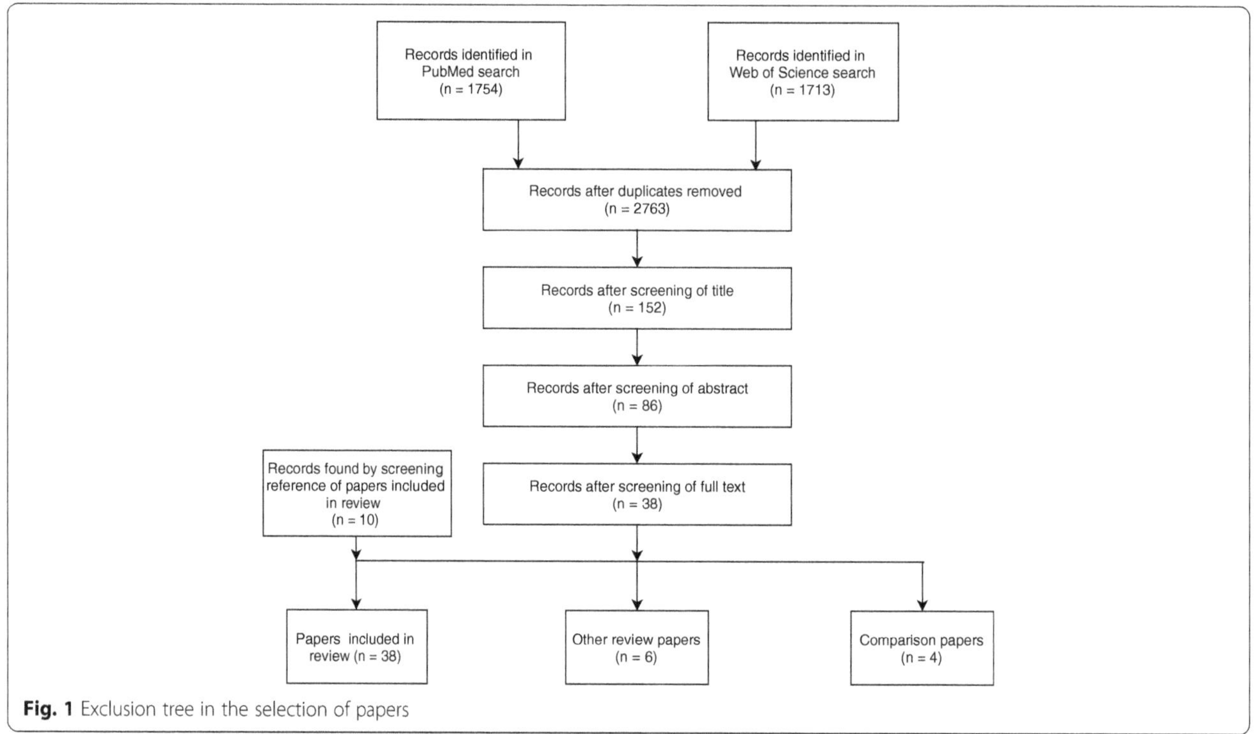

Fig. 1 Exclusion tree in the selection of papers

included the effect of antimicrobial compounds. Papers that focused on only the spread of a specific resistant bacterial pathogen were not included. In addition, papers based solely on statistical analysis were also excluded, as this review focuses on mathematical models.

Previously published reviews of mathematical models of AMR were identified during the review process. The reference lists of these reviews were scrutinised to identify additional papers that might fit the inclusion criteria. These are referred to as "papers identified by other means".

Analysing the papers

Three of the authors read the selected papers. Each person read a random sample of 2/3 of the papers (as described above), while ensuring that each paper was read by two authors. Information about the papers was extracted and sorted into five constructs (model description, modelling technique, modelling pathways, model specifications and model validation).

Relevant information for each of the five constructs was extracted from the papers. This information is described in Table 1. Furthermore, information on the following descriptive parameters was extracted from the papers: programming software, year of the publication of the paper, and the country of affiliation of the first author.

Model usefulness and documentation

We used the TRACE framework for good practice in model development and documentation developed by Grimm et al. [9] to evaluate the conformity of the models to the TRACE guidelines. These guidelines ensure that useful models are produced.

Studies were initially evaluated according to the constructs described in Table 1. Hereafter, studies that had verified the model and conducted sensitivity analysis – hence complying with two of the TRACE criteria [9] (Criteria 6 and 7) – were identified. These studies were further evaluated to assess whether they fulfilled the remaining criteria.

Results

Exclusion of papers

Studies that were excluded based on their title mainly included models of pathogen spread and the mode of action of antimicrobial compounds. The main reason for excluding studies based on the abstract or the full paper was that the study described statistical models of AMR spread and development. Another reason for exclusion was that the studies described a model of resistant bacteria without any susceptible counterpart, therefore merely describing a model of bacterial spread within a population. The exclusion of papers is described in Fig. 1.

Assessing the included papers

The vast majority of the models were population models (77%), while a small number were individual- or agent-based models. Only one was a nested model, in which individuals (pigs) and the bacterial populations inside them were modelled (Table 2).

Table 1 Description of the information extracted from the selected studies

Construct	Attributes	Levels	Comments
Model description	Modelled process	Spread of AMR Development of AMR Spread and development of AMR	Other types of AMR processes were for example fitness cost and difference in resistance due to the age of bacteria.
	Model type	Agent based Nested model Individual based Population Other models	Other model types were: Beverton-Holt, cellular automata, band-pass, or chemostat model.
	Population	Animal species Bacteria Humans	No specified host was used in cases where only the bacterial population was modelled.
	Environment	River Slurry Cellular automata Community Farm Hospital Human Animal species In vitro Not specified	Hospital refers to both human and veterinary hospitals.
Modelling techniques	Simulation / analytic	Simulation Analytic Analytic & simulation	
	Uncertainty display	Deterministic Stochastic Deterministic & stochastic	Both deterministic and stochastic were used for example in the case of nested models and papers comparing deterministic and stochastic models.
Modelling population interactions	Mixing of population	Homogenous mixing Heterogeneous mixing Homogenous & heterogeneous mixing Not relevant	Both heterogeneous and homogenous mixing refers to e.g. rivers and network models with homogenous mixing at the nodes but heterogeneous between nodes. Not relevant may refer to development of specific traits such as efflux pumps.
	Co-existence level[a]	No conversion Single strain Uni-directional Bi-directional	Uni-directional was defined as a one-way conversion from resistant strain/carrier to sensitive strain/carrier or vice versa, whereas bi-directional conversion was possible in case of a two-way conversion. In case of no conversion, only competition between strains was possible.
Model specification	AMR display	Genotypic AMR Phenotypic AMR Genotypic & phenotypic AMR Other types of AMR	Other types of AMR describing a more molecular AMR mechanism were for example modelling of efflux pumps or plasmids.
	Number of resistant strains	Single resistant strain Multiple resistant strains	Multiple resistance means that two or more strains of the same bacterial species resistant to antimicrobials were modelled
	Bacterial species	Specified Not specified	If specified, the specific species was noted
	Dosing of the antimicrobial	Constant dosing Other dosing	Other dosing was for example specific treatment strategy

Table 1 Description of the information extracted from the selected studies *(Continued)*

Construct	Attributes	Levels	Comments
			or spatial distribution
	Antimicrobial compound	Single, not specified Single, specified Multiple, not specified Multiple, specified	If specified, the specific compound was noted
	Immune system	Yes No Not relevant	Not relevant describes situations where the model did not incorporate a human or animal host with a functioning immune system.
Model validation	Model validation	Literature No validation	
	Sensitivity analysis	Yes No	
	Bifurcation analysis	Yes No	

AMR Antimicrobial resistance; [a]the co-existence level was described according to Spicknall et al. [8], modified to population leve

Analytical solutions were used in eight models, while numeric simulations were used in 16 models. In 14 models, analytical solutions were obtained using numeric simulations. There were 29 models for which the uncertainty was modelled deterministically, a further four were stochastic, and five used both stochastic and deterministic uncertainty display (Table 3).

It was not relevant to describe the mixing of the population for four of the papers, as they focused on development of AMR without population mixing. The majority

Table 2 Model description – results of the information extracted from the selected studies

Modelled process	Model type	Population	Environment	Reference no.
Development of AMR	Individual based	Bacteria	Not specified	[66]
	Population	Bacteria	Human	[53, 67]
			In vitro	[19, 58]
			Pig	[14, 51]
			River	[17]
			Not specified	[16, 49, 68, 29, 18]
		Human	Not specified	[32]
	Other types[a]	Bacteria	In vitro	[59]
			Not specified	[69]
Spread of AMR	Agent based	Bacteria	Not specified	[57]
	Individual based	Dog	Hospital	[13]
	Population	Bacteria	Slurry	[64]
			Not specified	[30]
		Human	Community	[31, 48]
			Hospital	[47]
		Pig	Farm	[54]
Development and spread of AMR	Agent based	Bacteria	In vitro	[60]
	Nested	Pig & bacteria	Farm	[27]
	Population	Bacteria	River	[63]
		Human	Hospital	[33, 46, 50, 56]
			Hospital & community	[20]
			Not specified	[15, 34, 55]
	Other types[a]	Bacteria	In vitro	[61]
			Cellular automata	[70]

[a]Beverton-Holt [69] and Chemostat [59], Cellular automata [70], Chemostat [61]; *AMR* antimicrobial resistance

Table 3 Modelling technique – results of the information extracted from the selected studies

Simulation or analytic	Uncertainty display	Reference no.
Analytic	Deterministic	[18, 29, 30, 34, 48, 49, 59, 61]
Simulation	Deterministic	[17, 19, 31, 33, 50, 54, 63, 64, 67, 70]
	Stochastic	[13, 51, 60, 66]
	Deterministic & stochastic	[20, 27]
Analytic and simulation	Deterministic	[14–16, 32, 46, 47, 53, 55, 58, 68, 69]
	Deterministic & stochastic	[57, 58]

of the models used a homogenous mixing of the population (25 papers, 66%). There was no conversion from resistant strain to sensitive or vice versa in seven of the published models (18%), of which five described only a single strain infection and five modelled more than one strain without conversion between resistant and sensitive strains (Table 4).

Phenotypic AMR in single strains was modelled in the majority (11 models, 29%) of the models. Only nine models included the effect of the immune system, and 11 of the models used a constant effect of antimicrobial compound (Table 5).

Validation of the models was not reported in 27 of the papers (71%). Three models were validated based on the literature and ten models were validated based on data. Sensitivity analysis was carried out in 27 papers, while 11 papers did not report conducting a sensitivity analysis. Four of the papers reported no validation, sensitivity analysis or bifurcation analysis (Table 6).

Table 4 Modelling pathway – results of the information extracted from the selected studies

Mixing of population	Co-existing level	Reference no.
Homogeneous	No conversion	[14, 51, 58]
	Single strain	[19, 29, 30]
	Uni-directional	[15, 31, 33, 46–48, 53, 57, 59, 64]
	Bi-directional	[18, 34, 50, 54–56, 66, 67]
Heterogeneous	No conversion	[16]
	Single strain	[60]
	Uni-directional	[70]
	Bi-directional	[13]
Homogeneous & heterogeneous	No conversion	[27]
	Uni-directional	[61]
	Bi-directional	[17, 20, 63]
Not relevant	Single strain	[69]
	Uni-directional	[32, 49, 68]

Model usefulness and documentation

The papers frequently lacked proper discussion and evaluation of the model assumptions, the usefulness of the data for input parameters and the implications of model conclusions in relation to real-life situations. Only eight papers [13–20] verified the model and conducted sensitivity analysis, thus complying with two of the TRACE criteria [9] (Criteria 6 and 7, Table 6). We identified three papers [14, 17, 18] that satisfied all TRACE criteria except element 5, as none of the studies confirmed the internal validity of the models. Furthermore, these three studies could have provided a better evaluation of the implications of data for input parameters and model assumptions (Table 7).

Description of comparison papers

A special class of papers relating to quantitative comparisons of mathematical models of AMR was identified. Two papers compared the predictions of individual-based models [21] and stochastic models [22] to deterministic differential equation models. Both papers concluded that the deterministic approximation is valid when the number of simulated individuals is sufficiently large and the research question is not driven by single events (i.e. extinction events).

One paper [23] compared SIR models of four, six, eight and 12 compartments to include dual infection and time lag between treatment and AMR development. The inclusion of dual infections covers situations where patients may recover to a state with a coexistence of strains or strain takeover by the sensitive or resistant strain, depending on parameters. These results were independent of the complexity of the model.

One paper [24] compared six different deterministic differential pharmacodynamic models and the ability of statistical methods to identify data simulated from the six models as belonging to the correct one. They concluded that datasets containing only counts of bacteria did not provide sufficient information to identify the correct model. Additional experiments must be undertaken to determine which class of pharmacodynamic models best describe the data.

Discussion

Recently, Heesterbeek et al. [25] reviewed the importance of mathematical modelling of infectious disease dynamics in terms of improving public health. The authors concluded that, mathematical models can provide inside that can be used in public health policies through the use of new data.

Table 5 Model specification – results of the information extracted from the selected studies

AMR display	Number of resistant strains	Bacterial species	Modelling of antimicrobial dosing	Antimicrobial compound	Immune system	Reference
Genotypic	Single	Not specified	Not constant	Single, not specified	Not relevant	[18]
Phenotypic	Single	Specified	Constant	Single, specified	Not relevant	[16]
				Multiple, specified	Yes	[32, 53]
			Not constant	Single, specified	No	[14, 34]
					Not relevant	[19, 58]
				Single, not specified	No	[13]
				Multiple, not specified	Yes	[15]
					No	[48]
					Not relevant	[64]
		Not specified	Constant	Single, specified	Not relevant	[30]
				Single, not specified	Yes	[49]
					No	[67]
			Not constant	Single, specified	Not relevant	[63]
				Single, not specified	Yes	[46, 70]
					No	[20, 31, 54]
					Not relevant	[57, 69]
				Multiple, specified	Not relevant	[17]
				Multiple, not specified	No	[35]
	Multiple	Specified	Constant	Single, not specified	No	[27]
			Not constant	Single, specified	No	[51]
				Multiple, specified	No	[47]
					Not relevant	[60]
		Not specified	Constant	Single, not specified	Not relevant	[61]
			Not constant	Multiple, not specified	Yes	[33, 50, 56]
					No	[55]
Geno- and phenotypic	Multiple	Not specified	Not constant	Single, not specified	Not relevant	[66]
Other	Single	Specified	Constant	Multiple, specified	Not relevant	[29]
		Not specified	Constant	Single, not specified	Not relevant	[59]
	Multiple	Not specified	Constant	Single, not specified	Not relevant	[68]

AMR antimicrobial resistance

AMR is a major threat to public health, and the fight against it could benefit from the use of mathematical modelling. It could play an important role in providing an insight into the dynamics of AMR, quantifying the effect of factors that influence it and providing tools for its control and prevention. Furthermore, modelling can present an opportunity to elucidate potential gaps in our knowledge.

The reviewed papers varied in their choice of model structure and complexity – from simple deterministic models to advanced mechanistic models (agent-based, individual and nested models). However, they generally provided little justification for the model type and structure that was chosen. In addition, the majority of studies focused on modelling only one unit (Table 2), a single strain of a pathogen (Table 5), assumed homogeneous mixing (Table 4), and ignored uncertainty and stochasticity in the development and/or spread of AMR (Table 3). AMR is a multifactorial problem with several elements – including external factors and interactions within and between populations (microbiota, animal and human populations) – able to affect its development and spread [26]. This creates nonlinearity, heterogeneity, and stochasticity that should be considered when mathematical models of AMR are developed. Opatowski et al. [7] wrote that models should take into account the specific pathogen characteristics such as the resistance mechanism of the pathogen and cooperation among species. They concluded that this would provide major

Table 6 Model validation – results of the information extracted from the selected studies

Validation model	Sensitivity analysis	Bifurcation analysis	Reference
Data	Yes	Yes	[20]
		No	[13, 14, 16, 19]
	No	No	[29, 30, 58, 63]
		Not relevant	[60]
Literature	Yes	Yes	[15]
		No	[17, 18]
None	Yes	Yes	[46–48, 53, 64, 66–69]
		No	[27, 31–33, 49, 50, 54, 55–57]
	No	Yes	[55, 61]
		No	[34, 51, 59, 70]

improvements of models.. However, in the 6 years since their review was published, only one paper has described a truly nested model [27] (Table 2), modelling multiple bacterial strains within individuals (pigs) that interact as a population with a heterogeneous structure. Unfortunately, this model was not validated and does not allow conversion of the pathogens. Furthermore, one article [28] published a framework to cope with multiple nested layers from the genetic composition of cells, to the environment of cells, the host of the cells, and the environment of the host. This type of models is clearly something to be striving for in the future as the AMR problem is highly complex, and the interaction on many levels require a deep understanding. It would also be very helpful if the community could commit to using this type of standard models, so that the huge work of parameterise these models could begin. That in the future we could stand on the shoulders of each other instead of trying to building new models for every single problem.

Mechanistic modelling using stochastic processes can describe complex heterogeneous structures and processes, multiple pathogens/genes simultaneously, and model biological interactions that may affect AMR such as the immune system, the dosing effect of antibiotics, the microbiome and variabilities involved in the system. In addition, these models can provide insights into the temporal dynamics of AMR, both in the individual and the population. Arepeva et al. [11] also point to the advantage of this class of models over simpler types of models such as deterministic differential equations. Nine models used analytical solutions to solve the modelled system (Table 2), providing extensive mathematical solutions with a limited interpretation of the applicability of the outcomes to real life. In fact, only two papers [29, 30] attempted to validate the models using data. Analytical solutions can be useful when trying to avoid time-consuming and computer-intensive simulations. Nevertheless, from a practical point of view, the high complexity of AMR and limited translation of analytical solutions to real life can call the usefulness of this approach to solve and/or limit the AMR problem into question.

Ideally, models of AMR should be validated by data. However, many of the published models represent hypothetical situations in hospitals or communities with no supporting data [31–35]. Such models are only useful in the event that a similar hospital or environment can be located. If this is the case, experiments or observational studies can be carried out to validate the models. In addition, there seems to be a lack of knowledge of how to implement different typical parameters and how to relate these to reality. For instance, what is the carrying capacity of a human patient for different types of AMR bacteria or genes, and how do levels of AMR relate to transmission rates under different circumstances in a hospital or community? This highlights the necessity for further fundamental and conceptual research to provide information and data to develop useful simulation models of AMR processes.

Table 7 Fulfilment of the TRACE elements

Study	Problem formulation	Model description	Data evaluation	Conceptual model evaluation	Implementation verification	Model output corroboration
Suthar et al., 2014 [13]	Yes	Yes	Yes	No	No	Yes
Nguyen et al., 2014 [14]	Yes	Yes	Yes	Yes	No	Yes
Ibargüen-Mondragón et al., 2016 [15]	Yes	Yes	No	No	No	No
Bhagunde, Nikolaou, and Tam, 2015 [16]	Yes	Yes	No	Not completely	No	Not completely
Hellweger, 2013 [17]	Yes	Yes	Yes	Yes	No	Yes
zur Wiesch, Engelstädter, and Sebastian Bonhoeffer, 2010 [18]	Yes	Yes	Yes	Yes	No	Yes
Tam et al., 2007 [19]	Yes	Yes	No	Not completely	No	Not completely
Kouyos, zur Wiesch, and Bonhoeffer, 2011 [20]	Yes	Not completely	Not completely	Not	No	Yes

For a complete description of the TRACE elements see Grimm et al. [9]. The two TRACE elements model output verification and model analysis were fulfilled by all eight studies as this was a selection criterion for the comparison with the TRACE elements

Validation is an essential factor when developing a mathematical model. Validation can be both internal (conducted to ensure that the model is doing what it should) and external (conducted to assess whether the model outcomes resemble real life). Models were externally validated in only 13 of the studies; ten studies used data and three were dependent on literature. The absence of validation in many of the published models (Table 5) could be due to a lack of usable data. There is a large gap in our knowledge when it comes to the dynamics of AMR inside a host, especially in terms of genotypic AMR. Interestingly, none of the studies indicated that internal validation had been conducted. Several methods can be used to internally validate the models, such as the rationalism method, tracing method and face validity [36]. Internal validation is important to ensure that the code is free from errors, satisfying the fifth criteria of the TRACE method [9]. It is possible that internal validation has been conducted, even if it is not mentioned in the paper. Nevertheless, we believe that it is important to describe the methods and steps used for internal validation in order to ensure confidence in the predictions. A lack of model validation may increase the risk of erroneous outcomes and conclusions, which in turn may reduce any confidence the scientific community and decision makers have in the predictions. Strict internal validation of the models must therefore be conducted and reported. Furthermore, additional research should be conducted to provide data to externally validate the models, resulting in models that can provide trustworthy recommendations. There exist papers on mathematical models where the TRACE criteria are fulfilled. A good example hereof is written by Foddai et al. [37].

The vast majority of the papers focused on modelling AMR in relation to humans, either directly by modelling human populations (in hospitals or communities) or in bacteria related directly to human health. Only four models relating to animals were conducted (Table 1). Animals might constitute a reservoir of AMR that can be spread to humans through their products (e.g. meat [38–41]), the environment (faeces used as fertilisers [41–43]), or direct contact [41, 44, 45], so more attention should be paid to improving our understanding of AMR dynamics within livestock production systems and the environment.

All studies included in this review report that an increase in antimicrobial use increases AMR in general. Some papers report that certain strategies show relatively smaller increases in AMR, which could be due to reducing contact rates or cycling different kinds of antimicrobial products [13, 15, 20, 27, 31–34, 46–56]. One paper reported a decrease in AMR when using an antimicrobial against which bacteria have no resistance [35]. However, as the authors report, such a property is transient and will diminish in time proportional to the extent to which that drug is used. Some papers construct several pathways to achieving AMR (i.e. hospital- versus community-acquired AMR) and deduce the parameter values at which the R0 (basic reproduction number, denoting how infectious the disease is) is above 1 [20, 31, 48, 52, 55, 35, 57]. However, no papers actually fit epidemiological data to determine parameters or validate their model. There are many studies looking at the epidemiological spread of specific resistant pathogens (e.g. MRSA), but these studies were excluded from this review, as we are interested in the spread of resistance rather than specific pathogens. In stating that there are no data of epidemiological spread, we mean spread of resistance between bacteria in an in vivo situation. There is an abundance of papers describing spread in in vitro experiments [19, 58–61], yet we believe that such parameters can at best be a starting point for estimating parameters in vivo, as the natural environment is much more complex and competitive than a petri dish.

To improve our understanding of AMR, we might need to specifically understand the mechanisms that generate resistance. Some papers in our review modelled specific mechanisms (i.e. efflux pumps, senescence, indoles, or influence of the normal flora) [29, 53, 59, 61]. However, only one of these papers was actually validated by data [29]. Modelling specific mechanisms might be a way to better understand the behaviours and interactions of bacteria using these methods, and it may also give us a better understanding of how AMR interacts when multidrug resistance is considered.

The environmental impact of AMR was modelled in four papers: three of the papers modelled rivers and described the accumulation and survival of AMR [17, 62, 63]. One of the papers also included the effects of metals on the development of AMR [17]. One paper described AMR bacteria growth in slurry [64], showing that AMR bacteria can thrive in this medium. The aggregation and possible growth of AMR bacteria in the environment might be of great concern if bacteria are exposed to a mixture of AM from several sources e.g. in rivers or slurry, they may acquire multiple resistances. If there is a chance that these can then transfer back into the animal or human population, these types of models may be very useful.

The studies originated from 16 different countries and were published in 30 different journals. This indicates that a relatively large number of journals are interested in modelling AMR. Furthermore, it highlights that mathematical modelling is a relevant subject for a broad section of the scientific community. When screening and excluding papers, we might have excluded papers based on a misinterpretation of the title or abstract. However, to minimise such mistakes, we strived to include papers in cases where there was any doubt.

The majority of the studies modelled phenotypic AMR, while few models represented genotypic AMR

(Table 5). Modelling genotypic AMR can be more complicated as many genes can be linked to a specific antibiotic, and the relationship between gene abundance and antibiotic use seems to be more complex than first anticipated [65]. Modelling genotypic AMR requires the relevant genes for the modelled AMR to be represented, as well as circumstances allowing for the genetic AMR to be expressed as phenotypic AMR, leading to a spread of the resistant pathogen within the population. Published models of genotypic AMR do not link this AMR type to the development of phenotypic AMR and the subsequent spread of the resistant pathogen between individuals [18]. This is perhaps due to a lack of information on the necessary circumstances for the phenotypic expression of genetic resistance determinants, thus emphasising the need for more research to better understand this process. Understanding the process is essential in the prevention of AMR development and spread.

In our opinion, the following elements should be considered when developing future models of AMR:

1) Modelling the biological processes mechanistically. This allows heterogeneous processes and structures to be modelled and provides an insight into the 'how and why' of AMR occurrence, transfer and persistence.
2) Incorporating the uncertainty and variability of the system using stochastic modelling.
3) Extensive sensitivity analysis and model validation (both internal and external) using data that can support model development, parameterisation and validation.

The current study provides a comprehensive review of published models of AMR spread and development since 2006. Although the study focuses on providing insights into the technical elements of and differences between the models, it also provides an insight into the elements that should be included when AMR is modelled.

Conclusions

Many mathematical models of AMR development and spread exist. However, there is still a lack of knowledge regarding the underlying mechanisms at work, thus limiting the true usefulness of the developed models. Furthermore, few models complied with the TRACE criteria. Future AMR models should elucidate the dynamics and variability of AMR occurrence and spread in order to investigate ways of effectively influencing these dynamics to prevent and control AMR. In addition, it is of utmost importance to focus research on providing data to parameterise and validate AMR models in order to extract useful conclusions from them. There is a need for more rigorous model development and testing and more abundant experimental and observational data to support model validation.

Abbreviation

AMR: Antimicrobial resistance

Funding

This study was funded by the Danish Veterinary and Food administration. The funding party played no role in the design of this study.

Authors' contributions

ACB, KG, and TH completed the review, ACB, KG, TH, NT and AF designed the study and wrote the manuscript. All authors approved the submission of the manuscript.

Consent for publication

The study did not require consent for publication.

Competing interests

The authors declare that they have no competing interests.

Author details

[1]Department of Applied Mathematics and Computer Science, Technical University of Denmark, Asmussens Allé Building 303B, 2800 Kgs. Lyngby, Denmark. [2]Division of Diagnostics & Scientific Advice, Technical University of Denmark, Kemitorvet Building 204, 2800 Kgs. Lyngby, Denmark. [3]Department of Biotechnology and Biomedicine, Technical University of Denmark, Kemitorvet Building 204, 2800 Kgs. Lyngby, Denmark.

References

1. Clatworthy AE, Pierson E, Hung DT. Targeting virulence: a new paradigm for antimicrobial therapy. Nat Chem Biol. 2007;3:541–8.
2. Neu HC. The crisis in antibiotic resistance. Science (80-). 1992;257:1064–73. https://doi.org/10.1126/science.257.5073.1064.
3. Gandra S, Barter DM, Laxminarayan R. Economic burden of antibiotic resistance: how much do we really know? Clin Microbiol Infect. 2014;20: 973–80. https://doi.org/10.1111/1469-0691.12798.
4. Martinez JL. Environmental pollution by antibiotics and by antibiotic resistance determinants. Environ Pollut. 2009;157:2893–902. https://doi.org/10.1016/j.envpol.2009.05.051.
5. Zhang T, Zhang X-X, Ye L. Plasmid metagenome reveals high levels of antibiotic resistance genes and Mobile genetic elements in activated sludge. PLoS One. 2011;6:e26041. https://doi.org/10.1371/journal.pone.0026041.
6. Miller JH, Novak JT, Knocke WR, Pruden A. Survival of antibiotic resistant bacteria and horizontal gene transfer control antibiotic resistance gene content in anaerobic digesters. Front Microbiol. 2016;7 MAR:1–11.
7. Opatowski L, Guillemot D, Boëlle P-Y, Temime L. Contribution of mathematical modeling to the fight against bacterial antibiotic resistance. Curr Opin Infect Dis. 2011;24:279–87. https://doi.org/10.1097/QCO.0b013e3283462362.
8. Spicknall IH, Foxman B, Marrs CF, Eisenberg JNS. A modeling framework for the evolution and spread of antibiotic resistance: literature review and model categorization. Am J Epidemiol. 2013;178:508–20.
9. Grimm V, Augusiak J, Focks A, Frank BM, Gabsi F, Johnston ASA, et al. Towards better modelling and decision support: documenting model development, testing, and analysis using TRACE. Ecol Model. 2014;280:129–39. https://doi.org/10.1016/j.ecolmodel.2014.01.018.
10. Temime L, Hejblum G, Setbon M, Valleron AJ. The rising impact of mathematical modelling in epidemiology: antibiotic resistance research as a

case study. Epidemiol Infect. 2008;136:289–98. https://doi.org/10.1017/S0950268807009442.
11. Arepeva M, Kolbin A, Kurylev A, Balykina J, Sidorenko S. What should be considered if you decide to build your own mathematical model for predicting the development of bacterial resistance? Recommendations based on a systematic review of the literature. Front Microbiol. 2015;6 APR.
12. Moher D, Liberati a, Tetzlaff J, Altman DG, Grp P. Preferred reporting items for systematic reviews and meta-analyses: the PRISMA statement (reprinted from annals of internal medicine). Phys Ther. 2009;89:873–80.
13. Suthar N, Roy S, Call DR, Besser TE, Davis MA. An individual-based model of transmission of resistant bacteria in a veterinary teaching hospital. PLoS One. 2014;9.
14. Nguyen TT, Guedj J, Chachaty E, de Gunzburg J, Andremont A, Mentré F. Mathematical modeling of bacterial kinetics to predict the impact of antibiotic colonic exposure and treatment duration on the amount of resistant Enterobacteria excreted. PLoS Comput Biol. 2014;10:1–10.
15. Ibargüen-Mondragón E, Romero-Leiton JP, Esteva L, Burbano-Rosero EM. Mathematical modeling of bacterial resistance to antibiotics by mutations and plasmids. J Biol Syst. 2016;24:129–46. https://doi.org/10.1142/S0218339016500078.
16. Bhagunde PR, Nikolaou M, Tam VH. Modeling heterogeneous bacterial populations exposed to antibiotics: the logistic-dynamics case. AICHE J. 2015;61:2385–93. https://doi.org/10.1002/aic.14882.
17. Hellweger FL. Simple model of tetracycline antibiotic resistance in aquatic environment: accounting for metal Coselection. J Environ Eng. 2013;139:913–21.
18. Zur Wiesch PS, Engelstädter J, Bonhoeffer S. Compensation of fitness costs and reversibility of antibiotic resistance mutations. Antimicrob Agents Chemother. 2010;54:2085–95.
19. Tam VH, Schilling AN, Poole K, Nikolaou M. Mathematical modelling response of Pseudomonas aeruginosa to meropenem. J Antimicrob Chemother. 2007;60:1302–9.
20. Kouyos RD, zur Wiesch PA, Bonhoeffer S. On being the right size: the impact of population size and stochastic effects on the evolution of drug resistance in hospitals and the community. PLoS Pathog. 2011;7.
21. D'Agata EMC, Magal P, Olivier D, Ruan S, Webb GF. Modeling antibiotic resistance in hospitals: the impact of minimizing treatment duration. J Theor Biol. 2007;249:487–99.
22. Boëlle P-Y, Thomas G. Resistance to antibiotics: limit theorems for a stochastic SIS model structured by level of resistance. J Math Biol. 2016;73:1353–78. https://doi.org/10.1007/s00285-016-0996-2.
23. Beams AB, Toth DJA, Khader K, Adler FR. Harnessing intra-host strain competition to limit antibiotic resistance: mathematical model results. Bull Math Biol. 2016;78:1828–46.
24. Jacobs M, Grégoire N, Couet W, Bulitta JB. Distinguishing antimicrobial models with different resistance mechanisms via population Pharmacodynamic modeling. PLoS Comput Biol. 2016;12:1–19.
25. Heesterbeek H, Anderson RM, Andreasen V, Bansal S, De Angelis D, Dye C, et al. Modeling infectious disease dynamics in the complex landscape of global health. Science (80-). 2015;347:aaa4339. https://doi.org/10.1126/science.aaa4339.
26. Zur Wiesch PA, Kouyos R, Engelstädter J, Regoes RR, Bonhoeffer S. Population biological principles of drug-resistance evolution in infectious diseases. Lancet Infect Dis. 2011;11:236–47.
27. Græsbøll K, Nielsen SS, Toft N, Christiansen LE. How fitness reduced, antimicrobial resistant bacteria survive and spread: a multiple pig - multiple bacterial strain model. PLoS One. 2014;9.
28. Campos M, Llorens C, Sempere JM, Futami R, Rodriguez I, Carrasco P, et al. A membrane computing simulator of trans-hierarchical antibiotic resistance evolution dynamics in nested ecological compartments (ARES). Biol Direct. 2015;10:1–13. https://doi.org/10.1186/s13062-015-0070-9.
29. Bootsma MCJ, van der Horst MA, Guryeva T, ter Kuile BH, Diekmann O. Modeling non-inherited antibiotic resistance. Bull Math Biol. 2012;74:1691–705.
30. Nikolaou M, Tam VH. A new modeling approach to the effect of antimicrobial agents on heterogeneous microbial populations. J Math Biol. 2006;52:154–82.
31. Levin BR, Baquero F, Johnsen PJ. A model-guided analysis and perspective on the evolution and epidemiology of antibiotic resistance and its future. Curr Opin Microbiol. 2014;19:83–9.
32. Daşbaşı B, Öztürk İ. Mathematical modelling of bacterial resistance to multiple antibiotics and immune system response. Springerplus. 2016;5:408. https://doi.org/10.1186/s40064-016-2017-8.
33. Joyner ML. Modeling the differences in the development of a new antibiotic class versus the development of a next generation antibiotic on the total resistance in a hospital setting. J Biol Syst. 2012;20:109–32. https://doi.org/10.1142/S0218339012500039.
34. McBryde ES, McElwain DLS. A mathematical model investigating the impact of an environmental reservoir on the prevalence and control of vancomycin-resistant enterococci. J Infect Dis. 2006;193:1473–4. https://doi.org/10.1086/503439.
35. Haber M, Levin BR, Kramarz P. Antibiotic control of antibiotic resistance in hospitals: a simulation study. BMC Infect Dis. 2010;10.
36. Halasa T, Nielen M, Huirne RBM, Hogeveen H. Stochastic bio-economic model of bovine intramammary infection. Livest Sci. 2009;124:295–305. https://doi.org/10.1016/j.livsci.2009.02.019.
37. Foddai A, Enøe C, Krogh K, Stockmarr A, Halasa T. Stochastic simulation modeling to determine time to detect bovine viral diarrhea antibodies in bulk tank milk. Prev Vet Med. 2014;117:149–59. https://doi.org/10.1016/j.prevetmed.2014.07.007.
38. World Health Organization. Tackling antibiotic resistance from a food safety perspective in Europe. WHO Libr Cat Publ Data. 2011;:1–88. www.euro.who.int/en/publications/abstracts/tackling-antibiotic-resistance-from-a-food-safety-perspective-in-europe.
39. Barza M. Potential mechanisms of increased disease in humans from antimicrobial resistance in food animals. Clin Infect Dis. 2002;34(Suppl 3):S123–5.
40. Hammerum AM, Heuer OE. Human health hazards from antimicrobial resistant *Escherichia coli* of animal origin. Clin Infect Dis. 2009;48:916–21. https://doi.org/10.1086/597292.
41. Marshall BM, Levy SB. Food animals and antimicrobials: impacts on human health. Clin Microbiol Rev. 2011;24:718–33. https://doi.org/10.1128/CMR.00002-11.
42. Sengeløv G, Agersø Y, Halling-Sørensen B, Baloda SB, Andersen JS, Jensen LB. Bacterial antibiotic resistance levels in Danish farmland as a result of treatment with pig manure slurry. Environ Int. 2003;28:587–95. https://doi.org/10.1016/S0160-4120(02)00084-3.
43. Agersø Y, Sengeløv G, Jensen LB. Development of a rapid method for direct detection of *tet*(M) genes in soil from Danish farmland. Environ Int. 2004;30:117–22. https://doi.org/10.1016/S0160-4120(03)00156-9.
44. Moodley A, Guardabassi L. Transmission of IncN plasmids carrying *bla*CTX-M-1 between commensal *Escherichia coli* in pigs and farm workers. Antimicrob Agents Chemother. 2009;53:1709–11. https://doi.org/10.1128/AAC.01014-08.
45. Nijsten R, London N, van den Bogaard A, Stobberingh E. Resistance in faecal *Escherichia coli* isolated from pigfarmers and abattoir workers. Epidemiol Infect. 1994;113:45–52 https://doi.org/10.1017/S0950268800051451.
46. Friedman A, Ziyadi N, Boushaba K. A model of drug resistance with infection by health care workers. Math Biosci Eng MBE. 2010;7:779–92. https://doi.org/10.3934/mbe.2010.7.779.
47. Wang X, Liu S, Guo H. A nosocomial-pathogens-infections model with impulsive antibiotics treatment on multiple bacteria. Appl Math Comput. 2017;296:64–87. https://doi.org/10.1016/j.amc.2016.10.013.
48. Rodrigues P, Gomes MGM, Rebelo C. Drug resistance in tuberculosis-a reinfection model. Theor Popul Biol. 2007;71:196–212.
49. Ibargüen-Mondragón E, Mosquera S, Cerón M, Burbano-Rosero EM, Hidalgo-Bonilla SP, Esteva L, et al. Mathematical modeling on bacterial resistance to multiple antibiotics caused by spontaneous mutations. Biosystems. 2014;117:60–7. https://doi.org/10.1016/j.biosystems.2014.01.005.
50. Joyner ML, Manning CC, Canter BN. Modeling the effects of introducing a new antibiotic in a hospital setting: a case study. Math Biosci Eng. 2012;9:601–25. https://doi.org/10.3934/mbe.2012.9.601.
51. Ahmad A, Zachariasen C, Christiansen LE, Græsbøll K, Toft N, Matthews L, et al. Modeling the growth dynamics of multiple Escherichia coli strains in the pig intestine following intramuscular ampicillin treatment. BMC Microbiol. 2016;16:205. https://doi.org/10.1186/s12866-016-0823-3.
52. Graef JR, Kong L, Wang M. Stationary solution of a stochastic nosocomial epidemic model in hospital intensive care units. Stoch Anal Appl. 2014;32:840–50.
53. Alavez-Ramírez J, Castellanos JRA, Esteva L, Flores JA, Fuentes-Allen JL, García-Ramos G, et al. Within-host population dynamics of antibiotic-resistant M. tuberculosis. Math Med Biol. 2007;24:35–56.
54. Abatih EN, Alban L, Ersbøll AK, Lo Fo Wong DM. Impact of antimicrobial usage on the transmission dynamics of antimicrobial resistant bacteria among pigs. J Theor Biol. 2009;256:561–73.
55. Sun H-R, Lu X, Ruan S. Qualitative analysis of models with different treatment protocols to prevent antibiotic resistance. Math Biosci. 2010;227:56–67. https://doi.org/10.1016/j.mbs.2010.06.002.
56. Obolski U, Hadany L. Implications of stress-induced genetic variation for minimizing multidrug resistance in bacteria. BMC Med. 2012;10.

57. Gehring R, Schumm P, Youssef M, Scoglio C. A network-based approach for resistance transmission in bacterial populations. J Theor Biol. 2010;262:97–106. https://doi.org/10.1016/j.jtbi.2009.09.002.
58. Yurtsev EA, Chao HX, Datta MS, Artemova T, Gore J. Bacterial cheating drives the population dynamics of cooperative antibiotic resistance plasmids. Mol Syst Biol. 2013;9:683. https://doi.org/10.1038/msb.2013.39.
59. de Leenheer P, Dockery J, Gedeon T, Pilyugin SS. Senescence and antibiotic resistance in an age-structured population model. J Math Biol. 2010;61:475–99.
60. Murphy JT, Walshe R, Devocelle M. Modeling the population dynamics of antibiotic-resistant bacteria: an agent-based approach. Int J Mod Phys C. 2009;20:435–57. https://doi.org/10.1142/S0129183109013765.
61. Wang W, Zou X. Modeling the role of altruism of antibiotic-resistant bacteria. J Math Biol. 2014;68:1317–39.
62. Mostefaoui IM. Mathematical analysis of a model describing the number of antibiotic resistant bacteria in a polluted river. Math Methods Appl Sci. 2014; 37:1956–73. https://doi.org/10.1002/mma.2949.
63. Hellweger FL, Ruan X, Sanchez S. A simple model of tetracycline antibiotic resistance in the aquatic environment (with application to the Poudre River). Int J Environ Res Public Health. 2011;8:480–97.
64. Baker M, Hobman JL, Dodd CER, Ramsden SJ, Stekel DJ. Mathematical modelling of antimicrobial resistance in agricultural waste highlights importance of gene transfer rate. FEMS Microbiol Ecol. 2016;92:1–10.
65. Birkegård AC, Halasa T, Græsbøll K, Clasen J, Folkesson A, Toft N. Association between selected antimicrobial resistance genes and antimicrobial exposure in Danish pig farms. Sci Rep. 2017;7:9683. https://doi.org/10.1038/s41598-017-10092-9.
66. Schulman LS. Bacterial resistance to antibodies: a model evolutionary study. J Theor Biol. 2017;417:61–7. https://doi.org/10.1016/j.jtbi.2017.01.022.
67. Kim J, Lee DH, Song YS, Kang SW, Kim SW. The within-host population dynamics of normal flora in the presence of an invading pathogen and antibiotic treatments. J Microbiol Biotechnol. 2007;17:146–53.
68. Song HX, Peng YY, Zhu ZF. Competition between plasmid-bearing and plasmid-free organisms in the host: population dynamics and antibiotic resistance. Med Princ Pract. 2006;15:436–42.
69. Nemzer LR. A model of band-pass phenotypic resistance in a modified Beverton-Holt framework. Math Biosci. 2014;252:7–13. https://doi.org/10.1016/j.mbs.2014.03.003.
70. Kier LB. Modeling bacterial infection phenomena. Curr Comput Aided Drug Des. 2015;11:321–4 https://doi.org/10.2174/1573409912666151218155921.

16

Epidemiology and microbiology of Gram-positive bloodstream infections in a tertiary-care hospital in Beijing, China: a 6-year retrospective study

Qiang Zhu[1†], Yan Yue[3†], Lichen Zhu[2], Jiewei Cui[1], Minghui Zhu[1], Liangan Chen[1], Zhen Yang[1] and Zhixin Liang[1*]

Abstract

Background: Gram-positive bacterial bloodstream infections (BSIs) are serious diseases associated with high morbidity and mortality. The following study examines the incidence, clinical characteristics and microbiological features, drug resistance situations and mortality associated with Gram-positive BSIs at a large Chinese tertiary-care hospital in Beijing, China.

Methods: A retrospective cohort study of patients with Gram-positive BSIs was performed between January 1, 2011, and June 31, 2017, at the Chinese People's Liberation Army General Hospital. The patients' data were collected and included in the reviewing electronic medical records.

Results: A total of 6887 episodes of Gram-positive BSIs occurred among 4275 patients over 6 years, and there were 3438 significant BSI episodes 69% of these cases were healthcare-associated, while 31% were community-associated. The overall incidence of Gram-positive BSIs fluctuated from 7.26 to 4.63 episodes per 1000 admissions over 6 years. Malignancy was the most common comorbidity and indwelling central intravenous catheter was the most common predisposing factor for BSI. *Staphylococci* were the major pathogen (65.5%), followed by *Enterococcus spp:*(17.5%), *Streptococcus spp.*(7.1%) and other bacterial pathogens (9.9%). The resistance rates of *Staphylococci* and *E.faecium* to penicillins were more than 90%. the vancomycin-resistant isolates were *E. faecium* (4. 1%) and *staphylococcus epidermidis* (0.13%); and only *E.faecalis* and *E.faecium* showed resistance to linezolid (3.8% and 3.1%). Between 2011 and 2017, the overall mortality of Gram-positive BSIs decreased from 6.27 to 4.75% ($X^2 = 0.912$, $p = 0.892$). Neverthess, the mortality in the ICU decreased from 60.46 to 47.82%, while in the general ward it increased from 39.54 to 52.18%.

Conclusions: The morbidity and mortality of Gram-positive BSIs have showed downward trends. Vancomycin and linezolid are still consider the best treatment for patients with Gram-positive BSIs.

Keywords: Gram-positive bacteria, Bloodstream infections, Epidemiology, Incidence, Resistance, Outcome

* Correspondence: liangzhixin301@163.com
[†]Qiang Zhu and Yan Yue contributed equally to this work.
[1]Department of Respiratory Medicine, Chinese PLA General Hospital, Fuxing Road No. 28, Beijing 100853, China
Full list of author information is available at the end of the article

Background

BSIs are serious diseases associated with high morbidity and mortality, which are diffcult to treat and ofen result in a heavy social and economic burden [1]. In China, BSIs account for one-third of healthcare-associated infection, followed by lower respiratory tract and urinary tract infections [2]. Acoording to a resent USA_based prevalence surey, Gram-positive pathogens were the most frequently isolated pathogens among BSIs [3]. Acoording to CHINET, the most commonly gram-positive in 2010 were *Staphylococci*, *Enterococcus spp.* and *Streptococcus spp.* [4, 5]. In addition, some studies have reported that the crude incidence of BSIs varies from country to country [6–8].

Over recent years, due to the widespread use of antibiotics, immunosuppressants and anti-tumour drugs, and the increase of invasive medical examinations and treatments, the epidemiology and antimicrobial resistance have been changing. Multidrug resistant patterns in Gram-positive bacteria have resulted in difficult-to-treat or even untreatable cases, which in tum caused the increase in mortality. E.g. recent ECDC data from 2013 indicated a global increase in methicillin-resistant *staphy lococcus aureus* (MRSA) (> 50%) isolated from blood, and a higher rate in vancomycin- resistant Gram-positive coccus in Europe [9–11]. Morever, *Enterococcus spp.* has shown increasing prevalence of acquired resistance to penicillins, aminoglycosides and vancomycin, which was observed in many countries [12, 13]. A report from Europe has shown that there were more than 1.2 million episodes of BSIs with 157,000 deaths per year, while between 57,500 and 677,000 episodes of BSIs were reported in North America causing some 79,000 to 94,000 deaths [14].

Although there are number of study on BSIs, few data reports have focus on Gram-positive bacteria- BSIs and the epidemiology and antimicrobial resistance of various BSIs in different periods and regions, thus making it very difficult to timely choose antibiotic treatment based on the empirical evidence. Therefore, the purpose of this study was to provide more data on the incidence, microbiological features, mortality and drug resistance data at our hospital.

Methods

We performed a retrospective cohort study in patients with Gram-positive bacterial bloodstream infections between January 1, 2011, and June 31, 2017 at the Chinese People's Liberation Army General Hospital (PLAGH), a 2200-bed tertiary-level healthcare facility in Beijing, China.

Eligible patients included all patients with at least one positive blood culture for Gram-positive bacteria. In patients with persistent BSIs caused by the same organism, only the first episode was included within the previous 30 days. If patients had 2 or more separate BSIs, each infection was considered individually. All patients were identified by searching the real-time nosocomial infection surveillance system (RT-NISS) [15]. This platform utilizes data from electronic medical record systems, such as sex, hospital ward, comorbidity, and microbiology results, with the application of clinically validated algorithms to identify and classify all of the patients' infections. The infection management and disease control department of PLAGH developed RT-NISS. In addition, since Gram-positive bacilli are not routinely identified at our hospital, patients with those types of bacteria were excluded them from the study.

Data collection

The patients' data were collected and included in the reviewing electronic medical records. We recorded the demographic data, including age and sex; the clinical data included predisposing factors, the hospitalization wards, and comorbidities. The microbiological data included species of Gram-positive bacteria, likely sources of BSIs (identified by treating doctors and/or physicians of the infection management and disease control department), and antimicrobial susceptibility results. We aslo collected annual admission data to calculate incidence rates, which are expressed as the number of BSI episodes per 10,00 hospital admissions.

Definitions

The diagnosis of Gram-positive bacterial BSIs had to meet the following criteria: 1) isolation of Gram-positive bacteria from one or more blood cultures; 2) having one of the following symptoms: fever (> 38 °C), chills, or hypotension; and 3) elimination of the possibility of contamination during the collection and cultivation of blood samples [16]. Healthcare-associated BSIs included episodes of bacteraemia occurring more than 48 h after admission and < 7 days after discharge in patients undergoing intensive outpatient therapy involving regular hospital contact. Healthcare-associated Gram-positive BSIs were defined as the first positive blood culture obtained ≥48 h after hospital admission and with no evidence of infection at admission [16]. An episode was defined as the positive isolation of the Gram-positive bacteria from at least one blood culture sample from a patient and without a prior blood culture isolating the same bacteria within the previous 30 days [6]. Onset of BSIs was defined as the date when the blood culture was collected. Poly-microbial BSIs were defined as two or more clinically important organisms isolated from one single blood culture sample or different blood culture samples within 48 h. Active agents were confirmed according to the antibiotic susceptibility testing.

Identification and antibiotic susceptibility testing

Blood was cultured using a BacT/ALERT 3D system (Becton-Dickinson, Sparks, MD, USA) in the microbiology laboratory. Species identification was performed using the VITEK 2 system (BioMérieux, Marcy l'Etoile, France). Antibiotic susceptibility testing was performed using the VITEK 2 system or the Kirby-Bauer Disk Diffusion method (Oxoid, UK) according to the recommendations proposed by the Clinical and Laboratory Standards Institute (CLSI) [17].

Statistical analysis

Categorical variables are expressed as frequency counts and percentages with 95% confidence intervals (95% CIs). Continuous variables are expressed as medians and inter-quartile ranges. The incidence and mortality of Gram-positive BSIs over these years were determined using chi-square test for trend. The comparison of categorical variables was performed using Pearson's chi-square test or Fisher's exact test, while the comparison of continuous variables was performed using the Mann-Whitney U test. The results with a 2-tailed p-value < 0.05 were considered statistically significant. All of the statistical analyses were performed using SPSS software, version 20.0 (IBM Corp, Armonk, NY, USA).

Results

Incidence and species distribution

In total, 6887 episodes of BSIs caused by Gram-positive bacteria occurred among 4275 patients during the 6-year study period. Among 4275 patients with Gram-positive BSIs, 527 were infectioned with two different species (> 30 days apart), and 881 had 2 or more BSI with the same species < 30 days apart. Only the results for the first cases among repeat results were included, so there were 3438 significant BSI episodes.

Among all BSI isolates, the most common Gram-positive bacterial species was *Staphylococcui* (65.5%), followed by *Enterococcus spp.* (17.5%), *Streptococcus spp.*(7.1%) and other bacterial pathogens (9.9%). The species proportions in each year are shown in Table 1. In addition, 69% of these cases were healthcare-associated infections, 31% were community acquired, and *Staphylococci* was the most common isolate. For all Gram-positive BSIs species, healthcare-associated infection was more common than community-acquired infection except for *Streptococcus.*

The overall incidence of Gram-positive BSIs was 6.94 episodes per 10,00 admissions, and the rate decreased from 7.26 to 4.63 episodes per 10,00 admissions(X^2 = 1.0, $p = 0.986$) over 6 years (7.26 in 2011, 7.83 in 2012, 6.57 in 2013, 6.41 in 2014, 7.21 in 2015, 7.95 in 2016, 4.63 in 2017). Respectively, the overall incidence in each year showed a downward trend in the intensive care unit ($X^2 = 0.812$, $p = 0.992$), while there was no obvious change in the general ward($X^2 = 1.02$, $p = 0.985$) (Fig. 1).

Demographic and clinical characteristics

A total of 6887 episodes of Gram-positive BSIs occurred among 4275 patients over the 6 years. Demographics and clinical data were available for 1330 of these clinically relevent episodes, as shown in Table 2. The median age was 53 years old (95% CI 51–55%), and 870 (65%, 95% CI 48–81%) of patients were male. The age distribution had a certain relationship with the distribution of strains ($p < 0.001$), with *Enterococcal* BSIs being associated with older age. Malignancy was the most common comorbidity (28%), followed by hypertension (15%). Moreover, The Gram-positive BSIs incidence was 11.5 patients per 10,00 in the medical ward every year, 9.5 patients per 10,00 in the surgical ward, and 63.3 patients per 10,00 in the ICU, and the distribution of these clinically-relevant episodes in surgical ward were statistically different from our study ($p < 0.05$). Central intravenous catheters were the most common predisposing factors (11%), followed by chemoradiotherapy (6%) and indwelling urinary catheters (4%).

Antimicrobial susceptibility and outcomes

Antimicrobial resistance levels for the most common organisms of the Gram-positive BSIs are shown in Table 3. *Staphylococci* showed a high level of resistance to penicillin, ampicillin, erythromycin, and ciprofloxacin; the resistance of MRSA to penicillin and ampicillin was 100%, and the resistance of MSSA to penicillin was 96.2% but

Table 1 The species ratio from 2011 to 2017(6-months' data)

organisms	year							
	2011(926)	2012(1102)	2013(897)	2014(970)	2015(1145)	2016(1338)	2017(509)	total(6887)
staphylococcus	608[a](65.7)[b]	697(63.3)	580(64.7)	632(65.2)	751(65.6)	937(70.1)	303(59.5)	4508(65.5)
enterococcus	182(19.7)	208(18.9)	136(15.2)	151(15.5)	202(17.6)	217(16.2)	114(22.4)	1210(17.5)
streptococcus	59(6.3)	87(7.9)	89(9.9)	67(6.9)	75(6.6)	66(4.9)	42(8.3)	485(7.1)
others	77(8.3)	110(9.9)	92(10.2)	120(12.4)	117(10.2)	118(8.8)	50(9.8)	684(9.9)

[a]: The bolded data indicates the total number
[b]:The percentage of that group

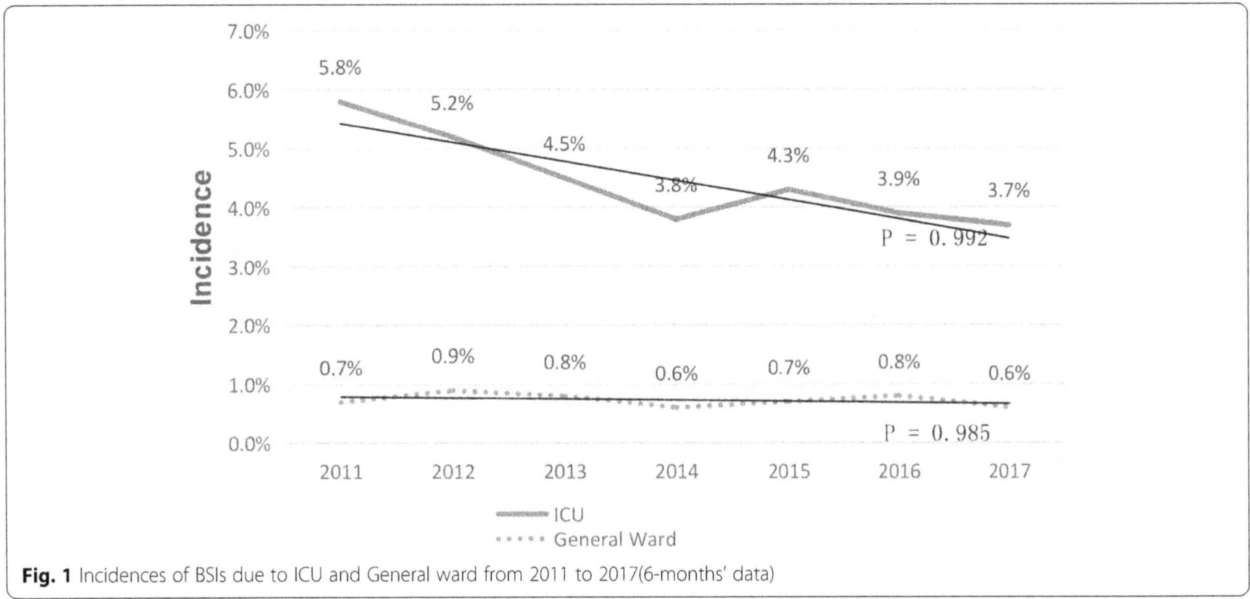

Fig. 1 Incidences of BSIs due to ICU and General ward from 2011 to 2017(6-months' data)

to ampicillin was 40.9%; *Staphylococci* was susceptible to gentamicin and tetracycline except for MRSA and *Staphylococcus haemolyticus*; only *Staphylococcus epidermidis* showed resistance to linezolid at a rate of 0.13% (1/756); and no vancomycin resistance was found. *E. faecalis* showed great sensitivity to penicillin, ampicillin, gentamicin, erythromycin, and ciprofloxacin, but *E. faecium* showed the opposite antibiotic resistance. The rates of Linezolid resistance of *E. faecalis* and *E.faecium* were 3.8% (5/132) and 3.1% (9/294), respectively, but only *E.faecium* showed resistance to vancomycin at a rate of 4.1% (12/294). There was no linezolid resistance or vancomycin resistance with *Streptococcus spp. viridians streptococci* that showed no resistance to penicillin, ampicillin, or clindamycin, but the rate of erythromycin resistance was 70.4%. However, *streptococcus pneumoniae* had a higher resistance rate than *viridians streptococci* in most of the antibiotics. In addition, since there is no national standard of the National Committee for Clinical Laboratory (NCCLS), it was not possible to judge the drug susceptibility of Gram-positive bacilli and others in the present study.

The mortality of Gram-positive bacterial bloodstream infections showed a downward trend from 2011 to 2017 (Fig. 2); The main pathogen causing death was *Staphylococci* (61.9%), followed by *Enterococcus spp.* (22.2%), *Streptococcus spp.* (7.6%) and others (6.3%). Mortality in patients infected with *Staphylococci* ($X^2 = 0.81$, $p = 0.991$) showed an increasing trend, while the mortality in patients infected with *Streptococcus spp.* ($X^2 = 14.62$, $p = 0.023$) and *Enterococcus spp.* ($X^2 = 4.0$, $p = 0.677$) showed a downward trend (Fig. 3). Between 2011 and 2017, the mortality in the ICU decreased from 60.46 to 47.82%, and that in the general ward increased from 39.54 to 52.18%.

Discussion

This study examined the incidence and characteristics of Gram-positive bloodstream infections in one of the largest tertiary-care hospitals in China. So far many studies have reported epidemiology, species distribution and antibiotic resistance of *Staphylococci, Enterococcus spp. Streptococcus spp.* Gram-positive bacilli and others [18–20], neverthless, only few studies have focused on Gram-positive bloodstream infections [21].

In our 6-year study, the incidence of Gram-positive BSIs switched order from 4.6 to 7.3 episodes per 10,00 admissions over 6 years. Acoording to our knowledge, thus far no such data, i.e. incidence rates of Gram-positive BSIs based on large retrospective studies have been reported. In the present study, a downward trend was observed in overall incidence in the ICU per year, while there was no obvious change on general ward. This might be explained with the increased importance of prevention and control infection among medical staff of ICU that was obvserved over recent years. Nevertheless, two recent studies haved reported an increase in the incidence of Gram-positive BSIs in general ward and ICUs [22, 23].

BSIs are commonly associated with comorbidities, such as malignancies, diabetes mellitus and infections [24, 6]. In the present study, we found that malignancy was the most common comorbidity, and the major predisposing factor for BSIs was indwelling central intravenous catheters; this data was consistent with previous results [25, 26]. Several studies have reported that the second most common factors is abdominal and lower respiratory tract infections [27, 18]; while we found that chemoradiotherapy was the second most common factor for BSIs. The observed differences might be due to the fact that the malignancy was the most common comorbidity with extensive use of

Table 2 Demographic and clinical characteristics of patients with BSIs

	Staphylococcus aureus(n = 227)	CoNS (N = 446)	enterococcus (n = 499)	Viri-dans streptococcus (n = 148)	Streptococcus pneumonia(n = 10)	total (n = 1330)	p-value
age	51(50–57)	53(51–55)	59(58–61)	52(50–54)	51(42–53)	53(51–55)	$p < 0.001$
Male	152(66,64–69)	284(64,58–69)	320(64,60–67)	108(73,71–74)	6(60,59–60)	870(65,48–81)	0.857
Female	75(34,30–35)	162(36,30–41)	179(36,32–39)	40(27,25–28)	4(40,39–40)	460(35,18–51)	0.455
Comorbidities							
Malignancy	68(30,27–32)	83(19,13–24)	175(35,31–38)	38(26,24–27)	6(60,59–60)	370(28,11–44)	$p < 0.001$
Trauma	15(7,4–9)	18(4,0–9)	20(4,0–7)	3(2,0–3)	1(10,9–10)	57(4,0–20)	0.408
Hypertension	35(15,12–17)	74(17,11–22)	69(14,10–17)	23(16,14–17)	2(20,19–20)	203(15,0–31)	0.994
Heart disease	15(7,4–9)	69(15,9–20)	38(8,4–11)	10(7,5–8)	1(10,9–10)	133(10,0–26)	0.007
Diabetes mellitus	25(11,8–13)	45(10,4–15)	54(11,7–14)	9(6,4–7)	3(30,29–30)	136(10,0–26)	0.007
Hematological disease	21(9,6–11)	12(3,0–8)	15(3,0–6)	8(5,3–6)	1(10,9–10)	57(4,0–20)	0.006
Hospital Ward							
Medical	117(52,49–54)	315(71,65–76)	305(61,56–63)	97(66,64–67)	10(100,99–100)	844(63,46–79)	0.219
Surgical	110(48,45–50)	131(29,23–34)	194(39,35–42)	51(34,32–35)	0(0,0–0)	486(37,20–53)	0.003
ICU	50(22,19–24)	122(27,21–32)	132(26,22–29)	28(19,17–20)	0(0,0–0)	332(25,9–41)	0.145
Predisposing factors							
central intravenous catheter	62(27,24–29)	42(9,3–14)	37(38,37–39)	4(3,1–4)	1(10,9–10)	146(11,0–27)	$p < 0.001$
indwelling urinary catheter	26(11,8–130	11(2,0–7)	18(18,17–19)	1(1,0–2)	0(0,0–0)	56(4,0–20)	$p < 0.001$
Immunosuppressive	22(10,7–12)	8(2,0–7)	8(8,7–9)	3(2,0–3)	2(20,19–20)	43(3,0–19)	$p < 0.001$
chemoradiotherapy	41(18,15–20)	21(5,0–10)	15(15,14–16)	4(3,1–4)	1(10,9–10)	82(6,0–22)	$p < 0.001$
endotracheal intubation	12(5,2–7)	11(2,0–7)	14(14,13–15)	1(1,0–2)	0(0,0–0)	38(3,0–19)	0.195
tracheostomy tube	6(3,0–5)	3(1,0–6)	6(6,5–7)	0(0,0–1)	0(0,0–0)	15(1,0–17)	0.211
Significant isolates							
Nosocomial	164(72,69–74)	312(70,64–75)	400(80,72–85)	50(34,32–35)	5(50,49–50)	931(70,53–86)	$p < 0.001$
Community acquired	63(28,25–30)	134(30,24–35)	99(20,31–38)	98(66,64–67)	5(50,49–50)	399(30,13–46)	$p < 0.001$

intravascular catheters for chemotherapy and the high rate of radiotherapy, which more commonly lead to BSIs.

In our study, 69% of infections were healthcare-associated while 31% were community-associated (69% VS 31%). We hypothesized that this occurred due to the following reasons: first, the study population was mainly focused on healthcare-associated infection, and blood collection and culturing was a routine examination for hospitalized patients with fever. Another reason was that the common predisposing factors of Gram-positive BSIs such as central intravenous catheters, immunosuppression, and chemoradiotherapy were mainly found with hospitalized patients in our study. Beyond that, we have found that a rate of Streptococcus pneumoniae infection in China is significantly lower compared to other developed countries [28]. Pneumococcal vaccine is routinely used to treat *streptococcus pneumonia* disease in developed countries, which might affect the morbidity and mortality [29]. Nevertheless, China is still facing great challenges, such as uncomplete network for monitoring infection with streptococcus pneumoniae and lack of relevant immune policy for standardized use of pneumococcal vaccine. Moreover, besides PPV23 there is no available vaccine in China.

In our study, *Staphylococci* was 100% sensitive to vancomycin and linezolid except for *Staphylococcus epidermidis*, for which the vancomycin resistance rate was 0.13%. These results were consistent with the studies by Fayez et al. [30]. However, Mamishi and colleagues have reported an obviously higher prevalence of resistance to penicillin by *Streptococcus pneumonia*, i.e. 42.86% in Asian countries [31]. The reason might be the wide use of the variety of interventional procedures, immunosuppressive agents and vancomycin, so it is necessary to strengthen monitoring drug resistance and rational use of antibiotics in clinical. All of the cases of *Staphylococci* showed more than 90% resistance to penicillin except for MRSA. However, Vasudeva has reported that all *Staphylococci* showed are 100% resistant to penicillin [32, 33]. This may be related to the different practical uses of β-lactam antibiotics in

Table 3 Rates of antimicrobial resistance among gram-positive bacteria most frequently isolated from patients with BSIs

Microbiology	Antimicrobial drug n_{ri}/n_{rt}(%resistant)								
	Penicillin	Ampicillin	Gentamicin	Erythomycin	Ciprofloxacin	Clindamycin	Linezolid	Vancomycin	Tetracycline
staphylococcus									
Staphylococcus aureus	96.2%(153/159)	40.9%(65/159)	32.7%(52/159)	57.9%(92/159)	34.6%(55/159)	51.6%(82/159)	–	–	30.8%(32/104)
CNS	96.4%(429/445)	74.4%(331/445)	20.4%(91/445)	85.6%(381/445)	47.0%(209/445)	69.2%(308/445	–	–	*
staphylococcus epidermidis	96.7%(731/756)	88.0%(665/756)	10.2%(77/756)	85.1%(643/756)	56.1%(424/756)	45.2%(342/756)	–	0.13%(1/756)	2.2%(15/685)
MRSA	100%(68/68)	100%(68/68)	47.1%(32/68)	75.0%(51/68)	86.8%(59/68)	75.0%(51/68)	–	–	38.2%(26/68)
Staphylococcus hominis	91.0%(832/914)	74.4%(680/914)	2.7%(24/914)	91.2%(834/914)	52.6%(481/914)	68.3%(624/914)	–	–	42.8%(345/806)
Staphylococcus haemolyticus	96.0%(117/122)	94.3%(115/122)	72.1%(88/122)	95.1%(116/122)	84.4%(103/122)	52.5%(64/122)	–	–	32.0%(39/122)
enterococcus									
E.faecalis	9.1%(12/132)	11.4%(15/132)	31.1%(41/132)	53.4%(31/58)	35.6%(47/132)	*	3.8%(5/132)	–	59.5%(47/79)
E.faecium	92.5%(272/294)	91.5%(269/294)	70.4%(207/294)	74.3%(139/187)	90.1%(265/294)	*	3.1%(9/294)	4.1%(12/294)	43.8%(89/203)
Streptococcus									
Viri-dans streptococcus	0%(0/32)	0%(0/48)	*	70.4%(23/24)	*	0%(0/24)	0%(0/25)	0%(0/25)	*
Streptococcus pneumonia	30%(3/10)	80%(8/10)	*	90%(9/10)	0%(0/3)	100%(1/1)	0%(0/10)	0%(0/10)	*

n_{ri} number of resistant isolates, n_{rt} number of isolates tested
-: without resistant; *: without test

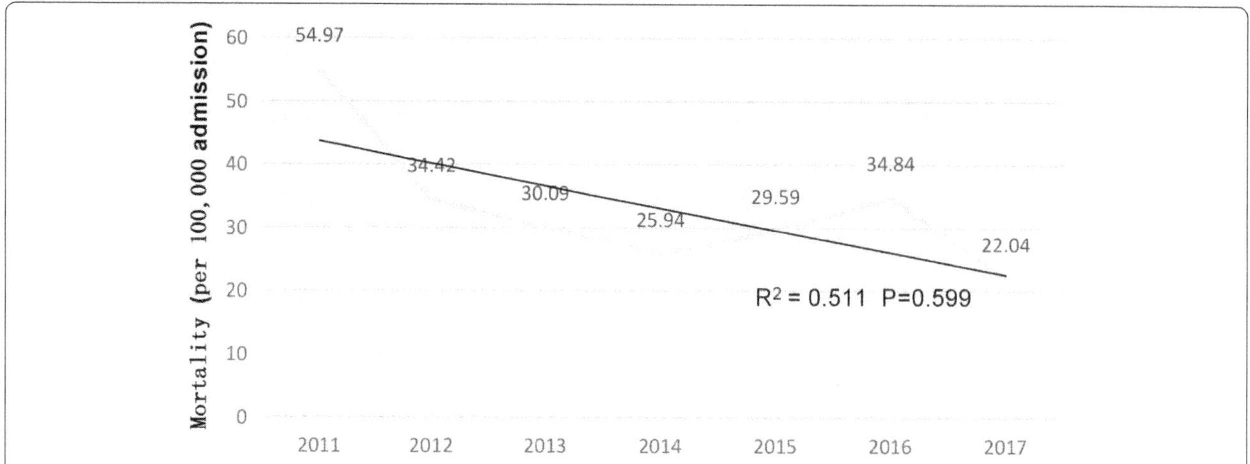

Fig. 2 Mortality of the Gram-positive bacterials BSIs from 2011 to 2017(6-months' data). The mortality from Gram-positive BSIs shows downward trend; the rate fluctuated from 54.97 to 22.04 episodes per 100,000 admissions during the 6 years

various areas, resulting in different drug resistance to bacteria. Mover, the resistance rates of *Staphylococci* to gentamicin and tetracycline were less than 50%, *Staphylococcus epidermis* which was consistent with the previous studies [21, 34]. Therefore, both gentamicin and tetracycline might be good treatment choice against *Staphylococci* used to decrease the overwhelmingly dependent on vancomycin and linezolid.

In our study, all of the vancomycin-resistant isolates were *E. faecium* (4.1%), which was lower compared to number of other studies from US and Europe [35, 36]. Both *E. faecalis* and *E. faecium* have shown resistance to linezolid (3.8% and 3.1%), which was similar to the results from two studies from China [18, 21], nonetheless, resistance to linezolid was rarely reported in foreign studies [37]. This may be explained with the species distribution and antimicrobial resistance that varies geographically. In addition, there were 219 (44%, 95%CI 38–50%) patients who were treated with effective antibiotics before obtaining the report of antibiotic susceptibility. Test reports have shown that patients with *E. faecalis* BSIs are more likely to receive effective treatment by the empirical use of antibiotics (61% vs 35%, $p = 0.013$). This may be explained by the low resistance rate of *E. faecalis* to many antimicrobial agents, such as penicillin (9.1%), ampicillin (11.4%), gentamicin (31.4%), and ciprofloxacin (35.6%).

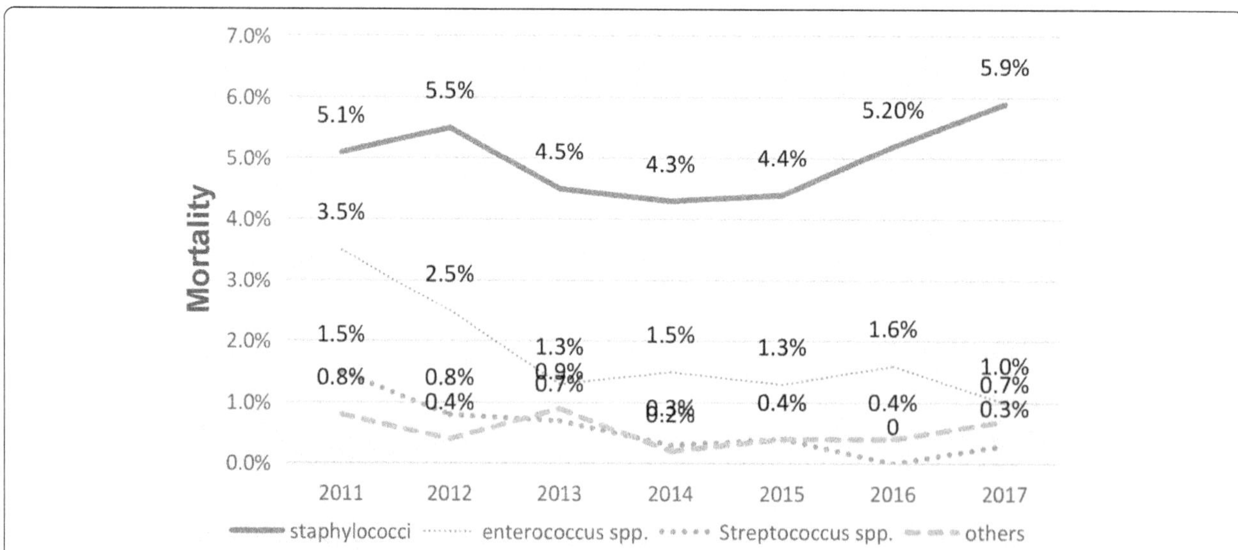

Fig. 3 Mortality of the major gram-positive bacterials BSIs from 2011 to 2017(6-months' data). The main pathogen causing death was *Staphylococci* (61.9%), followed by *Enterococcus spp.* (22.2%), *Streptococcus spp.* (7.6%) and others (6.3%). The mortality from *Staphylococci* ($X^2 = 0.81, p = 0.991$) shows an increasing trend, while the mortality from *Enterococcus spp.*($X^2 = 4.0, p = 0.677$) and *Streptococcus spp.*($X^2 = 14.62, p = 0.023$) shows a downward trend

In our study, there was no vancomycin and linezolid resistance to *streptococcus pneumoniae* and *viridians streptococci*, which was consistent with the studies done by Fayez and Marshall [30, 33]. *Viridians streptococci* was 100% sensitive to penicillin, but two other studies have reported that penicillin resistance rates have increased to more than 50% [38, 39]. The penicillin resistance rate of *Streptococcus pneumoniae* was 30%, similar to many European countries (20% to 50%), although much higher rates were reported in other Asian countries [40, 41], while there were only a few countries with lower rates (less than 10%) [9, 32, 42]. Therefore, the penicillin aslo resulted as a treatment choice for *Streptococcus spp.*

In our study, the crude mortality of Gram-positive BSIs and the mortality of *Enterococcus spp.* and *Streptococcus spp.* have shown a significant downward trend from 2011 to 2017. One possible reason might be that the number, correct timing and accuracy of blood cultures were all greater in a tertiary-care hospital thus medical workers could more correctly choose antibiotics in a timely manner. Further, there is a greater choice of antibiotics in non-tertiary hospitals. Another reason might be that tertiary-care hospitals have more complete strategy for strict control of infection that can reduce the mortality factors in BSIs. The mortality in the ICU has shown a decreased trend, while the general ward revealed contrary results. This could be explained by certain proportion of surgical and critically ill patients at our hospital, although many previous studies have shown that these patients have higher mortality rates than patients at the general ward [22, 23]. Nonetheless, the diagnosis and treatment technologies of ICU such as ventilator and ECMO have been rapidly developing rapidly over recent 5 years, and a variety of positive treatment measures have shown effective to improve cure rate and reduce mortality. Some other reasons that highlighted the importance of infection control measures among the medical staff of ICU are strict aseptic operations, good hand hygiene and similar. On the contrary, the use of indwelling central intravenous catheter seem to be increasing because of more chemotherapy and venous nutrition employed at general ward, while the consciousness of medical staff related to BSIs remained weak and the maintenance measures related to central intravenous catheter remained not enough strict. Aslo and the patients at general ward later received the empirical treatment thus further increasing the mortality.

There are several limitations in the present study that should be considered. First, the collection of clinical data depended on medical records rather than interviews and the comprehensive assessment of clinical symptoms. Second, there was an inevitable bias this was a single-centre study, and some of the results might have been affected by the small sample size. Finally, many drug susceptibility results could not be evaluated because of a lack of unified standards aslo and not all isolates underwent the same antimicrobial agent sensitivity tests, so many isolates lacked resistance comparisons with other isolates in the present study.

Conclusions

Gram-positive BSIs are the major cause of high morbidity and mortality, especially in patients with chronic disease and predisposing factors. However, in this study we found a decrease in morbidity and mortality, while the mortality at the general ward revealed the opposite trend. Although the resistance rates to vancomycin and linezolid among the Gram-positive BSIs increased, these antibiotics are still considered the best treatment options for patients with Gram-positive BSIs.

Abbreviations

BSIs: Gram-positive bacterial bloodstream infections; CHINET: China antimicrobial surveillance network; CLSI: The Clinical and Laboratory Standards Institute; ECOM: Extracorporeal membrane oxygenation; ICU: Intersive care unit; MRSA: Methicillin-resistant *staphylococcus aureus*; MSSA: Methicillin sensitive *staphyloccus aureus*; NCCLS: National Committee for Clinical Laboratory; PLAGH: Chinese People's Liberation Army General Hospital; RT-NISS: The real-time nosocomial infection surveillance system

Acknowledgements

We thank all of our colleagues at the Infection Management and Disease Control Department for making this study possible.

Authors' contributions

ZL conceived of this study and was responsible for the manuscript. QZ, YY collected the clinical data, interpreted the results, and wrote the manuscript. LZ, ZY, JC, and MZ, LC participated in data collection and critical revision of the manuscript. All authors read and approved the final manuscript.

Consent for publication

Not applicable

Competing interests

The authors declare that they have no competing interests.

Author details

[1]Department of Respiratory Medicine, Chinese PLA General Hospital, Fuxing Road No. 28, Beijing 100853, China. [2]Department of Respiratory Medicine, Affiliated Hospital of Nantong Third People's Hospital, Qingnian Central Street No. 99, Jiangsu Province 226000, China. [3]The postgraduate department, Chinese PLA General Hospital, Beijing 100853, China.

References

1. Pitter D, Tarara D, Wenzel RP. Nosocomial bloodstream infection in critically ill patients. Excess length of stay,extra costs,and attributable mortality. JAMA. 1994;217(20):1598–601.
2. Ding JG, Sun QF, Li KC, et al. Retrospective analysis of nosocomial infections in the intensive care unit of a tertiary hospital in china during 2003 to 2007. BMC Infect Dis. 2009;9(1):115.
3. Magill SS, Edwards JR, Bamberg W, Beldavs ZG, Dumyati G, Kainer MA, Lynfield R, Maloney M, Mcallister-Hollod L, Nadle J, et al. Emerging infections program healthcare associated infections and antimicrobial use prevalence survey team.Multistate point-prevalence survey of health care-associated infections. N Engl J Med. 2014;370:1198–208.

4. Zhu DM, Wang F, Hu FP, et al. CHINET 2010 surveillance of bacterial resistance in China. Chin J Infect Chemother. 2011;11:321–9.
5. GuangHui Li, DeMei Zhu, Fu Wang, et al. Bacterial distribution and susceptibility in bloodstream infections in China anti-biotic resistance surveillance program CHINET 2010. Chin J Infect Chemother. 2012;12(4): 251–58.
6. Wisplinghoff H, Bischoff T, Tallent SM, et al. Nosocomial bloodstream infections INUS hospitals:analysis of 24179 case from a prospective nationwide surveillance study. Clin Infect Dis. 2004;39(3):309–17.
7. Hortiwakul T, Nagij S, Chusri S, et al. Nosocomial bloodstream infections in Songklanagarind hospital:outcome and factors influenceing prognosis. J Med Assoc Thail. 2012;95(2):170–4.
8. Rodriguez-Creisems M, Alcaca L, Munoz P, et al. Bloodstream infections: evolution and trends in the microbiology workload,incidence,and etiology,1985-2006. Medicine. 2008;87(4):234–49.
9. EARS-Net: European centre for disease Prev Control (ECDC); Antimicrobial resistance interactive database (Internet);Stockholm (Sweden); ECDC (cited 2015 Oct 22).
10. Richter SS, Satola SW, Crispell EK, et al. Detection of Staphyloccus aureus isolates with heterogeneous intermidate-level resistance to Vancomycin in the United States. J Clin Microbiol. 2011;49:4203–7.
11. Jones RN. Microbiological features of Vancomycin in the 21st century: minium inhibitory concen-tration creep,bactericidal/static activity,and applied breakpoints to predict resistant strains. Clin Infect Dis. 2006; 42(1):13–24.
12. Bush LM, Calmon CCL, Wendeler M, Pitsakis P, Poupard J, Levsion ME, Johnosn CC. High-level penicillin resistance among isolates of enterococci implications for treatment of enterococci infections. Ann Inter Med. 1989;110(7):515–20.
13. Patterson JE, Zervos MJ. High-level gentamicin resistance in enterococci:microbiology,genetic basis,and epidemiology. Ren Infect Dis. 1990;12(4):644–52.
14. Goto M, Al-Hasan MN. Over all burden of bloodstream infection and nosocomial bloodstream infection in north American and Europe. Clin Microbiol Infect. 2013;19(6):501–7.
15. Du M, Xing Y, Suo J, Liu B, Jia N, Huo R, Chen C, Liu Y. Real-time automatic hospital-wide surveillance of nosocomial and outbreaks in a large chinese tertiary hospital. BMC Med Inform Decis Mak. 2014;14:9.
16. Garner JS, Jarvis WR, Emori TG, Horan TC. Hughs JM.CDC definitions for nosocomial infections. Am J Infect Control. 1988;16:128–40.
17. Humphries RM, Ambler J, Mitchell SL, Castanheira M, Dingle T, Hindler JA, Koeth L. Sei K; CLSI methods development and standardization working Group of the Subcommittee on antimicrobial susceptibility testing. J Clin Microbiol. 2018;26:56(4).
18. Zhang Y, Du M, Chang Y, Chen L-a. Incidence, clinical characteristics, and outcomes of nosocomial enterococcus spp. bloodstream infections in a tertiary-care hospital in Beijing, China: a four-year retrospective study. Antimicrob Resist Infect Control. 2017;6:73.
19. van der Mee-Marquet N, Domelier AS, Girard N, Quentin R. Epidemiology and typing of Staphylococcus aureus strains isolated from bloodstream infections. J Clin Microbiol. 2004;42(12):5650–7.
20. Berkowitz FE. The gram-positive bacilli:a review of microbiology,clinical aspects,and antimicrobial susceptibilities of a heterogenous group of bacteria. Pediatr Infect Dis J. 1994;13:1126–38.
21. Wu JN, et al. Epidemiology and microbiology of nosocomial bloodstream infections:analysis of 482 cases from a retrospective surveillance study. Zhejiang Univ-Sci B. 2015;16(1):70–7.
22. Bassetti M, Righi E, Carnelutti A. Bloodstream infections in the intensive care unit. Virulence. 2016;7(3):267–79.
23. Del Bono V, Giacobbe DR. Bloodstream infections in internal medicine. Virulence. 2016;7(3):353–65.
24. Billington EO, Phang SH, Gregson DB, Pitout JD, Ross T, Church DL, Laupland KB, Parkins MD. Incidence,risk factors and outcomes for enterococcus spp.blood stream infections:a population-based study. Int J Infect Dis. 2014;26:76–82.
25. Soufir L, Timist JF, Mache C, Carlet J, Chevrets RB. Attributable morbidity and mortality of catheter-related septicemia in critically ill patients:a mathed,risk-adjusted,cohort study. Infect Control Hosp Epidemiol. 1999;20:396–401.
26. Gahlot R, Nigam C, Kumar V, Yadav G, Anupurba S. Catheter-related bloodstream infections. Int J Crit Illn Inj Sci. 2014;4:162–7.
27. Valles J, Alvarez-Lerma F, Palomar M, Blanco A, Escor-esca A, Armestar F, Sirvent JM, Balasini C, Zaragoza R, Marin M. Study Group of infections disease of the spanish society of critical care Medicine.Health-care-associated bloodstream infections at admission to the ICU. Chest. 2011;139:810–5.
28. Laupland KB, Church DL. Population-based epidemiology and microbiology community-onset bloodstream infections. Clin Microbiol Rev. 2014;27(4):647–64.
29. Bonten MJM, Huijts SM, Bolkenbaas M, et al. Polysaccharid conjugate vaccine against pneumococcal pneumonia in adults. N Engl J Med. 2015;372(12):1114–25.
30. Fayyaz M, Mirza I, Ikram A, Hussain A, Ghafoor T, Shujat U. Pathogens causing bloodstream infections and their drug suscuptibility profile in immunocompromised. Coll Physicians Surg Pak. 2013;23:848–51.
31. Mamishi S, Moradkhani S, Mahmoudi S, Hosseinpour-sadeghi R, Pourakbari B. Penicillin-resistant trend of streptococcus pneumoniae in Asia: a systematic review.Iran J Microbiol. 2014;6:198–210.
32. Vasudeva N, Nirwan PS, Shirvastava P. Bloodstream infections and antimicrobial sensitivity patterns in a tertiary care hospital of India. Ther Adv Infect Dis. 2016;3(5):119–27.
33. Marshall S, Wilke W, Pfaller M, Jones R. Staphyloccus aureus and coagulase-negative staphylococci from blood stream infections:frequency of occurrence,antimicrobial suspectibility and molecular (mecA) characterization of oxacillin resistance in the SCOPE program. Diagn Microbiol Infect Dis. 1998;30:205–14.
34. Stuart JI, John MA, Milburn S, Diagre D, Wilson B, Hussain Z. Susceptibility patterns of coagulase negative staphyococci to several newer antimicrobial agents incomparison with vancomycin and oxacillin. Int J Anti-microb Agents. 2011;37:248–52.
35. Arias CA, Murray BE. The rise of the enterococcus:beyond vancomycin resistance. Nat Rev Microbiol. 2012;10:266–78.
36. Pinholt M, Osterggard C, Arpi M, Bruun NE, Schonheyder HC, Gradel KO, Sogaard M, Knudsen JD. Incidence,clinical characteristics and 30-day mortality on enterococcal bacteraemia in Denmark 2006-2009:a population-based cohort study. Clin Microbiol Infect. 2014;20(2):145–51.
37. Cattoir V, Leclercq R. Twenty-five years of shared life with vancomycin-resistant enterococci:is it time to divorce? J Antimicrob Chemother. 2013;68:731–42.
38. Balletto E, Mikulska M. Bacterial infections in hemato-poietic stem cell transplant recipients. Mediterr J Hematol Infect Dis. 2015;7:2015–45.
39. Pfaller MA, Jones RN, Marshall SA, Edmond MB, Wen-zel RP. Nosocomial streptococcal bloodstream infections in the SCOPE program:species occurrence and antimicrobial susceptibility. Diagn Microbiol Infect Dis. 1997;29:259–63.
40. Kaur A, Singh V. Bacterial isolates and their antibiotic sensitivity pattern in clinically suspected case of fever of unknown origin. K Science. 2014;16: 105–9.
41. Ahmed D, Nahid MA, et al. Bacterial etiology of bloodstream infections and antimicrobial resistance in Dhaka,Banfladesh,2005-2014. Antimicrob Resist Infect Control. 2017;6:2.
42. WHO Regional office for Europe. Central Asian and Eastern Europe surveillence of antimicrobial resistance. Ann Rep. 2014:58.

17

Factors associated with bacteraemia due to multidrug-resistant organisms among bacteraemic patients with multidrug-resistant organism carriage: a case control study

Hélène Mascitti[1], Clara Duran[1], Elisabeth-Marie Nemo[1], Frédérique Bouchand[2], Ruxandra Câlin[1], Alexis Descatha[1], Jean-Louis Gaillard[3], Christine Lawrence[3], Benjamin Davido[1], François Barbier[4] and Aurélien Dinh[1*]

Abstract

Background: Infections caused by multidrug-resistant organisms (MDRO) are emerging worldwide. Physicians are increasingly faced with the question of whether patients need empiric antibiotic treatment covering these pathogens. This question is especially essential among MDRO carriers. We aim to determine the occurrence of MDRO bacteraemia among bacteraemic patients colonized with MDRO, and the associated factors with MDRO bacteraemia among this population.

Methods: We performed a retrospective monocentric study among MDRO carriers hospitalized with bacteraemia between January 2013 and August 2016 in a French hospital. We compared characteristics of patients with MDRO and non-MDRO bacteraemia.

Results: Overall, 368 episodes of bacteraemia were reviewed; 98/368 (26.6%) occurred among MDRO carriers. Main colonizing bacteria were extended-spectrum beta-lactamase (ESBL)-producing *Escherichia coli* (40/98; 40.8%), ESBL-producing *Klebsiella pneumoniae* (35/98; 35.7%); methicillin-resistant *Staphylococcus aureus* (26/98; 26.5%) and multidrug-resistant *Pseudomonas aeruginosa* (PA) (12/98; 12.2%).
There was no significant difference considering population with MDRO bacteraemia vs. non-MDRO bacteraemia, except for immunosuppression [OR 2.86; $p = 0.0207$], severity of the episode [OR 3.13; $p = 0.0232$], carriage of PA [OR 5.24; $p = 0.0395$], and hospital-acquired infection [OR 2.49; $p = 0.034$].
In the multivariate analysis, factors significantly associated with MDRO bacteraemia among colonized patient were only immunosuppression [OR = 2.96; $p = 0.0354$] and the hospital-acquired origin of bacteraemia [OR = 2.62; $p = 0.0427$].

Conclusions: According to our study, occurrence of bacteraemia due to MDRO among MDRO carriers was high. Factors associated with MDRO bacteraemia were severity of the episode and hospital-acquired origin of the bacteraemia. Thus, during bacteraemia among patients colonized with MDRO, if such characteristics are present, broad-spectrum antimicrobial treatment is recommended.

Keywords: Multidrug-resistant organism, Antimicrobial, Bacteraemia, Carriage

* Correspondence: aurelien.dinh@aphp.fr
[1]Infectious disease unit, Raymond Poincaré University Hospital, AP-HP, Versailles Saint-Quentin University, 104 Bd R. Poincaré, 92380 Garches, France
Full list of author information is available at the end of the article

Background

There is currently an epidemiologic dramatic increase of multidrug-resistant organisms (MDRO) [1–5].

Infections caused by MDRO have been associated with severe adverse clinical outcomes, leading to increased mortality, prolonged hospital stay, and increased costs, mostly because of delayed effective therapy [6–9]. This dramatic spread takes place in both the community and hospital setting.

However, colonization and infection due to MDRO should be differentiated.

At this time, colonization with MDRO among patients is more frequent than infection.

But colonization with MDRO is a risk factor for infections due to MDRO, especially in transplanted patients and in intensive care unit [10–12].

If sepsis or sepsis-mimicking events occur among MDRO carriers, effective probabilistic broad-spectrum antibiotics are often prescribed in common practice [13]. Consequently, broad-spectrum antimicrobial treatments are increasingly used as empiric therapy among colonized patients. It could lead to unnecessary antibiotic exposure and selective pressure, creating more bacterial resistance.

This vicious circle is worryingly contributing to a rapid international dissemination of MDRO [14–16].

Physicians should therefore consider a prudent use of broad-spectrum antibiotics to limit new emergence of MDRO.

This requires updated studies to identify current risk factors for MDRO infection among MDRO carriers.

The primary objective of our study was to determine the occurrence of MDRO bacteraemia among bacteraemic patients colonized with MDRO, and which associated factors are predictive of bacteraemia due to MDRO among this population.

Methods

Settings and design

We performed a retrospective monocentric study among MDRO carriers (from any site: urine, respiratory, digestive, cutaneous), hospitalized with bacteraemia between January 2013 and August 2016 in our teaching hospital, according to STROBE statement [17]. We compared characteristics of patients with MDRO and non-MDRO bacteraemia.

Our university hospital is a disability referral centre for neurological impairment, including spinal cord injured patients. These patients are subject to high antimicrobial exposure because they might have a high rate of infections, especially urinary tract infections; they are also at increased risk of infection with multidrug-resistant bacteria [18–20]. The hospital has 255 acute-care facility beds (including 28 beds of intensive care unit) and 108 for rehabilitation, with around 8400 admissions annually. Average hospital stays are 6.9 days for acute care and 36.5 days for rehabilitation.

An active surveillance policy for MDRO carriage among high-risk patients is implemented: nasal swab for methicillin-resistant *Staphylococcus aureus* (MRSA), and rectal swab for Gram negative resistant bacteria and vancomycin-resistant enterococci.

Systematic screening is performed at hospital admission for all patients coming from acute or long-term care facilities, and for community patients previously known as carriers.

Moreover, weekly screening is performed in our intensive care and surgery departments.

All hospitalized patients with positive blood cultures for bacteria were identified from the microbiology laboratory database, and microbiological data was obtained and reviewed. Patients with MDRO carriage (at least one site) during the last 3 months until day of sepsis were included.

Medical charts were reviewed using a standardized data set to collect: demographic characteristics (age, sex, comorbidities, risk factors, etc); clinical, biological, and microbiological data (clinical and severity signs, laboratory tests, organisms identified), and outcomes of each episode.

Blood cultures were performed using aerobic and anaerobic blood culture vials incubated in a Bactec FX instrument (Bactec Ped+ and Lytic/10 Anaerobic/F, BD Diagnostics, Le Pont de Claix, France). The positive blood culture vials were subcultured on blood and chocolate Polyvitex agar plates. All isolates were then identified using MALDI-TOF mass spectrometry (Maldi Biotyper 3.0, Bruker Daltonique, Marnes la Vallée, France).

Antimicrobial susceptibility testing was carried out using the agar disk diffusion method (Bio-Rad) or an automated broth microdilution method (Phoenix, BD Diagnostics, Oxford, UK). The breakpoints used were those defined by the French Committee for Antimicrobial Susceptibility Testing (http://www.sfm-microbiologie.org/UserFiles/files/casfm/CASFM%20V1_0%20FEV_2018.pdf).

Definitions

Bacteraemia was defined as the association of at least one positive blood culture and a prescription of a systemic antibiotic treatment to treat bacteraemia. For common skin contaminants, such as coagulase-negative staphylococci or *Corynebacterium* sp., at least two different sets of blood cultures were required.

Polymicrobial bacteraemia was defined as having more than one organism found in the same bacteraemic episode.

MDRO status was determined for the *Enterobacteriaceae* group, *Acinetobacter* sp., *Pseudomonas aeruginosa*, and *Enterococcus* sp. as acquired non-susceptibility to at least one agent in three or more antimicrobial categories; for *Staphylococcus aureus* as resistance to methicillin [21].

High zone of prevalence of MDRO were southern Europe (Spain, Italy, Greece), North Africa and Asia according to European Centre for Disease Prevention and Control (ECDC) data (https://www.ecdc.europa.eu/en/home).

Hospital-acquired infection was determined as clinical signs of infection or infection arise at least 48 h after hospital admission.

Prior colonization was defined as isolation of MDRO from any site without any clinical signs of inflammation or sepsis, and antibiotic therapies targeting these MDRO, within a designated period of 3 months before the day of bacteraemia.

Prior antibiotic use was defined as the use of at least 1 dose of any antimicrobial treatment in a designated period of 3 months until the day before sepsis.

Immunosuppression included the following: diabetes mellitus, ongoing neoplasia, hemopathy, HIV, hypogamma globulinemia, immunosuppressive therapy (ie. corticotherapy > 20 mg/d, chemotherapy or immunosuppressive treatment such as cyclophosphamide, azathioprine and cyclosporine).

Primary site of infection were clinically suspected (by the physician in charge or reported on the medical chart) or bacteriologically documented with the same bacterial identification as that in the blood culture. Primary sites were categorized as urinary tract infection, catheter line-associated bacteraemia, osteoarticular infection, pulmonary tract infection, skin and soft tissue infection, intra-abdominal infection, and unknown when no primary site had been identified.

Severity was defined as the requirement of at least one of the following criteria: volume expansion, assisted (mechanical) ventilation, vasopressor requirement, and intensive care unit (ICU) admission during the episode.

Cure was defined as the absence of clinical and biological signs of infection at 1 month after end of antimicrobial treatment or at hospital discharge without any additional antimicrobial treatment.

Mortality was defined as dead status before 30 days after the end of antimicrobial treatment.

Statistical analysis

All continuous variables are presented as mean and standard deviation, and the categorical variables are presented as frequencies. Correlations between risk factors and MDRO bacteraemia among patients colonized with MDRO were determined by Student's t-test for continuous variables and the Pearson's $\chi 2$ test for categorical variables.

Univariate analysis and multivariate analysis were performed. Variable for multivariate analysis were all associated risks that had a *p*-value ≤ 0.05 and sex in the univariate analysis.

The relative risks of MDROs bacteraemia were estimated by calculating the adjusted odds ratios (OR) and corresponding 95% confidence intervals (CI).

All reported probability values (*P*-values) were based on two-sided tests, and a *P*-value of 0.05 was considered statistically significant. All analyses were performed using the Statistical Package for Social Science (SPSS) version 17.0 (SPSS, Chicago, IL, USA).

Results

During the study period, a mean of 198 ± 54 screening per month was performed, and mean positive results for MDRO per patient was 23 ± 5%, with 45% of extended-spectrum beta-lactamase (ESBL)-producers isolates.

In total, 368 episodes of bacteraemia were reviewed; 98 (26.6%) occurred among 77 MDRO carriers (Fig. 1). Eight bacteraemia episodes were plurimicrobial.

Considering the 98 episodes of bacteraemia among MDRO carriers, mean age was 55.8 years old, and sex ratio was 1.65. Prior antimicrobial treatment in the last 3 months occurred in 66 (67.3%) cases, 42 (42.9%) patients had an indwelling catheter, 33 (33.7%) were immunosuppressed, and 55 (56.1%) were considered as severe.

Main primary site of infections were urinary tract infections (25; 25.5%) and catheter-line associated infections (25; 25.5%); 12 (12.2%) patients presented primary bacteraemia.

Bacteraemia were hospital-acquired in 62 (63.3%) cases.

The rate of bacteraemia due to MDRO was 53.1% (*n* = 52) (Table 1). Among them, 41 (78.8%) episodes were due to multidrug-resistant *Enterobacteriaceae*, of which 22 (42.3%) were due to ESBL *Enterobacteriaceae*.

Overall, main colonizing bacteria were ESBL-producing *Escherichia coli* (EC) (*n* = 40; 40.8%), ESBL-producing *Klebsiella pneumoniae* (KP) (*n* = 35; 35.7%); MRSA (*n* = 26; 26.5%), and *Pseudomonas aeruginosa* (PA) (*n* = 12; 12.2%). Twenty-five patients (for 32 episodes) were carriers of several MDRO. Sites of carriage and microorganisms identified are presented in Table 2.

Among carriers with bacteraemia due to MDRO, a discordant identification between carriage and bacteraemia was found in 23 (44.2%) episodes (Table 3).

On the contrary, 29 (55.8%) episodes had a concordant identification, which were due to ESBL KP (*n* = 10), ESBL EC (*n* = 7), MRSA (*n* = 4), VIM-type carbapenemase-producing PA (n = 3), ESBL *Enterobacter cloacae* (*n* = 2), ceftaroline-resistant PA (*n* = 1), carbapenemase-producing *E. cloacae* (*n* = 1), and ceftaroline-resistant *Acinetobacter baumanii* (*n* = 1). Sites of carriage were rectal (*n* = 18), urinary (*n* = 14), respiratory (*n* = 11) and cutaneous (*n* = 7).

The global cure rate was 83/98 (84.6%).

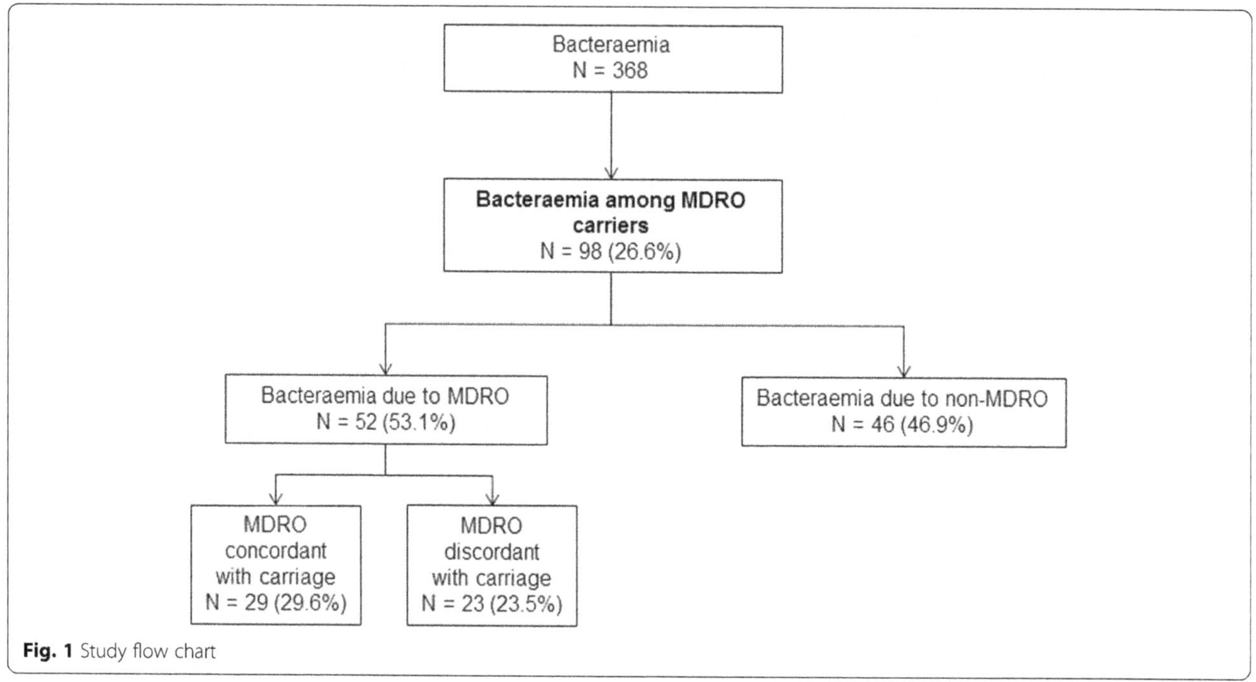

Fig. 1 Study flow chart

In univariate analysis, there was no significant difference considering population with MDRO bacteraemia vs. non-MDRO bacteraemia, except for immunosuppression [OR 2.86; $p = 0.0207$], severity of the episode [OR 3.13; $p = 0.0232$], carriage of *Pseudomonas aeruginosa* [OR 5.24; $p = 0.0395$], and hospital-acquired infection [OR 2.49; $p = 0.034$] (Table 4).

In the multivariate analysis (Table 4), factors significantly associated with MDRO bacteraemia among colonized patient were only immunosuppression [OR = 2.96; $p = 0.0354$], and the nosocomial origin of bacteraemia [OR = 2.62; $p = 0.0427$].

Discussion

In our study, the rate of MDRO bacteraemia among bacteraemic patients colonized with MDRO is high (53.1%).

Main factors associated with MDRO bacteraemia in those patients are immunosuppression, severity of the episode, colonization with *Pseudomonas aeruginosa,* and nosocomial infection in univariate analysis. In multivariate analysis, the only significant factors found are severity of the episode and the nosocomial origin of the infection.

The originality of our study is to focus on bacteraemic patient colonized with MDRO. Our main question is: when should we treat with probabilistic broad-spectrum antimicrobial treatment patients with known MDRO colonization and positive blood cultures?

Risk factor for MDRO/ESBL infections

Most studies focused on colonization and infections due to multidrug-resistant *Enterobacteriaceae,* in ICU, or among immunosuppressed patients.

For example, in a 6-year prospective study, Razazi et al. screened 6303 patients admitted in ICU [22]; 843 (13.4%) had ESBL *Enterobacteriaceae* carriage detected. Among those carriers, 111 (13%) patients developed ICU-acquired pneumonia, of whom only 48 (43%) had ESBL *Enterobacteriaceae* pneumonia (6% of carriers). Moreover, considering ventilator-acquired pneumonia in ICU patients, Bruyère et al. noted in their retrospective study that the positive predictive value of digestive ESBL *Enterobacteriaceae* colonization for ESBL *Enterobacteriaceae* pneumonia was also low (41.5%) [23].

More generally, in a prospective multicenter cohort study in ICU, Barbier et al. demonstrated that ESBL *Enterobacteriaceae* infections increased carbapenem consumption, length of stay and day 28 mortality [24]. Also, ESBL *Enterobacteriaceae* infections (16.4%) were rather infrequent in carriers.

In Holland, a study focused on the predictive value of prior colonization for third-generation cephalosporin-resistant *Enterobacteriaceae* for infection due to the same microorganism [25]. This study was performed in all medical wards of an hospital, ICU included. The authors noted that, among 9422 episodes, 1657 (17.6%) of colonized patients were bacteraemic, and 64 (3.8%) were colonized with third-generation cephalosporin-resistant *Enterobacteriaceae.*

In this study, the occurrence of MDRO bacteraemia was low, corresponding to usual epidemiological data in Holland. In our study, the rate of infection due to MDRO is higher which may be due to local epidemiology.

Finally, an Israelian cohort study, with 431 carriers of carbapenem-resistant *Klebsiella pneumonia* (CRKP)

Table 1 Main characteristics of multidrug-resistant organism carriers with bacteraemia

Variable	Non MDR bacteraemia (*n* = 46)	MDR bacteraemia (*n* = 52)	Odds Ratio	*P* value
Sex (male)	30 (65.2%)	31 (59.6%)	0.70 [0.35; 1.79]	0.5683
Recent (< 3 months) trip in zone with high MDRO prevalence[a]	6 (13.0%)	3 (5.8%)	0.41 [0.10; 1.74]	0.2250
Prior antimicrobial treatment in last 6 months	28 (60.9%)	38 (73.1%)	1.74 [0.74; 4.09]	0.2004
Urinary indwelling catheter	19 (41.3%)	23 (44.2%)	1.13 [0.51; 2.51]	0.7704
Immunosuppression	10 (21.7%)	23 (44.2%)	2.86 [1.17; 6.95]	*0.0207*
Severity	7 (15.2%)	19 (36.5%)	3.13 [1.17; 8.36]	*0.0232*
Primary site of infection				
UTI	10 (21.7%)	15 (28.8%)	1.46 [0.58; 3.67]	0.4218
Intra abdominal infection	6 (13.0%)	5 (9.6%)	0.71 [0.20; 2.50]	0.5929
Bone and joint infection	4 (8.7%)	0 (0.0%)	0.00 [0.00; I]	0.9710
Respiratory tract infection	2 (4.3%)	6 (11.5%)	2.87 [0.55; 14.98]	0.2113
Skin soft tissue infection	7 (15.2%)	4 (7.7%)	0.46 [0.13; 1.70]	0.2471
Catheter line associated infcetion	10 (21.7%)	15 (28.8%)	1.46 [0.58; 3.67]	0.4218
No primary site of infection	5 (10.9%)	7 (13.5%)	1.28 [0.38; 4.33]	0.6965
Colonization MDR pathogen				
Polymicrobial	15 (32.6%)	17 (32.7%)		
CRE	1 (2.2%)	2 (3.8%)		
ESBL *Escherichia coli*	23 (50.0%)	17 (32.7%)	0.49 [0.22; 1.09]	0.0814
Klebsiella spp.	18 (39.1%)	25 (48.1%)	1.44 [0.64; 3.22]	0.3738
ESBL *Klebsiella* spp.	17 (37.0%)	23 (44.2%)		
Carba-R *Klebsiella* spp.	1 (2.2%)	1 (1.9%)		
CASE *Klebsiella* spp.	0 (0.0%)	1 (1.9%)		
Citrobacter spp.	1 (2.2%)	2 (3.8%)	1.80 [0.16; 20.53]	0.6360
ESBL *Citrobacter* spp.	1 (2.2%)	2 (3.8%)		
Enterobacter spp.	5 (10.9%)	8 (15.4%)	1.63 [0.45; 5.98]	0.4590
ESBL *Enterobacter* spp.	5 (10.9%)	7 (13.5%)		
Carba-R *Enterobacter* spp.	0 (0.0%)	1 (1.9%)		
Acinetobacter baumanii	2 (4.3%)	3 (5.8%)	0.43 [0.04; 4.92]	0.4984
ESBL *A. baumanii*	1 (2.2%)	1 (1.9%)		
Carba-R *A. baumanii*	1 (2.2%)	1 (1.9%)		
Cefta-R *A. baumanii*	0 (0.0%)	1 (1.9%)		
Pseudomonas aeruginosa	2 (4.3%)	10 (19.2%)	5.24 [1.08; 25.32]	*0.0395*
ESBL *P. aeruginosa*	0 (0.0%)	1 (1.9%)		
Carba-R *P. aeruginosa*	0 (0.0%)	3 (5.8%)		
Cefta-R *P. aeruginosa*	2 (4.3%)	6 (11.5%)		
MRSA	11 (23.9%)	15 (28.8%)	1.29 [0.52; 3.19]	0.5814
VRE	1 (2.2%)	0 (0.0%)	0.88 [0.05; 14.51]	0.9300
Type of infections				
Nosocomial	24 (52.2%)	38 (73.1%)	2.49 [1.07; 5.78]	*0.0340*
Cure rate	39 (84.8%)	44 (84.6%)	0.99 [0.33; 2.97]	0.9817

[a]Geographic area with high incidence of extended-spectrum beta-lactamase-producing bacteria, CRE and VRE: Southern Europe (Spain, Italy, Greece), North Africa and Asia

Carba-R Carbapenem-resistant; *CASE* Cephalosporinase-producing; *Cefta-R* Ceftaroline-resistant; *CRE* Carbapenem-resistant Enterobacteriaceae; *ESBL* Extended-spectrum beta-lactamase; *MDR* Multidrug-resistant; *MRSA* Methicillin-resistant Staphylococcus aureus; *VRE* Vancomycin-resistant Enterococci

italicised valued are statistically significant

Table 2 Multidrug-resistant organism carriage according to site

	Urinary	Rectal	Respiratory	Cutaneous / Wound
ESBL *Enterobacteriaceae*	30	59	2	13
CRE (NDM + OXA types)	1	2	0	0
CASE *Enterobacteriaceae*	0	1	0	0
ESBL *Pseudomonas aeruginosa*	1	0	0	3
Carba-R *P. aeruginosa*	0	2	0	2
Cefta-R *P. aeruginosa*	0	2	3	0
ESBL *Acinetobacter baumanii*	0	1	0	0
OXA-23 *A. baumanii*	0	2	0	0
Cefta-R *A. baumanii*	0	1	0	0
MRSA	3	0	19	4
VRE	0	1	0	0

ESBL Extended-spectrum beta-lactamase; *CRE* Carbapenem-resistant *Enterobacteriaceae*; *CASE* Cephalosporinase; *Carba-R* Carbapenem-resistant; *Cefta-R* Ceftaroline-resistant; *MRSA* Methicillin-resistant *Staphylococcus aureus*; *VRE* Vancomycin-resistant Enterococci

Table 3 Discordant identification between carriage and blood culture

Carriage MDRO	Blood culture MDRO
ESBL *Escherichia coli*	MDR non-ESBL *E. coli*
ESBL *E. coli*	ESBL *K. pneumoniae*
ESBL *E. coli*	ESBL *K. pneumoniae*
CASE *Klebsiella pneumoniae*	MDR *K. pneumoniae*
ESBL *K. pneumoniae*	MDR non-ESBL *E. coli*
ESBL *K. pneumoniae*	MDR *K. pneumoniae*
ESBL *K. pneumoniae*	MDR *Proteus mirabilis*
ESBL *K. pneumoniae*	MDR *Serratia marcescens*
ESBL *K. pneumoniae*	Cefta-R *P. aeruginosa*
Cefta-R *Pseudomonas aeruginosa*	MDR non-ESBL *E. coli*
Cefta-R *P. aeruginosa*	MDR *Enterobacter cloacae*
ESBL *E. cloacae*	MDR *P. mirabilis*
ESBL *Acinetobacter baumanii*	MDR non-ESBL *E. coli*
Cefta-R *A. baumanii*	MDR *P. aeruginosa*
ESBL *Morganella morganii*	MDR Providencia stuartii
MRSA	MDR non-ESBL *E. coli*
MRSA	MDR non-ESBL *E. coli*
MRSA	ESBL *K. pneumoniae*
MRSA	MDR *Enterococcus faecium*
ESBL *E. coli*ESBL *K. pneumoniae*MRSA	MDR non-ESBL *E. coli*
ESBL *E. coli*ESBL *K. oxytoca* ESBL *Citrobacter* sp.ESBL *M. morganii* MRSA	MDR *P. mirabilis*
ESBL *E. coli*ESBL *K. pneumoniae*	MDR non-ESBL *E. coli*
ESBL *E. coli*MRSA	MDR non-ESBL *E. coli*

CASE Cephalosporinase-producing; *Cefta-R* Ceftaroline-resistant; *ESBL* Extended-spectrum beta-lactamase; *MDRO* Multidrug-resistant organism; *MRSA* Methicillin-resistant *Staphylococcus aureus*

Table 4 Multivariate analysis associated with multidrug-resistant organism bacteraemia

Variable	MDR bacteraemia	Univariate analysis		Multivariate analysis	
		Odds Ratio	*P* value	Odds Ratio	*P* value
Sex (male)	31/61 (50.8%)	0.70 [0.35; 1.79]	0.5683	1.04 [0.40; 2.70]	0.9403
Immunosuppression	23/33 (69.7%)	2.86 [1.17; 6.95]	*0.0207*	*2.96 [1.08; 8.13]*	*0.0354*
Severity	19/26 (73.1%)	3.13 [1.17; 8.36]	*0.0232*	2.32 [0.78; 6.88]	0.1303
Colonization MDR *Pseudomonas aeruginosa*	10/12 (83.3%)	5.24 [1.08; 25.32]	*0.0395*	2.95 [0.49; 17.77]	0.2386
Hospital-acquired	38/62 (61.3%)	2.49 [1.07; 5.78]	*0.034*	*2.62 [1.03; 6.64]*	*0.0427*

MDR Multidrug-resistant
italicised valued are statistically significant

included, noted that the rate of bloodstream infections (BSI) was 20% and rate of BSI due to Gram negative resistant bacteria was 80% (68/85) [26]. Among them, 19 BSI were due to CRKP and 20 to ESBL *Enterobacteriaceae*. However, in this study, no prognostic factors of CRKP BSI were identified.

The authors concluded that this raises the question regarding the use of probabilistic broad-spectrum antibiotic therapy for MDRO carriers who develop severe sepsis, as in our study.

Moreover, the authors also described frequent discordance between bacteria involved in carriage and in blood cultures [26].

Carriage of MDRO is generally the marker of high antibiotic exposure of the patient, which induces selective pressure on all flora. Yet, all MDRO are not screened, and usual screening techniques are not 100% sensitive. Therefore, a MDRO not identified during screening could be responsible for sepsis. But the indication of broad-spectrum antimicrobial treatment during sepsis among patients with MDRO carriage is still under debate, as patients do have a higher risk of MDRO infection, even if due to a different microorganism.

Risks associated with infection due to MDRO

Regarding infection due to MRSA, colonization by MRSA is a well-known risk factor [27–29], especially in critically ill neonates children [30].

Thus, risk factors for infection due to MDRO is a complex phenomenon due to various microbiological, clinical, demographic and anamnestic characteristics [22, 23, 31, 32].

Use of algorithm to limit unnecessary use of broad-spectrum antimicrobial treatment should be encouraged [31, 32], as the one suggested by M. Basseti and J. Rodriguez Baño, which includes simple and easy to collect criteria: severity of the episode, community-acquired character, previous colonization to MDRO, indwelling device, age and previous exposure to antibiotic [33].

Lastly, new rapid diagnosis tests for bacterial resistance could help to avoid unnecessary broad-spectrum antimicrobial treatment among bacteraemic population known to be colonized by MDRO [34–37].

Bias and weakness

The bias and weakness of our study are due to its monocentric and retrospective design, and limited sample size. Some data may be missing such as previous antimicrobial prescriptions due to memory bias. All patients were not systematically screened for MDRO at every site. Still, we studied several MDRO (ESBL bacteria, carbapenem-resistant *Enterobacteriaceae* and MRSA for example) and different sites of carriage which reflect every day practice in a tertiary care hospital. Finally, another limit of this work is that we were not able to identify patients with re-hospitalization or transferred from another hospital, which could imply an underestimation of the proportion of hospital-acquired infections.

Future research is needed to better understand the link between colonization and infection due to MDRO.

Conclusions

According to our study, occurrence of bacteraemia due to MDRO among bacteraemic MDRO carriers was high. However, concordance between carried bacteria and blood culture bacteria was not always consistent.

Factors associated with MDRO bacteraemia were severity of the episode and nosocomial origin of the bacteraemia.

Thus, during bacteraemia among patients colonized with MDRO, if characteristics above described are present, broad-spectrum antimicrobial treatment is recommended.

Abbreviations

BSI: bloodstream infections; CRKP: carbapenem-resistant *Klebsiella pneumonia*; EC: *Escherichia coli*; ECDC: European Centre for Disease Prevention and Control; ESBL: extended-spectrum beta-lactamase; HIV: human immunodeficiency virus; ICU: intensive care unit; KP: *Klebsiella pneumoniae*; MALDI-TOF: matrix assisted laser desorption ionisation - time of flight; MDRO: multidrug-resistant organisms; MRSA: methicillin-resistant *Staphylococcus aureus*; OR: odds ratio; PA: *Pseudomonas aeruginosa*.

Acknowledgments

The authors would like to thank Elodie Choisy from the infectious disease unit of Raymond Poincaré Hospital for her help and support.

Authors' contributions

ADi developed the study design. JLG and CL performed all laboratory tests. HM, CD and EMN were responsible for data collection. ADe performed statistical analysis. ADi and FBa were responsible for data analysis and data interpretation. CD, FBo, FBa and ADi drafted the first version of the manuscript. All authors revised and approved the final manuscript.

Consent for publication
Not applicable.

Competing interests
The authors declare that they have no competing interests.

Author details
[1]Infectious disease unit, Raymond Poincaré University Hospital, AP-HP, Versailles Saint-Quentin University, 104 Bd R. Poincaré, 92380 Garches, France. [2]Pharmacy department, Raymond Poincaré University Hospital, AP-HP, Versailles Saint-Quentin University, 104 Bd R. Poincaré, 92380 Garches, France. [3]Microbiological laboratory, Raymond Poincaré University Hospital, AP-HP, Versailles Saint-Quentin University, 104 Bd R. Poincaré, 92380 Garches, France. [4]Intensive care unit, Orléans Hospital, 14 Avenue de l'Hôpital, 45067 Orléans, France.

References
1. WHO. Antimicrobial resistance: global report on surveillance 2014 [Internet]. 2014 [cited 2018 Aug 21]. Available from: http://apps.who.int/iris/bitstream/handle/10665/112642/9789241564748_eng.pdf;jsessionid=99C1FBE19E0C74F2E8288949002DFE34?sequence=1
2. Drieux L, Brossier F, Duquesnoy O, Aubry A, Robert J, Sougakoff W, et al. Increase in hospital-acquired bloodstream infections caused by extended spectrum β-lactamase-producing Escherichia coli in a large French teaching hospital. Eur J Clin Microbiol Infect Dis. 2009;28:491–8.
3. Saurina G, Quale JM, Manikal VM, Oydna E, Landman D. Antimicrobial resistance in Enterobacteriaceae in Brooklyn, NY: epidemiology and relation to antibiotic usage patterns. J Antimicrob Chemother. 2000;45:895–8.
4. European Centre for Disease Prevention and Control (ECDC). Antimicrobial resistance surveillance in Europe 2016. Annual report of the European Antimicrobial Resistance Surveillance Network (EARS-Net) [Internet]. 2016 [cited 2018 Mar 26]. Available from: https://ecdc.europa.eu/sites/portal/files/documents/AMR-surveillance-Europe-2016.pdf
5. Centers for Disease Control and Prevention (CDC). Vital Signs: Carbapenem-Resistant Enterobacteriaceae. Morb Mortal Wkly Rep [Internet]. 2013 [cited 2018 Apr 2];62:165–70. Available from: https://www.cdc.gov/mmwr/preview/mmwrhtml/mm6209a3.htm
6. Lee SY, Kotapati S, Kuti JL, Nightingale CH, Nicolau DP. Impact of extended-Spectrum β-lactamase–producing Escherichia coli and Klebsiella species on clinical outcomes and hospital costs: a matched cohort study. Infect Control Hosp Epidemiol. 2006;27:1226–32.
7. Lautenbach E, Patel JB, Bilker WB, Edelstein PH, Fishman NO. Extended-Spectrum -lactamase-producing Escherichia coli and Klebsiella pneumoniae: risk factors for infection and impact of resistance on outcomes. Clin Infect Dis. 2001;32:1162–71.
8. Blot S, Depuydt P, Vogelaers D, Decruyenaere J, De WJ, Hoste E, et al. Colonization status and appropriate antibiotic therapy for nosocomial bacteremia caused by antibiotic-resistant gram-negative bacteria in an intensive care unit. Infect Control Hosp Epidemiol. 2005;26:575–9.
9. de Kraker MEA, Wolkewitz M, Davey PG, Koller W, Berger J, Nagler J, et al. Burden of antimicrobial resistance in European hospitals: excess mortality and length of hospital stay associated with bloodstream infections due to Escherichia coli resistant to third-generation cephalosporins. J Antimicrob Chemother. 2011;66:398–407.
10. Bonten MJ, Weinstein RA. The role of colonization in the pathogenesis of nosocomial infections. Infect Control Hosp Epidemiol. 1996;17:193–200.
11. Detsis M, Karanika S, Mylonakis E. ICU acquisition rate, risk factors, and clinical significance of digestive tract colonization with extended-Spectrum Beta-lactamase-producing Enterobacteriaceae: a systematic review and meta-analysis. Crit Care Med. 2017;45:705–14.
12. Gómez-Zorrilla S, Camoez M, Tubau F, Cañizares R, Periche E, Dominguez MA, et al. Prospective observational study of prior rectal colonization status as a predictor for subsequent development of Pseudomonas aeruginosa clinical infections. Antimicrob Agents Chemother. 2015;59:5213 9.
13. Barbier F, Bailly S, Schwebel C, Papazian L, Azoulay É, Kallel H, et al. Infection-related ventilator-associated complications in ICU patients colonised with extended-spectrum β-lactamase-producing Enterobacteriaceae. Intensive Care Med. 2018;44:616–26.
14. Karah N, Haldorsen B, Hermansen NO, Tveten Y, Ragnhildstveit E, Skutlaberg DH, et al. Emergence of OXA-carbapenemase- and 16S rRNA methylase-producing international clones of Acinetobacter baumannii in Norway. J Med Microbiol. 2011;60:515–21.
15. Chen S, Hu F, Xu X, Liu Y, Wu W, Zhu D, et al. High prevalence of KPC-2-type carbapenemase coupled with CTX-M-type extended-spectrum beta-lactamases in carbapenem-resistant Klebsiella pneumoniae in a teaching hospital in China. Antimicrob agents Chemother. American Society for Microbiology (ASM). 2011;55:2493–4.
16. Munoz-Price LS, Hayden MK, Lolans K, Won S, Calvert K, Lin M, et al. Successful control of an outbreak of Klebsiella pneumoniae Carbapenemase—Producing K. pneumoniae at a long-term acute care hospital. Infect Control Hosp Epidemiol. 2010;31:341–7.
17. STROBE Statement [Internet]. [cited 2018 Sep 18]. Available from: https://www.strobe-statement.org/index.php?id=strobe-home
18. Dinh A, Saliba M, Saadeh D, Bouchand F, Descatha A, Roux ALL, et al. Blood stream infections due to multidrug-resistant organisms among spinal cord-injured patients, epidemiology over 16 years and associated risks: a comparative study. Spinal Cord [Internet]. 2016 [cited 2017 Mar 11];54:720–725. Available from: http://www.nature.com/doifinder/10.1038/sc.2015.234
19. Esposito S, Leone S, Noviello S, Lanniello F, Fiore M. Antibiotic resistance in long-term care facilities. New Microbiol. 2007;30:326–31.
20. Couderc C, Jolivet S, Thiébaut ACM, Ligier C, Remy L, Alvarez A-S, et al. Fluoroquinolone use is a risk factor for methicillin-resistant Staphylococcus aureus Acquisition in Long-term Care Facilities: a nested case-case-control study. Clin Infect Dis. 2014;59:206–15.
21. Magiorakos A-P, Srinivasan A, Carey RB, Carmeli Y, Falagas ME, Giske CG, et al. Multidrug-resistant, extensively drug-resistant and pandrug-resistant bacteria: an international expert proposal for interim standard definitions for acquired resistance. Clin Microbiol Infect. 2012;18:268–81.
22. Razazi K, Mekontso Dessap A, Carteaux G, Jansen C, Decousser J-W, de Prost N, et al. Frequency, associated factors and outcome of multi-drug-resistant intensive care unit-acquired pneumonia among patients colonized with extended-spectrum β-lactamase-producing Enterobacteriaceae. Ann Intensive Care. 2017;7:61.
23. Bruyère R, Vigneron C, Bador J, Aho S, Toitot A, Quenot J, et al. Significance of prior digestive colonization with extended-Spectrum β-lactamase–producing Enterobacteriaceae in patients with ventilator-associated pneumonia. Crit care med. Crit Care Med. 2016;44:699–706.
24. Barbier F, Pommier C, Essaied W, Garrouste-Orgeas M, Schwebel C, Ruckly S, et al. Colonization and infection with extended-spectrum β-lactamase-producing Enterobacteriaceae in ICU patients: what impact on outcomes and carbapenem exposure? J Antimicrob Chemother. 2016;71:1088–97.
25. Rottier WC, Bamberg YRP, Dorigo-Zetsma JW, van der Linden PD, Ammerlaan HSM, Bonten MJM. Predictive value of prior colonization and antibiotic use for third-generation cephalosporin-resistant Enterobacteriaceae bacteremia in patients with sepsis. Clin Infect Dis. 2015;60:1622–30.
26. Amit S, Mishali H, Kotlovsky T, Schwaber MJ, Carmeli Y. Bloodstream infections among carriers of carbapenem-resistant Klebsiella pneumoniae: etiology, incidence and predictors. Clin Microbiol Infect. 2015;21:30–4.
27. Simor AE, Loeb M, CIDS/CAMM guidelines committee. The management of infection and colonization due to methicillin-resistant Staphylococcus aureus: A CIDS/CAMM position paper. Can J Infect Dis. 2004;15:39–48.
28. Stenehjem E, Rimland D. MRSA nasal colonization burden and risk of MRSA infection. Am J Infect Control. 2013;41:405–10.
29. Garrouste-Orgeas M, Timsit J-F, Kallel H, Ben AA, Dumay MF, Paoli B, et al. Colonization with methicillin-resistant Staphylococcus aureus in ICU patients morbidity, mortality, and Glycopeptide use. Infect Control Hosp Epidemiol. 2001;22:687–92.
30. Milstone AM, Goldner BW, Ross T, Shepard JW, Carroll KC, Perl TM. Methicillin-resistant Staphylococcus aureus colonization and risk of

subsequent infection in critically ill children: importance of preventing nosocomial methicillin-resistant Staphylococcus aureus transmission. Clin Infect Dis. 2011;53:853–9.

31. Tumbarello M, Trecarichi EM, Bassetti M, De Rosa FG, Spanu T, Di Meco E, et al. Identifying patients harboring extended-Spectrum-β-lactamase-producing Enterobacteriaceae on hospital admission: derivation and validation of a scoring system. Antimicrob Agents Chemother. 2011;55:3485–90.
32. Goodman KE, Lessler J, Cosgrove SE, Harris AD, Lautenbach E, Han JH, et al. A clinical decision tree to predict whether a Bacteremic patient is infected with an extended-Spectrum β-lactamase–producing organism. Clin Infect Dis. 2016;63:896–903.
33. Bassetti M, Baño JR. Should we take into account ESBLs in empirical antibiotic treatment? Intensive Care Med. 2016;42:2059–2062.
34. Renvoisé A, Decré D, Amarsy-Guerle R, Huang T-D, Jost C, Podglajen I, et al. Evaluation of the βLacta test, a rapid test detecting resistance to third-generation cephalosporins in clinical strains of Enterobacteriaceae. J Clin Microbiol. American Society for Microbiology (ASM). 2013;51:4012–7.
35. Gallah S, Decré D, Genel N, Arlet G. The β-Lacta test for direct detection of extended-spectrum-β-lactamase-producing Enterobacteriaceae in urine. J Clin Microbiol American Society for Microbiology (ASM). 2014;52:3792–4.
36. Delport JA, Strikwerda A, Armstrong A, Schaus D, John M. MALDI-ToF short incubation identification from blood cultures is associated with reduced length of hospitalization and a decrease in bacteremia associated mortality. Eur J Clin Microbiol Infect Dis. 2017;36:1181–6.
37. Beganovic M, Costello M, Wieczorkiewicz SM. Effect of Matrix-Assisted Laser Desorption Ionization-Time of Flight Mass Spectrometry (MALDI-TOF MS) Alone versus MALDI-TOF MS Combined with Real-Time Antimicrobial Stewardship Interventions on Time to Optimal Antimicrobial Therapy in Patients with Positive Blood Cultures. Munson E, editor. J Clin Microbiol. 2017;55:1437–45.

18

Clostridium difficile infection perceptions and practices

Laurel Legenza[1,2*], Susanne Barnett[1], Warren Rose[1], Nasia Safdar[3], Theresa Emmerling[1], Keng Hee Peh[1] and Renier Coetzee[2]

Abstract

Background: *Clostridium difficile* infection (CDI) is understudied in limited resource settings. In addition, provider awareness of CDI as a prevalent threat is unknown. An assessment of current facilitators and barriers to CDI identification, management, and prevention is needed in limited resource settings to design and evaluate quality improvement strategies to effectively minimize the risk of CDI.

Methods: Our study aimed to identify CDI perceptions and practices among healthcare providers in South African secondary hospitals to identify facilitators and barriers to providing quality CDI care. Qualitative interviews (11 physicians, 11 nurses, 4 pharmacists,) and two focus groups (7 nurses, 3 pharmacists) were conducted at three district level hospitals in the Cape Town Metropole. Semi-structured interviews elicited provider perceived facilitators, barriers, and opportunities to improve clinical workflow from patient presentation through CDI (1) Identification, (2) Diagnosis, (3) Treatment, and (4) Prevention. In addition, a summary provider CDI knowledge score was calculated for each interviewee for seven components of CDI and management.

Results: Major barriers identified were knowledge gaps in characteristics of *C. difficile* identification, diagnosis, treatment, and prevention. The median overall CDI knowledge score (scale 0–7) from individual interviews was 3 [interquartile range 0.25, 4.75]. Delays in *C. difficile* testing workflow were identified. Participants perceived supplies for CDI management and prevention were usually available; however, hand hygiene and use of contact precautions was inconsistent.

Conclusions: Our analysis provides a detailed description of the facilitators and barriers to CDI workflow and can be utilized to design quality improvement interventions among limited resource settings.

Keywords: Healthcare associated infection, Infection control, Qualitative study, Antimicrobial stewardship, Global health

Background

Clostridium difficile infection (CDI) is an increasingly important healthcare-associated infection associated with long hospitalisations and high patient morbidity and mortality [1]. CDI often results from normal gut bacterial disruption due to broad-spectrum antimicrobial use, allowing for overgrowth of toxigenic *C. difficile*. CDI outbreaks have been reported extensively in the United States (US) and Europe over the last two decades. CDI in these hospitals is prevalent supporting extensive CDI prevention and control measures. However, CDI is understudied in low and limited resource settings, including nearly all African countries. Where limited data exists, a study at a tertiary hospital in Cape Town, South Africa found 22% of stool samples from patients with suspected CDI diarrhoea were *C. difficile* positive [2]. In addition, patients in South Africa are disproportionately affected by HIV and tuberculosis (TB) and therefore also experience known CDI risk factors of prior hospital and antibiotic exposure—exposures that

* Correspondence: Legenza@wisc.edu
[1]University of Wisconsin-Madison School of Pharmacy, 777 Highland Ave, Madison, WI 53705, USA
[2]University of the Western Cape School of Pharmacy, Robert Sobukwe, Cape Town 7535, South Africa
Full list of author information is available at the end of the article

can uniquely contribute to an increased risk of CDI and poor outcomes [3, 4].

Treatment of CDI requires a comprehensive approach that includes infection prevention and control (IPC) measures to limit transmission and prevent outbreaks. Although no CDI IPC guidelines exist specific to African countries, the Infectious Diseases Society of America (IDSA) and European Society of Clinical Microbiology and Infectious Diseases guidelines consistently recommend IPC components of antimicrobial stewardship programs (ASP) which include effective environment cleaning, patient isolation, use of personal protective equipment such as gowns and gloves, surveillance, and education [5]. These evidence-based recommendations are key to effective CDI management. The feasibility of using these recommendations in populations with limited healthcare resources has not been established. In addition, healthcare provider knowledge of CDI and the guidance to effectively mitigate and manage patient populations at higher risk for CDI is unknown.

Provider knowledge of CDI and treatment measures are essential to both successfully manage CDI and prevent disease transmission. An assessment of current facilitators and barriers to CDI identification, management, and prevention is needed to design and evaluate improvement strategies to effectively minimize the risk of CDI. To our knowledge, no comprehensive study of barriers and facilitators to CDI workflow (identification, diagnosis, treatment, and prevention) in Sub-Saharan Africa exists. Our study aims to fill this gap by eliciting CDI perceptions and management practices among healthcare providers in South African secondary hospitals to uncover facilitators and barriers to providing quality CDI care.

Methods

Data collection

We utilized a qualitative approach to elicit health care providers' perceptions of barriers and facilitators to CDI management because it provides detailed process oriented results. We conducted semi-structured interviews and focus groups among clinical providers at three secondary hospitals in South Africa. A Systems Engineering Initiative for Patient Safety (SEIPS) model served as a framework for the interview guide. The SEIPS framework connects work systems to patient and organizational outcomes, while including interactions in the work system between available tools, people, tasks, the internal environment, and the organization [6]. The semi-structured interview assessed each subject's CDI knowledge and traced workflow from patient presentation with CDI symptoms through CDI 1.) Identification, 2.) Diagnosis, 3.) Treatment, and 4.) Prevention. Interview questions were structured to reveal facilitators and barriers to these CDI workflow steps and opportunities to improve CDI treatment. The interview guide included optional probes to use when appropriate to gather additional information. When participants revealed a lack of CDI knowledge from the preliminary questions, the interview was then modified to contain general questions about diarrhoea management. As a qualitative study, the interviewer could use information gathered from prior interviews to direct future interview discussions and build on emerging concepts. For example, asking for further detail and implications on processes mentioned with open-ended questions.

Participants

Providers working in three public secondary (district) level hospitals in the Western Cape, Cape Town Metropole, South Africa were invited to participate in this study. The three participating hospitals, averaging 265 inpatient beds overall, were previously selected to be included in a CDI quality improvement intervention. Our study aimed to interview, at minimum, 15 providers among five provider types including front-line nurses, nurse managers, pharmacists, junior physicians (registrars and medical officers), and senior physicians (consultants and department administrators). Semi-structured interviews and focus groups occurred August–November 2016.

Study investigators included healthcare providers from the US and South Africa with local hospital affiliations. The interviewers, a study investigator and a visiting US pharmacy resident, recruited front-line healthcare providers with convenience and snowball sampling, and recruited senior providers with purposive sampling. There were no participant exclusion criteria. Interviews were conducted as focus group discussions if preferred by participants. Participants were provided an informed consent document approved by the ethics committee prior to the interview and could decline participation at any time. Interviews were conducted by the interviewer in consultation rooms and offices. All interviews were conducted in English by one of the two interviewers with questions from a semi-structured interview guide and probing techniques by the interviewer. Interviews continued until thematic saturation was observed regarding barriers and facilitators for CDI treatment and management. The University of the Western Cape Research Ethics Committee granted approval for this qualitative study.

Data analysis

Interview audio recordings were transcribed verbatim and checked for accuracy. Data analysis included coding to factors determined a priori (including key workflow steps: 1) Identification, 2) Diagnosis, 3) Treatment, and 4) Prevention) as well as inductive coding to emerging themes [7]. Two individuals from a team of three coders (LL, TE, and KP) conducted each coding phase. Paired coding with two coders per phase was performed to minimize bias. Coding schema was created to reconcile local medical terminology. Discrepancies in coding were resolved by consensus. Kappa scores were calculated to assess coding agreement at a mid-point and at the conclusion of coding. While we had initially planned to map results with the SEIPS framework, CDI management knowledge was significantly lower than expected and insufficient to frame the results in terms of tools, people, tasks, the internal environment, and the organization. Alternatively, we mapped coded themes to the workflow structure identified from the interviews.

After identifying large discrepancies in health care provider knowledge regarding CDI during the interview process, a scoring system was developed to categorize participants' CDI knowledge from their interview responses (Table 1). The intent of the assessment was to quantify the unexpected differences. With the knowledge assessment, one knowledge point was possible from each of the following seven CDI-related components: signs and symptoms (e.g. diarrhoea), characteristics of bacteria (e.g. microbiology, virulence mechanism, disruption of normal flora, opportunistic), hand hygiene (e.g. soap and water needed to clean hands, not just alcohol), treatment (e.g. metronidazole, oral vancomycin, fecal transplant, contraindication with loperamide), contact precautions/ isolation (contagious), risk factors (e.g. healthcare exposure, antibiotic use, immunocompromised by medication or illness [cancer, HIV status, CD4 count < 200] proton pump inhibitor use), and diagnosis (e.g. stool sample and testing methods, polymerase chain reaction[PCR]/toxin detection). The following responses did not receive a point allocation: 1) only stating 'bacterial infection' for characteristics of bacteria, 2) stating a non-specific sign and symptoms of infection or illness without stating diarrhoea, 3) stating rehydration (electrolytes) without specific antibiotic treatment name. Total knowledge score from each individual interview was further classified into four categories: 'no knowledge' (0–1 point), 'limited knowledge' (2–3 points), 'moderate knowledge' (4–5 points), and 'advanced knowledge' (6–7 points). Each CDI knowledge category was also scored across all interviewees. Researchers conducted subgroup analysis of knowledge level based on occupation and performed analysis of individual CDI assessment knowledge categories by participant and occupation. The two focus group interviews were excluded from the knowledge assessment analysis due to potential knowledge score overestimation. However, dialogue from the group interviews was included in the qualitative analysis. All analyses were conducted using NVIVO software (Version 11, QSR International).

Table 1 *Clostridium difficile* knowledge assessment

Criteria for *Clostridium difficile* knowledge	Points
Signs and symptoms (diarrhoea)	1
States characteristics of bacteria (any mention of: microbiology, virulence mechanism, disruption of normal flora, opportunistic)	1
Soap and water needed to clean hands, not just alcohol	1
Treatment options (any mention of: metronidazole, oral vancomycin, fecal transplant, contraindication with loperamide)	1
Contact isolation needed (or contagious)	1
Risk factors (immunocompromised, antibiotic use, proton pump inhibitors)	1
Diagnosis (stool sample, testing methods [PCR/toxins])	1
Total points	=
No knowledge = 0–1[a] Limited knowledge = 2–3 Moderate knowledge = 4–5 Advanced knowledge = 6–7	

[a]Point allocation of 1 is considered no knowledge because there are multiple diseases associated with any one of the criteria, unless person states characteristics of bacteria

Results

A total of 26 semi-structured interviews were conducted with healthcare providers (11 nurses, 4 pharmacists, 11 physicians) of various rankings (Table 2). In addition, two focus groups were conducted; one with seven nurses and the second with three pharmacists, resulting in 36 study participants (Table 2). Kappa scores indicated high intercoder agreement (midpoint kappa = 0.71, final kappa 0.63). The median overall CDI knowledge score from the 26 individual interviews was 3 [interquartile range 0.25, 4.75]. Subgroup median knowledge scores and an analysis of responders' knowledge of each category are presented in Table 3. Inductive themes were coded for processes required for CDI workflow and organizational culture (beliefs and attitudes) regarding change (i.e. the ease of positive change at the organization or 'change culture') in order to inform future interventions. Healthcare provider responsibility and accountability for components of CDI management emerged as an organizational culture theme from the interviews. Thematic saturation of barriers and facilitators to CDI management was reached across the health care provider types (i.e. no additional themes emerged after iterative analysis of 26 interview and two focus group transcripts) [8]. CDI workflow steps are presented along with corresponding knowledge scores, barriers, and facilitators, (Section I: Workflow) and followed by organizational culture themes (Section II: Organizational Culture).

Table 2 Occupations and stated titles of healthcare providers interviewed

Healthcare Provider Occupation	Participants	Interviews
Nurse		
Operational managers or Assistant manager	4	4
Registered nurse or unspecified nurse	4	4
Infection Prevention and Control Nurse	2	2
Nurse Training Clinical Program Coordinator	1	1
Ward Nurses Focus Group Interview	7	1
Subtotal:	18	12
Pharmacist		
Pharmacist	4	4
Pharmacist Focus Group Interview	3	1
Subtotal:	7	5
Physician		
Head of Department	2	2
Consultant	1	1
Unspecified physician	1	1
Registrar	1	1
Medical officer	5	5
Intern	1	1
Subtotal:	11	11
Total (N)	36	28

Section I: Workflow

Figure 1 presents workflow depicted from interview results, along with facilitators and barriers to CDI management summarized in the context of the CDI workflow, including the previously identified steps of CDI identification, diagnosis, treatment, and prevention. When CDI is suspected, a stool sample is sent to an offsite laboratory for *C. difficile* identification by PCR. Following CDI diagnosis, treatment and infection prevention and control measures are initiated. Processes were consistent between healthcare providers with knowledge of the workflow step.

Identification and healthcare provider knowledge

CDI identification requires knowledge of the bacteria, risk factors and clinical suspicion when patients present with CDI signs and symptoms. A major barrier to identification is low CDI knowledge. Ten interviews (6 nurses, 4 pharmacists) scored as 'no CDI knowledge' (Table 3). One participant candidly revealed the lack of CDI knowledge.

> *"It's actually the first time that I hear about it, to be honest"* - Pharmacist

CDI signs and symptoms were most commonly known by healthcare providers ($n = 16$, 61.5%). Thirteen (50%) participants could not describe CDI risk factors that could prompt clinical inquiry for CDI; this knowledge gap creates a potential barrier for prompt identification. Two physicians reported extensive experience with CDI in the United Kingdom. A recurrent theme from the interviews among providers was that identification for

Table 3 *Clostridium difficile* infection (CDI) knowledge scores overall, by healthcare provider, and each CDI knowledge category

CDI knowledge sorted by healthcare provider

		Occupation			Overall
		Nurse ($n = 11$)	Physician (n = 11)	Pharmacist ($n = 4$)	All participants ($n = 26$)
Median Score (0–7), [1st, 3rd interquartile]		1 [0, 2.5]	5 [4, 6]	0.5 [0, 1]	3 [0.25, 4.75]
Knowledge Classification, n (%)					
No		6 (54.5)	0 (0.0)	4 (100.0)	10 (38.5)
Limited		4 (36.4)	0 (0.0)	0 (0.0)	4 (15.4)
Moderate		0 (0.0)	6 (54.5)	0 (0.0)	6 (23.1)
Advanced		1 (100.0)	5 (45.5)	0 (0.0)	6 (23.1)
Knowledge assessed in each CDI knowledge category					
Components of CDI knowledge assessment, n (%)					
1. Identification	1.1 Characteristics of bacteria	2 (18.2)	4 (36.4)	0 (0.0)	6 (23.1)
	1.2 Risk factors	3 (27.3)	10 (90.9)	0 (0.0)	13 (50.0)
	1.3 Signs and symptoms	3 (27.3)	11 (100.0)	2 (50.0)	16 (61.5)
2. Diagnosis	2.1 Diagnosis	1 (9.1)	10 (90.9)	0 (0.0)	11 (42.3)
3. Treatment	3.1 Treatment options	1 (9.1)	7 (63.6)	0 (0.0)	8 (30.8)
4. Prevention	4.1 Hand washing needed	4 (36.4)	7 (63.6)	0 (0.0)	11 (42.3)
	4.2 Need for contact isolation	4 (36.4)	8 (72.7)	0 (0.0)	12 (46.2)

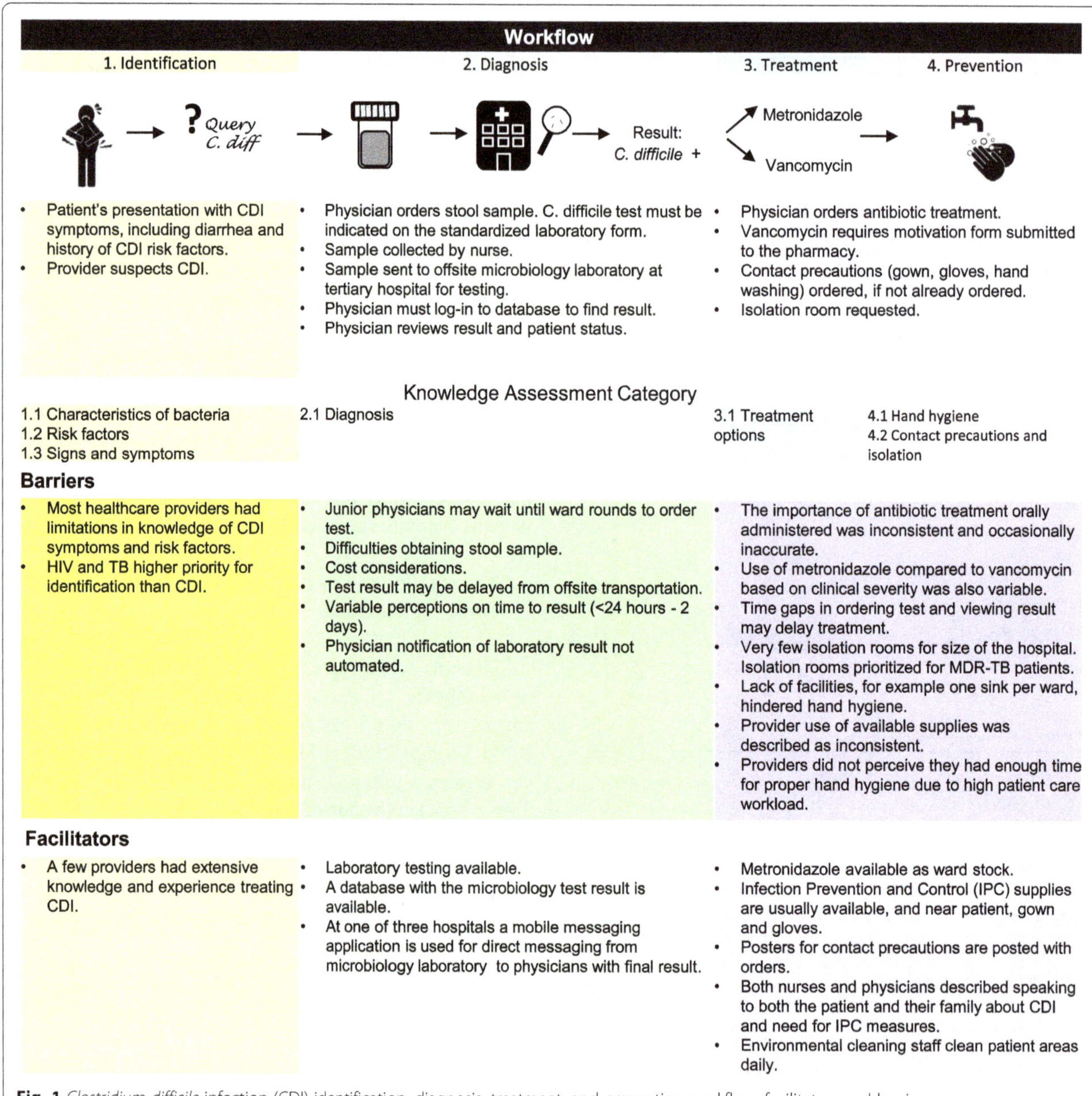

Fig. 1 *Clostridium difficile* infection (CDI) identification, diagnosis, treatment, and prevention workflow: facilitators and barriers

HIV and TB was prioritized over CDI. Physicians who have worked in the United Kingdom (U.K.) elaborated that the sense of urgency in South Africa for CDI was different than their previous experience due to competing attention of other prevalent disease.

> *"When I was in the UK [United Kingdom] years ago... [when] the manager mentioned C. diff the staff would jump up and down and get incredibly panicky... we just don't have that sense of urgency here... if you mention to someone in any hospital, they will go 'Okay, what is that?' [in cavalier tone]... however, if you tell them there is a patient with a potential XDR-TB [Extensively drug-resistant TB], then they may jump up and down. So the whole thing with C. diff it's a reality... ...a lot of people just think it's a disease with the elderly, but we have a lot of immunocompromised patients..."* - Physician

At one hospital, CDI awareness in senior staff only increased after an outbreak in the hospital. Awareness was lower for rotating junior staff who did not experience the outbreak.

> *"In terms of my junior staff, I think [CDI] ranks quite low. I think it's got to do with the way we've become*

aware last year. We've had more cases making us aware that it's highly infectious." - Physician

While some providers conjectured CDI to be a national problem, others did not, and no providers were aware of CDI magnitude in South Africa. Facilitating CDI identification were the senior providers with higher CDI knowledge. At one of the hospitals, an ASP was referenced as attributing to low incidence.

Diagnosis

After identification, to inform diagnosis, a stool sample from the patient is tested at a laboratory for *C. difficile*. While all hospitals in our study had laboratory testing available to conduct a *C. difficile* PCR test, testing occurred offsite as there was not capacity for the PCR test at the onsite laboratory. In order to test for *C. difficile*, physicians must indicate the test on a standardized laboratory form. Perception of time to result varied widely and was attributed to delays in initiating treatment. Additional barriers identified included staff difficulties obtaining stool samples due to staff shortages and non-standardized collection of laboratory samples. Laboratory test costs were occasionally cited as reasons to not test for *C. difficile*. Eleven interview participants described CDI diagnosis (42.3%, Table 3).

"Most of the time they are not tested, because they come from the emergency, and because our emergency is so busy, then the patient is pushed up to the ward. So then only when the patient is in the ward, and then we are actually reporting the [diarrhoea] to them [post call]. And then report that the patient is having diarrhoea; then that's the only time that they collect a stool specimen, and then after some, a couple of days, they get the results: the patient is positive. See... It could be about a week." - Nurse Focus Group

Other attributes identified in delaying the time to diagnosis include waiting for a physician to suggest the *C. difficile* test or until ward rounds to order it. To find results, physicians must proactively login to the database—usually from their personal mobile phones, as computer stations are not easily available. One of three hospitals uses a mobile messaging application for direct messaging from the microbiology laboratory to physicians with the goal of reducing the result notification time.

"I think the one resource that we've shown very well is the communication system. I think we chose the cheapest one we could find which is WhatsApp and that does make a difference in terms of managing your patients and getting a quicker diagnosis. The thing about WhatsApp is if a patient had a positive result, it would take the doctor another 2 days to figure it out that an infection exists. We actually have an alert system that works." - Physician

After observing the test result, the physician informs the nursing staff if the patient has a CDI. The IPC nurses are also informed of results and may, in turn, inform the medical team. However, there is not a timely and consistent pathway for this notification, especially during post-call hours. The IPC nurse sends physicians a report including positive *C. difficile* test results on a monthly basis.

Treatment

Antibiotic treatment options for antibiotic-associated diarrhoea included in South African treatment guidelines at the time of the interviews were oral metronidazole initially and oral vancomycin for diarrhoea not responsive to metronidazole; vancomycin must be oral to reach the infection. Of note, the interviews were conducted prior to the revised IDSA CDI guidelines in 2018 [3]. Eight (30.8%) respondents mentioned CDI treatment options, including treatment with metronidazole and vancomycin, though the importance of antibiotic treatment administered orally was reported inconsistently and occasionally inaccurately.

A few providers also discussed the clinical use of metronidazole compared to vancomycin, including patients' illness severity.

"So patients who don't respond to metronidazole would definitely be candidates for vancomycin or a metronidazole allergy." - Physician

Communication barriers were attributed to delays in treatment and included factors such as results being finalized while the physician was post call and drug order errors needing clarification.

Healthcare providers' high familiarity with metronidazole and its availability on the hospital floor as ward stock facilitated its use for CDI treatment. To order vancomycin and other antibiotics on the Essential Medicine List for Hospital Level Adults, providers needed to complete a pharmacy-approved motivation form that facilitates appropriate antibiotic use. Participants reported a time gap between ordering, sending the medication chart to the pharmacy, having the medication delivered to the ward, and administrating it to the patients. Some orders might be written up and not sent to the pharmacy. For stat orders, nurses may retrieve orders from the pharmacy. The pharmacies were closed during evenings and weekends. An emergency stock of inventory is kept in the emergency center. If the needed drug is unavailable, an on-call pharmacist is called-in to prepare it.

Occasionally medication was not administered and incorrectly documented as unavailable while drug was available in the emergency stock. Other reported barriers to patients receiving medications as ordered included: illegible handwriting, medication orders not including which ward an order came from, and physicians writing brand names when nurses only know the generic name. Additionally, sometimes a medication was given and not recorded; other times the patients missed doses because they were not present.

> *"The problem with this is ...that sometimes the results come back, the doctor is post call. Yes, and then he will only get the feedback the next day when he is actually coming to check on his patients. So that is the delay to start"*- Nurse Focus Group

Prevention: Contact precautions, hand hygiene, isolation, environmental cleaning

Contact precautions CDI prevention procedures include contact precautions (e.g. gown, gloves) to reduce the risk of *C. difficile* spreading to other patients. Twelve (46.2%) participants reported the need for strict contact precautions when CDI was suspected or diagnosed. Supplies and procedures for IPC (included posters displaying orders for contact precautions) were usually available but not always utilised. Supplies (including gowns, gloves, masks, and hand sanitizer) were available in close proximity to a patient once contact precautions were ordered. Staff education and timely notification of need for infection control were the most common barriers to IPC measures. Pressure from patient bed shortages can lead to patients being placed near each other. Contact precautions with the first suspicion of CDI was described at one of the hospitals.

> *"...any patient with diarrhoea is placed with contact precaution; until we know if they have been exposed to any antibiotics, we put them as high risk."* - Physician

At the three hospitals, the ward nurse in charge will enforce contact precautions with the nurses and the attending/consulting physicians will enforce junior physicians' contact precautions. The IPC team also enforces IPC practices. Both physicians and nurses inform patients about contact precautions; patients are told to inform their family members. While senior physicians reported informing patients of the need for IPC in the CDI setting, nurses considered themselves more approachable than the physicians and took a primary role in communicating with patients. One junior physician admitted his/her peers' shortfalling.

> *"I think that from all of it, that is where the biggest failing comes in—that we often don't tell patients enough of the stuff. So, I would like to think that once it's done there is a proper [communication] about the patient having things that can be transmitted, with words that they can understand and the importance of them not going around and touching lots of things and letting them know the reasons for gloving up and putting on gowns and stuff for their own peace of mind...It's apathy from the medical staff we forget to do these things..."* - Physician

Hand hygiene Facilitators and barriers to hand hygiene were related to the treatment of patients with CDI and additional infections. Hand hygiene practices for patients with CDI should include hand washing with soap and water to remove *C. difficile* spores that are not killed by alcohol hand sanitizers. Supplies, including paper towels, soap, and hand sanitizer, were frequently available but not always utilised. Some stated that insufficient supplies were a barrier; others said that supplies were always available. Eleven (42.3%) participants acknowledged the importance of washing hands with soap and water when treating patients with CDI (Table 3).

> *"...have to use soap and water, we take [the] de-germ [alcohol based hand sanitizer] away from bedside so they are forced to use soap and water."* - Physician

Some perceptions regarding this important hand hygiene practice were inaccurate.

> *"I would not say a normal hand soap is better for* C. diff, *I would say something alcohol based."* - Physician

Staffing shortages and high workload were described as reasons for inconsistent hand hygiene practices.

> *"Can I tell you, all over the basins is that sign [WHO's "5 Moments of Hand Hygiene"]... but we don't practice it...We don't follow five moments of Hand Hygiene. We follow it when we go home... You can't afford to take that 5 min."* – Nurse Focus Group

Participants described hand hygiene events (e.g. ultraviolent light, blue soap) in their hospitals that encouraged effective hand hygiene. Many stated that overcrowding and lack of facilities (e.g. one sink per ward) hindered hand hygiene as well as: the high ratio of patients to nurses, education limitations, and sometimes-empty alcohol and/or soap dispensers.

Isolation Infrastructure limitations were a major barrier to IPC, often preventing CDI patients from allocation to an isolation room. Isolation room availability ranged from two to four rooms. Isolation rooms were specifically prioritized for multidrug resistant tuberculosis (MDR-TB) patients, who may occupy the room for a month. CDI is viewed as a lower priority for isolation rooms.

> *"The fact that we have got a lot of immunocompromised patients in terms of our HIV rates and TB rates, a lot of our patients are at risk due to the use of antibiotics. In the UK we used to see a lot of elderly patients, but here you have got a different spectrum of patients, so C. diff is a huge risk... I think everyone focuses on MDR and very few people actually focus on C. diff ... C. diff is not something that is high on the radar."* - Physician

Challenges for IPC included patient education regarding IPC, especially patients leaving isolation, walking around the hospital, and using shared bathrooms.

> *"The big problem that we have in our wards is a lack of isolation facilities. For an entire hospital, we've got only four isolation rooms [that] do not include isolation bathrooms. So a C. diff patient would have to use the same toilet as other patients."* - Physician

Both nurses and physicians described speaking to patients and their family members about isolation. An elevated desire from patients to understand their condition was expressed when patients were moved to an isolation room.

> *"Sometimes you'll find the patient doesn't know what is going on, but when you move them into an isolation room then they want to know why."* - Nurse

Environmental cleaning The ward managers inform cleaning staff verbally about room cleaning needs. Under supervision, the cleaners complete a written checklist for the bathrooms and patient rooms. Cleaning is sometimes rushed due to high bed demand, and the staff nurses will help.

> *"It's just that we are busy so the beds are always in demand so sometimes there is no opportunity for cleaning because everything is rush, rush, rush, rush. When the patient is waiting on discharge, others are waiting for that bed so we don't have the opportunity to do the spring cleaning of the unit. We aren't always able to do it in a calm environment."* – Nurse

Section II: Organizational Culture

Themes related to organizational culture (beliefs and attitudes) and how leadership and administration respond to new ideas, specifically 'change culture', were analyzed in order to inform future interventions. Through this coding an additional organizational culture theme emerged related to healthcare provider responsibility and accountability.

Change culture: how leadership and administration respond to new ideas

The majority of respondents described leadership as being supportive of new ideas. Some respondents did not feel leadership was supportive of bottom-up ideas; others believed that ideas with evidence of positive impact would be supported. A few respondents noted a barrier to change related more to nursing staff and junior physician turnover than to administrative support. Progressive change is difficult when the same education concepts are repeated with rotating healthcare providers; institutional memory regarding CDI and CDI management was lost.

> *"Implementing change and practical change are very different, so we are able to change our practice so we can make lots of suggestions... but the difficulty comes in that our staff [is a] rotating staff."* - Physician

A nurse new to a leadership position anticipated facing challenges in changing long-standing practices.

> *"The people above me, the specialist physicians or consultants, are quite open to change. If you can show clearly that an idea is going to work, the department is open to change and improving things. As you get higher up the leadership chain, it becomes more difficult to introduce change. I do find that on the face of it, the managers seem to be okay and accepting and are happy to listen."* - Physician

Responsibility and accountability

While the interviewees described achievements of and challenges for patients and healthcare providers following IPC precautions, low adherence emerged as a compelling theme—sometimes in the context of IPC in general and for the treatment of TB, particularly when participants had limited CDI knowledge. Perception of the threats from infectious diseases and IPC prioritization also appear to be barriers to adherence when supplies are available. Accountability structures are not in place to properly encourage providers to remain knowledgeable about guidelines nor enforce IPC precautions.

"It seems we have many awareness days... we had spike last year, 2 years ago... we have had quite a few staff members contracted tuberculosis... people only get aware if their buddy gets it... It makes it real." - Physician

"Just to get the doctors to wear gloves—that for me is another thing where I can just say... like, 'Why are you not wearing gloves?' or, just tell them 'Your patient has TB. Can you put on your mask please?' ...together with the hand washing, and at the end of the day, it is part of the IPC principles to have full personal protection equipment available in the unit, but there's hand sanitizers, soap, and water, available in the unit, so no one has an excuse." - Physician

Informal structures for peer accountability were discussed as a helpful strategy from two interviews. First, accountability for hand hygiene occurred on the ASP ward round at one hospital. Second, an Operational Manager in the Operating Room (Theater) described nursing and cleaning staff who speak up about needs and follow cleaning expectations.

"The cleaning staff and the nursing staff is quite well informed as to what is supposed to happen, because sometimes they can tell you. 'Sister, this was not done yet; You can't really put your patient here'... Those are the people that I work with... that I come across, that will tell me. Doesn't matter if you are the cleaner, you can tell me, 'Sister, it's not ready yet.' You understand. It's that relationship that we have [of a] multidisciplinary team, to do what is expected of us." – Nurse

Discussion

Principal findings

This is the first qualitative study of CDI in Sub-Saharan Africa, and the results provide novel insight into CDI treatment and workflow in a limited resource setting. The context of CDI in Africa is especially important to consider given the high HIV and tuberculosis prevalence and high risk of *C. difficile* associated mortality in this population. This study reveals significant barriers and facilitators to CDI treatment in public district (secondary) level South African hospitals. Major barriers included knowledge gaps in CDI management, especially regarding awareness of the infection, transmission, treatment, and IPC practices among health care providers. Physician CDI knowledge was higher than nurse and pharmacist knowledge. The results reveal opportunities for healthcare provider education related to CDI. Our study affirms that healthcare providers have an awareness of evidence-based IPC precautions but barriers to following them include perceptions of priority and time availability.

Implications: perceptions and knowledge

Based on quantitative results from the overall CDI knowledge assessment, participants had limited CDI knowledge. Gaps in CDI knowledge may delay clinical suspicion and all workflow steps in CDI identification, diagnosis, treatment and prevention. While physicians scored higher, some physicians were less confident regarding when to order the *C. difficile* test resulting in delayed diagnosis. Physicians with high CDI knowledge noted an urgency surrounding CDI not observed in junior physicians and other healthcare providers.. This, together with a high risk of mortality in patients with positive *C. difficile* test results, underscores an urgent need for education and intervention tailored to relevant aspects of healthcare providers' job responsibilities.

Overall, participants scored well in areas of identifying CDI risk factors, signs, and symptoms. However, improvement is needed in terms of educating healthcare professionals in South Africa about other aspects of CDI. In the occupation subgroup analysis, nurses and pharmacists appear to be less knowledgeable about CDI characteristics, with response rates of 50% or less in all the knowledge assessment categories. The identified areas for potential development relevant to nurses and pharmacists are: CDI patients' need for contact isolation, the importance of hand washing instead of using alcohol gel in preventing the spread of CDI, and CDI treatment options. Nurses can also be educated to suspect CDI when monitoring bowel movements.

This study reveals a more complicated process for obtaining and administering vancomycin compared to metronidazole that may be hindering healthcare providers' use of vancomycin. In an epidemiology, treatment, and outcomes study in the same setting, vancomycin was rarely ordered (2%) as initial CDI treatment [4]. One strategy is to incorporate treatment options for CDI into pharmacist education and teach pharmacists what to look for on physician-submitted motivation forms. Pharmacist education about treatment options is especially important considering the role pharmacists have in the approval process for vancomycin use. The healthcare team should be educated on the clinical use of vancomycin for CDI with an emphasis on timely preparation and delivery.

How results relate to other studies

Our study affirms current literature's described need for improved CDI identification in settings with extensive CDI experience. Despite a history of substantial CDI outbreaks in Europe, a study identified persistent underdiagnoses of CDI when all diarrhoea samples were tested at 482 hospitals across 20 European countries; 23% of *C.*

difficile positive results were not identified at the local hospital. Authors attributed the underdiagnoses to a lack of clinical suspicion and suboptimal laboratory diagnostic methods [9]. Meanwhile, in the US, a regulatory climate that reduces hospital reimbursement for patients who develop hospital-acquired infections is driving efforts to refine testing protocols to avoid *C. difficile* over testing and inappropriate diagnosis [10]. These studies emphasize the importance of appropriate testing for diagnosis.

A global review of CDI guidelines found antimicrobial stewardship (ASPs) to be universally recognized as an essential evidence-based component of CDI IPC [5]. Continued development of interdisciplinary ASPs in limited resource settings is necessary to facilitate effective CDI management and IPC measures.

One barrier to hand hygiene identified in this study was the perception that there is insufficient time available for thorough hand cleaning. Indeed, in a study conducted in the US about healthcare providers' compliance with IPC practices for patients with CDI, full compliance was very low and time-consuming with a mean time for full compliance greater than 5 min for patients in single isolation rooms [11]. Patient care workload continues to be a barrier to full compliance with CDI contact precautions in high resource settings [12]. Therefore, improving full compliance of IPC practices in limited resource settings will require both a workload adjustment to allow more time per patient and education on the importance of CDI-related IPC practices.

Significant challenges for the implementation of IPC programs and practices exist in low and limited resource settings, including infrastructural constraints with a limited number of isolation rooms and variable staff compliance with hand hygiene practices. A similar qualitative study in India found perceived workload and nursing staff turnover to be barriers to infection control [13]. This relates to our study's previously referenced finding that perceived workload hindered infection control practices, especially regarding hand hygiene. Our respondents reported high turnover of both nursing staff and junior physicians as barriers to implementing change. The secondary hospitals included in our study did not have an IPC team as developed as the one in the tertiary hospital in India. The study in India also found participants reporting the availability of IPC supplies but experiencing challenges with compliance, while an international study of healthcare settings representing 30 countries identified inadequate supplies as a barrier to infection control of multidrug resistant organisms in some high and middle income countries [13, 14].

Limitations

As a qualitative study, the results are not generalizable to a larger population but may be transferable to similar settings. Visiting researchers' presence conducting the interviews may have affected responses; stated practices are not necessarily the reality of practice. While all interviews were conducted in English, English was a second language for some participants. This may have limited the respondents' understanding of some questions and ability to articulate responses. Furthermore, we may have underestimated facilitators to CDI management in an attempt to identify improvement opportunities. Our analysis was not a systematic audit of workflow and practices, and some inaccuracies may exist. To mitigate bias, multiple researchers of the study team reviewed the results. Finally, as we developed the knowledge assessment after the interviews were completed, the assessment is not yet validated and results are limited. Our knowledge assessment measured breadth of CDI knowledge and not depth. For example, some providers gave detailed explanations for some of the knowledge components, such as advantages of different testing protocols, yet these explanations were still only assigned one point for that component.

Conclusions

Our analysis provides a detailed description of the facilitators and barriers to CDI workflow, including the need for increased healthcare provider knowledge of CDI management. Interventions should increase CDI knowledge and utilization of the available systems and supplies by addressing the identified barriers and championing the identified facilitators. Increasing CDI knowledge alone is unlikely to be effective without addressing the need to create a sense of urgency around CDI and appropriate IPC practices. The results provide context for technical intervention and implementation strategies in low-resource public healthcare settings. This study serves as a baseline and supplements quantitative CDI patient data from ongoing CDI research including provider education and a clinical intervention to improve CDI quality of care in South Africa. The results of this workflow and provider knowledge analysis identify areas of need and are useful to design interventions to improve the quality of care for CDI patients in this population and similar limited resource settings.

Abbreviations

ASP: Antimicrobial stewardship programs; CDI: *Clostridium difficile* infection; IPC: Infection prevention and control; MDR(-TB): Multidrug resistant(–tuberculosis); PCR: Polymerase chain reaction; SEIPS: Systems Engineering Initiative for Patient Safety; TB: Tuberculosis; UK: United Kingdom; US: United States; XDR-TB: Extensively drug-resistant TB

Acknowledgements

We thank South African Department of Health for their collaboration. We also thank the Western Cape hospitals participating in this study. We appreciate the ongoing collaboration between the University of the Western Cape and the University of Wisconsin-Madison.

Funding
There was no funding for this study. LL was supported by an internal endowment at the University of Wisconsin-Madison.

Authors' contributions
LL designed the study, designed data collection, monitored data collection for the whole study, conducted interviews, transcribed audio, analysed the data, drafted and revised the paper. SB provided guidance on the study and revised the paper. WR provided guidance on the study and revised the paper. NS provided guidance on the study and revised the paper. TE transcribed audio, analysed data, and revised the paper. KHP transcribe audio, analysed data, and revised the paper. RC facilitated the collaborative project between the University of the Western Cape and the University of Wisconsin, provided guidance on the study and revised the paper. All authors read and approved the final manuscript.

Consent for publication
Not applicable.

Competing interests
The authors declare that they have no competing interests.

Author details
[1]University of Wisconsin-Madison School of Pharmacy, 777 Highland Ave, Madison, WI 53705, USA. [2]University of the Western Cape School of Pharmacy, Robert Sobukwe, Cape Town 7535, South Africa. [3]University of Wisconsin School of Medicine and Public Health, 750 Highland Ave, Madison, WI 53726, USA.

References
1. Steiner C, Barrett M, Sun Y. HCUP Projections: Clostridium Difficile Hospitalizations 2004-2015. Projections Report #2015-02 2015 [Available from: https://www.hcup-us.ahrq.gov/reports/projections/2015-02.pdf.
2. Rajabally N, Kullin B, Ebrahim K, Brock T, Weintraub A, Whitelaw A, et al. A comparison of Clostridium difficile diagnostic methods for identification of local strains in a South African centre. J Med Microbiol. 2016;65(4):320-7.
3. McDonald LC, Gerding DN, Johnson S, Bakken JS, Carroll KC, Coffin SE, et al. Clinical Practice Guidelines for Clostridium difficile Infection in Adults and Children: 2017 Update by the Infectious Diseases Society of America (IDSA) and Society for Healthcare Epidemiology of America (SHEA). Clin Infect Dis. 2018.
4. Legenza L, Barnett S, Rose W, Bianchini M, Safdar N, Coetzee R. Epidemiology and outcomes of Clostridium difficile infection among hospitalised patients: Results of a multicentre retrospective study in South Africa. BMJ Global Health. 2018;3(4).
5. Balsells E, Filipescu T, Kyaw MH, Wiuff C, Campbell H, Nair H. Infection prevention and control of Clostridium difficile: a global review of guidelines, strategies, and recommendations. J Glob Health. 2016;6(2):020410.
6. Carayon P, Schoofs Hundt A, Karsh BT, Gurses AP, Alvarado CJ, Smith M, et al. Work system design for patient safety: the SEIPS model. Qual Saf Health Care. 2006;(15 Suppl 1):i50-8.
7. Bradley EH, Curry LA, Devers KJ. Qualitative data analysis for health services research: developing taxonomy, themes, and theory. Health Serv Res. 2007; 42(4):1758-72.
8. Glaser BG. The discovery of grounded theory : strategies for qualitative research: New Brunswick, N.J. : Aldine Transaction, [1999] ©1999; 1999.
9. Davies KA, Longshaw CM, Davis GL, Bouza E, Barbut F, Barna Z, et al. Underdiagnosis of Clostridium difficile across Europe: the European, multicentre, prospective, biannual, point-prevalence study of Clostridium difficile infection in hospitalised patients with diarrhoea (EUCLID). Lancet Infect Dis. 2014;14(12):1208-19.
10. Fang FC, Polage CR, Wilcox MH. Point-Counterpoint: What Is the Optimal Approach for Detection of Clostridium difficile Infection? J Clin Microbiol. 2017;55(3):670-80.
11. Yanke E, Zellmer C, Van Hoof S, Moriarty H, Carayon P, Safdar N. Understanding the current state of infection prevention to prevent Clostridium difficile infection: a human factors and systems engineering approach. Am J Infect Control. 2015;43(3):241-7.
12. Yanke E, Moriarty H, Carayon P, Safdar N. A qualitative, interprofessional analysis of barriers to and facilitators of implementation of the Department of Veterans Affairs' Clostridium difficile prevention bundle using a human factors engineering approach. Am J Infect Control. 2018;46(3):276-84.
13. Barker AK, Brown K, Siraj D, Ahsan M, Sengupta S, Safdar N. Barriers and facilitators to infection control at a hospital in northern India: a qualitative study. Antimicrob Resist Infect Control. 2017;6:35.
14. Safdar N, Sengupta S, Musuuza JS, Juthani-Mehta M, Drees M, Abbo LM, et al. Status of the Prevention of Multidrug-Resistant Organisms in International Settings: A Survey of the Society for Healthcare Epidemiology of America Research Network. Infect Control Hosp Epidemiol. 2017;38(1):53-60.

High frequency and molecular epidemiology of metallo-β-lactamase-producing gram-negative bacilli in a tertiary care hospital in Lahore, Pakistan

Noor Ul Ain[1], Anam Iftikhar[1], Syeda Sadia Bukhari[1], Samyyia Abrar[1], Shahida Hussain[1], Muhammad Hayat Haider[1], Farhan Rasheed[2] and Saba Riaz[1,3*]

Abstract

Background: Metallo-β-lactamase (MBL)-producing isolates have a strong impact on diagnostic and therapeutic decisions. A high frequency of MBL-producing gram-negative bacilli has been reported worldwide. The current study was based on determining the incidence of MBL-producing imipenem-resistant clinical isolates and investigating the β-lactamase gene variants in strains conferring resistance to a carbapenem drug (imipenem).

Methods: A total of 924 gram negative isolates were recovered from a tertiary care hospital in Lahore, Pakistan, during a two-year period (July 2015 to February 2017). The initial selection of bacterial isolates was based on antibiotic susceptibility testing. Strains resistant to imipenem were processed for the molecular screening of β-lactamase genes. Statistical analysis for risk factor determination was based on age, gender, clinical specimen and type of infection.

Results: The rate of imipenem resistance was calculated to be 56.51%. Among the 142 strains processed, the phenotypic tests revealed that the incidence of MBLs was 63.38% and 86.61% based on the combination disc test and the modified Hodge test, respectively. The frequencies of bla_{TEM}, bla_{SHV}, bla_{OXA}, bla_{IMP-1}, and bla_{VIM} genes were calculated to be 46%, 34%, 24%, 12.5% and 7%, respectively. The co-expression of bla_{MBL} (bla_{IMP} and bla_{VIM}) and bla_{ESBL} (bla_{TEM}, bla_{SHV}, bla_{OXA}) was also detected through multiplex and singleplex PCR. bla_{OXA}, bla_{TEM} and bla_{SHV} coexisted in 82% of the isolates. Co-expression of ESBL and MBL genes was found in 7% of the isolates.

Conclusion: To our knowledge, this is the first report from Pakistan presenting the concomitant expression of bla_{OXA}, bla_{TEM} and bla_{SHV} with bla_{IMP-1} and bla_{VIM} in MBL-producing gram-negative bacilli.

Background

Dissemination of life-threatening infections caused by β-lactamase-producing pathogens is a major setback to antimicrobial therapy. The widespread use of carbapenems has resulted in the emergence of carbapenemases, conferring resistance against carbapenem drugs [1–3]. Resistance to carbapenems is worrisome because of the very limited therapeutic options available to treat resistant infections [4, 5]. The diverse mechanisms of resistance to imipenem include AmpC enzymes accompanied by membrane porin alterations and upregulation of efflux pumps [5, 6]. The second phenomenon is carbapenem hydrolysis by carbapenemases [7–9]. The epicentre for the emergence of carbapenemases and that of extended spectrum beta lactamases (ESBLs) were different, but the association of their genes is apparent through some studies, where ESBL genes are found to exist in MBL-producing isolates [10].

Among carbapenemases, metallo-β-lactamases (MBLs) are of prime importance for the region under study because of the emergence of new variants of MBL, such as New Delhi metallo-β-lactamase (NDM) [11] and various

* Correspondence: saba.mmg@pu.edu.pk
[1]Department of Microbiology and Molecular Genetics, University of the Punjab, Lahore 5400, Pakistan
[3]Citilab and Research Center, Lahore, Pakistan
Full list of author information is available at the end of the article

IMP variants from the subcontinent. MBLs belong to class B carbapenemases according to the Ambler classification system [12]. bla_{IMP}, bla_{NDM} and bla_{VIM} are important MBL gene clusters that are carried by mobile plasmids compatible with a vast array of clinically important pathogens [13, 14]. In addition, oxacillinases belonging to class D include serine β-lactamases and are known to be associated primarily with *Enterobacteriaceae* carbapenem-resistant epidemics.

With more than 37 types of IMP carbapenemases known [15], IMP-1 was the first to be reported in Japan in 1991[16]. IMP-4-type enzymes, first discovered in Hong Kong during the 2000s [17], were later found to be responsible for an outbreak in 2005 in Melbourne, Australia [18]. The dissemination of resistance genes from *Serratia* spp. and *Pseudomonas aeruginosa* to other members of *Enterobacteriaceae* caused these genes to become endemic in Australia. Approximately 20 different subtypes of IMP enzymes have been described to be associated with *Pseudomonas* spp., *Acinetobacter* spp. and *Enterobacteriaceae* infections throughout the globe [19].

The first case of VIM-1 enzyme-conferred resistance was reported in 1999 in Verona, Italy [20]. With reports of VIM-2 being highly prevalent in Europe, Asia, America and Africa [21], a recent global surveillance study reported four new variants of VIM [22]. After their discovery in New Delhi in 2009 [23], NDM-1-producing *Klebsiella pneumoniae* and *E. coli* have been widely reported throughout the globe, including various European countries as well as China, Kenya, Japan, Algeria and Syria [24–27]. A research study has indicated dissemination of the NDM-1 carbapenemase gene through horizontal gene transfer in Pakistan, India and the UK [28].

The rise in carbapenem resistance in Asian countries has been evident, as reported imipenem resistance rose from 20% in the Philippines [29] to 40% in Vietnam [30]. Recently, > 50% carbapenem-resistant *Klebsiella pneumoniae* isolates have been recorded in India [31]. With the first report of emergence among *Acinetobacter baumannii* clinical isolates in Scotland in 1985 [32], plasmid-borne OXA-48 carbapenemases were reported to be highly disseminated in isolates from 18 countries in Europe and Africa [33].

The resistance pattern of metallo-β-lactamases in Pakistan has not been widely studied. In Pakistan, imipenem was only rarely available prior to the year 2000 [34]. Later, carbapenem resistance was reported mainly in *P. aeruginosa* in Lahore and Karachi [35, 36]. A report from Rawalpindi confirmed that 78% of isolates were MBL producers, with major incidence of MBL production in *Acinetobacter baumannii* and *Pseudomonas aeruginosa* [37].

A very limited number of reports have been published from Pakistan that are based on molecular analysis of genes acquired by carbapenem-resistant isolates. This study aimed to determine the incidence of MBLs through phenotypic and genotypic analyses. Moreover, this study is based on the detection of the gene variants responsible for resistance to carbapenem drugs. To the best of our knowledge, this is the first study from Lahore on the molecular epidemiology and coexistence of bla_{ESBLs} and bla_{MBLs}.

Methods

Study design

Microbiological testing was conducted at the pathology laboratory of Allama Iqbal Medical College Lahore from July 2015 to July 2017. The study was approved by the Ethical Committee of Citilab and Research Centre Pakistan (CitiLab and Research Centre Ref # 30th – 15 CLRC/ 30th). The segment of the work based on molecular analysis was carried out at the Department of Microbiology and Molecular Genetics, University of the Punjab, Lahore.

Bacterial isolates

A total of 3000 samples were obtained from clinical samples. All clinical specimens were subjected to isolation and identification of significant pathogens according to CLSI procedures (CLSI 2015, 2016). Among 2000 cultures with positive growth, 924 gram negative isolates bacilli were further screened for acquisition of imipenem resistance. On the basis of antibiotic susceptibility patterns, 142 isolates resistant to imipenem were further analysed by molecular tools. Identification of bacterial isolates was performed on the basis of culture characteristics, gram staining and conventional biochemical tests. Confirmation of gram-negative isolates was performed by API 20 NE identification strips (bioMerieux, France). The identified strains were stored in 30% glycerol broth at – 70 °C. Isolates were obtained from wound infections ($n = 487$), urine samples ($n = 187$), sputum samples ($n = 90$), tips and catheters ($n = 47$), fluids and effusions ($n = 44$) and others, including tissue samples, bone samples, and vaginal swabs ($n = 57$) (Table 3).

Antimicrobial susceptibility testing

Antimicrobial susceptibility testing (AST) for all isolates was carried out by the Kirby-Bauer method [38] on Mueller-Hinton agar plates (Oxoid) as per Clinical and Laboratory Standard Institute (CLSI, 2016) recommendations. The antibiotic panel used in screening of the cultures was specific for gram-negative bacteria: penicillins (amoxicillin 30 μg, amoxicillin-clavulanic acid 40 μg, and piperacillin-tazobactam 30 μg), monobactam (aztreonam 30 μg), extended-spectrum cephalosporins (ceftriaxone 30 μg, cefepime 30 μg, cefotaxime 30 μg, cefoxitin 30 μg, and ceftazidime 30 μg), carbapenems (imipenem 30 μg), aminoglycosides (amikacin 30 μg and gentamicin 30 μg), quinolone (ciprofloxacin 30 μg) and trimethoprim-sulfamethoxazole (40 μg). The results of the susceptibility testing were used to calculate the multiple antibiotic resistance (MAR) index for the clinical isolates in order to estimate drug resistance trends and the emergence of new resistant isolates.

Phenotypic detection of MBLs

Phenotypic detection of MBLs was based on three tests according to the CLSI guidelines (2015–2016). The combination disc test, using a disc of imipenem and imipenem with incorporated EDTA, was performed as per the method used by *Wadekar, Anuradha* [39]. A modified Hodge test (MHT) was performed according to the method used by Kumar et al. [40]. The results for each type of isolate were interpreted according to the criteria defined in CLSI 2016. All antibiotics were obtained from Oxoid, Inc. (Canada). E-strips with IMI and IMP/EDTA were used for epsilometer confirmation of MBLs according to the manufacturer's instructions (Liofilchem®).

Molecular characterization of MBLs

DNA template preparation for PCR

The template DNA was extracted from isolates using previously described methods [41]. Briefly, a single colony of bacterial isolate was immersed in low TE, and the suspension was boiled for 10 min. The bacterial cell emulsion was centrifuged, and DNA in the supernatant was directly used as a template for PCR amplification.

Detection of ESBL and MBL genes

All of the positive MBL isolates based on phenotypic detection ($n = 123$) were further confirmed by singleplex and multiplex colony PCR. Multiplex PCR for bla_{TEM}, bla_{OXA} and bla_{SHV} detection was devised. The primer sequences used for the detection of bla_{TEM}, bla_{OXA} and bla_{SHV} genes have been previously reported [42]. Screening for isolates having the bla_{IMP-1} gene and bla_{VIM} gene was performed by singleplex PCR using previously reported primers [43, 44]. The PCR reaction was set up with a 25 μl mixture containing 10X PCR buffer, 2.5 mM mixture of dNTPs, 20 pmol each primer and 2.5 U of Taq polymerase. The amplification conditions were set with an initial denaturation at 95 °C proceeded by 35 cycles of 1 min denaturation at 95 °C, 1.5 min annealing (temperatures mentioned in Table 1), extension for 1 min and final extension for 10 min at 72 °C. The Mg concentration was maintained between 1 and 1.5 mM.

Statistical analysis

The collected demographic data were statistically analysed using the Statistical Package for Social Sciences (SPSS version 23). The proportions of *Acinetobacter* spp., *Pseudomonas* spp. and members of *Enterobacteriaceae* were calculated using the chi-square test and odds ratios (ORs). A p value of < 0.05 was considered statistically significant. The associations among the type of infection, age, gender and type of isolate were calculated.

Results

Distribution of clinical isolates

In this study, the resistance pattern of imipenem-resistant clinical isolates was assessed, and the incidence of MBL production among these isolates was determined. Moreover, the significant gene variants associated with the MBL phenotype were analysed. Demographic factors and sites of infection were major highlights of the statistical data analysis. Out of a total of 942 isolates, the total frequency of imipenem resistance was calculated to be 56.512% ($n = 512$). The highest resistance to imipenem was observed for *Acinetobacter* spp., at 61.89%. *Pseudomonas* spp. ranked second in terms of the acquisition of imipenem resistance, with a frequency of 61.89%, followed by *Klebsiella* spp. (50.26%) and *Escherichia coli* (37.97%). Males were found to be more prone to the acquisition of imipenem-resistant infections (60.69%) compared to females (39.31%). The infectivity rates varied between different age groups, with the maximum mean observed among individuals of the age group 20–40 years. The mean age of individuals acquiring MBL infection was 30 years. Wound infections were found to be the most dominant type of infection (51.70%), followed by urinary tract infections (19.86%), respiratory

Table 1 List of the Primers used for the detection of ESBL-Type variant ($bla_{OXA,}$ bla_{TEM} and bla_{SHV}) and MBL-type variants (bla_{IMP-1} and bla_{VIM})

Primers	Sequences	Annealing temperature (Tm °C)	References	Expected PCR product
bla_{IMP-1}	AGCGCAGCATATTGATTGC ACAACCAGATGCTGCCTTACC	53.6	[43]	587
Bla_{VIM}	ATGGTCGTTATGGCATATC TGGGCCGTGTCAGCCAGAT	57	[44]	510
Bla_{TEM}	CCCCGAAGAAGTCCTTTC ATCAGCAATAGTCCCAGC	55	[42]	500
Bla_{SHV}	AGGGCTTGACTGCCATTTTG ATTTGCGTGATTTCATTT	55	[42]	400
Bla_{OXA}	ATATCTCGCTTGTTGCATCTCC AAACCCTTCAGCTCATCC	55	[42]	600

tract infections (9.6%), and infections associated with in-dwelling catheters (5.2%).

Antibiotic susceptibility testing of MBL isolates

The panel of antibiotics recommended according to CLSI 2016 guidelines was applied for all isolates belonging to *Enterobacteriaceae, Pseudomonas* spp. and *Acinetobacter* spp. *Escherichia coli* and *Klebsiella* spp. exhibited susceptibility to gentamycin and piperacillin-tazobactam (23%), amikacin (16%) and sulfamethoxazole/trimethoprim (15%). All the generations of cephalosporins, carbapenem and monobactams showed a complete resistance pattern. *Pseudomonas* spp. and *Acinetobacter* spp. presented susceptibility to amikacin and aztreonam (12%), piperacillin-tazobactam (8%), sulfamethoxazole/trimethoprim and gentamycin (7%) and ciprofloxacin (3%). Multiple antibiotic resistance (MAR) index values for > 50% of the isolates fell in the range of 0.81–1.00, and 86% of the *Pseudomonas* spp. isolates fell in the range of 0.91–1.0. *E. coli* predominantly had a MAR index value of 0.91–1. A total of 75% of the *Klebsiella* spp. isolates had a MAR index value ranging between 0.81 and 1.

Phenotypic detection of MBLs

Out of the 906 isolates analysed, 142 randomly selected isolates were suspected to produce metallo-β-lactamases. Among these isolates, 63.38% ($n = 90$) revealed a positive combination disc test, whereas 36.61% ($n = 52$) remained non-determinable by CDST. A total of 86.61% ($n = 123$) of the isolates were confirmed to be MBL producers through the modified Hodge test with meropenem. However, the modified Hodge test with imipenem detected 78.17% ($n = 111$) of the isolates as positive for MBL production and 22.53% ($n = 32$) as negative for MBL production. A total of 68% ($n = 96\%$) of the strains were confirmed to exhibit the MBL phenotype through the epsilometer test (E-test).

Multiplex PCR for bla_{OXA}, bla_{TEM}, bla_{SHV}, bla_{IMP} and bla_{VIM}

The presence of bla_{OXA}, bla_{TEM} and bla_{SHV} genes was confirmed in 57.74% ($n = 82\%$) of MBL-producing strains by multiplex PCR. The existence of the bla_{TEM} gene in MBL-producing isolates was found to be the most prevalent, at 46%, followed by the bla_{SHV} gene (34%) and bla_{OXA} gene (24%). bla_{IMP-1} and bla_{VIM} genes were detected in 12.5% ($n = 18$) and 7% ($n = 10$) of strains, respectively. The coexistence of all these genes was determined by multiplex PCR. In total, 60% (49/82) of the MBL-positive strains were found to have the bla_{OXA}, bla_{TEM} and bla_{SHV} genes in coexistence with each other. The bla_{TEM} gene was found to coexist with bla_{OXA}-*type* variants in 21% ($n = 30$) of the MBL producers. The combination of bla_{TEM} and bla_{SHV} was detected to be the most common, as exhibited by 24% of the strains. The coexistence of bla_{OXA} and bla_{SHV} genes was observed in 12% of the total isolates. The three genes bla_{TEM}, bla_{OXA} and bla_{SHV} were found to coexist in 9% of the strains (Fig. 1).

Statistical analysis

Statistical analysis was performed with SPSS version 23.0 individually for all groups of isolates, including *Escherichia coli, Klebsiella* spp., *Acinetobacter* spp. and *Pseudomonas* spp. (Table 2). The associations among demographic variables, including age, gender and type of infections, were determined by calculating odd ratios and performing the chi-square test. A p-value of < 0.05 was considered statistically significant (Tables 2, 3, 4).

Discussion

Pakistan is a country where empirical drug therapy and misuse of antibiotics are common practice. Poor sanitation, filthy practices in clinical settings, and ill-informed health care workers are factors in the dissemination of nosocomial pathogensto the community. Routinely used second-generation drugs are quickly being replaced by drugs of last resort, and this situation is ultimately an enduring threat to mankind. According to one estimate, first-line antibiotic-resistant pathogens account for 25,692 neonatal deaths annually in Pakistan [45]. Resistance to carbapenems has been significantly observed in Asian countries, including Pakistan [30, 46, 47]. At

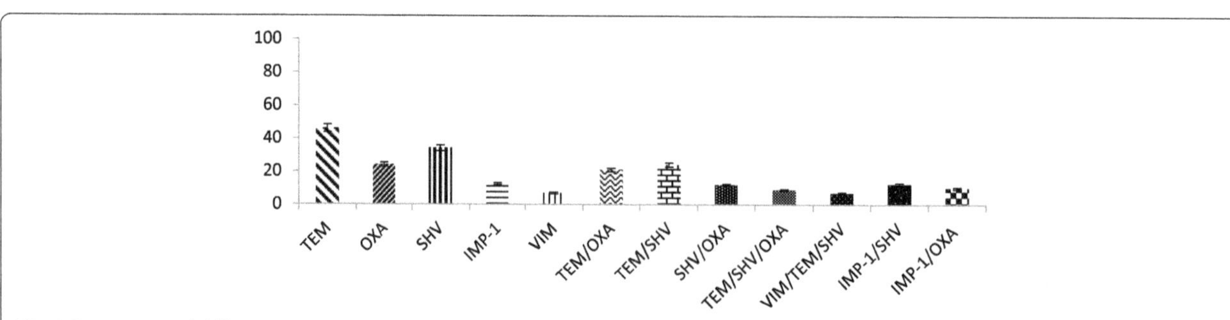

Fig. 1 Frequencies of different gene variants (*TEM, SHV, OXA, VIM, IMP*) in MBL producing clinical isolates. The presence of genes bla_{OXA}, bla_{TEM}, bla_{SHV} $bla_{IMP-1}$and $bla_{VIM}$was detected in MBL strains through PCR

Table 2 Comparison of Carbapenem resistant isolates between different age groups

Age (years)	No. of Isolates	Imipenem		Chi value	OR (95% CI)	*p*-value
		R	S			
Escherchia coli						
1–9	5	4 (80%)	1 (20%)	–	2.28 [0.23–22.87]	0.643
10–19	7	4 (57.14%)	3 (42.85%)		0.758 [0.157–3.66]	0.704
20–29	38	15 (39.47%)	23 (60.52%)	10.10	0.317 [0.153–0.657]	0.001
30–39	29	9 (31.03%)	20 (68.96%)	7.85	0.308 [0.132–0.723]	0.005
40–49	34	13 (38.23%)	21 (61.76%)	2.45	0.537 [0.245–1.176]	0.117
50–59	32	11 (34.37%)	21 (65.62%)	4.58	0.414 [0.182–0.940]	0.032
60–69	26	8 (30.76%)	18 (69.23%)	5.69	0.316 [0.120–0.831]	0.017
70–79	9	5 (55.55%)	4 (44.44%)	–	0.809 [0.177–3.69]	1.000
> 79	7	2 (28.57%)	5 (71.42%)	–	0.150 [0.018–1.237]	0.145
Acinetobacter spp.						
1–9	11	8 (66.66%)	4 (33.33%)	1.252	1.8 [0.638–5.072]	0.999
10–19	25	18 (72%)	7 (28%)	3.14	2.015 [0.92–4.41]	0.264
20–29	39	29 (74.35%)	10 (25.64%)	8.05	2.94 [1.37–6.33]	0.076
30–39	42	31 (73.80%)	11 (26.19%)	0.56	1.33 [0.633–2.79]	0.004
40–49	38	21 (55.26%)	17 (44.74%)	6.18	2.94 [1.28–6.73]	0.451
50–59	34	24 (70.58%)	10 (29.41%)	–	3.87 [1.26–11.81]	0.009
60–69	20	15 (75%)	5 (25%)	–	1.031 [0.23–4.53]	0.026
70–79	10	6 (60%)	4 (40%)	–		0.999
> 79	4	4 (100%)	0 (0%)			
Klebsiella spp.						
1–9	11	6 (54.54%)	5 (45.45)	0.870	0.505 [0.119–2.145]	0.351
10–19	10	6 (60%)	4 (40%)	–	0.857 [0.220–3.343]	1.000
20–29	40	22 (55%)	18 (45%)	1.040	0.695 [0.345–1.401]	0.824
30–39	41	19 (46.34%)	22 (53.65%)	1.52	0.645 [0.320–1.299]	0.218
40–49	26	15 (57.69%)	11 (42.30%)	0.749	1.458 [0.619–3.43]	0.387
50–59	26	8 (30.76%)	18 (69.23%)	5.230	0.356 [0.143–0.883]	0.022
60–69	19	9 (47.36%)	10 (52.63)	0.097	0.851 [0.309–2.343]	0.755
70–79	11	8 (72.72%)	3 (27.27%)	–	2.286 [0.493–10.605]	0.466
> 79	5	2 (40%)	3 (60%)	–	0.417 [0.051–3.435]	0.608
Pseudomonas spp.						
1–9	9	6 (66.67%)	3 (33.34%)	–	1.05 [0.22–5.13]	1.000
10–19	34	20 (58.83%)	14 (41.17%)	0.497	0.71 [0.28–1.82]	0.481
20–29	75	54 (72%)	21 (28%)	5.093	2.02 [1.09–3.74]	0.024
30–39	61	38 (62.29%)	23 (37.70%)	2.127	1.59 [0.85–3.00]	0.145
40–49	44	23 (52.27%)	21 (47.72)	0.130	1.14 [0.56–2.31]	0.718
50–59	51	30 (58.83%)	21 (41.17%)	1.917	1.63 [0.81–3.25]	0.166
60–69	25	14 (56%)	11 (44%)	0.410	1.35 [0.54–3.41]	0.522
70–79	6	3 (50%)	3 (50%)	–	0.63 [0.11–3.66]	0.670
> 79	2	2 (100%)	0	–	–	0.477

OR* Odd ratio& *p* value < 0.05 is considered as statistically significant

Table 3 Association of imipenem resistant isolates with type of clinical specimens

Isolate	Sample	(*N*)	Imipenem		Chi value	OR	*p*-value
			R	S			
Escherichia coli	Wound	65	22	43	23.013	0.276 [0.159–0.478]	0.000
	Fluids & Effusion	13	3	10	–	0.123 [0.027–0.553]	0.007
	Tips & Catheters	6	5	1	–	1.833 [0.192–17.48]	1.00
	Urine	79	34	45	0.894	0.756 [0.422–1.351]	0.344
	Sputum	12	5	7	0.096	0.824 [0.242–2.806]	0.757
	Others	14	4	10	–	0.403 [0.290–0.559]	0.070
Acinetobacter spp.	Wound	130	92	38	7.16	1.79 [1.16–2.75]	0.006
	Fluids & Effusion	13	11	2	–	6.67 [1.26–35.28]	0.021
	Tips & Catheters	22	17	5	0.171	1.32 [0.35–4.97]	0.679
	Urine	21	11	10	0.265	1.27 [0.51–3.15]	0.606
	Sputum	25	15	10	2.73	2.17 [0.85–5.50]	0.098
	Others	13	10	3	–	4.38 [1.05–18.17]	0.056
Klebsiella spp.	Wound	71	43	28	0.004	0.983 [0.59–1.64]	0.947
	Fluids & Effusion	11	6	5	0.031	0.88 [0.22–3.49]	0.861
	Tips & Catheters	10	7	3	–	0.75 [0.16–3.52]	0.700
	Urine	58	25	33	0.534	0.79 [0.43–1.48]	0.465
	Sputum	30	13	17	0.110	0.86 [0.36–2.06]	0.740
	Others	10	4	6	–	0.59 [0.15–2.35]	0.504
Pseudomonas spp.	Wound	221	142	79	1.84	1.29 [0.89–1.85]	0.174
	Fluids & Effusion	7	5	2	–	2.12 [0.36–12.38]	0.680
	Tips & Catheters	9	6	3	–	0.62 [0.13–2.99]	0.674
	Urine	29	19	10	4.669	2.44 [1.06–5.58]	0.031
	Sputum	23	9	14	0.547	0.69 [0.27–1.81]	0.459
	Others	20	11	9	0.210	1.29 [0.43–3.84]	0.647

OR* Odd ratio& *p* value < 0.05 is considered as statistically significant

present, numerous reports of MBL producers and ESBL producers from Pakistan present clinical catastrophes and alarming health issues [41, 48, 49]. The present study demonstrates the frequency of imipenem resistance among clinical isolates and the incidence of MBLS producers associated with imipenem resistance in connection with various demographic factors and types of infection. The frequency of imipenem resistance in our study was 56%, which is significantly higher than the data reported from Asian countries in the last decade (2002–2012), with one epidemiological study reporting 1.9% resistance to imipenem and 2.4% resistance to meropenem [4].

Table 4 Comparison of infection rate between male and female

Isolates	Gender	(*N*)	Imipenem		Chi value	OR*	*p*-value**
			R	S			
Escherichia coli	Male	106	41	65	0.0067	1.025 [0.57–1.85]	0.934
	Female	84	32	52			
Acinetobacter spp.	Male	136	94	42	41.05	4.51 [2.81–7.24]	0.0001
	Female	90	63	127			
Klebsiella spp.	Male	97	57	40	4.67	1.87 [1.058–3.328]	0.03
	Female	95	41	54			
Pseudomonas spp.	Male	203	125	78	0.0017	0.98 [0.61–1.59]	0.483
	Female	110	68	42			

OR* Odd ratio& *p* value < 0.05 is considered as statistically significant

Comparison of the antibiotic resistance profiles of all the pathogens with those reported in other recent studies has revealed relatively similar patterns. The resistance pattern of *Acinetobacter* spp. to imipenem in our study (61.89%) is in conformity with reports by Anwar et al., but a lower rate (77.5%) of imipenem resistance in this region was reported by Shamim et al. [50]. *Acinetobacter* spp., the pathogen renowned for hospital-acquired infections, was predominantly found to be associated with wound infections and was the causative agent of 92% infections associated with imipenem resistance. *Pseudomonas* spp. was the second most prominent pathogen associated with the acquisition of imipenem resistance, with a frequency of 61.89%, and has been noted in other reports from Pakistan, presenting imipenem resistance rates of 13.42% in 2011 and of 28% and 49.5% in 2015, thus demonstrating a sharp rise in the frequency of imipenem resistance [49, 51, 52]. The victims of *Pseudomonas* spp. infections were found predominantly in the group of patients with post-burn infections. This finding is in conformity with studies on invasive burn wound infections that document *P. aeruginosa* as a leading pathogen among gram-negative organisms [53, 54]. Wound infections were particularly found to be associated with *Acinetobacter* spp. (OR = 1.79 [1.16–2.75]) and *Pseudomonas* spp. *OR = 1.29 [0.89–1.85]).

The incidence of MBL among imipenem-resistant *Acinetobacter* spp. was calculated to be 89%, which is comparable to that reported in a study by Anwar et al., presenting a frequency of 83.3% MBLs among carbapenem-resistant isolates [55]. A total of 78% of the imipenem-resistant *Pseudomonas* spp. isolates were detected to be MBL producers by the MHT test, representing a lower incidence compared to the study by Shan et al. that stated the incidence rate to be 87.5% [49].

Our study demonstrates the OXA-type variants to be predominantly associated with resistance to imipenem. All of the isolates harbouring bla_{IMP} were also found to harbour bla_{TEM}. Despite the uncommon origin of two major groups of β-lactamases, bla_{ESBL} and bla_{MBL}, their association is imminent according to recent research [10]. We analysed the isolates for the coexistence of MBL-type and ESBL-type variants. The bla_{VIM} gene variant for MBL production was also found to be in coexistence with bla_{TEM} and bla_{SHV} in *Providencia stuartii* and *Enterobacter* spp. A total of 12.5% isolates were found to coexhibit the bla_{IMP-1} and bla_{SHV} genes, whereas 10% were positive for the bla_{OXA} gene along with the bla_{IMP-1} gene.

The abovementioned mechanism of coexistence of genes has been reported in *Klebsiella pneumoniae, Escherichia coli, Salmonella* spp. and *Enterobacter* spp. [56]. Plasmids containing the bla_{NDM-1} gene have been observed to coexhibit genes for CTX-M, TEM-1 and OXA-1 enzymes. Major ESBL and MBL genes, including bla_{CTX-M}, bla_{SHV}, bla_{TEM}, and bla_{OXA-51}, and genes for the VIM-family and IMP-family, have been reported to coexist in clinically resistant *Acinetobacter baumannii* in Iran [57]. However, one study concluded that there was no significant relationship between ESBL and MBL production genes [57]. Ertapenem-resistant, ESBL-producing *Klebsiella pneumoniae* isolates have been reported in Italy and shown to carry novel porin variants that contributed to the reduced susceptibility of isolates to meropenem and imipenem [58].

The coexistence of the genes for MBL and ESBL variants in our isolates indicates the simultaneity of the emergence of different variants of β-lactamases among pathogens in our clinical settings. This finding also suggests that the resistance against imipenem in our isolates is mediated by MBL-type enzymes along with the overproduction of ESBL-type enzymes, as suggested by other studies [5, 7]. To the best of our knowledge, this is the first study from Pakistan reporting the coexistence of bla_{IMP} with bla_{TEM}-type and *SHV*-type variants. None of the isolates was found to coexhibit all the tested genes (bla_{OXA}, bla_{TEM}, bla_{SHV}, bla_{IMP-1} and bla_{VIM}).

Conclusion

In conclusion, ESBL- and MBL-producing bacterial isolates are emerging very rapidly in the region. A great number of carbapenem-resistant clinical bacterial species are resistant to most of the commonly used antibiotics, demonstrating the rise of super-bacteria and their pan-resistance to antimicrobial therapy. Determining the resistance mechanisms and the root cause for their elimination are of great importance. It is also important to implement the routine screening of ESBLs and MBLs in laboratory procedures before antibiotic therapy begins. Further studies are required to specify other types of gene variants prevalent among clinical isolates in our region for the implication of medication in clinical settings.

Abbreviations

CDST: Combination disc test; DDST: Double disc synergy test; E test: Epsilometer test; ESBLs: Extended-spectrum β-lactamase-producing strains; ESBLs: Extended-spectrum β-lactamases; MBLs: Metallo-β-lactamases; MDR: Multidrug-resistant; MIC: Minimum inhibitory concentration

Acknowledgements

This work was funded by the Department of Microbiology and Molecular Genetics, University of the Punjab. The project was established in collaboration with Allama Iqbal Medical College, Lahore, for sample and data collection. The efforts of Mr. Muhammad Umar Farooq, Biostatistician & Incharge IT, Institute of Public Health (IPH), Lahore, is highly acknowledged for his efforts in performing the data analysis. The authors would like to thank Dr. Muhammad Faisal, CEO of Citilab and the research centre, for his valuable and collaborative suggestions.

Funding

No funding was received for this study.

Declaration
This study is part of the Ph.D. thesis of Noor-Ul-Ain.

Authors' contributions
NUA, SR, and FR designed the study. NUA, AI, SSB and SH performed the experimental work. AI, SSB, and MHH collected the data. NUA, SA, and MHH analysed the data. All authors read and approved the final manuscript.

Consent for publication
Not applicable.

Competing interests
The authors declare that they have no competing interests.

Author details
[1]Department of Microbiology and Molecular Genetics, University of the Punjab, Lahore 5400, Pakistan. [2]Department of Pathology, Allama Iqbal Medical College, Lahore, Pakistan. [3]Citilab and Research Center, Lahore, Pakistan.

References
1. Baran I, Aksu N. Phenotypic and genotypic characteristics of carbapenem-resistant Enterobacteriaceae in a tertiary-level reference hospital in Turkey. Ann Clin Microbiol Antimicrob. 2016;15(1):20.
2. Khalifa HO, et al. High carbapenem resistance in clinical gram-negative pathogens isolated in Egypt. Microb Drug Resist. 2017;23(7):838–44.
3. Mirsalehian A, et al. Determination of carbapenem resistance mechanism in clinical isolates of Pseudomonas aeruginosa isolated from burn patients, in Tehran, Iran. Journal of epidemiology and global health. 2017;7(3):155–9.
4. Xu Y, et al. Epidemiology of carbapenem resistant Enterobacteriaceae (CRE) during 2000-2012 in Asia. Journal of thoracic disease. 2015;7(3):376.
5. Satlin MJ, et al. Multicenter clinical and molecular epidemiological analysis of bacteremia due to carbapenem-resistant Enterobacteriaceae (CRE) in the CRE epicenter of the United States. Antimicrob Agents Chemother. 2017;61(4): e02349–16.
6. Wang, J.-T., et al., Carbapenem-nonsusceptible enterobacteriaceae in Taiwan. PLoS One, 2015. 10(3): p. e0121668.
7. Ye Y, et al. Mechanism for carbapenem resistance of clinical Enterobacteriaceae isolates. Experimental and Therapeutic Medicine. 2018;15(1):1143–9.
8. Dalmolin TV, et al. Detection and analysis of different interactions between resistance mechanisms and carbapenems in clinical isolates of Klebsiella pneumoniae. Braz J Microbiol. 2017;48(3):493–8.
9. Zafer MM, et al. Antimicrobial resistance pattern and their beta-lactamase encoding genes among Pseudomonas aeruginosa strains isolated from cancer patients. Biomed Res Int. 2014:2014.
10. Iraz M, et al. Distribution of β-lactamase genes among carbapenem-resistant Klebsiella pneumoniae strains isolated from patients in Turkey. Annals of laboratory medicine. 2015;35(6):595–601.
11. Yong D, et al. Characterization of a new metallo-β-lactamase gene, blaNDM-1, and a novel erythromycin esterase gene carried on a unique genetic structure in Klebsiella pneumoniae sequence type 14 from India. Antimicrob Agents Chemother. 2009;53(12):5046–54.
12. Bush K, Jacoby GA, Medeiros AA. A functional classification scheme for beta-lactamases and its correlation with molecular structure. Antimicrob Agents Chemother. 1995;39(6):1211.
13. Walsh TR. Clinically significant carbapenemases: an update. Curr Opin Infect Dis. 2008;21(4):367–71.
14. Nordmann P, Poirel L. Emerging carbapenemases in gram-negative aerobes. Clin Microbiol Infect. 2002;8(6):321–31.
15. Haruta S, et al. Functional analysis of the active site of a metallo-β-lactamase proliferating in Japan. Antimicrob Agents Chemother. 2000;44(9):2304–9.
16. Ito H, et al. Plasmid-mediated dissemination of the metallo-beta-lactamase gene blaIMP among clinically isolated strains of Serratia marcescens. Antimicrob Agents Chemother. 1995;39(4):824–9.
17. Hawkey PM, et al. Occurrence of a new metallo-β-lactamase IMP-4 carried on a conjugative plasmid in Citrobacter youngae from the People's Republic of China. FEMS Microbiol Lett. 2001;194(1):53–7.
18. Hawkey P. Multidrug-resistant gram-negative bacteria: a product of globalization. J Hosp Infect. 2015;89(4):241–7.
19. Munita JM, Arias CA. Mechanisms of antibiotic resistance. Microbiology spectrum. 2016;4(2).
20. Scoulica EV, et al. Spread of Bla VIM-1-producing. E coli in a university hospital in Greece Genetic analysis of the integron carrying the bla VIM-1 metallo-β-lactamase gene Diagnostic microbiology and infectious disease. 2004;48(3):167–72.
21. Cornaglia G, Giamarellou H, Rossolini GM. Metallo-β-lactamases: a last frontier for β-lactams? Lancet Infect Dis. 2011;11(5):381–93.
22. Kazmierczak, K.M., et al., Multi-year, multi-national survey of the incidence and global distribution of metallo-β-lactamase-producing Enterobacteriaceae and P. aeruginosa. Antimicrob Agents Chemother, 2015: p. AAC. 02379–15.
23. Rolain J, Parola P, Cornaglia G. New Delhi metallo-beta-lactamase (NDM-1): towards a new pandemia? Clin Microbiol Infect. 2010;16(12):1699–701.
24. Berrazeg M, et al. New Delhi Metallo-beta-lactamase around the world: an eReview using Google maps. Eurosurveillance. 2014;19(20):20809.
25. Pfeifer Y, et al. Molecular characterization of Bla NDM-1 in an Acinetobacter baumannii strain isolated in Germany in 2007. J Antimicrob Chemother. 2011;66(9):1998–2001.
26. Bonnin R, et al. Dissemination of New Delhi metallo-β-lactamase-1-producing Acinetobacter baumannii in Europe. Clin Microbiol Infect. 2012;18(9):E362–5.
27. Nakazawa Y, et al. A case of NDM-1-producing Acinetobacter baumannii transferred from India to Japan. J Infect Chemother. 2013;19(2):330–2.
28. Kumarasamy KK, et al. Emergence of a new antibiotic resistance mechanism in India, Pakistan, and the UK: a molecular, biological, and epidemiological study. Lancet Infect Dis. 2010;10(9):597–602.
29. Litzow JM, et al. High frequency of multidrug-resistant gram-negative rods in 2 neonatal intensive care units in the Philippines. Infection Control & Hospital Epidemiology. 2009;30(6):543–9.
30. Le NK, et al. High prevalence of hospital-acquired infections caused by gram-negative carbapenem resistant strains in Vietnamese pediatric ICUs: a multi-Centre point prevalence survey. Medicine. 2016;95(27).
31. Bhat V, et al. Bacteriological profile and antibiotic susceptibility patterns of clinical isolates in a tertiary care cancer center. Indian journal of medical and paediatric oncology: official journal of Indian Society of Medical & Paediatric Oncology. 2016;37(1):20.
32. Walther-Rasmussen J, Høiby N. OXA-type carbapenemases. J Antimicrob Chemother. 2006;57(3):373–83.
33. Bonnin RA, Poirel L, Nordmann P. AbaR-type transposon structures in Acinetobacter baumannii. J Antimicrob Chemother. 2011;67(1):234–6.
34. Khan M, et al. Emerging bacterial resistance patterns in febrile neutropenic patients: experience at a tertiary care hospital in Pakistan. JPMA. The Journal of the Pakistan Medical Association. 2004;54(7):357–60.
35. Irfan S, et al. Molecular and epidemiological characterisation of clinical isolates of carbapenemresistant Acinetobacter baumannii from public and private sector intensive care units in Karachi, Pakistan. J Hosp Infect. 2011;78(2):143–8.
36. Khan F, Khan A, Kazmi SU. Prevalence and susceptibility pattern of multi drug resistant clinical isolates of Pseudomonas aeruginosa in Karachi. Pakistan journal of medical sciences. 2014;30(5):951.
37. Kaleem F, et al. Frequency and susceptibility pattern of metallo-beta-lactamase producers in a hospital in Pakistan. The Journal of infection in developing countries. 2010;4(12):810–3.
38. Bauer A, et al. Antibiotic susceptibility testing by a standardized single disk method. Am J Clin Pathol. 1966;45(4):493.
39. Wadekar MD, Anuradha K, Venkatesha D. Phenotypic detection of ESBL and MBL in clinical isolates of Enterobacteriaceae. Int J Current Res Acad Rev. 2013;1(3):89–5.
40. Kumar S, Mehra S. Performance of modified Hodge test and combined disc test for detection of Carbapenemases in clinical isolates of Enterobacteriaceae. Int J Curr Microbiol App Sci. 2015;4(5):255–61.
41. Abrar S, et al. Distribution of CTX-M group I and group III β-lactamases produced by Escherichia coli and klebsiella pneumoniae in Lahore, Pakistan. Microb Pathog. 2017;103:8–12.
42. Colom K, et al. Simple and reliable multiplex PCR assay for detection of blaTEM, blaSHV and blaOXA–1 genes in Enterobacteriaceae. FEMS Microbiol Lett. 2003;223(2):147–51.

43. Shibata N, et al. PCR typing of genetic determinants for metallo-β-lactamases and integrases carried by gram-negative bacteria isolated in Japan, with focus on the class 3 integron. J Clin Microbiol. 2003;41(12):5407–13.
44. Galani I, et al. First identification of an Escherichia coli clinical isolate producing both metallo-β-lactamase VIM-2 and extended-spectrum β-lactamase IBC-1. Clin Microbiol Infect. 2004;10(8):757–60.
45. Laxminarayan R, Bhutta ZA. Antimicrobial resistance—a threat to neonate survival. Lancet Glob Health. 2016;4(10):e676–7.
46. Sekar R, et al. Carbapenem resistance in a rural part of southern India: Escherichia coli versus Klebsiella spp. Indian J Med Res. 2016;144(5):781.
47. Hu F-P, et al. Resistance trends among clinical isolates in China reported from CHINET surveillance of bacterial resistance, 2005–2014. Clin Microbiol Infect. 2016;22:S9–S14.
48. Ilyas M, et al. Frequency, susceptibility and co-existence of MBL, ESBL & AmpC positive Pseudomonas aeruginosa in tertiary care hospitals of Peshawar, KPK. In: Pakistan; 2015.
49. Shan S, Sajid S, Ahmad K. Detection of Bla IMP gene in Metallo-β-lactamase producing isolates of imipenem resistant Pseudomonas aeruginosa; an alarming threat. Journal of Microbiology Research. 2015;5(6):175–80.
50. Shamim S, Abbas M, Qazi MH. Prevalence of multidrug resistant Acinetobacter baumannii in hospitalized patients in Lahore. Pakistan Pakistan J Mol Med. 2015;2(1):23–8.
51. Ameen N, et al. Imipenem resistant Pseudomonas aeruginosa: the fall of the final quarterback. Pakistan journal of medical sciences. 2015;31(3):561.
52. Bashir D, et al. Detection of metallo-beta-lactamase (MBL) producing Pseudomonas aeruginosa at a tertiary care hospital in Kashmir. Afr J Microbiol Res. 2011;5(2):164–72.
53. Church D, et al. Burn wound infections. Clin Microbiol Rev. 2006;19(2):403–34.
54. AL-Aali KY. Microbial profile of burn wound infections in burn patients, Taif. Saudi Arabia Archives of Clinical Microbiology. 2016;7(2).
55. Anwar M, et al. Phenotypic detection of Metallo-Beta-lactamases in Carbapenem resistant Acinetobacter baumannii isolated from pediatric patients in Pakistan. Journal of pathogens. 2016:2016.
56. Nordmann P, Dortet L, Poirel L. Carbapenem resistance in Enterobacteriaceae: here is the storm! Trends Mol Med. 2012;18(5):263–72.
57. Safari M, et al. Prevalence of ESBL and MBL encoding genes in Acinetobacter baumannii strains isolated from patients of intensive care units (ICU). Saudi journal of biological sciences. 2015;22(4):424–9.
58. García-Fernández A, et al. An ertapenem-resistant extended-spectrum-β-lactamase-producing Klebsiella pneumoniae clone carries a novel OmpK36 porin variant. Antimicrob Agents Chemother. 2010;54(10):4178–84.

20

The importance of adjusting for enterococcus species when assessing the burden of vancomycin resistance: a cohort study including over 1000 cases of enterococcal bloodstream infections

Tobias Siegfried Kramer[1,2*], Cornelius Remschmidt[1,2], Sven Werner[3], Michael Behnke[1,2], Frank Schwab[1,2], Guido Werner[4,5], Petra Gastmeier[1,2] and Rasmus Leistner[1,2]

Abstract

Background: Infections caused by vancomycin-resistant enterococci (VRE) are on the rise worldwide. Few studies have tried to estimate the mortality burden as well as the financial burden of those infections and found that VRE are associated with increased mortality and higher hospital costs. However, it is unclear whether these worse outcomes are attributable to vancomycin resistance only or whether the enterococcal species (*Enterococcus faecium* or *Enterococcus faecalis*) play an important role. We therefore aimed to determine the burden of enterococci infections attributable to vancomycin resistance and pathogen species (*E. faecium* and *E. faecalis)* in cases of bloodstream infection (BSI).

Methods: We conducted a retrospective cohort study on patients with BSI caused by *Enterococcus faecium* or *Enterococcus faecalis* between 2008 and 2015 in three tertiary care hospitals. Data was collected on true hospital costs (in €), length of stay (LOS), basic demographic parameters, and underlying diseases including the results of the Charlson comorbidity index (CCI). We used univariate and multivariable regression analyses to compare risk factors for in-hospital mortality and length of stay (i) between vancomycin-susceptible *E. faecium*- (VSEm) and vancomycin-susceptible *E. faecalis*- (VSEf) cases and (ii) between vancomycin-susceptible *E. faecium*- (VSEm) *and* vancomycin-resistant *E. faecium-cases* (VREm). We calculated total hospital costs for VSEm, VSEf and VREm.

Results: Overall, we identified 1160 consecutive cases of BSI caused by enterococci: 596 (51.4%) cases of *E. faecium* BSI and 564 (48.6%) cases of *E. faecalis* BSI. 103 cases of *E. faecium* BSI (17.3%) and 1 case of *E. faecalis* BSI (0.2%) were infected by vancomycin-resistant isolates. Multivariable analyses revealed (i) that in addition to different underlying diseases *E. faecium* was an independent risk factor for in-hospital mortality and prolonged hospital stay and (ii) that vancomycin-resistance did not further increase the risk for the described outcomes among *E. faecium*-isolates. However, the overall hospital costs were significantly higher in VREm-BSI cases as compared to VSEm- and VSEf-BSI cases (80,465€ vs. 51,365€ vs. 31,122€ $p < 0.001$).

(Continued on next page)

* Correspondence: tobias.kramer@charite.de
[1]Charité Universitätsmedizin Berlin, Institute of Hygiene and Environmental Medicine, Berlin, Germany
[2]National Reference Center for the Surveillance of Nosocomial Infections, Berlin, Germany
Full list of author information is available at the end of the article

(Continued from previous page)

Conclusion: Our data indicates that in-hospital mortality and infection-attributed hospital stay in enterococci BSI might rather be influenced by Enterococcus species and underlying diseases than by vancomycin resistance. Therefore, future studies should consider adjusting for Enterococcus species in addition to vancomycin resistance in order to provide a conservative estimate for the burden of VRE infections.

Keywords: Bloodstream infection, Vancomycin-resistant enterococci, *Enterococcus faecium*

Introduction

Enterococcus spp. are part of the normal gastrointestinal flora. Among those pathogens, resistance to antimicrobial substances, notably to vancomycin, results in limited therapeutic options [1, 2]. In recent years, hospital-acquired infections (HAI) caused by vancomycin-resistant enterococci (VRE) have emerged as a relevant burden on patients and healthcare systems globally [3–5]. In order to reduce the spread of resistant strains in hospitals, infection control measures, e.g. contact precautions, have been proposed [6, 7]. To assess the efficiency of VRE prevention measures, the mortality- and financial burden of VRE infections has to be assessed. However, the methodological approach on assessing VRE-burden remains controversial [2, 8, 9] and only few studies have addressed economic aspects [10–15]. As costs are often not available as infection-attributable costs (costs after onset for infection) length of stay (LOS) after onset of infection is being used as a surrogate parameter [2, 8, 16].

Although analyses should compare VRE infections to VSE-infected patients when the attributable effect of vancomycin resistance is addressed, [2, 8, 16] prior studies also utilized comparisons to cohorts with non-enterococcus infections [17, 18] or cohorts without infection [8, 12, 19–24]. Since the course of enterococcal infections may also be influenced by the enterococcus subspecies itself [2, 8, 9, 25, 26], analyses not considering the pathogen species may therefore be biased as result of the different virulence of the pathogens.

In a large cohort of cases with bloodstream infection (BSI), we therefore studied the influence of vancomycin resistance and enterococcus subspecies on in-hospital mortality, hospital costs and length of hospital stay.

Methods

Setting, study design and data collection

The study was conducted at three different tertiary care hospitals of the Charité university hospital in Berlin, with 3011-beds in total [27]. After a confirmatory ethics vote was obtained from the Charité University Medicine ethics committee (internal processing key EA4/229/17), we performed a cohort study that included all cases of BSI caused by *Enterococcus faecalis* or *Enterococcus faecium* between January 1, 2008 and December 31, 2015. Cases were identified in the Charité microbiology database as hospitalized patients with blood cultures positive for one of these pathogens. Data on costs and hospital financial accounting was provided by the Charité Department of Financial Controlling as true hospital expenses in Euros. For all patients enrolled in this study, the following demographic and clinical characteristics were collected: age, sex, in-hospital death, length of hospital stay (LOS), day of BSI onset and stay on an intensive care unit (days). Length of stay in total and after BSI onset were defined as length of stay until death or discharge. The Charlson comorbidity index (CCI) was obtained on the basis of the patients' diagnosed comorbidities using the method of Charlson et al. and the adaptation for the ICD-10 by Thygesen et al. [28, 29]. The original 17 Charlson comorbidity categories were cumulated based on the affected organ system in the following ten disease categories: heart disease, cerebrovascular disease, neurologic disease, lung disease, rheumatic disease, gastrointestinal disease, liver disease, diabetes, renal disease and cancer/immunological disease.

Definitions and statistical methods

Cases were defined as patients with BSI caused by Enterococcus spp. *(Enterococcus faecalis* or *Enterococcus faecium)* during the study period. Each patient was included in the analysis once. Onset of BSI was defined as the date of the first blood culture positive for the respective pathogen. BSI was considered hospital-onset if it occurred after the third day of hospitalization. Mortality was assessed based on discharge alive or in-hospital death. Data on hospital costs were derived from true hospital costs (hospital expenses). The costs analyzed cover direct costs to the hospital of treatment and diagnostics as well as indirect hospital costs of activities without patient contact (e.g. administration, hospital maintenance). The estimated cost of individual cases was based on definite performances and on settlement keys (e.g. nurse working time per patient). Economic data was available on total hospital costs and on daily costs. A differentiation of costs before and after the infection was not available. However, as length of stay directly correlates with hospital costs, length of stay after onset for infection can be applied as proxy for infection attributable additional expenditures [2, 30, 31]. We therefore assessed the multiplicative effect on length of stay after BSI onset in a multivariable linear regression.

Descriptive, univariate analyses were performed for the total cohort, stratified by enterococcus species (i.e. vancomycin susceptible *E. faecium* vs. vancomycin susceptible *E. faecalis*) and by vancomycin susceptibility (i.e. vancomycin susceptible *enterococci* vs. vancomycin resistant enterococci). Since among E. faecalis-isolates only one isolate was resistant against vancomycin, only *E. faecium* (VSEm vs. VREm) were analyzed in the second analysis. Additionally, we compared in univariate analysis deceased patients and patients discharged alive. The median and the interquartile range (IQR) were calculated for continuous parameters; number and percentage were calculated for binary parameters. Univariate differences were tested using the Wilcoxon rank-sum test for continuous variables and the Chi-square test for binary variables.

The two linear regression analyses were performed for length of stay (LOS) after onset of enterococcal BSI by stepwise forward variable selection. The continuous parameters LOS after onset of BSI was log transformed to achieve normal distribution. Only surviving patients were included. Parameters considered in the full model were vancomycin resistance OR pathogen species (*E. faecium* or *E. faecalis*), sex, age and all underlying diseases assessed as described above. From the full model, parameters with the smallest Chi-square statistic and $p > 0.05$ in the type III test were removed. The regression coefficients were converted to the measures of effect using an exponential transformation and referred to as the multiplicative effect (ME) of investigated parameters. *P*-values < 0.05 were considered significant.

Multivariable, binary logistic regression was performed for in-hospital death by stepwise forward selection. The *p*-values for including a variable in the model was 0.05 and for excluding 0.06 respectively. Odds ratios (HR) with 95% confidence intervals (95% CI) were calculated. Parameters considered in the model were sex, age, pathogen species (*E. faecium* vs. *E. faecalis*) with the interaction of the vancomycin resistance and all underlying diseases assessed as described above.

All analyses were performed using SPSS (IBM SPSS statistics, Somer, NY, USA) and SAS (SAS Institute, Cary, NC, USA).

Microbiological methods

If a blood stream infection was suspected, blood cultures were drawn and incubated for up to seven days using standard blood culture tubes (BACTEC, Becton Dickinson Heidelberg Germany). If growth was detected, gram staining and culturing were performed. MALDI TOF MS and Vitek 2 automated system (Biomerieux Marcy l'etoile France) were used for identification and susceptibility testing of bacterial strains. They were interpreted using EUCAST definitions.

Results

We initially extracted $n = 24{,}086$ clinical isolates diagnosed with *Enterococcus faecium or Enterococcus faecalis* from the microbiology database. After excluding all

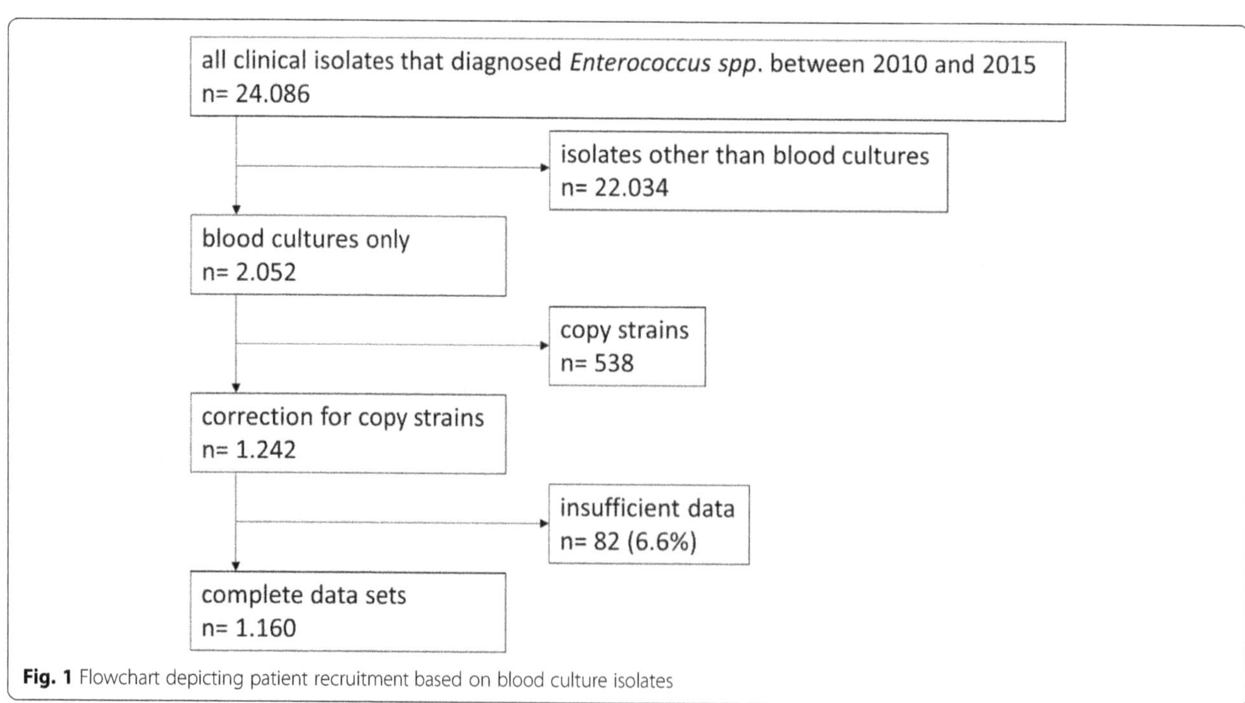

Fig. 1 Flowchart depicting patient recruitment based on blood culture isolates

Table 1 Univariate analysis of epidemiologic parameters, length of stay, and direct hospital costs of cases with blood stream infection caused by enterococcus spp. stratified by vancomycin resistance

Parameter	(A) VS-*E. faecium* (*n* = 493)	(B) VS-*E. faecalis* (*n* = 563)	*P-Value for A) vs. B)*		(C) VR-*E. faecium* (*n* = 103)	*P-Value for C) vs. A)*	
			P-Value	*OR (CI 95)*		*P-Value*	*OR (CI 95)*
In-hospital mortality	39.6% (195)	24.4% (132)	**0.000**	**2.137 (1.638-2.787)**	50.5% (52)	**0.041**	**1.558 (1.017–2.387)**
Male	58.6% (289)	63.1% (355)	0.141	0.830 (0.648-1.063)	66.0% (68)	0.163	1.371 (0.879–2.141)
Age in years, median (IQR)	67 (54–75)	64 (53–73)	0.059	n.a.	61 (52–70)	0.107	
Cardiac disease	28.2% (139)	29.0% (163)	0.786	0.964 (0.737-1.259)	26.2% (27)	0.683	0.905 (0.559-1.464)
Vascular disease	22.1% (109)	22.4% (126)	0.916	0.984 (0.736-1.317)	22.3% (23)	0.961	1.013 (0.608-1.687)
Pulmonary disease	20.1% (99)	23.1% (130)	0.236	0.837 (0.623-1.124)	21.4% (22)	0.769	1.081 (0.643-1.818)
Rheumatic disease	3.0% (15)	3.6% (20)	0.644	0.852 (0.431-1.683)	2.9% (3)	0.944	0.956 (0.272-3.364)
Gastrointestinal disease	5.5% (27)	3.7% (21)	0.174	1.495 (0.834-2.680)	5.8% (6)	0.888	1.068 (0.429-2.656)
Diabetes	22.9% (113)	32.0% (180)	**0.001**	**0,633 (0,481-0,833)**	19.4% (20)	0.437	0,810 (0.476-1.379)
Renal disease	59.0% (291)	52.8% (297)	**0.041**	**1.290 (1.011-1.647)**	70.9% (73)	**0.025**	**1.689 (1.065-2.679)**
Liver disease	29.6% (146)	19.9% (112)	**0.000**	**1.694 (1.276-2.249)**	42.7% (44)	**0.009**	**1.772 (1.146-2,74)**
Cancer/ immunological disease	48.1% (237)	36.1% (203)	**0.000**	**1.642 (1.283-2.101)**	53.4% (55)	0.325	1.238 (0.809-1.894)
Neurological disease	7.3% (36)	13.0% (73)	**0.003**	**0,529 (0,348-0,804)**	8.7% (9)	0.616	1.215 (0.566-2.608)
Charlson comorbidity index, median (IQR)	7 (4–9)	7 (4–9)	0.907	n.a.	7 (5–9)	0.377	n.a.
Length of stay as Median (IQR)							
LOS total (days)	42 (23–78)	32 (16–61)	**0.000**	n.a.	54 (36–85)	0.010	n.a.
LOS before BSI (days)	19 (9–34)	10 (2–25)	**0.000**	n.a.	27 (15–39)	**0.003**	n.a.
LOS after BSI (days)	18 (8–41)	16 (8–33)	0.308	n.a.	23 (8–45)	0.183	n.a.
LOS normal ward	15 (1–36)	11 (1–25)	**0.010**	n.a.	17 (0–44)	0.368	n.a.
LOS ICU	18 (1–49)	10 (1–40)	0.016	n.a.	24 (5–57)	0.050	n.a.
Hospital costs as median (IQR)							
Total hospital costs	51,365 (22,535-119,789)	31,122 (11,829-74,344)	**0.000**	n.a.	80,465 (47,887–157,447)	**0.000**	n.a.
Daily costs	1,237 (729–1,812)	1,014 (614–1,466)	**0.000**	n.a.	1,484 (1,095–2,186)	**0.000**	n.a.
Medical staff	7,600 (3169-16,468)	5,344 (1841-12,213)	**0.000**	n.a.	10,390 (6,364–20,983)	**0.002**	n.a.
Nursing staff	11,499 (4,476-26,237)	7,141 (2,610-21,591)	**0.000**	n.a.	16,661 (8,029–32,905)	**0.003**	n.a.
Assistant medical technicians	2,630 (1,028-5694)	1,906 (646–4,325)	**0.000**	n.a.	3,665 (1,397–6,795)	0.082	n.a.
Pharmacy	6,924 (2,200-20,922)	2,742 (636–7,865)	**0.000**	n.a.	17,145 (8,087–36,779)	**0.000**	n.a.
Expenses for implants/transplants	0 (0–412)	0 (0–170)	**0.005**	n.a.	20 (0–605)	0.767	n.a.
Medical supply	6,858 (2,820-15,057)	3,926 (− 1,338-9,782)	**0.000**	n.a.	9,878 (5,104–18,957)	**0.002**	n.a.
Medical infrastructure	1,893 (939–4,128)	1,473 (547–3,271)	**0.000**	n.a.	2,629 (1,611–5,219)	**0.001**	n.a.
Non-medical infrastructure	8,975 (4,215-18,206)	6,176 (2,576-14,049)	**0.000**	n.a.	12,244 (6,763–20,002)	**0.003**	n.a.

Categorical variables displayed as percentage and number; continuous variable displayed as median and interquartile range. **P*-value, categorical variables tested with Chi-square test, continuous variable tested with Wilcoxon rank sum test. *BSI* = blood stream infection, *IQR* = interquartile range, *OR* = odds ratio, *CI95* = 95% confidence interval. *VRE* = vancomycin-resistant enterococcus, *VSE* = vancomycin-susceptible enterococcus.
N.a. = not applicable
Bold entries represent statistically significant factors

isolates not derived from blood cultures and correcting for copy strains, 1242 patients with BSI caused by *E. faecium* or *E. faecalis* were included in the analysis (Fig. 1). Sufficient data on all relevant parameters was available for 96.4% of the patients. Overall, this accounted for 1160 patients, 91% with infections caused by VSE and 9% by VRE. Table 1 gives an overview of the parameters for all patients and shows the results of the (i) univariate comparison of VSEm vs. VSEf and (ii) the comparison of VSEm vs. VREm BSI cases. The highest in-hospital mortality rate was found among VREm cases (50.5%) followed by VSEm cases (39.6%) and VSEf cases (24.4%). Also regarding LOS, highest numbers were found among VREm cases (total LOS, 54 days) followed by VSEm (42 days) and VSEf (32 days). In all three groups, the Charlson comorbidity score was similar with a median of 7.

In multivariable analyses on LOS after BSI onset among vancomycin-susceptible enterococci cases, some chronic diseases and *E. faecium* statistically significant increased LOS as compared to *E. faecalis* (see Table 2). Vancomycin-resistance was not found to additionally increase LOS among *E. faecium* cases (see Table 2 and Fig. 2). Regarding in-hospital death, patients with *E. faecium*-BSI had a higher chance for death as compared to *E. faecalis*-cases when only vancomycin-susceptible cases were considered (see Table 3 and 4). Among *E. faecium* cases, vancomycin-resistant was not found to be an additional risk factor for death (Table 4).

Regarding economic aspects, almost all hospital costs were significantly higher in the VREm BSI cohort compared to the VSEm BSI and the VSEf cohort.

Discussion

During the last 15 years (since 2003), 4 meta-analyses on mortality- and financial burden of VRE infections [19, 22–24], and few recent studies on costs associated with VRE infections (not included in the meta-analyses) were published [13, 15, 32]. The studies demonstrate that vancomycin resistance is associated with overall worsened outcome (mortality, length of stay and hospital costs). However, although former studies indicated that *E. faecium* isolates might be more virulent than *E. faecalis* isolates irrespective of vancomycin resistance [2, 8, 9, 26], many of the above mentioned studies did not adjust for enterococcal subspecies. As Kaye et al. showed in 2004, this could lead to an overestimation of the outcome effects attributable to vancomycin resistance [9]. Some of the authors discussed this issue in their articles, arguing that meta-analyses cannot improve the quality of data published [22, 24].

In our analyses, in-hospital mortality and length of stay after BSI onset were independently associated with underlying diseases, age and *E. faecium* but not with vancomycin resistance.

Regarding mortality vancomycin resistance was associated with increased in-hospital mortality in the univariate analysis. This result is in agreement with recent studies including three meta-analyses [19, 22, 24]. However, after adjusting for underlying diseases, age, and species (*E. faecium* vs. *E. faecalis*), in-hospital mortality was no longer associated with VRE. There are several possible explanations for these differences with other studies.

Systemic enterococci infections mainly occur in patients with severe underlying diseases and comorbidities [33, 34] which also applies to our study cohort. Patients had a very high Charlson comorbidity score with a median of 7. In this regard, there was no significant difference between the cases infected with *E. faecalis*, *E. faecium* or vancomycin-resistant strains. Furthermore, infections caused by antimicrobial-resistant bacteria are often associated with increased morbidity and mortality [19]. These differences are explained by the delay in or even complete lack of an effective antibiotic treatment despite the availability of effective drugs [1, 24]. Prematunge et al. adjusted for appropriate antimicrobial

Table 2 Multivariable linear regression on length of stay of surviving patients after BSI onset

Parameter		VS-*E. faecium* vs. VS-*E. faecalis*					VS-*E. faecium* vs. VR-*E. faecium*				
		ME	Sig.	CI 95 (lower-upper)			ME	Sig.	CI 95 (lower-upper)		
Renal Disease		1.588	0000	1.891	–	3.868	1516	0.001	1.472	–	4.201
Age (years)		0.659	0000	0.969	–	0.987	Not significant				
Lung Disease		1.457	0000	1.800	–	4.342	1333	0.018	1.151	–	4.409
Gastrointestinal Disease		1.323	0001	1.959	–	11.025	Not significant				
Liver Disease		1.270	0.003	1.256	–	3.100	1370	0.009	1.226	–	4.155
Vascular Disease		1.216	0.016	1.104	–	2.622	Not significant				
Enterococcus species	*E. faecium*	1.258	0.004	1.170	–	2.324	Not applicable				
	E. faecalis	Reference = 1									

BSI = bloodstream infection, *CI95* = 95% confidence interval, *ME* multiplicative effect

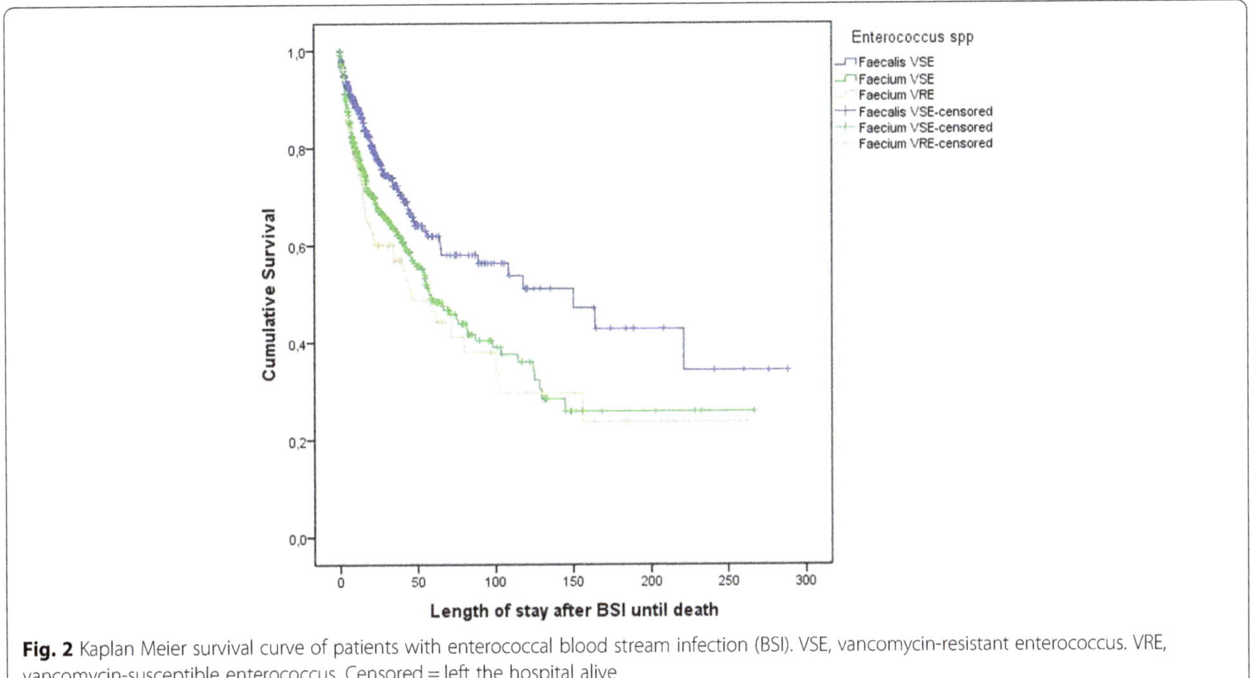

Fig. 2 Kaplan Meier survival curve of patients with enterococcal blood stream infection (BSI). VSE, vancomycin-resistant enterococcus. VRE, vancomycin-susceptible enterococcus. Censored = left the hospital alive

therapy but found that the differences remained [24]. Outcome differences resulting from varying pathogenicity of enterococci species is an alternative explanation [35, 36]. In the multivariable analysis we found only small differences for in-hospital mortality resulting from vancomycin resistance, differences which are insufficient to explain the univariate results. However, we observed significantly increased mortality associated with vancomycin-susceptible *E. faecium* compared to vancomycin-susceptible *E. faecalis.*

Possibly because *E. faecium* is the most common type of VRE worldwide and most *E. faecalis* isolates from infections are vancomycin-susceptible, it might be a limitation to most existing studies that this confounder is not

Table 3 Univariate analysis on risk factors for in-hospital death

Parameter	Discharge alive (*n* = 781)	In-hospital death (*n* = 379)	*P-value	OR (CI 95)
Vancomycin resistance	6.7% (52)	13.7% (52)	**< 0.001**	**2.273 (1.512-3.417)**
E. faecium	44.7% (349)	65.2% (247)	**< 0.001**	**2.311 (1.792-2.979)**
E. faecalis	55.3% (432)	34.8% (132)		**1 = Reference**
Male	61.2% (478)	62.0% (235)	0.792	1.037 (0.805-1.334)
Age (years), median (IQR)	64.0 (51–73)	66.0 (56–74)	**0.011**	n.a.
Heart disease	25.1% (196)	35.4% (134)	**< 0.001**	**1.641 (1.258-2.14)**
Vascular disease	19.6% (153)	27.7% (105)	**0.002**	**1,57 (1,18-2.091)**
Lung disease	19.6% (153)	26.1% (99)	**0.011**	**1.461 (1.093-1.952)**
Rheumatic disease	2.6% (20)	4.7% (18)	0.050	1.895 (0,99-3.626)
Gastrointestinal disease	4.1% (32)	5.8% (22)	0.195	1,44 (0,825-2.515)
Diabetes	26.8% (209)	27.4% (104)	0.807	1.033 (0,784-1.361)
Renal disease	46.9% (366)	78.1% (296)	**< 0.001**	**4.055 (3.061-5.371)**
Liver disease	18.2% (142)	42.2% (160)	**< 0.001**	**3.283 (2.498-4.314)**
Cancer/Immunological disease	41.4% (323)	45.4% (172)	0.194	1.176 (0,918-1.506)
Neurological disease	10.8% (84)	9.0% (34)	0.346	0,817 (0.537-1.241)

Categorical variables displayed as percentage and number; continuous variable displayed as median and interquartile range. *P-value, categorical variables tested with Chi-square test, continuous variable tested with Wilcoxon rank sum test. *BSI* = blood stream infection, *IQR* = interquartile range, *OR* = odds ratio, *CI95* = 95% confidence interval. *VRE* = vancomycin-resistant enterococcus, *VSE* = vancomycin-susceptible enterococcus. *N.a.* = not applicable
Bold entries represent statistically significant factors

Table 4 Results of multivariable binary logistic regression of risk factors for in-hospital death after enterococcal bloodstream infection

Parameter		VS-*E. faecium* vs. VS-*E. faecalis*			VS-*E. faecium* vs. VR-*E. faecium*		
		OR	*P*-value	CI95 (lower-upper)	OR	*P*-value	CI95 (lower-upper)
Age		1015	0,002	1005 – 1025	1016	0,010	1004 – 1029
Vascular disease		1407	0,042	1012 – 1956	Not significant		
Renal disease		3120	0,000	2274 – 4280	4005	0,000	2708 – 5922
Liver disease		2909	0,000	2109 – 4011	2390	0,000	1618 – 3529
Enterococcus species	VS-*E. faecium*	2023	0,000	1519 – 2695	Not applicable		
	VS-*E. faecalis*	Reference = 1			Not applicable		
Vancomycin-resistant		Not applicable			1.283	0.300	0.801 – 2.057
Vancomycin-susceptible		Not applicable			Reference = 1		

OR = odds ratio, *CI95* = 95% confidence interval

considered [10–16, 18–24, 32]. Prematunge et al. already pointed out in their 2016 meta-analysis, that it is possible that many observations on VRE-associated outcome are based on differences in the infection-causing species rather than on vancomycin resistance [24].

Attempts to assess the pathogenicity of enterococci go far back in time. In some of the previous studies, the pathogenic potential of commensal *E. faecium* was determined, whereas most of nowadays HAIs are caused by isolates of a different *E. faecium* lineage [37, 38]. These so-called hospital-associated strain types (formerly known as clonal complex CC17) differ from commensal human and animal isolates by a distinct core and accessory genome content. Ampicillin resistance is a phenotypic marker of these hospital-associated strain types [39–41]. It has been shown that AMP-R *E. faecium* isolates causing healthcare-associated infections are in fact more pathogenic than commensal variants [42, 43]. In a supplementary analysis (Additional file 1: Tables S1 and S2) we found that 95% of our *E. faecium* isolates were ampicillin-resistant (AMP-R), in contrast to only 1% of the *E. faecalis* isolates. Due to the uneven distribution of ampicillin resistance over the two pathogens we were not able to assess potential virulence differences between commensal and hospital-associated isolates. However, our results are supportive to previous population-based and molecular analyses of *E. faecium* from hospital-acquired infections.

Several reports have linked VRE infections with increased costs [13, 15, 19, 32]. In the univariate analyses, our data showed similar results as almost all costs were significantly higher in VREm-BSI patients than in patients with VSEm-BSI. Butler et al. reported that pharmacy costs are the second most relevant driver of increased costs, making up to 18% of the total amount [21]. In our cohort, the percentage of pharmaceutical costs for patients with VREm made up 21% of the total hospital costs while they made up only 9% of the costs of patents with BSI caused by VSEm (< 0,001). As we were not able to attribute costs to particular agents, these differences could be due to higher antibiotics costs or to differences in underlying conditions treated. For this reason, we analyzed the length of stay before and after onset of BSI. Our data showed increased lengths of stay overall and before onset of VREm-BSI, but not after. Interestingly, all BSIs were classified as HAIs as none occurred prior to day 3 after hospital admission. On average, the BSI episodes occurred on day 16 of hospitalization. Moreover, the same phenomenon was observed in the analysis of the infection-attributable LOS stratified by the two clinically relevant Enterococcus species. Cases with vancomycin susceptible *E. faecium* BSI were in-hospital longer before onset of infection than vancomycin susceptible *E. faecalis* cases. No difference in LOS was observed after onset of infection.

This study has several limitations. The cases were identified retrospectively through a microbiological database and 6.6% lacked sufficient data for this analysis. We did not have data on the course or severity of infection and the antibiotic treatment performed. We did not have separate data on true costs before and after the bloodstream infection. We did not perform molecular analyses on the enterococci isolates to assess their potential virulence traits.

Conclusion

In our study, vancomycin resistance in patients with *Enterococcus faecium* bloodstream infection was associated with increased total costs, length of stay before onset of infection, but not with infection-attributable LOS or in-hospital mortality. We observed that vancomycin-susceptible *E. faecium* infections were more strongly associated with increased LOS and mortality than vancomycin susceptible *E. faecalis* infections and might indicate higher virulence of *E. faecium* as compared to *E. faecalis.* In order to avoid overestimation of VRE-attributable effects, in addition to vancomycin-resistance species should be taken into consideration in future studies assessing the burden of VRE infections.

Abbreviations
95% CI: 95% confidence interval; BSI: blood stream infection; CCI: Charlson comorbidity index; HAI: hospital acquired infection; HR: Hazard ratios; IQR: interquartile range; LOS: length of stay; ME: multiplicative effect; VRE: vancomycin-resistant enterococcus; VREm: vancomycin resistant *Enterococcus faecium*; VSE: vancomycin-susceptible enterococcus; VSEf: vancomycin susceptible *E. faecalis*; VSEm: vancomycin susceptible *Enterococcus faecium*

Acknowledgements
We acknowledge support from the German Research Foundation (DFG).

Funding
No external funding was received for this study.

Authors' contributions
TSK, CR, PG and RL were responsible for the study design. RL supervised the study. MB, SW and RL were responsible for data collection and data cleaning. FS and RL conducted the statistical analysis. GW helped writing the manuscript and contributed significantly to the discussion. All authors interpreted the data, gave important intellectual content and revised the manuscript critically. All authors read and approved the final manuscript.

Consent for publication
Not applicable.

Competing interests
The authors declare that they have no competing interests.

Author details
[1]Charité Universitätsmedizin Berlin, Institute of Hygiene and Environmental Medicine, Berlin, Germany. [2]National Reference Center for the Surveillance of Nosocomial Infections, Berlin, Germany. [3]Department of Medical and Financial Controlling, Charité Universitätsmedizin Berlin, Berlin, Germany. [4]Robert Koch Institute, FG13 Nosocomial Pathogens and Antibiotic Resistance, Wernigerode, Germany. [5]National Reference Centre for Staphylococci and Enterococci, Berlin, Germany.

References
1. Zasowski EJ, Claeys KC, Lagnf AM, Davis SL, Rybak MJ. Time is of the essence: the impact of delayed antibiotic therapy on patient outcomes in hospital-onset Enterococcal bloodstream infections. Clin Infect Dis. 2016;62:1242–50.
2. Maragakis LL, Perencevich EN, Cosgrove SE. Clinical and economic burden of antimicrobial resistance. Expert Rev Anti-Infect Ther. 2008;6:751–63.
3. Bonten MJ, Willems R, Weinstein RA. Vancomycin-resistant enterococci: why are they here, and where do they come from? Lancet Infect Dis. 2001;1:314–25.
4. WHO publishes list of bacteria for which new antibiotics are urgently needed [http://www.who.int/mediacentre/news/releases/2017/bacteria-antibiotics-needed/en/]. Accessed 5 Mar 2018.
5. Gastmeier P, Schroder C, Behnke M, Meyer E, Geffers C. Dramatic increase in vancomycin-resistant enterococci in Germany. J Antimicrob Chemother. 2014;69:1660–4.
6. Simon A, Christiansen B. Adaptation and development of German recommendations on the prevention and control of nosocomial infections due to multiresistant pathogens. Gesundheitsforschung Gesundheitsschutz. 2012;55:1427–31.
7. Muto CA, Jernigan JA, Ostrowsky BE, Richet HM, Jarvis WR, Boyce JM, Farr BM. SHEA guideline for preventing nosocomial transmission of multidrug-resistant strains of Staphylococcus aureus and enterococcus. Infect Control Hosp Epidemiol. 2003;24:362–86.
8. Cosgrove SE. The relationship between antimicrobial resistance and patient outcomes: mortality, length of hospital stay, and health care costs. Clin Infect Dis. 2006;42(Suppl 2):S82–9.
9. Kaye KS, Engemann JJ, Mozaffari E, Carmeli Y. Reference group choice and antibiotic resistance outcomes. Emerg Infect Dis. 2004;10:1125–8.
10. Lloyd-Smith P, Younger J, Lloyd-Smith E, Green H, Leung V, Romney MG. Economic analysis of vancomycin-resistant enterococci at a Canadian hospital: assessing attributable cost and length of stay. J Hosp Infect. 2013;85:54–9.
11. Hayakawa K, Martin ET, Gudur UM, Marchaim D, Dalle D, Alshabani K, Muppavarapu KS, Jaydev F, Bathina P, Sundaragiri PR, et al. Impact of different antimicrobial therapies on clinical and fiscal outcomes of patients with bacteremia due to vancomycin-resistant enterococci. Antimicrob Agents Chemother. 2014;58:3968–75.
12. Cheah AL, Spelman T, Liew D, Peel T, Howden BP, Spelman D, Grayson ML, Nation RL, Kong DC. Enterococcal bacteraemia: factors influencing mortality, length of stay and costs of hospitalization. Clin Microbiol Infect. 2013;19:E181–9.
13. Lloyd-Smith P. Controlling for endogeneity in attributable costs of vancomycin-resistant enterococci from a Canadian hospital. Am J Infect Control. 2017;45:e161–4.
14. Pelz RK, Lipsett PA, Swoboda SM, Diener-West M, Powe NR, Brower RG, Perl TM, Hammond JM, Hendrix CW. Vancomycin-sensitive and vancomycin-resistant enterococcal infections in the ICU: attributable costs and outcomes. Intensive Care Med. 2002;28:692–7.
15. Puchter L, Chaberny IF, Schwab F, Vonberg R-P, Bange F-C, Ebadi E. Economic burden of nosocomial infections caused by vancomycin-resistant enterococci. Antimicrob Resist Infect Control. 2018;7:1.
16. Gandra S, Barter D, Laxminarayan R. Economic burden of antibiotic resistance: how much do we really know? Clin Microbiol Infect. 2014;20:973–9.
17. Bach PB, Malak SF, Jurcic J, Gelfand SE, Eagan J, Little C, Sepkowitz KA. Impact of infection by vancomycin-resistant enterococcus on survival and resource utilization for patients with leukemia. Infect Control Hosp Epidemiol. 2002;23:471–4.
18. Russell DL, Flood A, Zaroda TE, Acosta C, Riley MM, Busuttil RW, Pegues DA. Outcomes of colonization with MRSA and VRE among liver transplant candidates and recipients. Am J Transplant Off J Am Soc Transplant Am Soc Transplant Surg. 2008;8:1737–43.
19. Chiang HY, Perencevich EN, Nair R, Nelson RE, Samore M, Khader K, Chorazy ML, Herwaldt LA, Blevins A, Ward MA, Schweizer ML. Incidence and outcomes associated with infections caused by vancomycin-resistant enterococci in the United States: systematic literature review and meta-analysis. Infect Control Hosp Epidemiol. 2017;38:203–15.
20. McNeil SA, Malani PN, Chenoweth CE, Fontana RJ, Magee JC, Punch JD, Mackin ML, Kauffman CA. Vancomycin-resistant enterococcal colonization and infection in liver transplant candidates and recipients: a prospective surveillance study. Clin Infect Dis. 2006;42:195–203.
21. Butler AM, Olsen MA, Merz LR, Guth RM, Woeltje KF, Camins BC, Fraser VJ. Attributable costs of enterococcal bloodstream infections in a nonsurgical hospital cohort. Infect Control Hosp Epidemiol. 2010;31:28–35.
22. DiazGranados CA, Zimmer SM, Klein M, Jernigan JA. Comparison of mortality associated with vancomycin-resistant and vancomycin-susceptible enterococcal bloodstream infections: a meta-analysis. Clin Infect Dis. 2005;41:327–33.
23. Salgado CD, Farr BM. Outcomes associated with vancomycin-resistant enterococci: a meta-analysis. Infect Control Hosp Epidemiol. 2003;24:690–8.
24. Prematunge C, MacDougall C, Johnstone J, Adomako K, Lam F, Robertson J, Garber G. VRE and VSE bacteremia outcomes in the era of effective VRE therapy: a systematic review and meta-analysis. Infect Control Hosp Epidemiol. 2016;37:26–35.
25. Murray BE. Vancomycin-resistant enterococcal infections. N Engl J Med. 2000;342:710–21.
26. Noskin GA, Peterson LR, Warren JR. Enterococcus faecium and enterococcus faecalis bacteremia: acquisition and outcome. Clin Infect Dis. 1995;20:296–301.

27. Jahresbericht. 2015. [https://www.charite.de/fileadmin/user_upload/portal_relaunch/Mediathek/publikationen/jahresberichte/Charite_Jahresbericht_2015_EN.pdf]. Accessed 27 Mar 2018.
28. Charlson ME, Pompei P, Ales KL, MacKenzie CR. A new method of classifying prognostic comorbidity in longitudinal studies: development and validation. J Chronic Dis. 1987;40:373–83.
29. Thygesen SK, Christiansen CF, Christensen S, Lash TL, Sorensen HT. The predictive value of ICD-10 diagnostic coding used to assess Charlson comorbidity index conditions in the population-based Danish National Registry of patients. BMC Med Res Methodol. 2011;11:83.
30. Schulgen G, Kropec A, Kappstein I, Daschner F, Schumacher M. Estimation of extra hospital stay attributable to nosocomial infections: heterogeneity and timing of events. J Clin Epidemiol. 2000;53:409–17.
31. Barnett AG, Beyersmann J, Allignol A, Rosenthal VD, Graves N, Wolkewitz M. The time-dependent bias and its effect on extra length of stay due to nosocomial infection. Value Health. 2011;14:381–6.
32. Jiang HL, Zhou Z, Wang LS, Fang Y, Li YH, Chu CI. The risk factors, costs, and survival analysis of invasive VRE infections at a medical Center in Eastern Taiwan. Int J Infect Dis. 2017;54:18–24.
33. Guzman Prieto AM, van Schaik W, Rogers MR, Coque TM, Baquero F, Corander J, Willems RJ. Global emergence and dissemination of enterococci as nosocomial pathogens: attack of the clones? Front Microbiol. 2016;7:788.
34. von Baum H, Ober JF, Wendt C, Wenzel RP, Edmond MB. Antibiotic-resistant bloodstream infections in hospitalized patients: specific risk factors in a high-risk population? Infection. 2005;33:320–6.
35. Arias CA, Murray BE. The rise of the enterococcus: beyond vancomycin resistance. Nat Rev Microbiol. 2012;10:266–78.
36. Sava IG, Heikens E, Huebner J. Pathogenesis and immunity in enterococcal infections. Clin Microbiol Infect. 2010;16:533–40.
37. Gao W, Howden BP, Stinear TP. Evolution of virulence in enterococcus faecium, a hospital-adapted opportunistic pathogen. Curr Opin Microbiol. 2018;41:76–82.
38. Lebreton F, van Schaik W, McGuire AM, Godfrey P, Griggs A, Mazumdar V, Corander J, Cheng L, Saif S, Young S. Emergence of epidemic multidrug-resistant enterococcus faecium from animal and commensal strains. MBio. 2013;4:e00534–13.
39. Lester CH, Sandvang D, Olsen SS, Schønheyder HC, Jarløv JO, Bangsborg J, Hansen DS, Jensen TG, Frimodt-Møller N, Hammerum AM. Emergence of ampicillin-resistant enterococcus faecium in Danish hospitals. J Antimicrob Chemother. 2008;62:1203–6.
40. Top J, Willems R, Blok H, De Regt M, Jalink K, Troelstra A, Goorhuis B, Bonten M. Ecological replacement of enterococcus faecalis by multiresistant clonal complex 17 enterococcus faecium. Clin Microbiol Infect. 2007;13:316–9.
41. Freitas AR, Novais C, Duarte B, Pereira AP, Coque TM, Peixe L. High rates of colonisation by ampicillin-resistant enterococci in residents of long-term care facilities in Porto, Portugal. Int J Antimicrob Agents. 2018;51:503–7.
42. Zou J, Shankar N. Surface protein Esp enhances pro-inflammatory cytokine expression through NF-κB activation during enterococcal infection. Innate immunity. 2016;22:31–9.
43. Sillanpää J, Nallapareddy SR, Singh KV, Prakash VP, Fothergill T, Ton-that H, Murray BE. Characterization of the ebpfm pilus-encoding operon of enterococcus faecium and its role in biofilm formation and virulence in a murine model of urinary tract infection. Virulence. 2010;1:236–46.

21

Extended spectrum beta-lactamase mediated resistance in carriage and clinical gram-negative ESKAPE bacteria: a comparative study between a district and tertiary hospital in South Africa

Raspail Carrel Founou[1,2*], Luria Leslie Founou[1,3] and Sabiha Yusuf Essack[1]

Abstract

Background: Gram-negative ESKAPE bacteria are increasingly implicated in several difficult-to-treat infections in developed and developing countries. They are listed by the World Health Organization as resistant bacteria of critical priority in research.

Objectives: To determine the risk factors, prevalence, phenotypic profiles, genetic diversity and clonal relatedness of extended-spectrum β-lactamase (ESBL)-producing multi-drug resistant (MDR) Gram-negative ESKAPE bacteria in the faecal carriage and clinical samples from patients in an urban, tertiary and a rural, district hospital in uMgungundlovu District, KwaZulu-Natal, South Africa.

Methods: This study took place in a district and tertiary hospital during a two-months period from May to June 2017 in uMgungundlovu district, South Africa. Rectal swabs collected from hospitalized patients, at admission, after 48 h and at discharge (whenever possible) formed the carriage sample while clinical isolates routinely processed in the microbiological laboratory during the sampling period were also collected and formed the clinical sample. Gram-negative ESKAPE bacteria were screened for ESBL production on selective MacConkey agar and confirmed using ROSCO kits. Minimum inhibitory concentrations were determined, and real-time and multiplex polymerase chain reaction were used to ascertain the presence of $bla_{\text{CTX-M}}$ group-1-2-9, $bla_{\text{CTX-M}}$ group 8/25, bla_{SHV}, bla_{TEM}, $bla_{\text{OXA-1-like}}$, bla_{KPC}, bla_{VIM}, bla_{IMP}, bla_{GES} and AmpC genes. Genomic fingerprinting was also performed using ERIC-PCR. Risk factors for ESBL-mediating MDR Gram-negative ESKAPE colonization were ascertained by univariate and multivariate logistic regression analyses.

(Continued on next page)

* Correspondence: czangue@yahoo.fr
[1]Antimicrobial Research Unit, School of Health Sciences, College of Health Sciences, University of KwaZulu-Natal, Durban 4000, South Africa
[2]Department of Clinical Microbiology, Centre of Expertise and Biological Diagnostic of Cameroon, (CEDBCAM), Yaoundé, Cameroon
Full list of author information is available at the end of the article

(Continued from previous page)

Results: Overall prevalence of carriage of ESBL-mediating MDR Gram-negative ESKAPE was 37.21% (16/43), 42.31% (11/26) and 57.14% (4/7) at admission, after 48 h and at discharge respectively. The prevalence of ESBL-mediating MDR Gram-negative ESKAPE bacteria in faecal carriage (46%) was higher than clinical samples (28%). Colonization was mainly associated with the referral from district to tertiary hospital with high statistical significance (OR: 14.40, 95% CI 0.98–210.84). *bla*$_{CTX\text{-}M\text{-}group\text{-}9}$, *bla*$_{CTX\text{-}M\text{-}group\text{-}1}$ and *bla*$_{SHV}$ were the main resistance genes identified. Several patients carried more than two different isolates. A *Klebsiella pneumoniae* (K1) clone was circulating within wards and between hospitals.

Conclusion: The study highlights the high prevalence of ESBL-mediating MDR Gram-negative ESKAPE bacteria in carriage and clinical samples among hospitalized patients in uMgungundlovu, South Africa. The wide dissemination of these resistant ESKAPE bacteria in hospitals necessitates improvements in routine screening and reinforcement of infection, prevention and control measures.

Keywords: Antibiotic resistance, ESKAPE bacteria, ESBLs, Carriage, Clonality, Hospitalized patients

Introduction

The selective pressure exerted using antibiotics and aggravated by the dearth of new active substances in the current therapeutic pipeline has led to a considerable increase in antibiotic resistance (ABR) worldwide [1, 2]. A small group of bacteria, i.e., *Enterococcus spp., Staphylococcus aureus, Klebsiella pneumoniae, Acinetobacter baumannii, Pseudomonas aeruginosa* and *Enterobacter spp.*, termed "ESKAPE" due to their ability to escape the activity of and develop high levels of resistance to multiple antibiotics, have recently gained global attention [3–5]. Of the six infamous ESKAPE pathogens, the four Gram-negative bacteria, i.e., *K. pneumoniae, A. baumannii, P. aeruginosa*, and *Enterobacter spp.*, have been associated with four major types of multi-drug resistance (MDR), namely extended-spectrum β-lactamase (ESBL)-producing *K. pneumoniae* and *Enterobacter spp.*, carbapenemase-producing *A. baumannii* and metallo-β-lactamase producing *P. aeruginosa* (MBL-PA) which limit therapeutic options and negatively affect clinical outcomes [3–6]. Several resistance genes have been associated with the emergence of ESBL-mediating MDR Gram-negative ESKAPE bacteria globally. The bacterial production of enzyme hydrolysing antibiotics, particularly β-lactam antibiotics, is the most common mechanism of resistance in Gram-negative ESKAPE. Beta-lactamase enzymes have emerged following chromosomal mutation and acquisition of resistance genes carried on diverse mobile genetic elements (MGEs) such as plasmids, integrons, insertion sequences, transposons, genomic islands and bacteriophages [7]. The common transferability of resistance amongst bacteria will likely be associated with increasing rates of MDR infections and carriage, although some gaps remain as to the dissemination of multi-drug resistant bacteria in the community and among hospitalized patients.

MDR is increasingly being detected in numerous Gram-negative bacteria because of the extensive antibiotic use in communities and hospitals. Despite considerable efforts for their containment, ESBL-mediating multi-drug resistant Gram-negative ESKAPE bacteria are increasingly implicated in several difficult-to-treat infections in both developed and developing countries [5, 6, 8, 9] and were recently listed by the World Health Organization (WHO) as resistant bacteria of critical priority in research [3, 7, 8, 10]. Hospitals remain the main reservoir while immune-compromised patients such as those suffering from diabetes, chronic lung, kidney and cardiovascular diseases and cancers are the most affected. Whilst a better understanding on the impact of faecal carriage of ESBL-mediated resistance to Gram-negative ESKAPE bacteria is required, carriage is recognized as a potential risk for transmission and on subsequent development of infections especially in healthcare settings in developing countries due to inadequate infection, prevention and control measures.

In the African continent, antimicrobial resistance issue in general and MDR particularly, has not been adequately illustrated yet due limited financial resources. Knowledge of the burden of multidrug-resistant bacteria in South Africa could thus be valuable both to raise awareness on the necessity to prevent the spread of resistant infections in communities and hospitals, and to ameliorate empirical antibiotic therapy and clinical practice. This study seeks to compare the prevalence of faecal carriage of ESBL-mediated MDR Gram-negative ESKAPE bacteria among patients hospitalized in an urban, tertiary and a rural, district hospital in uMgungundlovu District, South Africa. In addition, the study is an attempt to provide insight into the risk factors associated with this carriage. Finally, the study assesses the phenotypic and genotypic characteristics and clonal relatedness of carriage and clinical ESBL-mediated MDR Gram-negative ESKAPE bacteria.

Materials and methods

Study population and settings

This study was conducted in a rural, district and urban, tertiary hospital, encoded for ethical reasons as H1 and

H2, respectively, during 2 months from May 2017 to June 2017 in uMgungundlovu district, South Africa. The district hospital (H1) represents the smallest level of hospital and provides four services including obstetrics and gynaecology, paediatrics and child health, general surgery and general medicine with 141 beds. In contrast, the tertiary hospital (H2) offers several specialties, receives referral patients according to a nationally agreed referral plan and has approximately 505 beds.

Patient enrolment and questionnaire survey

Total sampling was performed for the recruitment of participants i.e. all patients older than 18 years old, hospitalized in medical or surgical ward of the hospitals H1 and H2, and willing to participate were included in the study. Oral and written informed consent was obtained from all study participants after explanation of the procedure and purpose of the study. Patient information was gleaned from questionnaires completed by patients and data from patient records. Information was codified prior to analysis to maintain confidentiality.

Sample collection

Sample collection took place in both surgical and general medical wards during a two-month period, 1 month at each of the hospitals. Rectal swabs that were collected aseptically with Amies swabs from symptomatic in-patients, at three-time points, at admission, after 48 h and at discharge (whenever possible) formed the carriage sample. Isolates from symptomatic patients originating from tissue, blood, urine, intravenous catheters, and sputum routinely processed in the microbiological laboratory during the sampling period formed the clinical sample.

Definitions of terms

The specimen (blood, urine, sputum, tissue, intravenous catheter tips, fluid/aspirate and superficial swab) collected for diagnostic purpose from a symptomatic hospitalized patient was considered clinical sample. The clinical isolates were recovered from clinical samples obtained from patients hospitalized in various units of the selected hospitals. In contrast, carriage sample was the rectal swab collected from hospitalized patients at different time-points (admission, after 48 h and at discharge) out of diagnostic tests performed at hospitals.

Laboratory analysis

Identification of gram-negative ESKAPE bacteria

During the sample collection, all rectal swabs were cultured onto MacConkey agar with and without cefotaxime (2 mg/L). After incubation for 18-24 h at 37 °C, each morphotype growing on MacConkey with cefotaxime (MCA + CTX) was subjected to Gram staining, catalase and oxidase tests, followed by biochemical identification with API 20E (bioMérieux, Marcy l'Etoile, France) and Vitek® 2 System (bioMérieux, Marcy l'Etoile, France) using the GN card according to the manufacturer's instructions. Pure colonies were stored into Tryptone Soya Broth supplemented with 30% glycerol at – 20 °C for future use.

Phenotypic screening

All growing colonies were phenotypically screened for ESBL, AmpC, KPC, MBL, and OXA-48 production using ROSCO DIAGNOSTICA (Taastrup, Denmark) using 0.5 McFarland on Mueller-Hinton agar according to the manufacturer's instructions.

Antimicrobial susceptibility testing

Minimum inhibitory concentrations (MICs) were determined via broth microdilution for all presumptive ESBLs and/or AmpCs, and/or MBL producers. Ampicillin, cefoxitin, cefuroxime, cefotaxime, ceftazidime, meropenem, imipenem, ertapenem, amikacin, gentamicin, ciprofloxacin, tigecycline, tetracycline, doxycycline, nitrofurantoin, and colistin constituted the antibiotic panel for carriage isolates. The Vitek® 2 System and Vitek® 2 Gram-negative Susceptibility card (AST-N255) were used to determining the MICs of clinical isolates. The results of MIC tests were interpreted according to the European Committee on Antimicrobial Susceptibility Testing (EUCAST) breakpoints [11] and the MDR which is the resistance to three or more classes of antibiotics was also assessed. *Escherichia coli* ATCC 25922, *K. pneumoniae* ATCC 700603 and *K. pneumoniae* ATCC 51503 were used as controls.

Genomic characterization

Genomic extraction

Genomic DNA of selected strains were extracted using GenElute Bacterial Genomic DNA Kit (Sigma-Aldrich, St. Louis, MO, USA) according to the manufacturer's instructions. Genomic DNA was stored at – 20 °C for future use.

Multiplex polymerase chain reaction (M-PCR)

The isolates were subjected to molecular testing using conventional and M-PCR assays to identify $bla_{\text{CTX-M}}$ group 8/25 ($bla_{\text{CTX-M-gp8/25}}$), bla_{SHV}, bla_{TEM}, $bla_{\text{OXA-1-like}}$, $bla_{\text{OXA-48}}$, bla_{KPC}, bla_{VIM}, bla_{IMP} and bla_{GES} genes as previously described [12] (Additional file 1: Table S1).

Real-time polymerase chain reaction (RT-PCR)

RT-PCR was performed to ascertain bla_{AmpC}, $bla_{\text{CTX-M-group-1}}$ ($bla_{\text{CTX-M-gp1}}$), $bla_{\text{CTX-M-group-2}}$ ($bla_{\text{CTX-M-gp2}}$) and $bla_{\text{CTX-M-group-9}}$ ($bla_{\text{CTX-M-gp9}}$) resistance genes. Results were analysed on a programmable automate QuantStudio5™ (Applied Biosystems, CA, USA) using the Taqman Universal Master Mix 2× (Applied Biosystems, CA, USA) and ready-made assays (Thermo Scientific, CA, USA). Thermal temperature running conditions were as follows: UNG activation at 50 °C for 2 min, initial denaturation at 95 °C for 10 min, 30 cycles of denaturation at 95 °C for 10 s, annealing/extension at 60 °C for 1 min and a final extension at 60 °C for 30 s. The results were interpreted with QuantStudio™ design and analysis software version 1.4 (Applied Biosystems, CA, USA).

Genomic fingerprinting

Enterobacterial Repetitive Intergenic Consensus-Polymerase Chain Reaction (ERIC-PCR) was used to establish the link of different strains within and between hospitals, wards, carriage and clinical samples as well as across sampling points. The primers ERIC1 5'ATGTAAGCTC CTGGGGATTCAC3' and ERIC2 5'AAGTAAGTGAC TGGGGTGAGCG3' [13] were used and PCR reactions were carried out in a 10 μl volume containing 5 μl of Dream*Taq* Green Polymerase Master Mix 2X (Thermo Fisher Scientific, Johannesburg, South Africa), 2.8 μl of nuclease free water, 0.1 μl of each primer (100 μM), and 2 μl of DNA template. The reactions were carried out with the following cycling conditions: initial denaturation at 94 °C for 3 min, 30 cycles consisting of a denaturation step at 94 °C for 30 s, annealing at 50 °C for 1 min, extension at 65 °C for 8 min, a final extension step at 65 °C for 16 min and final storage at 4 °C. The generated amplicons were resolved by horizontal electrophoresis on 1.5% (wt/vol) Tris-Borate-EDTA (Merck, Germany) agarose gels together with the Quick-load®1-kb (Biolabs, New England) and run in an electric field of 110 V for 2 h 30 min. Electrophoresis gels were visualized by a UV light trans-illuminator, images were captured using a Gel Doc™ XR+ system (BioRad Laboratories, CA, Foster City, USA) and analysed by Image Lab™ Software (version 4.0, BioRad Laboratories, CA, Foster City, USA).

ERIC-PCR profiles were normalized using the Quick-load®1-kb (Biolabs, New England) DNA molecular weight marker as the external standard. For cluster analysis, data were exported to Bionumerics software (version 7.6, Applied Maths, TX, USA). Strains were allocated to different clusters by calculating the similarity coefficient from the homology matrix using the Jaccard method. Dendrograms were constructed based on the average linkages of the matrix and using the Unweighted Pair-Group Method (UPGMA). Optimization and band tolerance were set at 1% (version 7.6, Applied Maths, TX, USA) and 80% similarity cut-off was used to define clusters.

Data analysis

Data was coded and entered on an Excel spreadsheet (Microsoft Office 2016) and analysed using STATA (version 14.0, STATA Corporation, TX, USA). Risk factors for ESBL-mediating MDR Gram-negative ESKAPE colonization were ascertained by univariate and multivariate logistic regression analyses. Prevalence of MDR carriage was compared between categories (viz. hospital, ward and time-point) using the chi-square and Fisher's exact test as appropriate. A p-value < 0.05 was regarded as statistically significant.

Results

Population characteristics

A total of 75 hospitalized patients were contacted, amongst whom, 45 (60%) agreed to participate, answered the questionnaire and provided samples. Out of the 45 patients enrolled, faecal carriage was collected from 21 female and 24 were males, and the district hospital ($n = 27$) accounted more participant than the tertiary hospital ($n = 18$). The main reasons of hospitalization were cancer, cellulitis, hypoglycaemia, renal failure, diabetes, breath disorder, surgery and wound, in both hospitals. The patient's follow-up rate was 96%, 58% and 16% of rectal swabs collected at admission, after 48 h and at discharge, respectively.

The overall prevalence of carriage was 37.21% (16/43), 42.31% (11/26) and 57.14% (4/7) at admission, after 48 h and at discharge, respectively, with males being more colonized than females as were patients referred from another hospital (Table 1). Patients in the tertiary hospital were more likely to be colonized by MDR ESKAPE bacteria at admission (50%) and discharge (66.66%) than those of the district hospital (Table 1). Furthermore, patients admitted to the general medical ward were more colonized in the district hospital at all time-points whereas, in the tertiary hospital, the prevalence in the surgical ward was higher at admission and discharge. In parallel, the prevalence of MDR ESKAPE bacteria in faecal carriage (46%) was higher than clinical samples (28%).

Risk factors for MDR gram-negative ESKAPE bacteria carriage

Patients referred from the district to the tertiary hospital had an increased the risk of being colonized by resistant bacteria at admission (OR = 9, 95% CI 4.68–17.30) and after 48 h (OR = 4; 95% CI 1.50–10.66, Table 2). Similarly, the gender (male) increases the odds of being colonized at admission and after 48 h in district hospital (Table 2).

The multivariate analysis further confirmed that referral from district to tertiary hospital was significantly associated with MDR Gram-negative ESKAPE bacteria at admission (OR = 14.40, 95% CI 1. 0.98–210.84) and after 48 h (OR = 5.72, 95% CI 0.17–189.00) as was the gender for these two time-points in the district hospital (Table 3).

Table 1 Fecal carriage of resistant Gram-negative ESKAPE bacteria isolated from hospitalized patients in a rural district and a tertiary urban hospital

Variables	District Rural Hospital $n = 27$						Tertiary Urban Hospital $n = 18$					
	Admission, (%)	p	After 48 h, (%)	p	At discharge, (%)	P	Admission, (%)	p	After 48 h, (%)	p	At discharge, (%)	P
Overall	29.63	....	47.05	.....	50	....	50	...	33.33	...	66.66	...
Socio-demographic factors												
Gender												
Female	21.4	0.333	33	0.229	50	....	40	0.590	50	0.571	50	0.386
Male	38.4		63		0		55		29		100	
Clinical history												
Previous hospitalization (within one year)												
Yes	13	0.206	0	0.012	0	0.248	20	0.106	25	0.635	100	0.386
No	37		67		66.67		64		40		50	
Antibiotic use (during hospital stay)												
Yes	27.78	0.766	33.33	0.402	50	1.000	33	0.522	33	1.000	100	0.386
No	33.33		54.55		50		54		33		50	
Transferred from another hospital												
Yes	100	0.116	0	...	0	....	75	0.046	50	0.343	100	0.386
No	27		47		50		25		20		50	
Hospital ward												
Medicine	40	0.187	56	0.457	50	1.000	40	0.590	40	0.635	50	0.386
Surgery	17		38		50		55		25		100	

Out of the 45 patients enrolled, some refused rectal sampling, some were discharged or transferred after 48 h, while other could not be sampled due to their condition, leading to variability in number

Prevalence of MDR gram-negative ESKAPE bacteria

Out of 159 non-duplicates resistant Gram-negative bacteria isolated, 31 (19.50%) were MDR Gram-negative ESKAPE bacteria of which 21 (67.74%) were clinical isolates (11 tissue, 2 bloods, 3 urines, 3 intravenous catheters, 2 sputum) obtained after 48 h from hospitalized patients (15 males and 6 females) with symptomatic infections in different departments (medicine, surgery, intensive care units). Ten (32.26%) MDR Gram-negative ESKAPE bacteria were isolated from the rectal swab of in-patients (6 females, 4 males). In the district hospital, seven isolates were identified, five (71.43%) in carriage and two (28.57%) in clinical samples. *K. pneumoniae* ($n = 2$) and *E. aerogenes* ($n = 2$) were the main bacterial species isolated in carriage samples while *E. cloacae* ($n = 2$) was the sole clinical isolates. In contrast, in the tertiary hospital, five (20.83%) isolates were identified in carriage and 19 (79.16%) in clinical samples. The main pathogen identified in carriage was *E. aerogenes* ($n = 2$) while *P. aeruginosa* ($n = 7$) and *A. baumannii* ($n = 7$) were the main clinical isolates.

Table 2 Risk factors associated with faecal carriage of ESBL-producing Gram-negative ESKAPE bacteria (Univariate Logistic regression)

Variables	District hospital		Tertiary hospital	
	Admission	After 48 h	Admission	After 48 h
	OR (95% CI)	OR (95% CI)	OR (95% CI)	OR (95% CI)
Gender (F or M)	2.29 (0.42–12.50)	3.33 (0.45–24.44)	1.8 (0.21–15.40)	0.4 (0.16–10.02)
Antibiotic use (Yes or No)	1.3 (0.23–7.32)	0.42 (0.05–3.31)	0.43 (0.03–5.98)	1
Co-morbidity	1.05 (0.61–1.83)	1.03 (0.48–2.24)	1.05 (0.61–1.83)	1.03 (0.48–2.24)
Previous hospitalization	0.24 (0.02–2.40)	1	0.14 (0.01–1.76)	0.5 (0.03–8.95)
Transferred from another hospital	1	1	9 (0.93–86.52)	4 (0.21–75.67)
Ward (Medicine or Surgery)	0.3 (0.05–1.88)	0.48 (0.07–3.35)	1.8 (0.21–15.40)	0.5 (0.03–8.95)

Table 3 Predictive risk factors associated with fecal carriage of MDR Gram-negative ESKAPE bacteria in a district and tertiary hospital (Multivariate Logistic regression)

Variables	District Hospital		Tertiary Hospital	
	Admission; OR (95% CI)	After 48 h; OR (95% CI)	Admission; OR (95% CI)	After 48 h; OR (95% CI)
Gender (F or M)	7.12 (0.54–93.75)	3.61 (0.34–37.83)	1.21 (0.09–15.61)	0.29 (0.005–16.27)
Antibiotic use (Yes or No)	4.73 (0.28–80.57)	0.93 (0.08–11.40)	0.26 (0.007–9.01)	0.41 (0.009–17.46)
Transferred from another hospital	1	1	14.40 (0.98–210.84)	5.72 (0.17–189.00)
Hospital Ward (Medicine or Surgery)	0.08 (0.004–1.39)	0.42 (0.05–3.81)	2.09 (0.10–42.29)	1.14 (0.03–49.14)

Antimicrobial resistance profiles

In the tertiary hospital, especially in the medical ward, isolates expressed high resistance to ampicillin (100%), cefuroxime (100%) and cefotaxime (100%) in both carriage and clinical samples (Table 4). Similarly, in the surgical ward of the same hospital, clinical samples showed high resistance to ampicillin (100%), cefuroxime (100%), cefotaxime (88%), cefoxitin (88%), and nitrofurantoin (55%) while the unique carriage isolate was resistant to all the panel of antibiotics tested.

In the district hospital, the isolate identified in carriage samples in the surgical ward displayed maximum resistance (100%) to all antibiotics except colistin while those detected in medical ward exhibited high level of resistance to ampicillin (100%), cefuroxime (100%), cefotaxime (100%), ceftazidime (100%), cefoxitin (100%), amikacin (100%), gentamicin (100%), nitrofurantoin (100%) and tigecycline (100%) (Table 4).

Genetic diversity of isolated MDR strains

Overall, the predominant ESBL genes were $bla_{CTX\text{-}M\text{-}gp9}$ (90%, 28/31), $bla_{CTX\text{-}M\text{-}gp1}$ (71%, 22/31), bla_{SHV} (42%, 13/31), $bla_{CTX\text{-}M\text{-}gp8/25}$ (36%, 11/31), $bla_{OXA\text{-}1\text{-}Like}$ (29%, 9/31) and bla_{TEM} (23%, 7/31) for both carriage and clinical samples. In the tertiary hospital, $bla_{CTX\text{-}M\text{-}gp9}$ (100%), $bla_{CTX\text{-}M\text{-}gp1}$ (87.5%), bla_{KPC} (75%) and bla_{VIM} (50%) were the main resistance genes detected in *A. baumannii* while *K. pneumoniae* strains harboured mainly $bla_{CTX\text{-}M\text{-}gp8/25}$ (66.6%), bla_{TEM} (66.6%), bla_{SHV} (66.6%), $bla_{CTX\text{-}M\text{-}gp9}$ (50%) and $bla_{CTX\text{-}M\text{-}gp1}$ (50%) (Table 5). It is noteworthy to mention that all isolates harboured at least two resistance genes and a maximum of seven genes were detected in one *E. aerogenes* (G702R2B5) isolate (Fig. 1b). In the district hospital, $bla_{CTX\text{-}M\text{-}gp9}$ (100%), bla_{SHV} (100%), and bla_{TEM} (100%) were the predominant genes in *K. pneumoniae* whereas $bla_{CTX\text{-}M\text{-}gp9}$ (100%), $bla_{OXA\text{-}1\text{-}Like}$ (50%), $bla_{CTX\text{-}M\text{-}gp1}$ (50%) and $bla_{CTX\text{-}M\text{-}gp8/25}$ (50%) were the main genes identified in *E. cloacae* (Table 5).

Genomic fingerprint

ERIC-profiles revealed some associations within species and suggest a likely transmission of resistant ESKAPE bacteria across patients, wards and hospitals (Additional file 2: Table S2). For *K. pneumoniae*, one main cluster showing high genetic similarities was observed (Fig. 1a). *K. pneumoniae* strains A111R1B2 and A105R2B2 detected among two patients at admission for the former and after 48 h for the latter, in the medical ward of the district hospital showed 100% of similarity and shared common ancestors with one carriage and three clinical strains isolated in the tertiary hospital (Fig. 1a and Additional file 2: Table S2). Similarly, one pair of *E. aerogenes*, A105R1B5 and G702R1B5 isolated from two patients in the medical ward of the district and tertiary hospital, both at admission, also exhibited 100% of similarity and shared a common ancestor with another strain G702R2B5 collected after 48 h (Fig. 1b). Although, *A. baumannii* (Fig. 1c) and *P. aeruginosa* (Fig. 1d) were more genetically diverse, some isolates shared a common ancestor within and between the carriage and clinical samples.

Discussion

The overall prevalence of carriage at admission was 37.21% (16/43) and we found that 42.31% (11/26) and 57.14% (4/7) were still MDR ESKAPE carriers after 48 h and at discharge. Notwithstanding the small sample size, our results showed that the carriage of MDR Gram-negative ESKPAPE bacteria increased with the hospital length of stay. Our results are consistent with a Norwegian prospective cohort study carried out from 2009 to 2011 investigating the risk factors for and duration of prolonged faecal carriage of ESBL-producing *K. pneumoniae* amongst patients with community acquired urinary tract infections which revealed high prevalence of ESBL faecal carriage (ranging from 15 to 61%) at six different time points [14].

At hospital level, the rate of carriage at admission in the district hospital (30%) compared with the tertiary hospital (50%) suggests that patients admitted to the tertiary hospital are likely to be more colonized by MDR Gram-negative ESKAPE bacteria than those of the district healthcare facility (Table 1). Our findings could be explained by the fact that all patients admitted to this level of the hospital are generally transferred from lower level healthcare facilities of the South African health system. This is further confirmed by the increased odds of being colonized in the univariate and multivariate analysis.

Table 4 Resistance to selected antibiotics in ESBL-producing Gram-negative ESKAPE bacteria isolated from carriage and clinical samples in a district and tertiary hospital

Antibiotics	Tertiary hospital								District hospital					
	Medical ward				Surgical ward				Medical ward				Surgical ward	
	Carriage		Clinical		Carriage		Clinical		Carriage		Clinical		Carriage	
	MIC (μg/ml) range	No. resistant isolates (%)	MIC (μg/ml) range	No. resistant isolates (%)	MIC (μg/ml) range	No. resistant isolates (%)	MIC (μg/ml) range	No. resistant isolates (%)	MIC (μg/ml) range	No. resistant isolates (%)	MIC (μg/ml) range	No. resistant isolates (%)	MIC (μg/ml) range	No. resistant isolates (%)
Ampicillin	≥512	4 (100)	≥32	11 (100)	≥512	1 (100)	16–32	8 (100)	≥512	4 (100)	16- ≥ 32	2 (100)	≥512	1 (100)
Cefoxitin	8–512	3 (75)	4	7 (64)	16	1 (100)	8- ≥ 64	7 (88)	128 ≥ 512	4 (100)	≥64	2 (100)	≥512	1 (100)
Cefuroxime	≥512	4 (100)	≥64	11 (100)	128	1 (100)	8–64	8 (100)	256 ≥ 512	4 (100)	16- ≥ 64	2 (100)	≥512	1 (100)
Cefotaxime	≥512	4 (100)	≥64	11 (100)	128	1 (100)	1- ≥ 64	7 (88)	32- ≥ 512	4 (100)	< 1–32	2 (100)	≥512	1 (100)
Ceftazidime	512	4 (100)	≥64	8 (73)	256	1 (100)	1- ≥ 64	4 (50)	32- ≥ 512	4 (100)	≤1–16	2 (100)	≥512	1 (100)
Meropenem	0.5–2	2(50)	0.25	3 (27)	2	1 (100)	0.25 ≥ 16	4 (50)	0.25–16	2 (50)	0.25	0 (0)	16	1 (100)
Imipenem	4–8	4 (100)	0.25	3 (27)	16	1 (100)	0.5- ≥ 16	3 (37.3)	2–32	2 (50)	0.25–1	0 (0)	64	1 (100)
Ertapenem	1–2	4 (100)	0.5	0 (0)	16	1 (100)	≤0.5	0 (0)	0.25–8	3 (75)	0.5	0 (0)	64	1 (100)
Amikacin	8–128	4 (100)	8	2 (18)	64	1 (100)	2- ≥ 64	4 (50)	8–128	2 (100)	2	0 (0)	≥512	1 (100)
Gentamicin	128	4 (100)	≥16	8 (73)	8	1 (100)	1- ≥ 16	4 (50)	4–16	4 (100)	1	0 (0)	≥512	1 (100)
Ciprofloxacin	64–512	4 (100)	≥4	6 (55)	32	1 (100)	0.25- ≥ 4	5 (45)	0.5–64	3 (75)	≤0.25	0 (0)	32	1 (100)
Tigecycline	16–64	4 (100)	1	4 (36)	16	1 (100)	0.5- ≥ 8	3 (37.3)	2–64	4 (100)	1	0 (0)	8	1 (100)
Nitrofurantoin	≥512	4 (100)	128	9 (82)	≥512	1 (100)	≥512	6 (55)	≥512	4 (100)	16- ≥ 512	0 (0)	≥512	1 (100)
Colistin	8–512	4 (100)	0.5	0 (0)	8	1 (100)	≤0.5	0(0)	0(0)	0(0)	≤0.5	0 (0)	≤0.5	0

Table 5 Resistance genes in ESBL-producing Gram-negative ESKAPE bacteria

Bacteria	No. of strains, *n* = 31 (%)	Resistance genes, *n* (%)									
		AmpC	TEM	SHV	CTX-M group-1	CTX-M group-9	CTX-M Group 8/25	IMP	VIM	KPC	OXA-1-like
Tertiary hospital (*n* = 24)											
K. pneumoniae	6 (25)	2 (33.3)	4 (66.6)	4 (66.6)	3 (50)	3 (50)	4 (66.6)	1 (16.6)	1 (16.6)	1 (16.6)	2 (33.33)
A. baumannii	8 (33.3)	3 (37.5)	/	3 (37.5)	7 (87.5)	8 (100)	/	/	4 (50)	6 (75)	2 (25)
P. aeruginosa	7 (29.5)	1 (14.28)	/	/	7 (100)	7 (100)	/	/	/	/	/
E. aerogenes	2 (8.33)	2 (100)	/	2 (100)	/	2 (100)	2 (100)	/	/	/	2 (100)
E. cloacae	1 (4.16)	/	/	/	1 (100)	1 (100)	1 (100)	1 (100)	/	1 (100)	/
District hospital (n = 7)											
K. pneumoniae	2 (28.57)	/	2 (100)	2 (100)	1 (50)	2 (100)	1 (50)	/	/	/	2 (33.33)
P. aeruginosa	1 (14.28)	/	/	/	1 (100)	1 (100)	/	/	/	/	/
E. aerogenes	2 (28.57)	1 (50)	1 (50)	1 (50)	1 (50)	2 (100)	2 (100)	/	/	/	/
E. cloacae	2 (28.57)	1 (50)	/	1 (50)	1 (50)	2 (100)	1 (50)	/	/	/	1 (50)

Similarly, at discharge, patients of the tertiary hospital (67%) were more colonized than those of the district hospital (50%). This could be explained by the complexity of cases associated with invasive medical procedures and greater antibiotic use in the tertiary hospital. However, after 48 h, the prevalence of carriage was higher in patients in the district hospital (47%) compared with the tertiary hospital (33%) intimating. This contrast could point out sub-optimal infection prevention and control measures in this level of healthcare setting. Besides, tertiary hospital with its more complicated cases and subsequent higher antibiotic use would have likely created greater selection pressure for resistance, but an anomalously greater resistance was observed in carriage samples in the district hospital. The small sample numbers preclude nonetheless definitive conclusions about carriage rates and resistance patterns.

The prevalence of MDR Gram-negative ESKAPE bacteria in faecal carriage (46%) was higher than that of clinical samples (28%) during the study period. Faecal carriage of resistant bacteria has been demonstrated to precede infections and consequently, such high prevalence of asymptomatic faecal carriage is of critical significance. Our results concur with a study from France where the prevalence of MDR Gram-negative bacilli isolated from stool samples was higher than that of clinical samples during a non-outbreak situation in a French Hospital [15]. They are however higher than a report from Mahomed and Coovadia (2014) which demonstrated 4.7% of faecal carriage of ESBL producing *Enterobacteriaceae* amongst children from the community in KwaZulu-Natal, South Africa [16]. Our findings may be an underestimation because of different diagnostic, stewardship practices, preference for empirical treatment and budget constraints such that not every infection generates a microbiological sample.

During the two-months period, 21 clinically relevant MDR Gram-negative ESKAPE bacteria out of 74 isolates were identified in both hospitals. Moreover, the prevalence of MDR *A. baumannii* and *P. aeruginosa* were 41.61% (10 out of 21 MDR Gram-negative ESKAPE bacteria) and 33.33% (7 out of 21 MDR Gram-negative ESKAPE bacteria) in clinical samples, respectively. The isolation of three *A. baumannii* strains, cluster A1, from tissue of three different patients (ED01498924, ED01498793, ED01498924) in surgery, consolidate the likely dissemination of this cluster within this ward in the tertiary hospital (Additional file 2: Table S2 and Fig. 1c).

In carriage samples, MDR *K. pneumoniae* and *Enterobacter spp.* were the predominant bacteria in both hospitals. This is consistent with a South African study where *K. pneumoniae* was the main pathogen identified in stool samples of children from the community of KwaZulu-Natal, South Africa [16]. Similarly, a 68% prevalence of ESBL-producing *Enterobacteriaceae* faecal carriage was shown amongst Egyptian patients with community-acquired gastrointestinal complaints [17].

An interesting finding was the inter-hospital and interpatient spread of *K. pneumoniae* (cluster K1) in carriage, which were isolated from two patients (A105R2B2 and A111R1B2) hospitalized in general medicine in district hospital, sharing common ancestor with a patient (G702R3B2) from tertiary hospital (Additional file 2: Table S2). Interestingly, the isolated strains were identified in the medical ward and at different time-points, confirming the dissemination of this cluster across hospitals. In addition, *K. pneumoniae* strains from the same cluster (K1) were detected in urine (ED01500733) and sputum (ED01502268) of clinically ill patients hospitalized in intensive care unit (ICU) and medical ward in the tertiary hospital, respectively. This suggests that

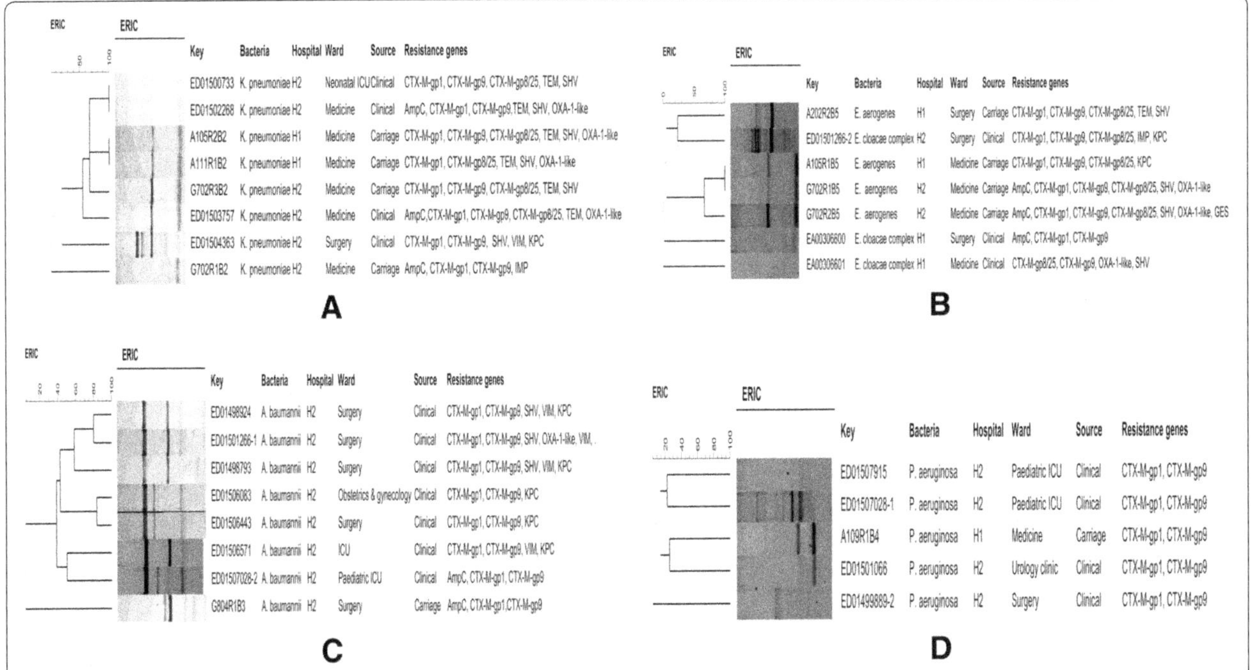

Fig. 1 Dendrograms of ESBL-producing of Gram-negative ESKAPE bacteria isolated from carriage and clinical samples from hospitalized patients. **a** *K. pneumoniae*, (**b**) *E. aerogenes* and *cloacae*, (**c**) *A. baumannii*, (**d**) *P. aeruginosa*

the *K. pneumoniae* K1 strains is circulating within wards and hospitals, and consequently could probably be source of nosocomial infections in hospitals.

Two patients, A105R1B5 and G702R1B5 also carried *Enterobacter spp.* (cluster E2) at admission in both district and tertiary hospitals, specifically in the medical wards (Additional file 2: Table S2) intimating the emergence of these strains in the community with subsequent entry into the district hospital, as the first level of care, and followed by spread to the tertiary hospital through referral. This result is consistent with our analyses which demonstrated that in the district hospital, the main risk factors were antibiotic use and gender while the referral and hospital ward were the principal risk factors at tertiary level (Tables 2 and 3).

Overall, the predominant ESBLs detected in carriage were $bla_{\text{CTX-M-gp9}}$ (90%), bla_{SHV} (60%), $bla_{\text{CTX-M-gp1}}$(50%), bla_{TEM} (40%) and $bla_{\text{OXA-1-like}}$ (40%). CTX-M is predominantly reported in community-acquired infections which would be more prevalent in the district hospital as the first level of care. These results are consistent with global reports. For instance, $bla_{\text{CTX-M-group}}$ were recently observed in adults in a community in Netherlands and ambulatory patients in Egypt with both gastrointestinal complaints [17, 18]. Similarly, studies from Guinee-Bissau, Niger, Gabon and Tanzania, reported high prevalence of ESBL faecal carriage with $bla_{\text{CTX-M}}$, bla_{TEM} and bla_{SHV} being the main genes identified [19–21]. The prevalence of AmpC was also higher in carriage (40%) compared to clinical samples (23.80%). Finally, carbapenemases were identified in clinical samples for in these hospitals, specifically, KPC and VIM in clinical *A. baumannii* isolates as well as IMP in a carriage *K. pneumoniae* isolate. An *E. aerogenes* isolate further showed bla_{GES} along with $bla_{\text{CTX-M-gp1}}$, $bla_{\text{CTX-M-gp9}}$, $bla_{\text{CTX-M-gp8/25}}$, bla_{SHV} and $bla_{\text{OXA-1-like}}$ in a carriage sample. The faecal carriage of MDR Gram-negative ESKAPE bacteria appears to be a source of cross-transmission between patients. The substantial genetic similarity within and between carriage and clinical isolates as well as wards and hospital settings reveal their potential implications in future outbreak situations that may occur either in hospitals or in communities. Efforts should thus be made amongst communities and asymptomatic patients for better containment of antibiotic resistance dissemination.

Gender, antibiotic use, type of healthcare settings and referral from another hospital were the main risk factors identified. These results suggest that routine screening for MDR Gram-negative ESKAPE bacteria at admission should be implemented, and infection, prevention and control measures reinforced to prevent potential outbreaks by these resistant pathogens [22].

Conclusion

This study highlights the high prevalence of ESBL-mediating MDR Gram-negative ESKAPE bacteria in carriage and clinical samples among hospitalized patients in uMgungundlovu. It is imperative to implement regular screening and surveillance of MDR Gram-negative ESKAPE bacteria in communities and hospitals, to monitor epidemiological changes, ascertain socio-economic impact and inform antibiotic treatment. These screening and surveillance measures coupled with strict infection prevention and control programmes and antimicrobial stewardship programmes (ASP) are essential to address antibiotic resistance in these settings.

Acknowledgments

The authors would like to express their profound gratitude to Professor Mlisana Koleka, Dr. Sumayya Haffejee and Mrs. Nadira Moodley of the National Health Laboratory of South Africa for their collaboration and for providing us with clinical strains. The Infection, Prevention and Control officers, Mrs. Thandi Masango, Mrs. Jennifer Grace Green and Mrs. Zelda Reddy, are also gratefully acknowledged for their considerable assistance during the sample collection in both hospitals.

Funding

This work was supported by the Antimicrobial Research Unit (ARU) and a scholarship awarded to R.C. Founou and L.L. Founou by the College of Health Sciences (CHS) of the University of KwaZulu-Natal. The National Research Foundation funded this study through the NRF Incentive Funding for Rated Researchers (Grant No. 85595), the NRF Competitive Grant for Rated Researchers (Grant no.: 106063) and the DST/NRF South African Research Chair in Antibiotic Resistance and One Health (Grant No. 98342) awarded to SY Essack. Any opinions, findings and conclusions, or recommendations expressed in this study are those of the authors, and therefore do not represent the official position of the funders. The funders had no role in the study design, data collection and analysis, preparation of the manuscript nor decision to publish.

Authors' contributions

RF co-conceptualized the study, undertook sample collection, laboratory and statistical analyses, prepared tables and figures, interpreted results and drafted the manuscript. LF undertook sample collection and laboratory analyses and vetted the results. SE co-conceptualized the study, undertook vetting of the results and critically reviewed the manuscript. All authors read and approved the manuscript.

Consent for publication

Not applicable.

Competing interests

Professor Essack is a member of the Global Respiratory Infection Partnership sponsored by an unrestricted educational grant from Reckitt and Benckiser. All other authors declare that there is no competing financial interest.

Author details

[1]Antimicrobial Research Unit, School of Health Sciences, College of Health Sciences, University of KwaZulu-Natal, Durban 4000, South Africa. [2]Department of Clinical Microbiology, Centre of Expertise and Biological Diagnostic of Cameroon, (CEDBCAM), Yaoundé, Cameroon. [3]Department of Food Safety and Environmental Microbiology, Centre of Expertise and Biological Diagnostic of Cameroon, (CEDBCAM), Yaoundé, Cameroon.

References

1. O'Neill J. Tackling drug-resistant infections globally: final report and recommendations. Rev Antimicrob Resist. 2016.
2. World Health Organization. Antimicrobial resistance global report on surveillance. Geneva: World Health Organization; 2014.
3. Rice LB. Federal funding for the study of antimicrobial resistance in nosocomial pathogens: no eskape. J Infect Dis. 2008;197(8):1079–81.
4. Almasaudi SB. *Acinetobacter spp.* as nosocomial pathogens: epidemiology and resistance features. Saudi J Biol Sci. 2016; In Press. doi: https://doi.org/10.1016/j.sjbs.2016.02.009.
5. Pedleton JN, Gorman SP, Gilmore BF. Clinical relevance of the ESKAPE pathogens. Expert Rev Anti-Infect Ther. 2013;11(3):297–308.
6. Lim C, Takahashi E, Hongsuwan M, Wuthiekanun V, Thamlikitkul V, Hinjoy S, Day NP, Peacock SJ, Limmathurotsakul D. Epidemiology and burden of multidrug-resistant bacterial infection in a developing country. elife. 2016;5. https://doi.org/10.7554/eLife.18082.
7. Dantas G, Sommer MOA. How to fight Back against antibiotic resistance. Am Sci. 2014;102:42–51.
8. Slavcovici A, Maier C. Antimicrobial resistance of ESKAPE-pathogens in culture-positive pneumonia. FARMACIA. 2015;63(2):201–5.
9. Founou RC, Founou LL, Essack SY. Clinical and economic impact of antibiotic resistance in developing countries: a systematic review and meta-analysis. PLoS One. 2017;12(12):e0189621.
10. World Health Organization. Global priority list of antibiotic-resistance Bacteria to guide research, discovery, and development of new antibiotics. Geneva: World Health Organization; 2017.
11. EUCAST. Breakpoint tables for interpretation of MICs and zone diameters. 2017. Available from http://www.eucast.org/clinical_breakpoints/.
12. Dallenne C, Costa AD, Decre D, Favier C, Arlet G. Development of a set of multiplex PCR assays for the detection of genes encoding important b-lactamases in Enterobacteriaceae. J Antimicrob Chemother. 2010;65(3):490–5. https://doi.org/10.1093/jac/dkp498.
13. Versalovic J, Koeuth T. Distribution of repetitive DNA sequences in eubacteria and application to fingerprinting of bacterial genomes. Nucleic Acids Res. 1991;19(24):6823–31.
14. Jorgensen SB, Soraas A, Sundsfjord A, Liestøl K, Leegaard TM, Jenum PA. Faecal carriage of extended spectrum beta-lactamase producing *Escherichia coli* and *Klebsiella pneumoniae* after urinary tract infection - a three-year prospective cohort study. PLoS One. 2017;12(3):e0173510.
15. Vidal-Navarro L, Pfeiffer C, Bouziges N, Sotto A, Lavigne JP. Faecal carriage of multidrug-resistant gram-negative bacilli during a non-outbreak situation in a French university hospital. J Antimicrob Chemother. 2010;65(11):2455–8. https://doi.org/10.1093/jac/dkq333.
16. Mahomed S, Coovadia MY. Faecal carriage of extended Spectrum Beta-lactamase producing *Escherichia coli* and *Klebsiella pneumoniae* in children from the community of Kwadedangendlale, KwaZulu-Natal, South Africa. Int J Infect Control. 2014;11(3):1–8. https://doi.org/10.3396/ijic.v11i3.14391.
17. Abdallah HM, Alnaiemi N, Reuland EA, Wintermans BB, Koek A, Abdelwahab AM, Samy A, Abdelsalam KW, Vandenbroucke-Grauls CMJE. Faecal carriage of extended-spectrum β-lactamase- and carbapenemase-producing *Enterobacteriaceae* in Egyptian patients with community-onset gastrointestinal complaints: a hospital -based cross-sectional study. Antimicrob Resist Infect Control. 2017;6(1):62. https://doi.org/10.1186/s13756-017-0219-7.
18. Reuland EA, Naiemi N, Kaiser AM, Heck M, Kluytmans JA, Savelkoul PH, Elders PJ, Vandenbroucke-Grauls CM. Prevalence and risk factors for carriage of ESBL-producing *Enterobacteriaceae* in Amsterdam. J Antimicrob Chemother. 2016;71(4):1076–82. https://doi.org/10.1093/jac/dkv441.
19. Isendahl J, Turlej-Rogacka A, Manjuba C, Rodrigues A, Giske CG, Nauclér P. Fecal carriage of ESBL-producing *E. coli* and *K. pneumoniae* in children in Guinea-Bissau: a hospital-based cross-sectional study. PLoS One. 2012;7:e51981.
20. Woerther PL, Angebault C, Jacquier H, Hugede HC, Janssens AC, Sayadi S, El Mniai A, Armand-Lefèvre L, Ruppé E, Barbier F, Raskine L, Page AL, Rekeneire DN, Andremont A. Massive increase, spread, and exchange of extended spectrum beta-lactamase-encoding genes among intestinal *Enterobacteriaceae* in hospitalized children with severe acute malnutrition in Niger. Clin Infect Dis. 2011;53(7):677–85. https://doi.org/10.1093/cid/cir522.
21. Schaumburg F, Alabi A, Kokou C, Grobusch MP, Köck R, Kaba H, Becker K, Adegnika AA, Kremsner PG, Peters G, Mellmann A. High burden of extended-spectrum beta-lactamase-producing *Enterobacteriaceae* in Gabon. J Antimicrob Chemother. 2013;68(9):2140–3. https://doi.org/10.1093/jac/dkt164.

Spread of the florfenicol resistance *floR* gene among clinical *Klebsiella pneumoniae* isolates in China

Junwan Lu[1,2†], Jinfang Zhang[2†], Lei Xu[2], Yabo Liu[2], Pingping Li[2], Tingyuan Zhu[2], Cong Cheng[1*], Shunfei Lu[1], Teng Xu[2], Huiguang Yi[2], Kewei Li[2], Wu Zhou[1], Peizhen Li[2], Liyan Ni[3] and Qiyu Bao[2*]

Abstract

Background: Florfenicol is a derivative of chloramphenicol that is used only for the treatment of animal diseases. A key resistance gene for florfenicol, *floR*, can spread among bacteria of the same and different species or genera through horizontal gene transfer. To analyze the potential transmission of resistance genes between animal and human pathogens, we investigated *floR* in *Klebsiella pneumoniae* isolates from patient samples. *floR* in human pathogens may originate from animal pathogens and would reflect the risk to human health of using antimicrobial agents in animals.

Methods: PCR was used to identify *floR*-positive strains. The *floR* genes were cloned, and the minimum inhibitory concentrations (MICs) were determined to assess the relative resistance levels of the genes and strains. Sequencing and comparative genomics methods were used to analyze *floR* gene-related sequence structure as well as the molecular mechanism of resistance dissemination.

Results: Of the strains evaluated, 20.42% (67/328) were resistant to florfenicol, and 86.96% (20/23) of the *floR*-positive strains demonstrated high resistance to florfenicol with MICs ≥512 μg/mL. Conjugation experiments showed that transferrable plasmids carried the *floR* gene in three isolates. Sequencing analysis of a plasmid approximately 125 kb in size (pKP18–125) indicated that the *floR* gene was flanked by multiple copies of mobile genetic elements. Comparative genomics analysis of a 9-kb transposon-like fragment of pKP18–125 showed that an approximately 2-kb sequence encoding *lysR-floR-virD2* was conserved in the majority (79.01%, 83/105) of *floR* sequences collected from NCBI nucleotide database. Interestingly, the most similar sequence was a 7-kb fragment of plasmid pEC012 from an *Escherichia coli* strain isolated from a chicken.

Conclusions: Identified on a transferable plasmid in the human pathogen *K. pneumoniae*, the *floR* gene may be disseminated through horizontal gene transfer from animal pathogens. Studies on the molecular mechanism of resistance gene dissemination in different bacterial species of animal origin could provide useful information for preventing or controlling the spread of resistance between animal and human pathogens.

Keywords: Florfenicol, *floR*, *Klebsiella pneumoniae*, Plasmid, Human pathogen

* Correspondence: 113246570@qq.com; baoqy@genomics.cn
†Junwan Lu and Jinfang Zhang contributed equally to this work.
[1]School of Medicine and Health, Lishui University, Lishui 323000, China
[2]School of Laboratory Medicine and Life Sciences/Institute of Biomedical Informatics, Wenzhou Medical University, Wenzhou 325035, China
Full list of author information is available at the end of the article

Background

Florfenicol, which is only used to treat animal infections, is a derivative of chloramphenicol that is active against chloramphenicol-resistant isolates [1]. Resistance to chloramphenicol occurs mainly through the production of inactivating enzymes called chloramphenicol acetyl transferases (CATs) [2] and chloramphenicol exporters, such as CmlA [3]. Over the past decade, most reports have demonstrated that the bacteria causing animal respiratory diseases show high resistance levels to chloramphenicol but are susceptible to florfenicol [4]. However, the resistance levels and number of bacteria that are resistant to florfenicol have increased due to the widespread use of florfenicol in the treatment of animal diseases [5–7]. A study on 1001 bacterial isolates showed that the resistance rates for trimethoprim/sulfamethoxazole and tetracycline were 3.0% and 14.7% in *Actinobacillus pleuropneumoniae* and 6.0% and 81.8% in *S. suis*, respectively, while the resistance rate for florfenicol was < 1% for all strains [8]. Other reports have cited different resistance rates. In Australia, 2.0% and 6.0% of *A. pleuropneumoniae* and *Pasteurella multocida* strains isolated from pig respiratory infections were resistant to florfenicol, respectively [9]. The resistance rate of *E. coli* strains from canine urinary tract infections to florfenicol was higher than that of other pathogens: 31.6% (36/114) [5].

The first florfenicol resistance gene, *pp-flo* (renamed *flo*), was identified on a plasmid in the fish pathogen *Photobacterium damselae* subsp. *piscicida* in 1996 [10]. The *floR* gene is closely related (97% identity) to the *flo* gene [11], and their proteins share 47% amino acid sequence identity with the CmlA protein. The *floR* gene was first reported in 1999 on the chromosome of the worldwide epidemic strain *Salmonella enterica* serovar Typhimurium DT104 [11]. The primary source of human DT104 infections was thought to be animal populations, with both direct contact and foodborne modes of transmission [12]. The IncC plasmid R55, which was initially described to be capable of conferring non-enzymatic chloramphenicol resistance in the 1970s, was then identified in *Klebsiella pneumoniae* [13]. Currently, nine florfenicol resistance genes [*floR*, *floRv*, *floSt*, *fexA*, *fexB*, *pexA*, *cfr*, *optrA* and *estDL136*] have been identified. With the exception of *cfr* and *estDL136*, which encode a 23S rRNA methyltransferase and a hydrolase, respectively, all of the genes encode exporters [14–18]. The *floR* gene and its analogs have mainly been identified in gram-negative bacteria, whereas the other resistance genes have mainly been detected in gram-positive bacteria [15–17].

Similar to other resistance genes, *floR* has been identified on both chromosomes and plasmids and has often been associated with mobile genetic elements and genomic islands [19, 20]. Mobile genetic elements enable translocation of the *floR* gene between DNA molecules, such as chromosomes and plasmids. A plasmid carrying the *floR* gene can spread among bacteria of the same and different species or genera via conjugation or transformation, thereby disseminating resistance [21]. Bacteria generally obtain multiple resistance genes through the horizontal transfer of plasmids carrying resistance genes [22].

K. pneumoniae, which is a member of the *Enterobacteriaceae*, is an opportunistic pathogen for both animals and humans. This bacterium is pervasive in the natural environment and benignly colonizes the gastrointestinal tracts of healthy humans and animals. However, the bacterium is also capable of causing a wide range of diseases in humans and different animal species [23]. *K. pneumoniae* strains are a common cause of health-care associated infections including pneumonia, urinary tract infections (UTIs), and bloodstream infections for critically ill and immunocompromised patients. These strains also infect healthy people in community settings, causing severe infections including pyogenic liver abscess, endophthalmitis, and meningitis [24]. For example, in animals, *K. pneumoniae* strains are well documented to cause mastitis and wounds in cattle [25]; endometritis, cystitis, and liver abscess in horses; tracheitis and wounds in birds; cystitis, phlebitis and otitis externa in dogs; and cystitis in cats [26]. *K. pneumoniae* has also been associated with classical foodborne disease outbreaks [19]. Notably, the prevalence of antibiotic resistance is increasing among *Enterobacteriaceae*, including *K. pneumoniae* [23, 27]. In this study, we used multiple genetic approaches to investigate the *floR* gene in *K. pneumoniae* isolates of human origin and to further demonstrate the potential transmission of this resistance determinant between animal and human pathogens.

Methods

Bacterial strains

The 328 non-duplicate *K. pneumoniae* strains used in this work were isolated from patient samples at the First Affiliated Hospital of Wenzhou Medical University in Wenzhou, China, from 2010 to 2014. This sample set included all *K. pneumoniae* strains collected during this time frame. Among these isolates, 55 were isolated in 2010, 109 in 2011, 55 in 2013 and 109 in 2014. The strains were identified using the Vitek-60 microorganism auto-analysis system (BioMerieux Corporate, Craponne, France).

PCR amplification of the *floR* gene

Total genomic DNA was extracted from the 328 isolates using AxyPrep Bacterial Genomic DNA Miniprep kits (Axygen Scientific, Union City, CA, USA). Template DNA was screened for the *floR* gene using a PCR method. According to the conserved *floR* gene-related regions of the *K. pneumoniae* genome obtained from a pool of strains mainly from this work [28], *floR* gene screening primers were designed and named $P_{SCR\text{-}F}$ and $P_{SCR\text{-}R\text{-}A/G}$, which correspond to the cm101 and cm115 primer sequences, respectively [29]. The sequence of the forward primer $P_{SCR\text{-}F}$ was 5'-TTTGGTCCGCTCTC AGAC-3′. Two variants of the reverse primer were used due to a single nucleotide polymorphism (A/G) identified in the region where the primer was designed: 5'-CGAGAAGAAG**A**CGAAGAAG-3′ ($P_{SCR\text{-}R\text{-}A}$) and 5'-CGAGAAGAAG**G**CGAAGAAG-3′ ($P_{SCR\text{-}R\text{-}G}$). These primers yield a product 496 bp in length. PCR amplification was carried out under the following conditions: an initial denaturation of 5 min at 95 °C; 35 cycles of denaturation (94 °C for 45 s), annealing (58 °C for 45 s), and extension (72 °C for 90 s); and a final extension step at 72 °C for 10 min [29]. The PCR products were purified using a MinElute PCR Purification kit (QIAGEN China, Shanghai, China) and sequenced by Sanger sequencing (in this work, all the PCR products and cloned fragments were sequenced by Sanger sequencing). The nucleotide sequences were analyzed and compared using the BLAST program (http://www.ncbi.nlm.nih.gov/BLAST).

Antimicrobial susceptibility testing

Antimicrobial susceptibility testing performed via the agar dilution method in accordance with the guidelines of the Clinical and Laboratory Standards Institute (CLSI document M100-S27, 2017) was used to determine the minimum inhibitory concentrations (MICs) [30]. The resistance threshold values (32 μg/mL) for both chloramphenicol and florfenicol were chosen according to the guidelines of CLSI document M100-S27 (2017) [30] and a publication for *E. coli* [31], respectively. *E. coli* ATCC 25922 was used as a quality control strain.

Pulsed-field gel electrophoresis (PFGE)

To assess the epidemiology of clinical isolates with *floR* genes, genomic DNA from *K. pneumoniae* isolates harboring *floR* genes was prepared for PFGE typing and digested with 40 U of *Xba* I (Takara, Dalian, China). The protocol and the *Xba* I restriction patterns of genomic DNA from the isolates were analyzed and interpreted according to initial criteria [32]. The Bio-Rad Quantity One program was used to analyze the PFGE results, and a minimum spanning tree was constructed using a categorical coefficient with unweighted pair group method with arithmetic mean (UPGMA) clustering [33].

Plasmid DNA extraction and sequencing

For plasmid (pKP18–125) sequencing, the transconjugant KP18/EC600 was incubated overnight in 5 mL of Luria-Bertani broth at 37 °C for approximately 16 h to an optimum optical density (OD_{600}) of 1.5 ± 0.2. The plasmid was then extracted using the alkaline lysis method as described previously [34]. Plasmid DNA was sequenced via Illumina HiSeq-2000 and Pacific Bioscience sequencing methods at the Beijing Genomics Institute (Beijing, China). Reads derived from the HiSeq-2000 sequencing were initially assembled de novo using SOAPdenovo software to obtain contigs of the plasmid. Pacific Bioscience sequencing reads of approximately 10–20 kb in length were mapped onto the primary assembly to scaffold the contigs. The gaps were filled either by remapping the short reads from HiSeq-2000 sequencing or by PCR product sequencing of the gaps. Glimmer software was used to predict protein-coding genes with potential open reading frames (ORF) > 150 bp [35]. Gview was used to construct basic plasmid features [36]. BLASTX was used to annotate the predicted protein-coding genes against the non-redundant protein database using an e-value threshold of 1e-5.

Collection and processing of *floR* gene-related sequences

In addition to the pKP18–125 sequence, other sequences containing the *floR* gene were obtained from the NCBI nucleotide database using *floR*, *pp-flo*, *flo*, *cmlA-like*, *floRv* and *floSt* as key terms. The resulting sequences were filtered, and only sequences containing a complete *floR* gene more than 9 kb in length (with approximately 4 kb both upstream and downstream of the *floR* gene) were retained. Multiple sequence alignments were performed using mafft with the 9-kb *floR* gene-related fragment of pKP18–125 (KY082186) as a reference [32], and the sequences were clustered with an identity of 80%. The sequence with greatest similarity to the other sequences in each cluster was chosen as a candidate for orthologous analysis. Orthologous groups of genes from the candidate sequences were identified using BLASTP and InParanoid [37]. The sequence retrieval, statistical analyses and other bioinformatics tools used in this study were accomplished using Python and Biopython scripts [38].

Cloning experiments

To identify and clone *floR* genes, we PCR amplified a fragment including the *floR* ORF sequence and its upstream 354-bp potential promotor region from strains positive for the *floR* gene. A set of PCR primers ($P_{ORF\text{-}F}$ and $P_{ORF\text{-}R}$) was designed using the *K. pneumoniae* plasmid pR55 sequence (JQ010984.1) as a reference. The primer sequences of $P_{ORF\text{-}F}$ and $P_{ORF\text{-}R}$ were 5'-GTCG AGAAATCCCATGAGTTCA-3′ and 5'-CAGACAGGA TACCGACATTCAC-3′, respectively. The PCR products were eluted from agarose gels and ligated into the pMD18 vector (TaKaRa, Dalian, China). Each recombinant plasmid (pMD18-*floR*) was transformed into *E. coli*

JM109 using the calcium chloride method, after which the bacterial colonies were grown on Luria-Bertani agar plates supplemented with ampicillin (100 μg/mL). The recombinant plasmids were isolated and digested with restriction enzymes to confirm insertion of a *floR* fragment of approximately 1600 bp in length. Each cloned *floR* fragment was analyzed by Sanger sequencing from a purified transformant and was further compared to the reference *floR* gene (JQ010984.1) using the BLASTN program.

Conjugation experiments

To examine the conjugation potential of resistance gene-harboring pKP18–125, we used rifampin-resistant EC600 as a recipient strain in a biparental mating, which was performed overnight at 37 °C on sterile nitrocellulose filters as previously described [39]. The transconjugants were selected on Mueller-Hinton agar plates containing 1200 μg/mL of rifampin and 16 μg/mL of florfenicol [40]. Plasmid DNA was extracted from transconjugants, and the presence of the *floR* gene was verified by PCR and PCR product sequencing. The plasmid (pKP18–125) of one transconjugant (KP18/EC600) was sequenced in full to verify that the *floR* gene was encoded on this transferable plasmid.

Results

floR gene detection and sequencing

Approximately 7.01% (23/328) of the isolates were positive for *floR* (Table 1). Of the 23 *floR*-positive strains, 4, 8, 4 and 7 strains were isolated in 2010, 2011, 2013 and 2014, respectively. The positive rates were similar among the strains collected from different years (7.27% [4/55] in 2010, 7.34% [8/109] in 2011, 7.27% [4/55] in 2013 and 6.42% [7/109] in 2014). Twenty-two fragments containing the *floR* ORF and their upstream potential promotor regions were successfully cloned; all the cloned ORF sequences shared approximately 99% nucleotide sequence identity. No amino acid variants were identified in the cloned ORFs.

Florfenicol and chloramphenicol MICs of the strains

The MICs of florfenicol and chloramphenicol were determined for the 328 clinical isolates, 3 transconjugants and transformants with cloned *floR* genes. The MIC results showed that 57 of the 328 clinical isolates (17.38%) were resistant to both florfenicol and chloramphenicol, whereas 67 (20.42%) and 113 (34.45%) of the strains were resistant to florfenicol and chloramphenicol, respectively. A total of 7.62% (25/328) and 11.59% (38/328) of the strains were resistant to florfenicol and chloramphenicol, respectively, with MIC values ≥512 μg/mL, and 64.93% (213/328) of the strains were susceptible, with MIC values < 32 μg/mL for both antibacterial agents.

The strains positive for the *floR* gene had much higher MIC values for both florfenicol and chloramphenicol than the *floR*-negative strains. Of the 23 *floR*-positive strains, 95.65% (22/23) showed high MIC values to florfenicol (≥512 μg/mL) (Table 2). Among the 305 strains negative for the *floR* gene, only 14.43% of the strains (44/305) showed resistance to florfenicol, and only 1.64% (5/305) of the strains had MIC values ≥512 μg/mL. The MIC values between the transformants with cloned *floR* genes and the clinical isolates were similar (Table 2).

A transferable plasmid carrying the *floR* gene

The results of the conjugation experiments for the 23 *floR*-positive clinical isolates showed that plasmids in

Table 1 Strains and plasmids used in this study

Strain or plasmid	Relevant characteristic(s)[a]	Reference or source
Strain		
KP1 - KP23	23 strains carrying the *floR* gene from 328 clinically isolated *K. pneumoniae* samples	this study
JM109	*Escherichia coli* JM109 was used as a host for the PCR product cloning	
EC600	*Escherichia coli* C600 *was* used as a host in conjugation experiments; Rf^r	
ATCC25922	*Escherichia coli* ATCC25922 is an FDA clinical isolate	
E. coli carrying plasmid		
pMD18-*floR*s/JM109	JM109 carrying the pMD18 vector encoding *floR* gene regions from 22 *floR* gene-positive strains	This study
pKP5/EC600	The transconjugant with KP5 plasmid transferred into EC600	This study
pKP6/EC600	The transconjugant with KP6 plasmid transferred into EC600	This study
pKP18/EC600	The transconjugant with KP18 plasmid transferred into EC600	This study
Plasmid		
pKP18–125	KP18 plasmid transferred into EC600 by conjugation and sequenced	This study
pMD18	Cloning vector for the PCR products of *floR* genes; Ap^r	TaKaRa

[a]*Rf* rifampin, *Ap* ampicillin

Table 2 MIC values for the *floR*-positive *K. pneumoniae* strains, transformants expressing cloned *floR* genes and transconjugants (μg/mL)

	Florfenicol			Chloramphenicol		
Name	Clinical isolate	Transformant	Transconjugant	Clinical isolate	Transformant	Transconjugant
KP5	1024	512	512	256	128	512
KP6	1024	256	512	512	256	512
KP18	> 1024	512	512	512	128	256
KP23	64			256		
KP4, 14, 19, 22	512			256		
KP21	512			128		
KP3, 8, 15	1024			1024		
KP10, 12, 13	1024			256		
KP11, 20	1024			128		
KP2, 7, 9, 16, 17	> 1024			> 1024		
KP1	> 1024			512		
ATCC25922	4					
JM109	4					
EC600	4					

three donor strains (KP5, KP6 and KP18) were successfully transferred to the recipient. PFGE analysis showed that the wild-type donors KP5, KP6 and KP18 harbored 2, 4 and 2 plasmids, respectively. However, each of the transconjugants (KP5/EC600, KP6/EC600 and KP18/EC600) only harbored the largest plasmid of the donor cells. The results of PCR product sequencing confirmed that *floR* genes were located on the transferred plasmids. The MIC results showed that the florfenicol and chloramphenicol resistance levels of the transconjugants were similar to those of the donor strains (Table 2).

Clonal relatedness of the *floR*-positive *K. pneumoniae* strains identified by PFGE

PFGE patterns with ≥80% identity were interpreted as closely or possibly related to the outbreak isolates. Of the 23 strains detected, 22 had good fingerprints; one strain (KP21) without clear bands could not be compared. Only two strains (KP5 and KP6) showed similar

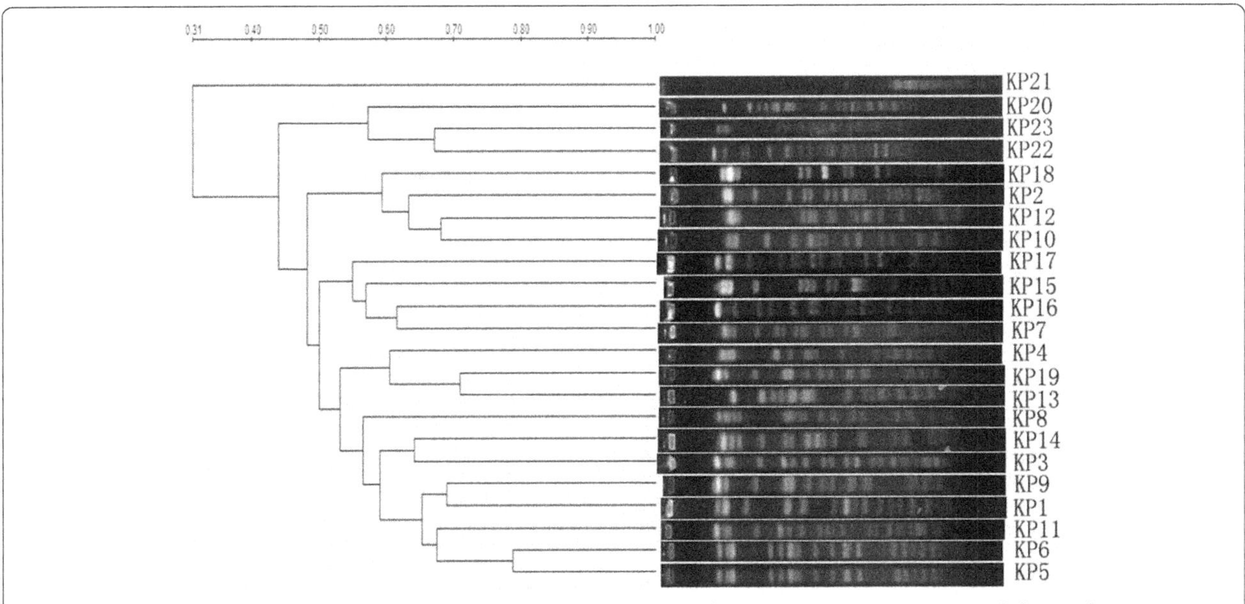

Fig. 1 Pulsed-field gel electrophoresis of *XbaI*-digested genomic DNA from the 22 *floR*-positive *K. pneumoniae* strains. Only one cluster, composed of KP5 and KP6, was determined to be clonally related

fingerprint patterns, whereas the remaining 20 strains had different genotypes (Fig. 1). KP5 was isolated from a sputum sample of a male patient in the Department of Neurosurgery in March 2014, while KP6 came from a sputum sample of a female patient in the intensive care unit (ICU) in the Department of Brain Surgery in April 2014.

Structure and comparative genomics analysis of *floR* gene-related regions

pKP18–125 was 125,329 bp in length. Annotation determined that the plasmid carried one replicon belonging to incompatibility group FII (IncFII) and harbored 164 coding sequences (CDs). The plasmid genome can be divided into 4 regions according to the functions of the ORFs as follows: the variable region, the conjugation region, the transfer leading region and the replication region. The variable region is approximately 40 kb in length and encodes 42 ORFs, including approximately 20 genes related to drug resistance, 13 recombination-related genes or structures (i.e., integrase and transposase genes and insertion sequences [ISs]) and 9 genes of unknown function. According to the structure of the mobile genetic elements, this region could be roughly divided into six units, including one class 1 integron and five transposons. The *floR* gene was located in a transposon-like fragment approximately 9 kb in length (accession number: KY082186) consisting of a conserved gene cluster of *lysR-floR-virD2*, 5 *tnp* units and two direct repeats (DRs). In this work, we mainly analyzed the structural characteristics of the 9-kb *floR* gene-related transposon-like fragment (Fig. 2).

Overall, a total of 105 DNA sequences of approximately 9 kb in length with the *floR* gene in their center were retrieved from all *floR* gene-containing sequences in the NCBI nucleotide database. Of these sequences, 45 were from complete or partial bacterial chromosomes, and 60 were from plasmid sequences. Through a multiple sequence alignment, 27 clusters with identities greater than 80% were obtained. According to the similarity of the core sequences adjacent to the *floR* gene, the sequences of these 27 clusters were orthologously analyzed and further clustered into 4 groups (G1- G4), with each group containing 2 subgroups (e.g., G1a and G1b). Group 1 consisted of only 2 sequences (KY082186 and KT282968) that shared approximately 7 kb in common (Fig. 1 and Table S1).

Eight representative sequences from the eight subgroups (one from each subgroup) are illustrated in Fig. 2 with their accession numbers. Sequences similar to the representative sequences are shown in Additional file 1: Table S1. The results of this orthologous analysis revealed that an approximately 2-kb sequence encoding *lysR-floR-virD2* was conserved and present in the majority of the sequences (79.0%, 83/105). Many of these sequences also shared the same upstream DR and complete or truncated downstream *tnp* unit (Fig. 1). The 9-kb *floR* gene-related transposon-like fragment of pKP18–125 in this study showed highest similarity to a 7-kb fragment from the plasmid pEC012 (KT282968). Interestingly, although pKP18–125 was isolated from a *K. pneumoniae* strain from a patient in South China, pEC012

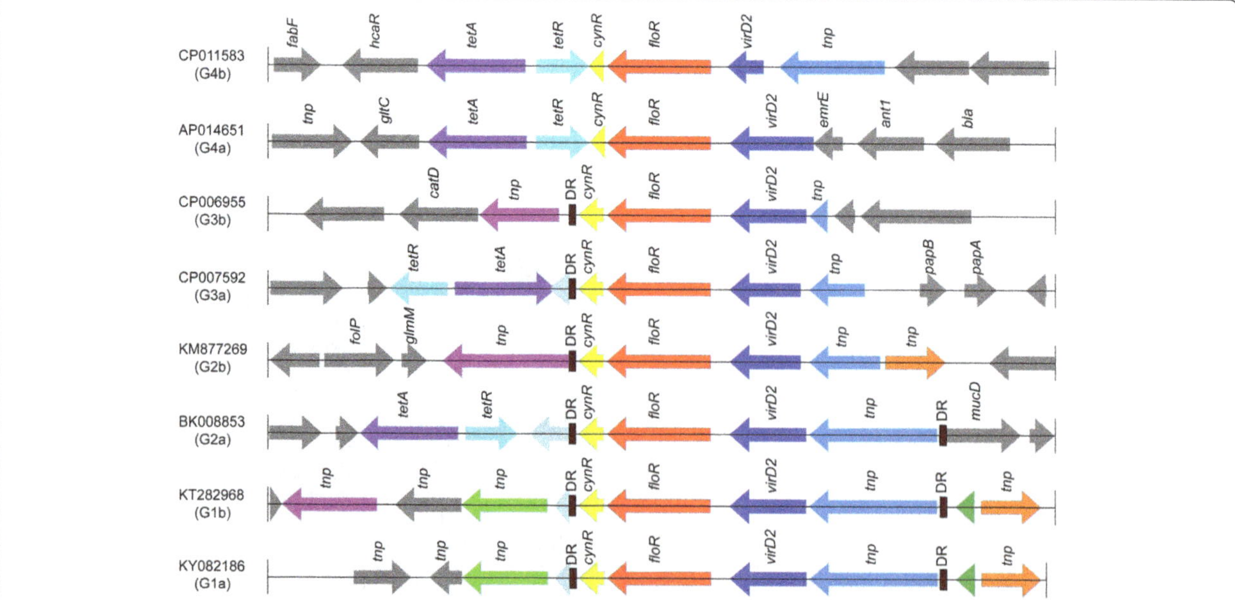

Fig. 2 Structure of the *floR* gene-related regions. Eight representative sequences from the four groups (one from each subgroup) are presented with their accession numbers. The arrows represent sequence units, and the same units are shown in the same color. The names of the sequence units are indicated over the arrows, with the sequence units of unknown function left blank

was found in an *E. coli* isolate from a chicken in North China [41].

Discussion

In this study, we found that among all the clinical *K. pneumoniae* isolates detected, 20.42% (67/328) were resistant to florfenicol, of which 7.01% (23/328) carried the *floR* gene, but 13.41% (44/328) were free of the *floR* gene. A similar report demonstrated a *floR* gene positivity rate of only 21.8% (26/119) among 119 florfenicol-resistant gram-negative bacilli from several freshwater Chilean salmon farms [42]. Our MIC results for the 328 strains demonstrated that the *floR* gene played a key role in the resistance of these bacteria to florfenicol. The *floR*-positive strains had a much higher resistance rate (23/23, 100%) and much higher MIC values for florfenicol (22/23, 95.65% with MIC values ≥512 μg/mL) than the *floR*-negative strains, which had a resistance rate of 14.43% (44/305) with only 1.64% (5/305) of the strains having MIC values ≥512 μg/mL. At present, of the nine florfenicol resistance genes, the *floR* gene is the only known florfenicol resistance gene that has been identified in *K. pneumoniae* strains of either human or animal origin [43]. Five genes (*fexA*, *fexB*, *pexA*, *optrA* and *cfr*) were mainly identified in gram-positive bacteria [15–17]. The *cfr* gene has also been occasionally identified in *E. coli* or *Proteus vulgaris* [44, 45] and *fexA* and *pexA* were once identified in *E. coli* [44]. The other three genes have only been identified in certain gram-negative bacteria (*floRv* in *Stenotrophomonas maltophilia* [46], *floSt* in *Salmonella* [47] and *estDL136* in *E.coli* [44]). We hypothesize that other mechanisms, such as exporters and enzymes, in addition to the known florfenicol resistance genes, may also be responsible for florfenicol resistance in gram-negative bacteria including *K. pneumoniae*.

The *floR* genes were located on both chromosomes and plasmids amidst various mobile genetic elements, indicating that horizontal transfer of the *floR* gene occurred among bacteria of different species. The *floR* gene was identified first on the chromosome of *S. typhimurium* DT104 (*Salmonella typhimurium* DT104) and then on a plasmid of *E. coli* isolate BN10660 [48] and was also identified on the IncC plasmid R55 harbored by *K. pneumoniae* [13] and on other sources [17, 43]. In *S. typhimurium* DT104, the *floR* gene was included in a 12.5-kb region with multiple resistance genes. The *tetR* and *tetA* tetracycline resistance genes were located downstream of the *floR* gene and were flanked by two integrons. One integron contained an *aadA2* gene and an incomplete *sulI* resistance gene, and the other harbored a β-lactamase gene and a complete *sulI* gene [49]. In pKP18–125, the downstream region was a class 1 integron that contained 5 resistance genes (*acc(6′)*, *arr2*, etc.) and was different from the 12.5-kb region of the *S. typhimurium* DT104 chromosome. Interestingly, the sequence most similar to the *floR*-containing fragment on pKP18–125 from a clinical *Klebsiella pneumoniae* isolate was located on pEC012 (KT282968), a plasmid from an *E. coli* strain isolated from a chicken [50]. This finding suggests that horizontal transfer of the *floR*-containing fragment occurred between bacteria of animal and human origins.

Our PFGE analysis revealed that two *floR*-positive strains (KP5 and KP6) had similar PFGE profiles. They were isolated from the same sample type (sputum) but were found in different hospitalized patients during different time periods. Some *K. pneumoniae* strains carrying resistance genes were previously reported to have caused outbreaks in European countries, indicating the potential risk of the spread of resistance genes through bacterial outbreaks, especially those caused by bacteria with resistance plasmids [51]. Although the relationship between the two strains carrying *floR* is still in question, effort should be made to avoid any pathogen outbreaks in hospital environments.

Conclusions

Our study demonstrated that 20.42% (67/328) of the clinical *K. pneumoniae* isolates were resistant to florfenicol, but only 7.01% (23/328) carried the *floR* gene. The *floR* gene was related to a transposon-like sequence and located on a conjugative plasmid. The most similar sequence to the *floR*-containing fragment on pKP18–125 was that a fragment on pEC012 in an *E. coli* strain isolated from a chicken. This finding indicates that resistance genes in animal pathogens might be disseminated to human pathogens. The dissemination of resistance genes from animals to humans reflects the risk to human health of antimicrobial agent use in animals. In addition, these results highlight the critical need to consistently implement effective strategies to prevent transmission and infection. Combating antibiotic-resistant bacteria supports patient care, agriculture, economic growth and national security.

Abbreviations

Ap: Ampicillin; BLAST: Basic local alignment search tool; ICU: Intensive care unit; MICs: Minimum inhibitory concentrations; PFGE: Pulsed-field gel electrophoresis; Rf: Rifampin

Acknowledgments

The authors would like to acknowledge all study participants and individuals who contributed to the study.

Funding

This work was funded by grants from the Natural Science Foundation of Zhejiang Province (LY14C060005 and LQ17H190001), the Science and Technology Foundation of Zhejiang Province (2015C33196) and the National Natural Science Foundation of China (81401702, 81501808 and 81501780).

Authors' contributions

JL, JZ, LX, YL, TZ and SL collected the strains and performed the experiments. KL, WZ and LN analyzed the experimental results. PL, TX and HY performed the bioinformatics analysis. JL, CC and QB wrote the manuscript. CC and QB designed the experiments. All authors read and approved the final manuscript.

Consent for publication

Not applicable.

Competing interests

The authors declare that they have no competing interests.

Author details

[1]School of Medicine and Health, Lishui University, Lishui 323000, China. [2]School of Laboratory Medicine and Life Sciences/Institute of Biomedical Informatics, Wenzhou Medical University, Wenzhou 325035, China. [3]The Second Affiliated Hospital, Wenzhou Medical University, Wenzhou 325035, China.

References

1. Apley MD. Clinical evidence for individual animal therapy for papillomatous digital dermatitis (hairy heel wart) and infectious bovine pododermatitis (foot rot). Vet Clin North Am Food Anim Pract. 2015;31:81–95. https://doi.org/10.1016/j.cvfa.2014.11.009.
2. Gaffney D, Foster T. Chloramphenicol acetyltransferases determined by R plasmids from gram-negative bacteria. J Gen Microbiol. 1978;109:351–8.
3. Schwarz S, Kehrenberg C, Doublet B, Cloeckaert A. Molecular basis of bacterial resistance to chloramphenicol and florfenicol. FEMS Microbiol Rev. 2004;28:519–42. https://doi.org/10.1016/j.femsre.2004.04.001.
4. Kucerova Z, Hradecka H, Nechvatalova K, Nedbalcova K. Antimicrobial susceptibility of Actinobacillus pleuropneumoniae isolates from clinical outbreaks of porcine respiratory diseases. Vet Microbiol. 2011;150:203–6. https://doi.org/10.1016/j.vetmic.2011.01.016.
5. Chang SK, Lo DY, Wei HW, Kuo HC. Antimicrobial resistance of Escherichia coli isolates from canine urinary tract infections. J Vet Med Sci. 2015;77:59–65. https://doi.org/10.1292/jvms.13-0281.
6. Geng Y, Wang KY, Huang XL, Chen DF, Li CW, Ren SY, et al. Streptococcus agalactiae, an emerging pathogen for cultured ya-fish, Schizothorax prenanti, in China. Transbound Emerg Dis. 2012;59:369–75. https://doi.org/10.1111/j.1865-1682.2011.01280.x.
7. Sun F, Zhou D, Wang Q, Feng J, Feng W, Luo W, et al. Genetic characterization of a novel blaDIM-2-carrying megaplasmid p12969-DIM from clinical Pseudomonas putida. J Antimicrob Chemother. 2016;71:909–12. https://doi.org/10.1093/jac/dkv426.
8. de Jong A, Thomas V, Simjee S, Moyaert H, El Garch F, Maher K, et al. Antimicrobial susceptibility monitoring of respiratory tract pathogens isolated from diseased cattle and pigs across Europe: the VetPath study. Vet Microbiol. 2014;172:202–15. https://doi.org/10.1016/j.vetmic.2014.04.008.
9. Dayao DA, Gibson JS, Blackall PJ, Turni C. Antimicrobial resistance in bacteria associated with porcine respiratory disease in Australia. Vet Microbiol. 2014;171:232–5. https://doi.org/10.1016/j.vetmic.2014.03.014.
10. Kim E, Aoki T. Sequence analysis of the florfenicol resistance gene encoded in the transferable R-plasmid of a fish pathogen, Pasteurella piscicida. Microbiol Immunol. 1996;40:665–9.
11. Arcangioli MA, Leroy-Setrin S, Martel JL, Chaslus-Dancla E. A new chloramphenicol and florfenicol resistance gene flanked by two integron structures in Salmonella typhimurium DT104. FEMS Microbiol Lett. 1999;174:327–32.
12. Mather AE, Reid SW, Maskell DJ, Parkhill J, Fookes MC, Harris SR, et al. Distinguishable epidemics of multidrug-resistant Salmonella typhimurium DT104 in different hosts. Science. 2013;341:1514–7. https://doi.org/10.1126/science.1240578.
13. Cloeckaert A, Baucheron S, Chaslus-Dancla E. Nonenzymatic chloramphenicol resistance mediated by IncC plasmid R55 is encoded by a floR gene variant. Antimicrob Agents Chemother. 2001;45:2381–2. https://doi.org/10.1128/AAC.45.8.2381-2382.2001
14. Wang Y, Zhang W, Wang J, Wu C, Shen Z, Fu X, et al. Distribution of the multidrug resistance gene cfr in Staphylococcus species isolates from swine farms in China. Antimicrob Agents Chemother. 2012;56:1485–90. https://doi.org/10.1128/AAC.05827-11.
15. Lang KS, Anderson JM, Schwarz S, Williamson L, Handelsman J, Singer RS. Novel florfenicol and chloramphenicol resistance gene discovered in Alaskan soil by using functional metagenomics. Appl Environ Microbiol. 2010;76:5321–6. https://doi.org/10.1128/AEM.00323-10.
16. Couto N, Belas A, Rodrigues C, Schwarz S, Pomba C. Acquisition of the fexA and cfr genes in Staphylococcus pseudintermedius during florfenicol treatment of canine pyoderma. J Glob Antimicrob Resist. 2016;7:126–7. https://doi.org/10.1016/j.jgar.2016.08.008.
17. Liu H, Wang Y, Wu C, Schwarz S, Shen Z, Jeon B, et al. A novel phenicol exporter gene, fexB, found in enterococci of animal origin. J Antimicrob Chemother. 2012;67:322–5. https://doi.org/10.1093/jac/dkr481.
18. Tao W, Lee MH, Wu J, Kim NH, Kim JC, Chung E, et al. Inactivation of chloramphenicol and florfenicol by a novel chloramphenicol hydrolase. Appl Environ Microbiol. 2012;78:6295–301. https://doi.org/10.1128/AEM.01154-12.
19. Gabida M, Gombe NT, Chemhuru M, Takundwa L, Bangure D, Tshimanga M. Foodborne illness among factory workers, Gweru, Zimbabwe, 2012: a retrospective cohort study. BMC Res Notes. 2015;8:493. https://doi.org/10.1186/s13104-015-1512-2.
20. Lai J, Wang Y, Shen J, Li R, Han J, Foley SL, et al. Unique class 1 integron and multiple resistance genes co-located on IncHI2 plasmid is associated with the emerging multidrug resistance of Salmonella Indiana isolated from chicken in China. Foodborne Pathog Dis. 2013;10:581–8. https://doi.org/10.1089/fpd.2012.1455.
21. da Silva GC, Rossi CC, Santana MF, Langford PR, Bosse JT, Bazzolli DMS. p518, a small floR plasmid from a south American isolate of Actinobacillus pleuropneumoniae. Vet Microbiol. 2017;204:129–32. https://doi.org/10.1016/j.vetmic.2017.04.019.
22. Anantham S, Harmer CJ, Hall RM. p39R861-4, a type 2 a/C2 plasmid carrying a segment from the a/C1 plasmid RA1. Microb Drug Resist. 2015;21:571–6. https://doi.org/10.1089/mdr.2015.0133.
23. Davis GS, Price LB. Recent research examining links among Klebsiella pneumoniae from food, food animals, and human extraintestinal infections. Curr Environ Health Rep. 2016;3:128–35. https://doi.org/10.1007/s40572-016-0089-9.
24. Martin RM, Bachman MA. Colonization, infection, and the accessory genome of Klebsiella pneumoniae. Front Cell Infect Microbiol. 2018;8:4. https://doi.org/10.3389/fcimb.2018.00004.
25. Kikuchi N, Kagota C, Nomura T, Hiramune T, Takahashi T, Yanagawa R. Plasmid profiles of Klebsiella pneumoniae isolated from bovine mastitis. Vet Microbiol. 1995;47:9–15.
26. Brisse S, Duijkeren E. Identification and antimicrobial susceptibility of 100 Klebsiella animal clinical isolates. Vet Microbiol. 2005;105:307–12. https://doi.org/10.1016/j.vetmic.2004.11.010.
27. Tzouvelekis LS, Markogiannakis A, Psichogiou M, Tassios PT, Daikos GL. Carbapenemases in Klebsiella pneumoniae and other Enterobacteriaceae: an evolving crisis of global dimensions. Clin Microbiol Rev. 2012;25:682–707. https://doi.org/10.1128/CMR.05035-11.
28. Ying J, Wang H, Bao B, Zhang Y, Zhang J, Zhang C, et al. Molecular variation and horizontal gene transfer of the homocysteine methyltransferase gene mmuM and its distribution in clinical pathogens. Int J Biol Sci. 2015;11:11–21. https://doi.org/10.7150/ijbs.10320.
29. Arcangioli MA, Leroy-Setrin S, Martel JL, Chaslus-Dancla E. Evolution of chloramphenicol resistance, with emergence of cross-resistance to florfenicol, in bovine Salmonella typhimurium strains implicates definitive phage type (DT) 104. J Med Microbiol. 2000;49:103–10. https://doi.org/10.1099/0022-1317-49-1-103.
30. Clinical and Laboratory Standards Institute. Performance standards for antimicrobial susceptibility testing; 27th informational supplement. In: Document; 2017. p. M100–S27.
31. Wasyl D, Hoszowski A, Zajac M, Szulowski K. Antimicrobial resistance in commensal Escherichia coli isolated from animals at slaughter. Front Microbiol. 2013;4:221. https://doi.org/10.3389/fmicb.2013.00221.
32. Katoh K, Standley DM. MAFFT multiple sequence alignment software version 7: improvements in performance and usability. Mol Biol Evol. 2013;30:772 80. https://doi.org/10.1093/molbev/mst010

33. Roussel S, Felix B, Vingadassalon N, Grout J, Hennekinne JA, Guillier L, et al. Staphylococcus aureus strains associated with food poisoning outbreaks in France: comparison of different molecular typing methods, including MLVA. Front Microbiol. 2015;6:882. https://doi.org/10.3389/fmicb.2015.00882.
34. Yi H, Xi Y, Liu J, Wang J, Wu J, Xu T, et al. Sequence analysis of pKF3-70 in Klebsiella pneumoniae: probable origin from R100-like plasmid of Escherichia coli. PLoS One. 2010;5:e8601. https://doi.org/10.1371/journal.pone.0008601.
35. Delcher AL, Bratke KA, Powers EC, Salzberg SL. Identifying bacterial genes and endosymbiont DNA with glimmer. Bioinformatics. 2007;23:673–9. https://doi.org/10.1093/bioinformatics/btm009.
36. Petkau A, Stuart-Edwards M, Stothard P, Van Domselaar G. Interactive microbial genome visualization with GView. Bioinformatics. 2010;26:3125–6. https://doi.org/10.1093/bioinformatics/btq588.
37. Remm M, Storm CE, Sonnhammer EL. Automatic clustering of orthologs and in-paralogs from pairwise species comparisons. J Mol Biol. 2001;314: 1041–52. https://doi.org/10.1006/jmbi.2000.5197.
38. Hu L, Zhong Q, Tu J, Xu Y, Qin Z, Parsons C, et al. Emergence of blaNDM-1 among Klebsiella pneumoniae ST15 and novel ST1031 clinical isolates in China. Diagn Microbiol Infect Dis. 2013;75:373–6. https://doi.org/10.1016/j.diagmicrobio.2013.01.006.
39. Xu T, Ying J, Yao X, Song Y, Ma P, Bao B, et al. Identification and characterization of two novel Bla(KLUC) resistance genes through large-scale resistance plasmids sequencing. PLoS One. 2012;7:e47197. https://doi.org/10.1371/journal.pone.0047197.
40. Rice LB, Carias LL, Bonomo RA, Shlaes DM. Molecular genetics of resistance to both ceftazidime and beta-lactam-beta-lactamase inhibitor combinations in Klebsiella pneumoniae and in vivo response to beta-lactam therapy. J Infect Dis. 1996;173:151–8.
41. Li XS, Wang GQ, Du XD, Cui BA, Zhang SM, Shen JZ. Antimicrobial susceptibility and molecular detection of chloramphenicol and florfenicol resistance among Escherichia coli isolates from diseased chickens. J Vet Sci. 2007;8:243–7.
42. Fernandez-Alarcon C, Miranda CD, Singer RS, Lopez Y, Rojas R, Bello H, et al. Detection of the floR gene in a diversity of florfenicol resistant gram-negative bacilli from freshwater salmon farms in Chile. Zoonoses Public Health. 2010;57:181–8. https://doi.org/10.1111/j.1863-2378.2009.01243.x.
43. Gordon L, Cloeckaert A, Doublet B, Schwarz S, Bouju-Albert A, Ganiere JP, et al. Complete sequence of the floR-carrying multiresistance plasmid pAB5S9 from freshwater Aeromonas bestiarum. J Antimicrob Chemother. 2008;62: 65–71. https://doi.org/10.1093/jac/dkn166.
44. Zhang A, Yang Y, Wang H, Lei C, Xu C, Guan Z, et al. Prevalence of sulfonamide and Florfenicol resistance genes in Escherichia Coli isolated from yaks (Bos Grunniens) and herdsmen in the Tibetan pasture. J Wildl Dis. 2015;51:626–33. https://doi.org/10.7589/2014-09-234.
45. Wang Y, Wang Y, Wu CM, Schwarz S, Shen Z, Zhang W, et al. Detection of the staphylococcal multiresistance gene cfr in Proteus vulgaris of food animal origin. J Antimicrob Chemother. 2011;66:2521–6. https://doi.org/10.1093/jac/dkr322.
46. He T, Shen J, Schwarz S, Wu C, Wang Y. Characterization of a genomic island in Stenotrophomonas maltophilia that carries a novel floR gene variant. J Antimicrob Chemother. 2015;70:1031–6. https://doi.org/10.1093/jac/dku491.
47. Alessiani A, Sacchini L, Pontieri E, Gavini J, Di Giannatale E. Molecular typing of Salmonella enterica subspecies enterica serovar Typhimurium isolated in Abruzzo region (Italy) from 2008 to 2010. Vet Ital. 2014;50:31–9. https://doi.org/10.12834/VetIt.1304.07.
48. Cloeckaert A, Baucheron S, Flaujac G, Schwarz S, Kehrenberg C, Martel JL, et al. Plasmid-mediated florfenicol resistance encoded by the floR gene in Escherichia coli isolated from cattle. Antimicrob Agents Chemother. 2000;44:2858–60.
49. Cloeckaert A, Sidi Boumedine K, Flaujac G, Imberechts H, D'Hooghe I, Chaslus-Dancla E. Occurrence of a Salmonella enterica serovar typhimurium DT104-like antibiotic resistance gene cluster including the floR gene in S. enterica serovar agona. Antimicrob Agents Chemother. 2000;44:1359–61.
50. Pan YS, Zong ZY, Yuan L, Du XD, Huang H, Zhong XH, et al. Complete sequence of pEC012, a multidrug-resistant IncI1 ST71 plasmid carrying Bla CTX-M-65, rmtB, fosA3, floR, and oqxAB in an avian Escherichia coli ST117 strain. Front Microbiol. 2016;7:1117. https://doi.org/10.3389/fmicb.2016.01117.
51. Hong JS, Yoon EJ, Lee H, Jeong SH, Lee K. Clonal dissemination of Pseudomonas aeruginosa sequence type 235 isolates carrying blaIMP-6 and emergence of blaGES-24 and blaIMP-10 on novel Genomic Islands PAGI-15 and -16 in South Korea. Antimicrob Agents Chemother. 2016;60:7216–23. https://doi.org/10.1128/AAC.01601-16.

Antibiotic consumption and antimicrobial resistance in Poland; findings and implications

Jadwiga Wojkowska-Mach[1†], Brian Godman[2,3,4,5], Amanda Glassman[6], Amanj Kurdi[2,7], Andrzej Pilc[8,9], Anna Rozanska[1], Szymon Skoczyński[10], Marta Wałaszek[11] and Tomasz Bochenek[9*†]

Abstract

Background: The problem of inappropriate use of antibiotics and the resulting growth in antimicrobial resistance (AMR) has implications for Poland and the world. The objective of this paper was to compare and contrast antibiotic resistance and antibiotic utilisation in Poland in recent years versus other European countries, including agreed quality indicators, alongside current AMR patterns and ongoing policies and initiatives in Poland to influence and improve antibiotic prescribing.

Methods: A quantitative ten-year analysis (2007–2016) of the use of antibiotics based on European Centre for Disease Prevention and Control (ECDC) data combined with a literature review on AMR rates and antimicrobial stewardship initiatives.

Results: The system of monitoring AMR and appropriate strategies to address AMR rates remain underdeveloped in Poland. The role of microbiological diagnostics and efforts to prevent infections is currently underestimated by physicians. Overall, Poland had one of the highest rates of total consumption of antibiotics in the analysed European countries. Total consumption of antibacterials for systemic use and relative consumption of beta-lactamase sensitive penicillins were characterized by small but statistically significant average annual increases between 2007 and 2016 (from 22.2 DIDs to 23.9 DIDs and from 0.8 to 1.3%, respectively).

Conclusions: The integrated activities around appropriate antibiotic prescribing in the pre- and post-graduate training of physicians and dentists seem to be particularly important, as well as changes in policies on prescribing antibiotics within ambulatory care. AMR and appropriate prescribing of antibiotics should be the focus of health policy actions in Poland.

Keywords: Antibiotic consumption, Antimicrobial resistance, Antimicrobial resistance surveillance, European Union, Health policy, Poland

Background

General

Antibiotics have significantly improved the prognoses of patients with infectious diseases, reducing morbidity and mortality. However, the use of antibiotics is invariably associated with the risk of resistance development, with numerous studies confirming the association between increasing use of antibiotics and enhanced antimicrobial resistance (AMR) [1–6]. Increasing AMR rates are not helped by concerns regarding the choice of antibiotic or duration of therapy, which can be incorrect in up to 50% of cases [3, 7], as well as the extent of irrational prescribing of antibiotics for essentially viral infections [3], or the increasing use of antibiotics in agriculture [7]. Acute upper respiratory tract infections (URTIs), which are the most common infections in ambulatory care, are essentially viral in origin but with high rates of inappropriate antibiotic use across countries [3, 8–10].

* Correspondence: t.bochenek@uj.edu.pl

[†]Jadwiga Wojkowska-Mach and Tomasz Bochenek contributed equally to this work.

[9]Department of Drug Management, Faculty of Health Sciences, Jagiellonian University Medical College, Grzegorzecka 20 Str., 31-531, Krakow, Poland

Full list of author information is available at the end of the article

As a result of growing concerns, we are seeing an increasing number of programmes and activities across countries, including European countries, to enhance appropriate antibiotic use to reduce AMR rates. These include the development of Antimicrobial Stewardship Program (ASP), as well as educational activities among physicians and pharmacists [8, 11–17]. ASPs include analysis of the consumption of antibiotics over time alongside instigation and monitoring of activities to improve appropriate use.

However, whilst the European Surveillance of Antimicrobial Consumption (ESAC) network, and more recently the European Centre for Disease Prevention and Control (ECDC) [18, 19] and WHO Europe [20], have researched antibiotic utilisation across Europe including Poland, as well as assessed quality indicators for antibiotic utilisation, there is currently limited patient-level data to improve antibiotic prescribing in Poland. Physicians are one of the key stakeholders to improve future antibiotic use in Poland, with limited if any purchasing of antibiotics without a prescription due to current restrictions.

We are aware of concerns with antibiotic prescribing in Poland. A study published in 2008 showed that between 2002 and 2005, at least 64.3% of the studied population were prescribed antibiotics [21]. Panasiuk et al. reported that 78.5% of adults with acute URTIs had antibiotics as empirical first-line treatment [22]. Overall anti-infectives (Anatomical Therapeutic Chemical class: ATC J01-J07X) constituted approximately 5% of pharmaceutical reimbursement in ambulatory care in Poland in 2010, with amoxicillin with clavulanic acid among the top 25 reimbursed medicines with the greatest sales [23]. However, between 2004 and 2008, Poland's total antibiotic use was comparable to the median European level [24].

There have been initiatives in Poland to improve physician antibiotic prescribing through guidelines, with the most recent guidelines published in 2016 [25]. However, there have been concerns whether these have been properly disseminated and implemented, especially given current individualism within the Polish healthcare system, acceptance of authority ('power distance'), and physicians wishing to avoid uncertainty [26]. In addition, current short medical consultations do not allow for establishing a close relationship between physicians and their patients, including educating patients regarding the appropriate use of antibiotics. There are also concerns with the lack of National Health Fund (NHF) activity to improve the prescribing of antibiotics among physicians in Poland unlike co-ordinated activities in, for instance, the Republic of Srpska [14], as well as former Soviet Union Republics, such as Azerbaijan [17].

There are also concerns with the rate of hospital acquired infections in Poland [27], which need addressing alongside generally improving antibiotic utilization in Poland to reduce AMR rates.

Antimicrobial resistance patterns across Europe and activities to reduce AMR

The gathering and analysis of information on drug resistance of bacterial strains among European countries is facilitated by the Healthcare-Associated Infections Surveillance Network (HAI-Net) [28] within the European Centre for Disease Prevention and Control (ECDC). Detailed data on drug resistance of selected bacterial strains and groups of antibiotics are gathered within the European Antimicrobial Resistance Surveillance Network (EARS-Net) [29].

As discussed, there are several ongoing activities across countries to reduce rising AMR rates given ongoing concerns. Identified objectives within the WHO Global Plan on Antimicrobial Resistance [30] included sharing knowledge and evidence, as well as instigating programmes to optimise antibiotic use through education and other activities. This is particularly important in Poland, where the incidence of various types of infections, including surgical site infections [31] and bloodstream infections associated with central venous catheters, appear higher than in neighbouring countries [27].

We are aware there needs to be greater documentation and discussions about current activities in Poland to improve antibiotic use. This includes assessing the quality of antibiotic use in ambulatory care against agreed indicators, including the use of combination penicillins, third- and fourth-generation cephalosporins, as well as fluoroquinolones, as these are considered by the WHO and others as critically important antibiotics to monitor [20, 32, 33].

Consequently, the objective of this paper was to compare and contrast antibiotic resistance and antibiotic utilisation in Poland in recent years versus other European countries, including agreed quality indicators, alongside current AMR patterns and ongoing policies and initiatives in Poland to influence antibiotic prescribing. The findings will help guide the development of future pertinent policies to improve antibiotic prescribing in Poland, given current concerns.

Methods

A quantitative research was conducted on ECDC findings and combined with a literature review to document current antibiotic resistance rates in Poland, as well as initiatives to improve antibiotic prescribing. The literature review was not a systematic review; however, it included most cited expert publications. Simple statistical analyses were performed to help identify any trends where pertinent. We have used such approaches in previous publications to assess the influence of current antibiotic strategies as well as help plan future activities [13, 14, 16, 17]. Table 1 presents the measures which were used to assess the quality of antibiotic prescribing in Poland, in ambulatory care, during the past 10 years (i.e. from 2007 to 2016) based on ECDC, WHO and other suggested indicators among the J01 ATC class [19, 21, 32–34]. Linear regression analysis was used to assess any significant changes in the trends of the quality indicator measures (continuous variable) over the study period from 2007 to 2016; hence five regression models were conducted; one model per each quality indicator measure, but with time as the independent factor in all of the five models.

Ambulatory care, including general practitioner prescribing and out-patient dispensing (children and adult patients), was chosen for comparative purposes, as this contains the highest proportion of antibiotic use in Poland. In 2016, antibiotic consumption was 23.98 Defined Daily Doses per 1000 inhabitants per day (DIDs) within ambulatory (community) care, while only 1.36 DIDs within hospital sector [19]. In addition, comparative figures are available across Europe in recent years via ECDC. The only exceptions are Cyprus and Romania, where the authorities provided total consumption data, i.e. including in-patient use, as they were unable to separate out the different components.

The findings for Poland in 2016 were also compared with other European countries including those with the highest and lowest values for each indicator, with a special emphasis on neighbouring CEE countries, to again provide future guidance. Descriptive statistics were used to summarise the study variables. Univariate linear regression was used to evaluate any annual trend change in the study outcomes during the study period.

Results

Specific actions to prevent AMR in Poland

The coordinated system of monitoring AMR rates among patients in Poland has been implemented since 1997 with the establishment of the National Reference Centre for Antimicrobial Susceptibility Testing (NRCAST). Since 2002, information on antimicrobial utilisation across sectors, including hospitals and ambulatory care, has also been gathered via NRCAST. This organisation is also in charge of identification and susceptibility testing of bacterial strains from serious and difficult to diagnose infections, with a special focus on certain pathogens such as Methicillin-resistant *Staphylococcus aureus* (MRSA), and monitoring of the spread of resistant strains in hospitals and ambulatory care across Poland. NRCAST also provides data to the European Antimicrobial Resistance Surveillance Network (EARSS-Net) as well as ECDC.

In 2004, the Ministry of Health (MoH) established the National Programme for the Protection of Antibiotics (NPPA) coordinated by the National Institute of Medicines. with the main goal: to monitor AMR in Poland. The MoH is also the main stakeholder in charge of policy development to help prevent or reduce AMR in Poland as well as providing the legal framework for hospital infection control. The Chief Sanitary Inspectorate is responsible for suggesting potential initiatives where concerns exist. In practice, activity of the MoH in the area of AMR monitoring and prevention has been limited, principally left to the State Consultant for Microbiology and the Chief Sanitary Inspectorate to formulate policies on AMR. As far as the NHF's involvement is concerned, usually only limited activities have been undertaken to date to help improve antibiotic use with appreciable autonomy among physicians. Having said this, pneumococcal vaccination became compulsory in

Table 1 Indicators used to assess the quality of antibiotic prescribing

Indicator's description	Indicator's acronym or shortened name
Consumption of antibacterials for systemic use (J01) expressed in defined daily doses per 1000 inhabitants per day (DIDs)	Total consumption J01
Consumption of beta-lactamase sensitive penicillins (J01 CE) expressed as percentage of the total consumption of antibacterials for systemic use (J01); i.e. relative consumption of beta-lactamase sensitive penicillins	J01 CE%
Consumption of combination of penicillins, including beta-lactamase inhibitor (J01CR) expressed as percentage of the total consumption of antibacterials for systemic use (J01); i.e. relative consumption of combination of penicillins, including beta-lactamase inhibitor	J01CR%
Consumption of third- and fourth-generation cephalosporins (J01(DD + DE)) expressed as percentage of the total consumption of antibacterials for systemic use (J01); i.e. relative consumption of third- and fourth-generation cephalosporins	J01DD + DE%
Consumption of fluoroquinolones (J01MA) expressed as percentage of the total consumption of antibacterials for systemic use (J01); i.e. relative consumption of fluoroquinolones	J01MA%
Ratio of the consumption of broad-spectrum (J01(CR + DC + DD+(F-FA01))) to the consumption of narrow-spectrum penicillins, cephalosporins and macrolides (J01(CE + DB + FA01))	J01B/N%

Poland in January 2017. The roles of other Polish health care system stakeholders in policy formulation to prevent or reduce AMR are principally advisory ones.

Current resistance patterns in Poland

Infections in Polish patients illustrate the relationship between high utilisation and high levels of resistance, i.e. the high consumption of trimethoprim and sulfamethoxazole [35] has been accompanied by high levels of antibiotic resistance [5]. Having said this, the prevalence of MRSA in Poland in 2013 was 16%, with prevalence rates exceeding 25% in many EU Member States [35].

Concerns with current AMR rates in Poland are confirmed by data on *Acinetobacter baumannii* infection (ACI), which are some of the most important opportunistic pathogens responsible for the most severe infections characterised by the high level of resistance to commonly used antibiotics. More than 75% of ACI strains of *A. baumannii* isolated from pneumonia cases among hospitalised patients in southern Poland were resistant to 14 out of 16 antimicrobials tested [36], with approximately 60% of *A. baumannii* strains from patients with invasive infections, pneumonia, bloodstream infections and meningitis, resistant to all antimicrobials tested with the exception of colistin. The extensively-drug resistant strains accounted for 80.8% of isolates tested [37]. The largest AMR outbreak in Poland in recent years was observed between 2012 and 2014 in two major cities (Warsaw and Poznan). It concerned New Delhi metallo-β-lactamase (NDM)-producing Enterobacteriaceae. Out of 374 cases of infection/colonisation with NDM-positive Enterobacteriaceae identified in that period, 370 cases were associated with a *Klebsiella pneumoniae* outbreak [38].

Concerns with AMR are exacerbated by the fact that the current surveillance systems in Poland do not currently function optimally. Examples include concerns with data on MRSA epidemiology both in the general population of hospitalised patients, as well as new-borns with very low birth weight [39]. Interestingly, along with a high level of MRSA prevalence at 15% among adult patients in general hospitals, considerable heterogeneity of strains has been detected.

Empiric use of antibiotics vs. routine testing as well as prevention

Efforts in Poland to contain AMR should ideally rely on microbiological tests to guide current treatment as well as provide guidance on optimal empiric treatment when the need arises. A good example is the Polish Neonatological Network where data is gathered from Neonatal Intensive Care Units (NICU) on infection surveillance among newborns with very low birth weights [39]. The analysis of antibiotic utilisation in MRSA infections compared with methicillin-sensitive *Staphylococcus aureus* (MSSA) infections revealed that average therapy durations were 11.2 and 12.3 days respectively [39]. Concurrently, the level of glycopeptides' use was high in both MRSA and MSSA infections, providing a rationale for the introduction of quick molecular tests into routine clinical practice, especially in NICUs [40].

Despite situations such as this, the role of microbiological diagnostics to reduce empiric use of antibiotics as well as efforts to prevent infection is currently underestimated by physicians in Poland [38, 41, 42]. Nowadays, there is a greater focus on treatment rather than prevention, since in Poland, unlike some Western European countries, diagnostic laboratories are organised separately from hospital structures, with most microbiologists not directly involved in treatment decisions. This is particularly problematic for nosocomial infections.

In addition, usually health care providers (hospitals, family physicians) must pay for microbiologic diagnostic tests from their budgets and ambulatory care patients must pay for tests out of pocket. Both of these can be a concern. Consequently, most community acquired infections are currently treated empirically.

Quantitative analysis of antibiotic prescribing quality indicators in ambulatory care

Table 2 contains details of the pertinent antibiotic prescribing quality indicators in ambulatory care in Poland

Table 2 Key ambulatory care antibiotic prescribing quality indicators for Poland 2007 to 2016

Indicator – ECDC code	2007	2008	2009	2010	2011	2012	2013	2014	2015	2016	*P*-value*	% change 2016/2007
Total utilisation J01	22.2	20.8	23.6	21.1	21.1	22.9	23.6	22.8	26.2	23.9	0.0357	8.3
J01 CE%	0.8%	0.8%	0.6%	0.7%	0.5%	0.7%	0.7%	0.9%	1.3%	1.3%	0.0391	62.5
J01CR%	18.7%	21.7%	20.9%	21.3%	30.3%	16.9%	16.5%	16.6%	17.0%	18.5%	0.2949	−1.07
J01DD + DE%	< 0.1%	< 0.1%	< 0.1%	< 0.1%	< 0.1%	< 0.1%	< 0.1%	< 0.1%	< 0.1%	< 0.1%		NA
J01MA%	5.2%	5.8%	5.3%	5.8%	5.6%	5.3%	5.0%	5.3%	5.3%	5.9%	0.9867	13.5
J01B/N%	30.3%	32.5%	36.3%	37.1%	57.6%	36.9%	34.9%	29.0%	24. 8%	25.8%	0.3771	−14.9

Note: *p-value obtained from the linear regression model
Legend: explanation of acronyms is provided in Table 1

during the past 10 years. Total consumption of antibacterials for systemic use and consumption of fluoroquinolones expressed as percentage of the total consumption of antibacterials for systemic use (i.e. relative consumption of fluoroquinolones) were characterized by small increases between 2007 and 2016 (8.3 and 13.5%, respectively), with a significant average annual increase of 3.6% ($p = 0.0357$) for total antibiotic consumption. Relative consumption of beta-lactamase sensitive penicillins revealed a much bigger increase in the analyzed period (62.5%), with a significant average annual increase of 0.0006% ($p = 0.0391$). The relative consumption of combination of penicillins, including beta-lactamase inhibitor, as well as a ratio of the consumption of broad-spectrum to the consumption of narrow-spectrum penicillins, cephalosporins and macrolides decreased in the analyzed period by 1.07 and 14.9% respectively.

The total consumption of antibiotics in the surveyed European countries ranged in 2016 from 10 DIDs in the Netherlands to 36 DIDs in Greece (median 12 DIDs), while Poland had one of the highest consumption rates, exceeding the European median (expressed in DIDs) more than twice (Fig. 1). Only some countries of Southern Europe had higher consumption rates, while in the remaining 78.3% countries the consumption rates were lower than in Poland.

However, interpretation of the other assessed indices does not bring unequivocally negative conclusions. There has been a sizeable increase in consumption of beta-lactamase sensitive penicillins (J01 CE) from a very low share of total antibiotic consumption in previous years (Table 2). The current share of these antibiotics in treatment is on a notably low level when compared with other European countries (Fig. 2). Encouragingly, the consumption of combination penicillins (J01CR), third- and fourth-generation cephalosporins (J01(DD + DE)) and fluoroquinolones (J01MA) is on a relatively low level (Figs. 3, 4, 5). Poland is among the European countries with the lowest share of these antibiotics within overall antibiotic consumption, especially with regard to third- and fourth-generation cephalosporins. On the other hand, in ambulatory care wide-spectrum antibiotics are used relatively more often (ratio J01(CR + DC + DD+(F-FA01) to J01(CE + DB + FA01)) – Fig. 6 (explanation of acronyms is provided in Table 1, see also Abbreviations). However, the situation has improved in comparison to the past years. In 2007 the share of wide-spectrum antibiotics was 30.3%, while in 2016 it was 25.8% (Table 2).

Discussion

There is currently a variable situation regarding antibiotic prescribing in Poland. Poland is at the high end of antibiotic utilization in recent years; at almost 24 DIDs in 2016, appreciably higher than Estonia, Latvia or Slovenia. In addition, consumption grew significantly by about 8% between 2007 and 2016; however, appreciably lower than the 36% increase in total worldwide antibiotic consumption during the past decade [6]. There are also concerns with the low level of prescribing of beta-lactamase sensitive penicillins in Poland, compared for instance with Slovakia, Finland, Slovenia or Sweden. However, encouragingly prescribing rates for these penicillins have been growing in recent years. Encouragingly as well, there was relatively low consumption of combination penicillins and third- and fourth-generation cephalosporins in Poland, with a slight decrease over the years.

There was also a relatively low level of fluoroquinolone consumption in Poland versus other European countries (at 5.9% in 2016). However, there are concerns regarding the growth of fluoroquinolone prescribing in Poland in recent years, expressed as a percentage of the total antibiotic consumption (Table 2). The use of fluoroquinolones, due

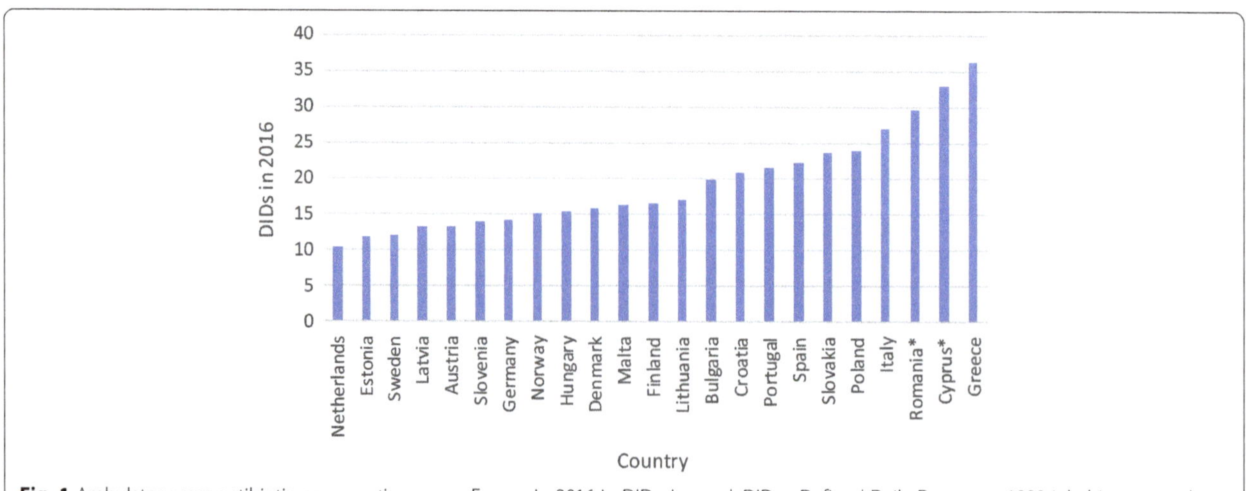

Fig. 1 Ambulatory care antibiotic consumption across Europe in 2016 in DIDs. Legend: DIDs - Defined Daily Doses per 1000 inhabitants per day; *only total consumption data available

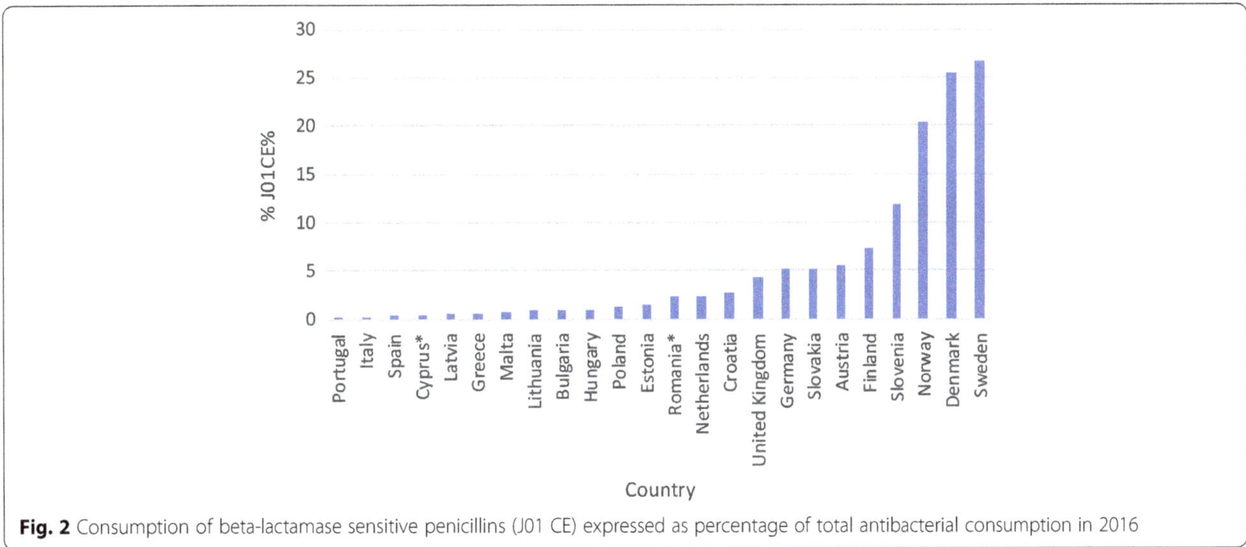

Fig. 2 Consumption of beta-lactamase sensitive penicillins (J01 CE) expressed as percentage of total antibacterial consumption in 2016

to their numerous side effects, should be limited to situations where there are no other therapeutic options available. One of the most important side effects of the use of fluoroquinolones is (among others) *Clostridium difficile* infections (CDI) [11]. The Polish hospitals reported almost the highest crude incidence density of community-associated CDI incidence densities (1.4 cases/10,000 patient-days) in Europe (EU/EEA mean was only 0.8 cases/10,000 patient-days) [43]. Consequently, there is an urgent need to educate physicians in Poland about the appropriate use of fluoroquinolones, unless this is a consequence of high antimicrobial resistance in Poland to other antibiotics. This will be investigated further in future research projects.

There are also concerns at the extent of prescribing of broad versus narrow spectrum antibiotics in Poland, their consumption ratios in 2016 being very high level at 25.81% of total antibiotic consumption versus for instance 0.68% in Finland. Fortunately, this ratio is decreasing in Poland.

This variable picture regarding current antibiotic utilisation patterns in Poland may well reflect the relative lack of educational activities by the NHF and the MoH among physicians. We do know that there is a lack of preparedness among physicians in Poland for educational activities in the field of rational antibiotic therapy. In addition, we are aware that research in area of medical education has shown that problem-based learning curricula are rarely introduced in a country with a high 'power distance' and 'uncertainty avoidance', which currently includes Poland [44]. This is confirmed by both high total consumption antibiotics versus other European countries and a high proportion (ratio) of broad-spectrum antibiotics. The notion of power distance refers to the degree of hierarchy in a

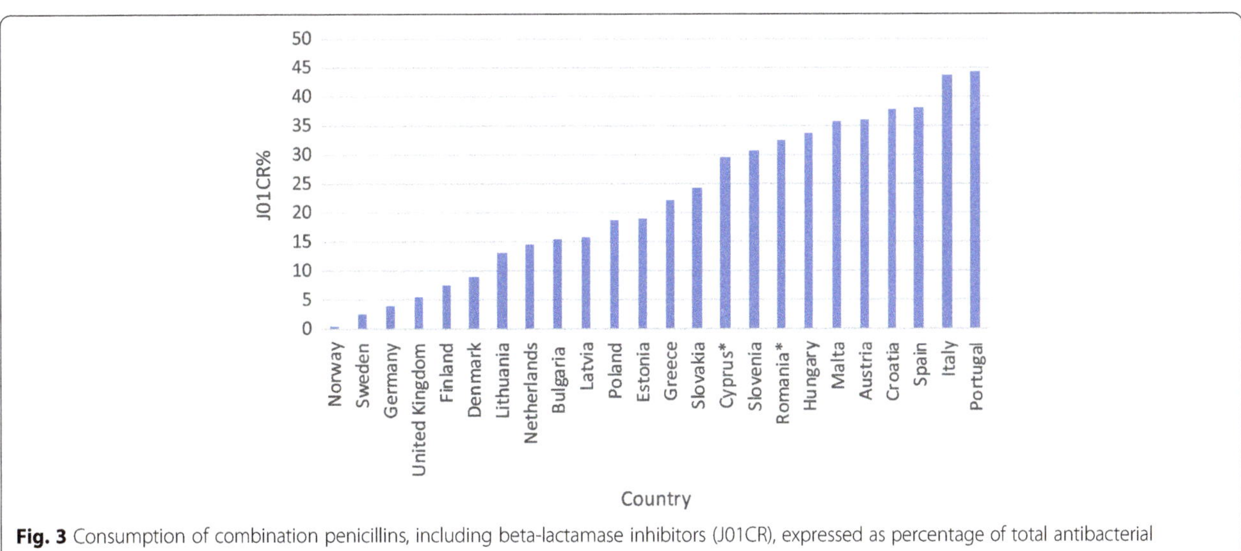

Fig. 3 Consumption of combination penicillins, including beta-lactamase inhibitors (J01CR), expressed as percentage of total antibacterial consumption in 2016

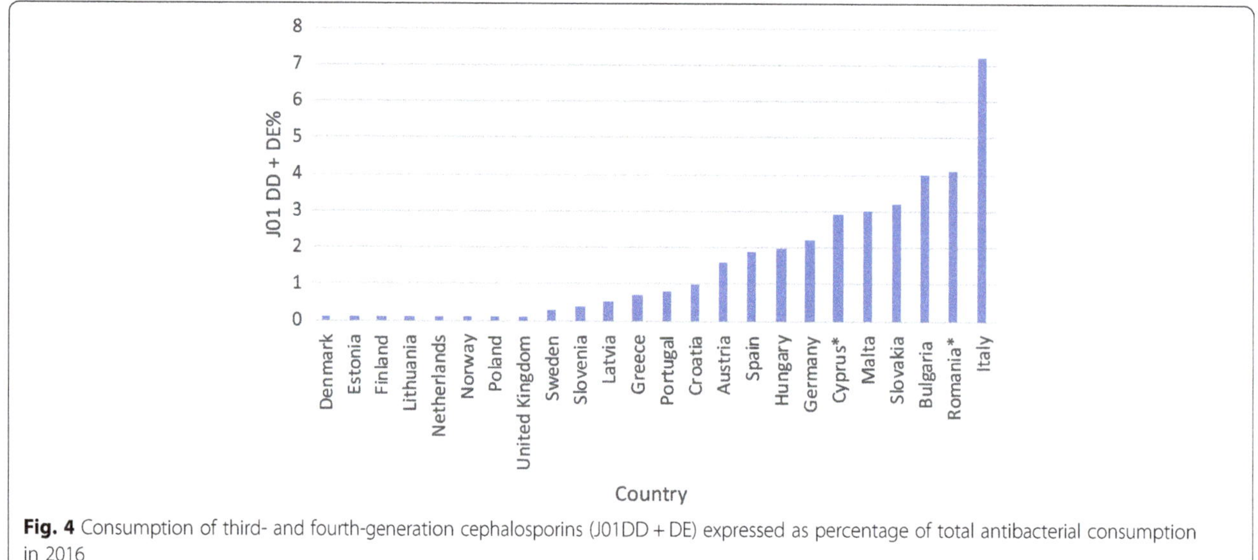

Fig. 4 Consumption of third- and fourth-generation cephalosporins (J01DD + DE) expressed as percentage of total antibacterial consumption in 2016

country and it has been defined by Hofstede as the extent to which the less powerful members of organizations and institutions accept and expect that power is distributed unequally [45]. The notion of uncertainty avoidance deals with a society's tolerance for uncertainty and ambiguity. A higher score indicates that people feel uncomfortable in novel, unknown or surprising situations [45].

Overall, integrated activities around appropriate antibiotic prescribing in the pre- and post-graduate training of physicians and dentists should be particularly important. Currently, the concept of antimicrobial stewardship (AMS) is not included in the curricula of studies and specializations except for specialization for microbiologists. However, in the Polish health care system there are very few physicians-microbiologists (only 110 professionally active in 2018). There could also be the involvement of other specialists in hospitals, such as hospital pharmacists, as part of Drugs and Therapeutic Committees helping with the implementation and monitoring of AMS programs [46].

Other direct measures, which could be recommended for implementation in Poland, include the introduction of limitations in antibiotic prescribing within ambulatory care in Poland, through their stratification, similar to the Republic of Srpska (Bosnia and Herzegovina) or Slovenia, or a basic positive list of medicines with reference prices and a supplementary list which includes more expensive medicines [13, 16]. In the Republic of Srpska amoxicillin, benzathine-phenoxymethylpenicillin, cefalexin, doxycycline, erythromycin, phenoxymethylpenicillin, and sulfamethoxazole with trimethoprim are reimbursed between 90 to 100%; with norfloxacin reimbursed 50%; with 100% co-payment for all other antibiotics [16]. In Slovenia, the national health insurance

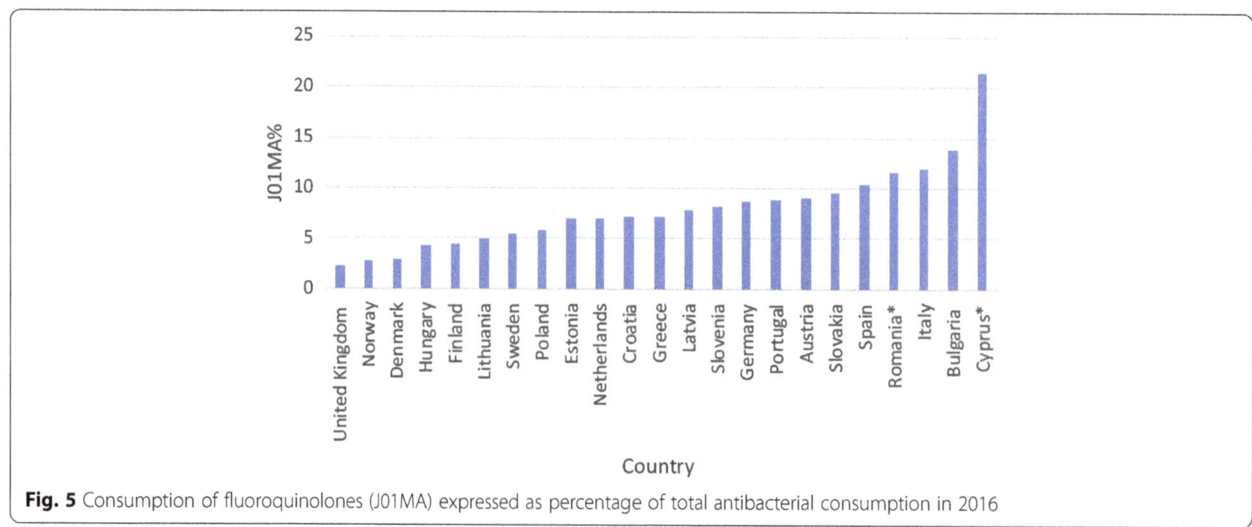

Fig. 5 Consumption of fluoroquinolones (J01MA) expressed as percentage of total antibacterial consumption in 2016

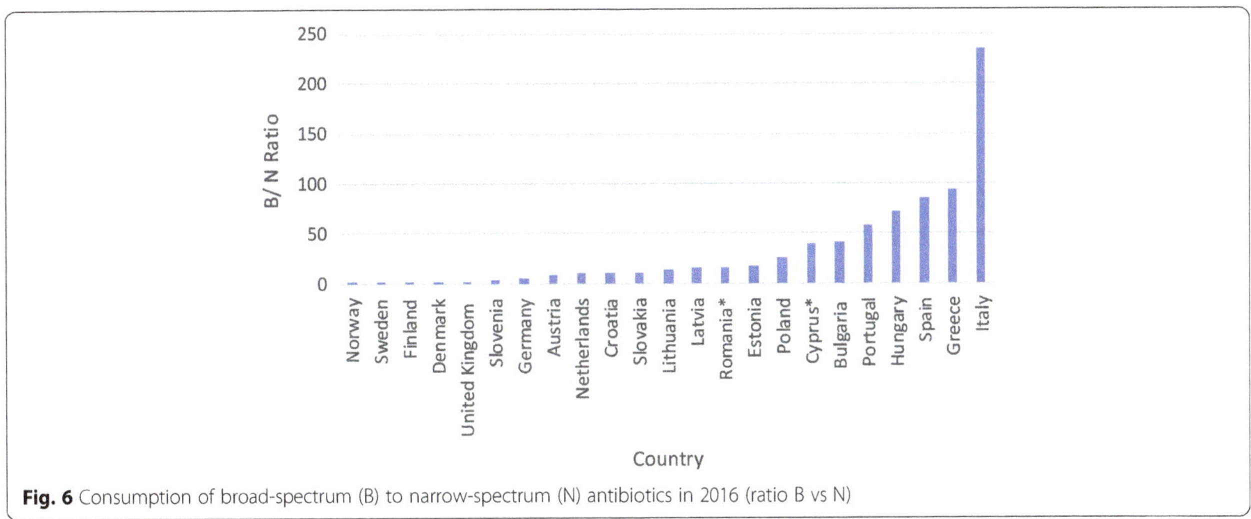

Fig. 6 Consumption of broad-spectrum (B) to narrow-spectrum (N) antibiotics in 2016 (ratio B vs N)

company has instigated prescribing restrictions for amoxicillin/clavulanic acid, third-generation cephalosporins, fluoroquinolones and the macrolides together with their place in therapy i.e., first, second or third line, to enhance antibiotic prescribing [13]. Such activities can potentially be applied in Poland to reduce excessive prescribing of broad-spectrum antibiotics.

Promoting and spreading knowledge on antibiotics, as medicines designated for combatting bacterial infections but ineffective against viruses, is urgently needed. The education campaigns should be targeted not only at physicians, but also patients, especially because other factors should be taken into consideration. These include the relative cost of prescribed antibiotic and the cost of medical consultations. Educational programmes, including academic detailing and providing decision support systems, have improved antibiotic use, although some of the results have been modest [8, 47, 48]. Feedback to physicians, especially high prescribers of antibiotics, has also worked well [49]. Enhancing physician communication skills, as well as the availability of point-of-care testing, can also reduce inappropriate prescribing of antibiotics for acute respiratory tract infections [50, 51]. Although not confirmed by prospective studies, it might be expected that in countries where medical consultations and the cost of antibiotics is high, there will be a lower likelihood for excessive use of antibiotics. Unfortunately, from this perspective, prices of commonly prescribed antibiotics are usually low in Poland, which may result in increased consumption and secondary antibiotic resistance. In contrast, ambulatory patients usually must pay out-of-pocket for microbiological diagnostic tests, which are very often more expensive than prescribed antibiotics. This may result in underutilization of diagnostic testing due to financial reasons.

Consequently, other avenues will be important for improving antibiotic utilization. The provision of health services is overwhelmingly focused on the treatment of infections rather than their prevention in Poland. This applies to many elements of infection control programmes, regarding both nosocomial and non-hospital infections. Notably, hand hygiene should be mentioned, since the existing level of knowledge of its rules is not sufficient among medical personnel and the compliance with recommendations is rather low in Poland. Intensive educational campaigns, addressed to both medical and social workers, are highly required. The more specific procedures, aiming to prevent certain forms of infections (e.g. 'bundle strategies' for prevention of device-associated infections in intensive care units, including small sets of evidence-based practices which have been proven to improve patient outcomes, when applied together) should be actively promoted and implemented. A more effective interdisciplinary education and cooperation between physicians and staff of microbiological laboratories are necessary, and implementation of fast and modern diagnostic methods is crucial. AMR surveillance is largely underdeveloped, and the scale of AMR in Poland may be underestimated. This is despite a relatively high consumption of antibiotics and some alarming trends for certain bacteriological strains. These are considerations for the future.

Conclusions

Whilst the coordinated system of monitoring AMR rates in Poland was initiated almost 20 years ago, it remains underdeveloped, similarly to appropriate strategies to address AMR. The role of microbiological diagnostics, and efforts to prevent infections, is currently underestimated by physicians, who put a greater emphasis on treatment rather than prevention.

Total consumption of antibacterials for systemic use and relative consumption of beta-lactamase sensitive penicillins were characterized by small but statistically significant average annual increases between 2007 and 2016. Overall, Poland has one of the highest rates of total consumption of antibiotics among European countries. Although indicators such as the prevalence of MRSA are within the average values observed in the EU, in case of *P. aeruginosa*, *K. pneumoniae* and *Acinetobacter* there is over 50% resistance to fluoroquinolones, in invasive infections cases in Poland (highest prevalence rates among the EU countries).

Since the limited educational activities among physicians and dentists may play an important role in the current antibiotic consumption patterns, integrated actions focusing on appropriate antibiotic prescribing in the pre- and post-graduate training should be instigated and followed up at national level. The introduction of limitations in antibiotic prescribing within ambulatory care, through their stratification, is also recommended. Education campaigns targeted also to patients are urgently needed as well. Overall, taking actions to improve antibiotic utilisation should be in focus of health policy actions in Poland.

Abbreviations

AMR: antimicrobial resistance; AMS: antimicrobial stewardship; ASP: Antimicrobial Stewardship Program; ATC: Anatomical Therapeutic Chemical; CDI: *Clostridium difficile* infections; CEE: Central and Eastern European; DDD: defined daily dose; DIDs: DDDs per 1000 inhabitants per day; EARSS-Net: European Antimicrobial Resistance Surveillance Network; ECDC: European Centre for Disease Prevention and Control; ESAC: European Surveillance of Antimicrobial Consumption; HAI-Net: Healthcare-Associated Infections Surveillance Network; J01 CE: beta-lactamase sensitive penicillins; J01(CE + DB + FA01): narrow-spectrum penicillins, cephalosporins and macrolides; J01(CR + DC + DD+(F-FA01)): broad-spectrum antibacterials; J01(DD + DE): third- and fourth-generation cephalosporins; J01CR: combination of penicillins, including beta-lactamase inhibitor; J01-J07X: antiinfectives for systemic use; J01MA: fluoroquinolones; MoH: Ministry of Health; MRSA: methicillin-resistant *Staphylococcus aureus*; MSSA: methicillin-sensitive *Staphylococcus aureus*; NDM: New Delhi metallo-β-lactamase; NHF: National Health Fund; NICU: Neonatal Intensive Care Units; NRCAST: National Reference Centre for Antimicrobial Susceptibility Testing; SE: Southern European; URTI: upper respiratory tract infections; WHO: World Health Organization

Acknowledgements

Not applicable.

Funding

No funding was supporting this research.

Authors' contributions

JWM conceptualized and designed the study, analyzed and interpreted the data, drafted the manuscript; BG conceptualized and designed the study, analyzed and interpreted the data, reviewed and revised the manuscript; AG drafted the manuscript, AK analyzed and interpreted the data, AP drafted the manuscript, AR drafted the manuscript, SS drafted the manuscript, MW drafted the manuscript, TB conceptualized and designed the study, analyzed and interpreted the data, drafted, reviewed and revised the manuscript, was the corresponding author. All authors approved the final manuscript as submitted and agree to be accountable for all aspects of the work.

Consent for publication

Not applicable.

Competing interests

The authors declare that they have no competing interests.

Author details

[1]Department of Microbiology, Faculty of Medicine, Jagiellonian University Medical College, Czysta 18 Str., 31-121, Krakow, Poland. [2]Strathclyde Institute of Pharmacy and Biomedical Sciences, Strathclyde University, G4 ORE, Glasgow, UK. [3]Health Economics Centre, Liverpool University Management School, Chatham Street, Liverpool, UK. [4]Department of Laboratory Medicine, Division of Clinical Pharmacology, Karolinska Institute, Karolinska University Hospital Huddinge, SE-141 86 Stockholm, Sweden. [5]Department of Public Health Pharmacy and Management, School of Pharmacy, Sefako Makgatho Health Sciences University, Garankuwa, South Africa. [6]Center for Global Development, 2055 L Street NW, Washington, DC 20036, USA. [7]Department of Pharmacology, College of Pharmacy, Hawler Medical University, Erbil, Iraq. [8]Department of Neurobiology, Institute of Pharmacology, Polish Academy of Sciences, Krakow, Poland. [9]Department of Drug Management, Faculty of Health Sciences, Jagiellonian University Medical College, Grzegorzecka 20 Str., 31-531, Krakow, Poland. [10]Department of Pneumonology, School of Medicine in Katowice, Medical University of Silesia, Katowice, Poland. [11]Department of Nursing, Institute of Health Sciences, State Higher Vocational School in Tarnów, Tarnów, Poland.

References

1. Chambers HF. The changing epidemiology of Staphylococcus aureus? Emerg Infect Dis. 2001;7(2):178–82.
2. Watanabe M, Iyobe S, Inoue M, et al. Transferable imipenem resistance in Pseudomonas aeruginosa. Antimicrob Agent Chemother. 1991;35:147–51.
3. Llor C, Bjerrum L. Antimicrobial resistance: risk associated with antibiotic overuse and initiatives to reduce the problem. Ther Adv Drug Saf. 2014;5(6): 229–41. https://doi.org/10.1177/2042098614554919.
4. Caron WP, Mousa SA. Prevention strategies for antimicrobial resistance: a systemic review of the literature. Infect Drug Resist. 2010;3:25–33.
5. Pomorska-Wesołowska M, Różańska A, Natkaniec J, Gryglewska B, Szczypta A, Dzikowska M, et al. Longevity and gender as the risk factors of methicillin-resistant Staphylococcus aureus infections in southern Poland. BMC Geriatr. 2017;17:51. https://doi.org/10.1186/s12877-017-0442-3.
6. Laxminarayan R, Matsoso P, Pant S, Brower C, Røttingen JA, Klugman K, et al. Access to effective antimicrobials: a worldwide challenge. Lancet. 2016;387(10014):168–75. https://doi.org/10.1016/S0140-6736(15)00474-2.
7. Ventola CL. The antibiotic resistance crisis: part 1: causes and threats. Pharmacy and Therapeutics. 2015;40(4):277–83.
8. Dyar OJ, Beovic B, Vlahovic-Palcevski V, Verheij T, Pulcini C. How can we improve antibiotic prescribing in primary care? Expert Rev Anti-Infect Ther. 2016;14(4):403–13. https://doi.org/10.1586/14787210.2016.1151353.
9. Harris AM, Hicks LA, Qaseem A. Appropriate antibiotic use for acute respiratory tract infection in adults: advice for high-value care from the American College of Physicians and the Centers for Disease Control and Prevention. Ann Intern Med. 2016;164(6):425–34. https://doi.org/10.7326/M15-1840.
10. McCaig LF, Besser RE, Hughes JM. Trends in antimicrobial prescribing rates for children and adolescents. JAMA. 2002;287(23):3096–102.
11. Barlam TF, Cosgrove SE, Abbo LM, MacDougall C, Schuetz AN, Septimus EJ, et al. Implementing an antibiotic stewardship program: guidelines by the Infectious Diseases Society of America and the Society for Healthcare Epidemiology of America. Clin Infect Dis. 2016;62:e51–77. https://doi.org/10.1093/cid/ciw118.
12. Pulcini C. Antibiotic stewardship: update and perspectives. Clin Microbiol Infect. 2017;23(11):791–2. https://doi.org/10.1016/j.cmi.2017.08.020.
13. Furst J, Cizman M, Mrak J, Kos D, Campbell S, Coenen S, et al. The influence of a sustained multifaceted approach to improve antibiotic prescribing in

Slovenia during the past decade: findings and implications. Expert Rev Anti-Infect Ther. 2015;13(2):279–89. https://doi.org/10.1586/14787210.2015.990381.

14. Markovic-Pekovic V, Grubisa N, Burger J, Bojanic L, Godman B. Initiatives to reduce nonprescription sales and dispensing of antibiotics: findings and implications. J Res Pharm Pract. 2017;6(2):120–5. https://doi.org/10.4103/jrpp.JRPP_17_12.
15. Dar OA, Hasan R, Schlundt J, Harbarth S, Caleo G, Dar FK, et al. Exploring the evidence base for national and regional policy interventions to combat resistance. Lancet. 2016;387(10015):285–95. https://doi.org/10.1016/S0140-6736(15)00520-6.
16. Bojanić L, Marković-Peković V, Škrbić R, Stojaković N, Đermanović M, Bojanić J, et al. Recent initiatives in the republic of Srpska to enhance appropriate use of antibiotics in ambulatory care; their influence and implications. Front Pharmacol. 2018;9:442. https://doi.org/10.3389/fphar.2018.00442.
17. Abilova V, Kurdi A, Godman B. Ongoing initiatives in Azerbaijan to improve the use of antibiotics; findings and implications. Expert Rev Anti-Infect Ther. 2018;16(1):77–84. https://doi.org/10.1080/14787210.2018.1417835.
18. ECDC. European Surveillance of Antimicrobial Consumption Network (ESAC-Net). http://www.ecdc.europa.eu/en/activities/surveillance/ESAC-Net/Pages/index.aspx Accessed 10 July 2018.
19. ECDC. Quality indicators for antibiotic consumption in the community in Europe. https://ecdc.europa.eu/en/antimicrobial-consumption/surveillance-and-disease-data/database Accessed 10 July 2018.
20. WHO. Antimicrobial Medicines Consumption (AMC) Network. 2017. http://www.euro.who.int/en/publications/abstracts/antimicrobial-medicines-consumption-amc-network-amc-data-20112014-2017 Accessed 10 July 2018.
21. Dziurda D, Polak S, Skowron A, Kuschill-Dziurda J, Brandys J. Analysis of non-hospital antibacterial pharmacotherapy in Poland. Int J Infect Dis. 2008;12:483–9. https://doi.org/10.1016/j.ijid.2007.12.014.
22. Panasiuk L, Lukas W, Paprzycki P, Verheij T, Godycki-Ćwirko M, Chlabicz S. Antibiotics in the treatment of upper respiratory tract infections in Poland. Is there any improvement? J Clin Pharm Therapeutics. 2010;35:665–9. https://doi.org/10.1111/j.1365-2710.2009.01136.x.
23. NHF National Health Fund. Report on expenditures of the NHF in pharmaceutical reimbursement in 2010. 2010 http://www.nfz.gov.pl/download/gfx/nfz/pl/defaultstronaopisowa/349/14/1/refundacja_2010.pdf. Accessed 10 July 2018.
24. Chlabicz M, Chlabicz S, Marcinowicz L, Rogowska-Szadkowska D, Pytel-Krolczuk B, Leszczyńska K. Outpatient use of systemic antibiotics in Poland: 2004-2008. Przegl Epidemiol. 2014;68(3):435–47.
25. Hryniewicz W, Albrecht P, Radzikowski A et al. Rekomendacje postępowania w pozaszpitalnych zakażeniach układu oddechowego. Narodowy Program Ochrony Antybiotyków na lata 2011–2015. http://www.antybiotyki.edu.pl/pdf/Rekomendacje2016.pdf Accessed 10 July 2018.
26. Meeuwesen L, van den Brink-Muinen A, Hofstede G. Can dimensions of national culture predict cross-national differences in medical communication? Patient Educ Couns. 2009;75(1):58–66. https://doi.org/10.1016/j.pec.2008.09.015.
27. Walaszek M, Rozanska A, Bulanda M, Wojkowska-Mach J. Polish Society of Hospital Infections T. alarming results of nosocomial bloodstream infections surveillance in polish intensive care units. Przeg Epidemiol. 2018;72(1):33–44.
28. ECDC. European Center for Disease Prevention and Control. Healthcare-associated Infections Surveillance Network (HAI-Net). http://ecdc.europa.eu/en/healthtopics/Healthcare-associated_infections/HAI-Net/Pages/HAI-Net-surveillance-network.aspx Accessed 10 July 2018.
29. ECDC. European Center for Disease Prevention and Control. Surveillance and disease data for antimicrobial resistance. http://ecdc.europa.eu/en/healthtopics/antimicrobial-resistance-and-consumption/antimicrobial_resistance/EARS-Net/Pages/EARS-Net.aspx Accessed 10 July 2018.
30. WHO. World Health Organization. Global Action Plan on Antimicrobial Resistance. 2015. http://www.wpro.who.int/entity/drug_resistance/resources/global_action_plan_eng.pdf Accessed 10 July 2018.
31. Wójkowska-Mach J, Jaje E, Romaniszyn D, Kasparek M, Frańczuk B, Bulanda M, Heczko PB, et al. Comparison of SSI rate in endoarthoplasty of hip and knee in a Cracow patient population and the importance of postdischarge surveillance. Infection. 2008;36:36–40. https://doi.org/10.1007/s15010-007-6339-x.
32. Adriaenssens N, Coenen S, Tonkin-Crine S, Verheij TJ, Little P, Goossens H. European surveillance of antimicrobial consumption (ESAC): disease-specific quality indicators for outpatient antibiotic prescribing. BMJ Qual Saf. 2011;20(9):764–72.
33. Adriaenssens N, Coenen S, Versporten A, Muller A, Vankerckhoven V, Goossens H. European Surveillance of Antimicrobial Consumption (ESAC): quality appraisal of antibiotic use in Europe. J Antimicrob Chemother. 2011;66 Suppl 6:vi71–7. doi: https://doi.org/10.1093/jac/dkr459.
34. WHO. World Health Organization. ATC/DDD Index 2017. WHO ATC system. https://www.whocc.no/atc_ddd_index/. Accessed 10 July 2018.
35. ECDC. European Center for Disease Control and Prevention. Annual surveillance reports and protocols - antimicrobial consumption. 2015. https://ecdc.europa.eu/en/antimicrobial-consumption/surveillance-and-disease-data/report-protocol Accessed 10 July 2018.
36. Chmielarczyk A, Pilarczyk-Żurek M, Kamińska W, Pobiega M, Romaniszyn D, Ziółkowski G, et al. Molecular epidemiology and drug resistance of Acinetobacter baumannii isolated from hospitals in southern Poland: ICU as a risk factor for XDR strains. Microb Drug Resist. 2016;22(4):328–35. https://doi.org/10.1089/mdr.2015.0224.
37. Chmielarczyk A, Pomorska-Wesołowska M, Szczypta A, Romaniszyn D, Pobiega M. Molecular analysis of methicillin-resistant Staphylococcus aureus strains isolated from different types of infections from patients hospitalized in 12 regional, non-teaching hospitals in southern Poland. J Hosp Infect. 2017;95(3):259–67. https://doi.org/10.1016/j.jhin.2016.10.024.
38. Izdebski R, Baraniak A, Zabicka D, Machulska M, Urbanowicz P, Fiett J, et al. Enterobacteriaceae producing OXA-48-like carbapenemases in Poland, 2013-January 2017. J Antimicrob Chemother. 2017. https://doi.org/10.1093/jac/dkx457.
39. Romaniszyn D, Różańska A, Chmielarczyk A, Pobiega M, Adamski P, Helwich E, et al. Epidemiology, antibiotic consumption and molecular characterisation of Staphylococcus aureus infections – data from the polish neonatology surveillance network, 2009-2012. BMC Infect Dis. 2015;15:169. https://doi.org/10.1186/s12879-015-0890-3.
40. Różańska A, Wójkowska-Mach J, Adamski P, et al. Antibiotic consumption in laboratory confirmed vs. non-confirmed bloodstream infections among Very Low Birth Weight Neonates in Poland. Ann Clin Microbiol Antimicrob. 2017;16(1):20. https://doi.org/10.1186/s12941-017-0196-y.
41. Stefanoff P, Rogalska J, Czech M, Staszewska E, Rosinska M. Antimicrobial prescriptions for acute gastrointestinal infections: uncovering the iceberg. Epidemiol Infect. 2013;141(4):859–67. https://doi.org/10.1017/S0950268812001173.
42. Wojkowska-Mach J, Gryglewska B, Romaniszyn D, Natkaniec J, Pobiega M, Adamski P, et al. Age and other risk factors of pneumonia among residents of polish long-term care facilities. Int J Infect Dis. 2013;17(1):e37–43. https://doi.org/10.1016/j.ijid.2012.07.020.
43. ECDC. Clostridium difficile infections - Annual Epidemiological Report for 2016. https://ecdc.europa.eu/en/publications-data/clostridium-difficile-infections-annual-epidemiological-report-2016 Accessed 10 July 2018.
44. Jippes M, Majoor GD. Influence of national culture on the adoption of integrated and problem-based curricula in Europe. Med Educ. 2008;42(3):279–85. https://doi.org/10.1111/j.1365-2923.2007.02993.x.
45. Deschepper R, Grigoryan L, Lundborg CS, Hofstede G, Cohen J, Kelen GV, Deliens L, Haaijer-Ruskamp FM. Are Cultural dimensions relevant for explaining cross-national differences in antibiotic use in Europe? BMC Health Serv Res. 2008;6(8):123.
46. Schellack N, Bronkhorst E, Coetzee R, Godman B, Gous AGS, Kolman S, et al. SASOCP position statement on the pharmacist's role in antibiotic stewardship. South Afr J Infect Dis. 2018;33(1):28–35.
47. McDonagh MS, Peterson K, Winthrop K, Cantor A, Lazur BH, Buckley DI. Interventions to reduce inappropriate prescribing of antibiotics for acute respiratory tract infections: summary and update of a systematic review. J Int Med Res. 2018;46(8):3337–57.
48. Formoso G, Paltrinieri B, Marata AM, Gagliotti C, Pan A, Moro ML, et al. Feasibility and effectiveness of a low-cost campaign on antibiotic prescribing in Italy: community level, controlled, non-randomised trial. BMJ. 2013;347:f5391.
49. Hallsworth M, Chadborn T, Sallis A, Sanders M, Berry D, Greaves F, et al. Provision of social norm feedback to high prescribers of antibiotics in general practice: a pragmatic national randomised controlled trial. Lancet. 2016;387(10029):1743–52.
50. Köchling A, Löffler C, Reinsch S, Hornung A, Böhmer F, Altiner A, et al. Reduction of antibiotic prescriptions for acute respiratory tract infections in primary care: a systematic review. Implement Sci. 2018;13(1):47.
51. Mangione-Smith R, Zhou C, Robinson JD, Taylor JA, Elliott MN, Heritage J. Communication practices and antibiotic use for acute respiratory tract infections in children. Ann Fam Med. 2015;13(3):221–7.

24

Healthcare-associated infections in intensive care units in Taiwan, South Korea, and Japan: recent trends based on national surveillance reports

Cho-Han Chiang[1†], Sung-Ching Pan[2†], Tyan-Shin Yang[1], Keisuke Matsuda[3], Hong Bin Kim[4,5], Young Hwa Choi[6], Satoshi Hori[7], Jann-Tay Wang[1,2,8], Wang-Huei Sheng[1,2,8], Yee-Chun Chen[1,2,8,9*], Feng-Yee Chang[10] and Shan-Chwen Chang[1,2]

Abstract

Background: Sustainable systematic interventions are important for infection prevention and control (IPC). Data from surveillance of healthcare-associated infections (HAI) provides feedback for implementation of IPC programs. To address the paucity of such data in Asia, we searched for national HAI surveillance and IPC programs in this region.

Methods: Data were analysed from national surveillance reports of three Asian countries: Taiwan, South Korea and Japan from 2008 to 2015. National IPC programs were identified.

Results: There were differences among the countries in surveillance protocols, hospital coverage rates, and national IPC policies and programs. Nevertheless, there was a 53.0% reduction in overall HAI over the 8-year period. This consisted of a decrease from 9.34 to 5.03 infections per 1000 patient-days in Taiwan, from 7.56 to 2.76 in Korea, and from 4.41 to 2.74 in Japan (Poisson regression, all $p < 0.05$). Across the three countries, *Escherichia coli* and *Candida albicans* were the major pathogens for urinary tract infection. *Staphylococcus aureus, Acinetobacter baumannii* and *Enterococcus faecium* were common bloodstream pathogens. For pneumonia, *S. aureus, A. baumannii, Pseudomonas aeruginosa*, and *Klebsiella pneumoniae* were the predominant pathogens, with considerable country differences. There was a 64.6% decrease in the number of isolates of methicillin-resistant *S. aureus*, 38.4% decrease in carbapenem-resistant *P. aeruginosa* and 49.2% decrease in carbapenem-resistant *A. baumannii* (CRAB) in Taiwan (all $p < 0.05$), and similarly in Korea with the exception of CRAB (30.5 and 50.4% reduction, respectively, both $p < 0.05$).

Conclusion: We found a significant decrease in HAI across the three countries in association with sequential multifaceted interventions such as hand hygiene, care bundles, and antimicrobial stewardships. Further regional collaboration could be forged to develop joint strategies to prevent HAI.

Keywords: Healthcare-associated infections, National surveillance, Antimicrobial resistance, National policy, Infection prevention and control program

* Correspondence: yeechunchen@gmail.com
[†]Cho-Han Chiang and Sung-Ching Pan contributed equally to this work.
[1]College of Medicine, National Taiwan University, Taipei, Taiwan
[2]Department of Internal Medicine, National Taiwan University Hospital, Taipei, Taiwan
Full list of author information is available at the end of the article

Background

The European Healthcare-associated Infections Surveillance Network (HAI-net) is one of the most coordinated and comprehensive surveillance systems that monitors healthcare-associated infections (HAI). By centralizing data on antimicrobial use, HAI incidence, and HAI point prevalence, HAI-net builds a regional landscape that allows inter-country comparison and provides feedback for implementation of regional infection prevention and control (IPC) guidelines [1].

With its high burden of HAI, Asia stands to benefit by learning from such a surveillance network. A recent meta-analysis reported a pooled HAI incidence density of 20 cases per 1000 intensive care unit-days in Southeast Asia [2]; studies in India and China found pooled ventilator-associated pneumonia of 9.4 and 20.8 cases per 1000 ventilator-days, respectively [3, 4]. Establishing surveillance in Asian countries, either as national or regional collaborations, might help relevant stakeholders to identify systemic gaps and establish improvements in IPC.

The current understanding of HAI surveillance in Asia remains limited despite the relatively large numbers of IPC conducted in Asia [2, 5]. Likewise, national scale data documenting the regional HAI epidemiology in Asia is scarce [2]. To better understand the current state of HAI surveillance and IPC programs in Asia, we searched for data on existing national HAI surveillance programs. Three Asian countries: Taiwan [6, 7], South Korea [8–10], and Japan [11] were found to conduct nationwide HAI surveillance systems. The present study is based on data derived from open access reports from the surveillance systems of these countries. They include temporal trends of HAI in intensive care units (ICUs), the major causative pathogens and antimicrobial resistance (AMR). Nationally implemented IPC policies were also reviewed to gain insights on important interventions instituted in these three countries.

Methods

Study design and source of data

We performed a Google and PubMed search to determine the existing national HAI surveillance systems in Asian countries using the following terms "national nosocomial infection surveillance" or "national healthcare-associated infection surveillance" in combination with specific country names. The inclusion criteria were: English language, open access data or PubMed publications, annual data containing either point prevalence or yearly surveillance for 5 or more years. Data from the national HAI surveillance systems were retrospectively retrieved and analysed.

National surveillance systems of Taiwan, South Korea, and Japan

Three national HAI surveillance systems met the study criteria. These were the Taiwan Nosocomial Infection Surveillance (TNIS), Korean National Healthcare-associated Infection Surveillance (KONIS), and Japan Nosocomial Infection Surveillance (JANIS). Each system prospectively collects data on the incidence, causative pathogens, and antimicrobial resistance of HAI in ICUs. HAI data are stratified by infection site: urinary tract infection (UTI), bloodstream infection (BSI), hospital-acquired pneumonia (HAP); by device-use: catheter-associated urinary tract infection (CAUTI), central line-associated bloodstream infection (CLABSI), and ventilator-associated pneumonia (VAP); and by type of hospital (in Taiwan and South Korea). These HAI cases and categories are in accord with the definitions of the US National Healthcare Safety Network (NHSN) system with minor modifications to account for differences in clinical or laboratory practice and national policies.

Data collection

Demographic data for each country were retrieved from the World Bank and their respective national authorities. Hospital and ICU composition of each surveillance system were recorded from their official web portals. Annual data of overall HAI, device-associated HAI, causative pathogens, and rates of AMR of important bacteria were also retrieved from the three surveillance systems. We selected the study period as 2008 to 2015 because data for this period were accessible across all three systems. National-scale IPC policies and programs were obtained by online search or in consultation with experts from the three countries.

Data analysis

Incidence densities of overall HAI were determined as pooled means of UTI, BSI, and HAP rates, and calculated as overall HAI episodes per 1000 patient-days. Analysis of device-associated HAI included CAUTI, CLABSI, and VAP. For Taiwan and Korea, incidence densities of device-associated HAI were calculated as device-associated infection episodes per 1000 device-days. For Japan, device-associated HAI were analysed by device-associated infection episodes per 1000 patient-days which made Japanese data incompatible with data from other countries. Causative pathogens were classified at the species level. AMR proportions of selected pathogens were calculated as number of antimicrobial-resistant isolates divided by the total number of isolates of the same species.

Statistical analysis

A Poisson regression model was used to assess the temporal trends of HAI incidence. Linear regression was used to analyse the trends in AMR isolates, using the STATA statistical program (version 14.0 Texas, USA). A P value < 0.05 was considered statistically significant.

Results

Characteristics of Taiwan, South Korea and Japan's National Surveillance Systems

The characteristics of the national HAI surveillance systems of Taiwan, South Korea, and Japan are summarised in Table 1 [6, 8, 11]. The type, size and proportion of hospitals enrolled in the national surveillance varied among the countries. Taiwan included medical centres and regional hospitals classified according to hospital accreditation. Most of them had hospital beds of 300 beds or more. Korea and Japan included hospitals with more than 300 and 200 beds, respectively. The hospital coverage and participation rates were 21.2 and 100.0% in Taiwan, 18.0 and 38.6% in Korea, and 1.9 and 6.8% in Japan, respectively. A total of 472, 169 and 163 ICUs were enrolled in Taiwan, Korea and Japan, respectively. The number of participating hospitals and ICUs in all three countries during the study period has expanded (Additional file 1: Table S1) [6, 8, 11]. Categorization of HAI was different in JANIS, which presented only UTI, CLABSI and VAP. Infection incidence was also calculated differently as episodes per 1000 patient-days.

National infection control policies or programs and HAI trends across Taiwan, South Korea, and Japan

Numerous independent changes, aimed at improving surveillance and compliance, were made for national IPC policies, programs, or practices in each country (Fig. 1). Additional file 2: Table S2 summarised the details of national IPC programs in the past two decades by country. For example, during the study period hand hygiene, care bundles, hospital environment hygiene program and antimicrobial stewardship were the main interventions implemented in Taiwan. The hand hygiene program adapted the WHO multimodal strategies with particular emphasis on alcohol-based hand rub at the point of care. The care bundles program aimed to prevent CAUTI, CLABSI, and VAP. On the other hand, Korea and Japan enforced IPC practices by legislating and mandating IPC in hospitals. Incentives in terms of reimbursement 1.8–2.7 US dollars and 10 US dollars per admission were given to hospitals who met IPC standards in Korea and Japan, respectively. All three countries mandated assignment of infection control personnel. They also implemented formal and structured antimicrobial stewardship programs, which include surveillance of AMR pathogens and regulations of antimicrobial use.

Overall HAI rates

All three countries experienced a significant reduction of approximately 50% in HAI rates by the end of the study period. The incidence density in Taiwan decreased by 46.2% from 9.3 to 5.0 infections per 1000 patient-days; in Korea HAI declined by 63.1% from 7.6 to 2.8, and in Japan by 38.6% from 4.4 to 2.7 (Poisson regression, all $p < 0.05$) (Fig. 1).

There was a significant reduction in device-associated HAI at all sites of infection in Taiwan and Korea ($p < 0.05$) (Fig. 2). Japan had low rates of CAUTI and CLABSI (presented as infections per 1000 patient-days) that persisted over the 8-year period. The most remarkable change was noted for CAUTI in Korea, with an 81.3% decrease from 4.8 to 0.9 infections per 1000 device-days ($P < 0.05$). All three countries experienced a similar trend in VAP during the study period with a 57.7% reduction from 2.6 to 1.1 infections per 1000 device-days in Taiwan.

Causative pathogens

The distributions of the top five (or four for Japan) causative pathogens according to country and site of infection in 2015 are shown in Table 2. For Taiwan and Korea, UTI, BSI and HAP data were presented; for Japan, UTI, CLABSI and VAP data were presented. A more comprehensive list of pathogens is shown in Additional file 3: Table S3, Additional file 4: Table S4, and Additional file 5: Table S5.

Escherichia coli and *Candida albicans* were included in the top five organisms causing UTI in all three countries. *E. coli* and *C. albicans* constituted 19.8 and 16.9%, 17.6 and 12.6, 37.6 and 7.9% of UTI for Taiwan, Korea, and Japan, respectively (Table 2). Along with *Candida albicans*, non-*albicans Candida* species and yeast-like organisms constituted 31.4% of the urinary tract pathogens in Taiwan. In Korea, 23.4% of the UTI were due to *Candida* species (Additional file 3: Table S3).

Staphylococcus aureus was a major pathogen of BSI. The rates were 14.2% in Korea, 13.0% in Japan, and 6.5% in Taiwan (Table 2). Along with *S. aureus*, *Staphylococcus epidermidis and* coagulase-negative staphylococci constituted 38.8% of the CLABSI isolates in Japan. There were major differences among the countries in the distribution of other predominant pathogens. *Acinetobacter baumannii* and *E. faecium* were the predominant BSI pathogens in Taiwan and Korea. Major *Candida* species constituted 12.1% of the BSI isolates in Taiwan and 12.9% in Korea (Additional file 4: Table S4).

S. aureus, *P. aeruginosa* and *K. pneumoniae* were the predominant pathogens for HAP across all three countries (Table 2). Interestingly, *A. baumannii* was predominant in Taiwan and Korea but not in Japan, similar to the observation for BSI. For Taiwan and Korea, these four pathogens comprised 65.7 and 81.2% of the HAP isolates, respectively.

Antimicrobial resistance

Higher AMR rates were noted in Korea than in Taiwan (Fig. 3). The data for Japan were incomplete for several study years and are not shown in the figures. There was

Table 1 Demographics and national surveillance systems of Taiwan, South Korea and Japan

Parameter	Taiwan	South Korea	Japan
Country background			
Population[a]	23,433,753[b]	50,746,659[c]	127,276,000[d]
Income bracket[e]	High income	High income	High income
GDP, US dollars	571,736 million[f]	1,530,750.92 million[g]	4,872,136.95 million[g]
Share of GDP on national health expenditure	6.3%[f]	7.6%[h]	10.7%[h]
Number of hospitals[a]	486[i]	534[j]	7426[k]
Surveillance system	Taiwan Nosocomial Infection Surveillance (TNIS)	Korean National Healthcare-associated Infection Surveillance System (KONIS)	Japan Nosocomial Infection Surveillance (JANIS)
Year established	2001	2006	2000
Authority	Centers for Disease Control, Ministry of Health and Welfare, Taiwan	Korea Centers for Disease Control and Prevention	Ministry of Health, Labor and Welfare, Japan
ICU Surveillance[a]			
Number of hospitals enrolled	103	96	143
Number of ICUs enrolled	472	169	163
Types of hospitals enrolled (total number in the country)	Medical Centers and Regional hospitals [l] ($n = 103$)	Bed size > 900, 700–899, 300–699 ($n = 249$)[n]	Bed size > 200 ($n = 2100$)
Hospital coverage rate	21.2% (103/486)	18.0% (96/534)	1.9% (143/7426)
Hospital participation rate[m]	100.0% (103/103)	38.6% (96/249)	6.8% (143/2100)
Mandated standard ratio of infection control personnel	1 dedicated full-time certificated IC nurse per 300 beds (basic) or per 250 beds (optimal) 1 FTE qualified IC doctor per 500 beds (basic) or per 300 beds (optimal)[o] For hospitals > 500 beds: 1 FTE IC medical technician (basic) or 1 dedicated full-time certificated IC medical technician (optimal); 1 FTE IC medical technician for hospitals with 300–499 beds (optimal)	1 dedicated full-time IC nurse per 200 beds (basic) or per 150 beds (optimal)[n] 1 qualified IC doctor per 300 beds	1 dedicated full-time certificated IC nurse (at > 0.8 FTE)[p] 1 part-time IC doctor (at > 0.5 FTE) 1 part-time IC medical technician and 1 part-time pharmacist (at > 0.5 FTE) Additional manpower for antimicrobial stewardship[p]
Healthcare-associated infection data provided			
Site-specific HAIs	UTI, BSI, HAP: episode per 1000 patient-day	UTI, BSI, HAP: episode per 1000 patient-day	UTI: episode per 1000 patient-day
Device-associated HAIs	CAUTI, CLABSI, VAP: episode per 1000 device-day	CAUTI, CLABSI, VAP: episode per 1000 device-day	CLABSI, VAP: episode per 1000 patient-day
Causative pathogens	Top 10 of the most common pathogens	99% of all the causative pathogens	Top 5 of the most common pathogens[q]
Antimicrobial-resistant pathogens	MRSA, VRE, CRAB, CRPA, CRE, CREC, CRKP	MRSA, VRE, IRAB, IRPA, CefR-KP, CipR-KP, CefR-EC, CipR-EC	MRSA

Abbreviations: BSI bloodstream infections, *CAUTI* catheter-associated urinary tract infection, *CefR-EC* cefotaxime-resistant *Escherichia coli*, *CefR-KP* cefotaxime-resistant *Klebsiella pneumoniae*, *CipR-EC* ciprofloxacin-resistant *E. coli*, *CipR-KP* ciprofloxacin-resistant *K. pneumoniae*, *CLABSI* central line-associated bloodstream infections, *CRAB* carbapanem (imipenem or meropenem)-resistant *Acinetobacter baumannii*, *CRE* carbapanem (imipenem, meropenem, or ertapenem)-resistant Enterobacteriaceae, *CREC* carbapanem (imipenem, meropenem, or ertapenem)-resistant *E. coli*, *CRKP* carbapanem (imipenem, meropenem, or ertapenem)-resistant *K. pneumoniae*, *CRPA* carbapanem (imipenem or meropenem)-resistant *Pseudomonas aeruginosa*, *FTE* full-time equivalent, *GDP* gross domestic product, *HAI* Healthcare-associated infections, *HAP* hospital-acquired pneumonia, *IC* infection control, *IRAB* imipenem-resistant *A. baumannii*, *IRPA* imipenem-resistant *P. aerugonisa*, *MRSA* methicillin-resistant *Staphylococcus aureus*, *MSSA* methicillin-susceptible *S. aureus*, *UTI* urinary tract infections, *VAP* ventilator-associated pneumonia, *VRE* vancomycin-resistant enterococci (*Enterococcus faecalis* or *E. faecium*)

[a]2014 data

[b]Data retrieved from http://www1.stat.gov.tw/ct.asp?xItem=15408&CtNode=4692&mp=3. Assessed 14 April 2018.

[c]Data retrieved from https://data.worldbank.org/country/korea-rep. Assessed 14 April 2018

[d]Data retrieved from https://data.worldbank.org/country/japan?view=chart. Assessed 14 April 2018

[e]Data retrieved from World Bank Country and Lending Groups at https://datahelpdesk.worldbank.org/knowledgebase/articles/906519-world-bank-country-and-lending-groups. Accessed 10 September 2018. For the current 2019 fiscal year, high-income economies are those with a gross national income per capita, calculated using the World Bank Atlas method of $12,056 or more

[f]2016 data. Raw data NT dollars 17,152,093 million, converted to US dollars by ratio 30:1. Retrieved from https://www.mohw.gov.tw/lp-3781-2.html. Accessed 10 September 2018
[g]2017 data based on World Bank national accounts data, and Organization for Economic Co-operation and Development (OECD) National Accounts data. Retrieved from https://data.worldbank.org/indicator/NY.GDP.MKTP.CD. Accessed 10 September 2018
[h]2017 data based on Organization for Economic Co-operation and Development (OECD) estimated data for Japan and provisional data for Korea. Retrieved from https://stats.oecd.org/Index.aspx?DataSetCode=SHA. Accessed 10 September 2018
[i]Data retrieved from https://www.mohw.gov.tw/dl-40542-045687b7-aa43-458c-ab70-e8ff24c5b1b3.html. Accessed 10 September 2018
[j]Data retrieved from http://kosis.kr/eng/statisticsList/statisticsList_01List.jsp?vwcd=MT_ETITLE&parentId=D#SubCont. Accessed 10 September 2018
[k]Data retrieved from http://www.mhlw.go.jp/english/database/db-hh/2-2.html. Accessed 10 September 2018
[l]The data for Taiwan included medical centers and regional hospitals, which were classified according to hospital accreditation and covered only acute care hospitals
[m]The hospital coverage rate was calculated as the number of participating hospitals divided by the total number of hospitals in the same year in each country. The hospital participation rate was calculated as the number of participating hospitals divided by the total number of hospitals to be enrolled in each surveillance system
[n]In terms of surveillance, the requirement for participation in KONIS was 1 full-time infection control nurse over 200-bed size hospital. Regarding the mandatory personnel requirement, this regulation has been launched as a financial incentive program since 2016, as described in Additional file 2: Table S2
[o]Data available at https://www.cdc.gov.tw/professional/info.aspx?treeid=beac9c103df952c4&nowtreeid=bd387fa55fef03f0&tid=FED32554F2B55D11. Accessed September 10, 2018
[p]Infection prevention and control incentive through reimbursement policies was revised in 2010, 2012 and 2018, as described in Additional file 2: Table S2. Since 2012, each hospital is reimbursed 1000 JPY (about 10 USD) per patient per admission if it fulfills the Ministry of Health, Labor and Welfare requirements which mandated one dedicated full-time certificated ICN (at > 0.8 FTE), one part-time ICD (at > 0.5 FTE), one part-time IC pharmacist and one part-time medical technician/microbiologist (at > 0.5 FTE). Since 2018, reimbursement policies per admission included three parts. It provides 3900 JPY (about 39 USD) per admission for infection prevention and control incentive at a major hospital, or 1000 JPY for a small hospital. Additional 1000 JPY was reimbursed if this hospital participates a local IPC network incentive. Another 1000 JPY was reimbursed for AS incentive. For hospitals with AS incentive, it mandates the following manpower in addition to 2012 requirements: one part-time doctor mainly for AS (at > 0.5 FTE), one full-time ICP either a certificated ICN or IC pharmacist or medical technician
[q]MRSA and MSSA are listed as separate pathogens

a significant decrease in the number of isolates of methicillin-resistant *S. aureus* (MRSA) from 2008 to 2015. This included a 64.6% reduction in Taiwan and 30.5% in Korea ($p < 0.05$) (Fig. 3a). The proportion of MRSA among all *S. aureus* isolates in 2015 remained high in Korea (83.1%), while it decreased in Taiwan by 12.3% from 79.9% in 2008 to 70.1% over the 8-year period. There was also a significant decrease in the number of isolates of carbapenem-resistant *P. aeruginosa* (CRPA) during the study period with a reduction of 50.4% in Korea and 38.4% in Taiwan ($p < 0.05$) (Fig. 3b).

Carbapenem-resistant *A. baumannii* (CRAB) was more commonly isolated in Taiwan than in South Korea. The number of CRAB isolates initially increased in Taiwan and then decreased significantly with a total reduction of 49.2% from 2010 to 2015 ($p < 0.05$). In contrast, the number of CRAB isolates in Korea increased by 91.8% by the end of the study period (Fig. 3c). The proportion of CRAB among *A. baumannii* isolates was higher in Korea than in Taiwan, and increased from 2008 to 2015 in both countries.

Discussion

In the current study, we described the surveillance and IPC programs of Taiwan, South Korea and Japan. A variation in surveillance protocol, such as HAI case definition and surveillance items was found among the three countries although these protocols were similar to those employed by the HAI-net and NHSN. There were also common IPC strategies shared by the three countries, but each with special emphasis on different aspects of IPC. We also compared the rates of HAI and the most common causative pathogens as reported by the three surveillance systems. There was a 53% decline in overall HAI in the surveyed ICUs of all three countries over the 8-year period. The overall incidence densities of HAI in Taiwan, Korea, and Japan in 2015 were 5.0, 2.8, and 2.7 per 1000 patient-days, respectively. These rates are comparable to HAI-net (2.6 per 1000 patient-days), and substantially lower than those of developing countries, as shown in Table 3 [2, 12–15].

We believe that essential elements that contributed to the sustained decrease in the incidence of HAI in Taiwan, Korea and Japan were the national surveillance programs combined with improvement in IPC practices [16]. In Korea, there was a significant decline in device-associated HAI in association with the implementation of the KONIS program [17]. National IPC programs such as hand hygiene, care bundles, antimicrobial stewardships, and environmental hygiene have been shown to effectively reduce HAI and infections caused by AMR pathogens [7, 18–20]. In Taiwan, hand hygiene program over a 4-year period were found to reduce HAI in ICU by 17.2% and BSI by 12.7% [20], and care bundles to further reduce CAUTI and CLABSI by 22.7 and 12.2%, respectively [21, 22]. In Korea, a multicentre study found that VAP rate decreased from 4.08 to 1.16 cases per 1000 ventilator-days following 3 months of bundle intervention [23]. Evidence-based IPC practices have been shown to be cost-saving and effective in preventing HAI [20, 24]. Adoption of these practices to reduce HAI burden might be helpful for many Asian countries, which are facing problems such as rising healthcare costs and inefficient healthcare insurance systems [25].

Appointment of infection control professionals or infection control committees is a common strategy across the three countries (Fig. 1, Additional file 2: Table S2). In Japan, one serious fundamental obstacle before 2010 was the lack of personnel dedicated to IPC. In 2010, Japan revised medical reimbursement system and provided 10

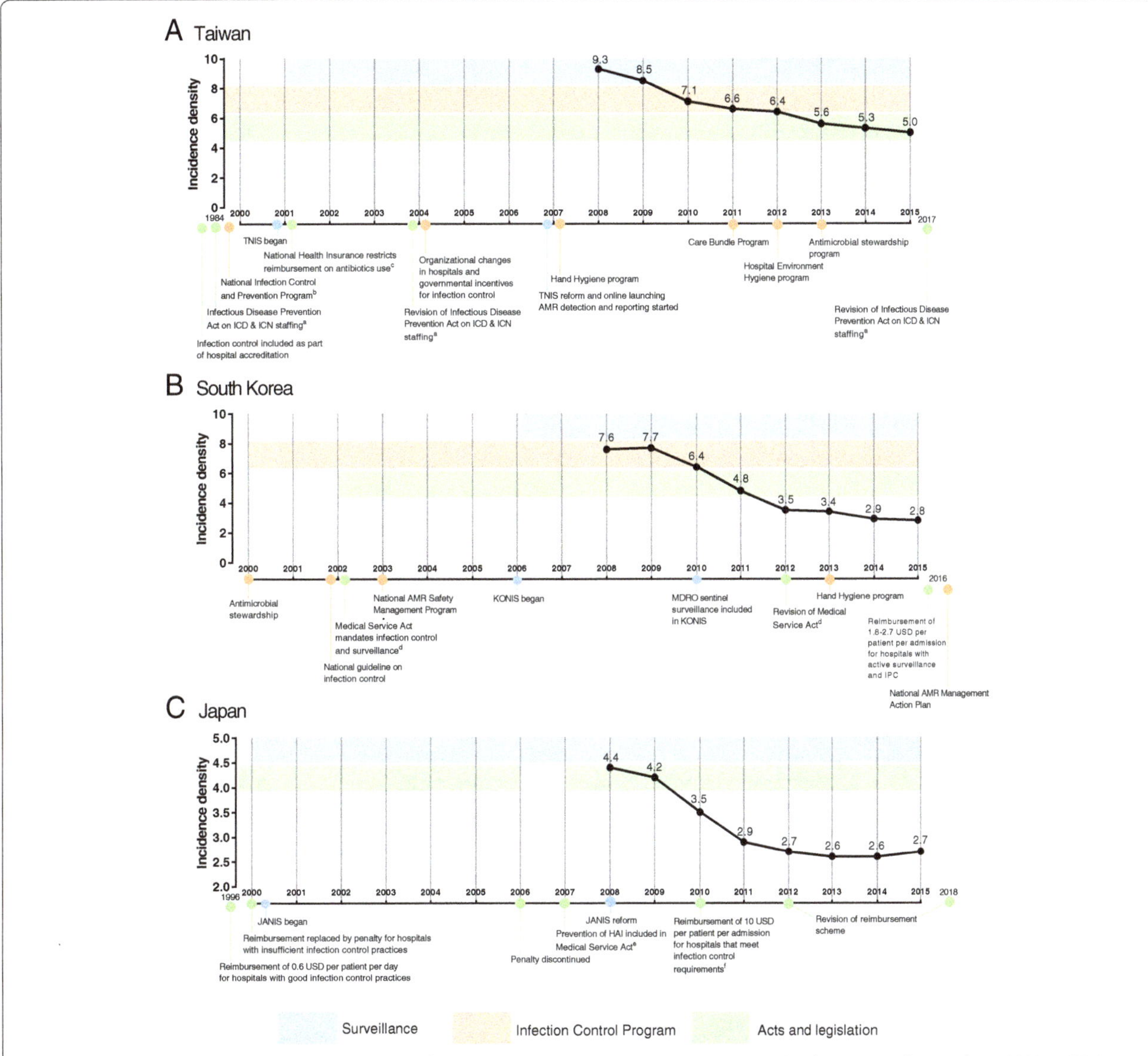

Fig. 1 Incidence densities of healthcare-associated infections in intensive care units across Taiwan, South Korea, and Japan from 2008 to 2015. Abbreviations: AMR: antimicrobial-resistance; HAI: healthcare-associated infections; ICN: infection control nurse; ICP: infection control personnel; IPC: infection prevention and control; JANIS: Japan Nosocomial Infection Surveillance; ICD: infection control doctor; KONIS: Korean National Healthcare-associated Infection Surveillance; MDRO: multi-drug resistant organisms; TNIS: Taiwan Nosocomial Infection Surveillance. [a] In 1984, every teaching hospital in Taiwan was required to have one ICN per 300 hospital beds. In 2004, hospitals with more than 500 beds are required to have at least one ICD, and hospitals with more than 300 beds are required to have at least one ICN per 250 beds. In 2017, hospitals with more than 500 beds are encouraged to have one ICD for every 300 beds and one ICN for every 250 beds (Table 1). [b] Included training healthcare staff, establishing infection control committees, and formulating hospital policies. [c] Restricts use of antimicrobials in ambulatory patients with upper respiratory infections but without evidence of bacterial infection. [d] Act 29 specifies that IPC are the duties of hospitals with more than 300 beds. Act 47 mandates IPC as part of hospital accreditation. In 2012, hospitals with more than 200 beds are required to appoint an infection control committee and at least one full-time experienced staff (Table 1). [e] Japanese medical law obligated all health care institutions to implement operational safety measures against HAI, which includes IPC guidelines, IPC training, and disease reporting. [f] Hospitals should have an infection control team that consists of ICN, ICD, infection control pharmacist and infection control microbiology technologist. Hospitals should also have an IPC policy and antimicrobial stewardship program (Table 1). **a** Taiwan; **b** South Korea; **c** Japan

USD per patient per admission if a hospital payed the annual cost for the designated work hours for infection control personnel which included certificated nurse, doctor, pharmacist and medical technician/microbiologist. IPC incentives through reimbursement policies were revised in 2012 and 2018, as described in Additional file 2: Table S2. Such a scheme encourages hospitals dedicated certificated personnel to participate in IPC (Table 1). Other than manpower, personnel training and resource infrastructure are essential for surveillance and prevention of HAI [26, 27].

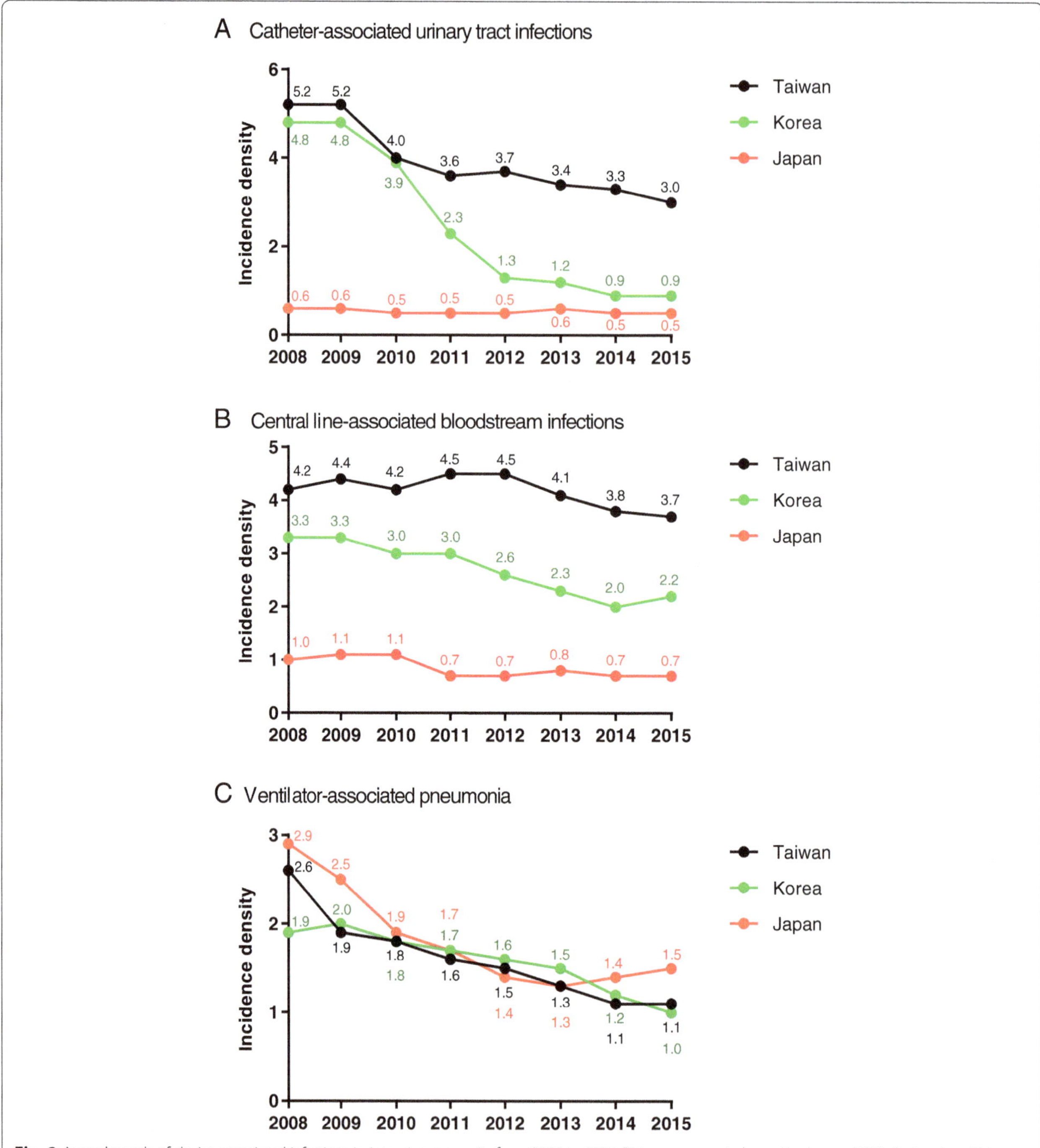

Fig. 2 Annual trends of device-associated infections in intensive care units from 2008 to 2015. Data are presented as episodes per 1000 device-days (Taiwan, Korea) or episodes per 1000 patient-days (Japan; data comprised urinary tract infections, central line-associated bloodstream infections and ventilator-associated pneumonia). **a** Catheter-associated urinary tract infections; **b** Central line-associated bloodstream infections; **c** Ventilator-associated pneumonia

During the study period, financial incentives to support IPC programs were employed by Korea and Japan. Japan switched its reimbursement system to a penalty system in 2000, and then changed it back to the current reward system in 2010. This suggests that a supportive environment that encourages IPC practices might be better than one that punishes for wrongdoing, and should be fostered by national authorities for effective prevention of HAI [27]. Correspondingly, such a difference in reimbursement may have well influenced the outcomes of HAI in Taiwan, Korea and Japan.

Changes in case definition might have contributed to the observed HAI trends. For example, the newer definition for UTI established in 2009 would probably have

Table 2 Common causative pathogens of healthcare-associated infections in intensive care units enrolled in the national surveillance systems of Taiwan, South Korea, and Japan in 2015

Rank	Organism	Proportion	Organism	Proportion	Organism	Proportion
Urinary Tract Infections[a]	Taiwan ($N = 3990$)		South Korea ($N = 760$)		Japan ($N = 202$)	
1	*Escherichia coli*	19.8%	*Escherichia coli*	17.6%	*Escherichia coli*	37.6%
2	*Candida albicans*	16.9%	*Candida albicans*	12.6%	*Pseudomonas aeruginosa*	16.3%
3	*Enterococcus faecium*	8.5%	*Enterococcus faecalis*	9.5%	*Candida albicans*	7.9%
4	*Pseudomonas aeruginosa*	7.4%	*Enterococcus faecium*	9.3%	*Klebsiella pneumoniae*	6.9%
5	*Klebsiella pneumoniae*	7.3%	*Klebsiella pneumoniae*	8.6%	*Enterococcus faecalis*	6.4%
Bloodstream Infections	Taiwan ($N = 4138$)		South Korea ($N = 1288$)		Japan[b] ($N = 268$)	
1	*Acinetobacter baumannii*	10.4%	*Enterococcus faecium*	14.7%	*Staphylococcus epidermidis*	15.7%
2	*Klebsiella pneumoniae*	9.6%	*Staphylococcus aureus*	14.2%	*Staphylococcus aureus*	13.0%
3	*Enterococcus faecium*	7.2%	*Acinetobacter baumannii*	12.6%	Coagulase negative staphylococci	10.1%
4	*Staphylococcus aureus*	6.5%	Coagulase negative staphylococci	12.0%	*Serratia marcescens*	5.6%
5	*Candida albicans*	6.2%	*Enterococcus faecalis*	7.3%		
Pneumonia	Taiwan ($N = 1397$)		South Korea ($N = 554$)		Japan[c] ($N = 650$)	
1	*Pseudomonas aeruginosa*	22.5%	*Acinetobacter baumannii*	34.5%	*Staphylococcus aureus*	21.8%
2	*Acinetobacter baumannii*	18.0%	*Staphylococcus aureus*	28.5%	*Pseudomonas aeruginosa*	18.6%
3	*Klebsiella pneumoniae*	16.2%	*Klebsiella pneumoniae*	9.4%	*Klebsiella pneumoniae*	7.8%
4	*Staphylococcus aureus*	9.0%	*Pseudomonas aeruginosa*	8.8%	*Stenotrophomonas maltophilia*	6.8%
5	*Enterobacter species*	6.2%	*Enterobacter aerogenes*	3.2%		

[a]The National Healthcare Safety Network definition of catheter-associated urinary tract infections was updated in 2015, and excluded *Candida*, yeasts or molds as potential pathogens. Nevertheless, TNIS, KONIS and JANIS kept these pathogens and data are provided
[b]Japan's data on bloodstream infection represents central line-associated bloodstream infections
[c]Japan's data on pneumonia represents ventilator-associated pneumonia

excluded cases that might have been classified as HAI under the older definition [28]. Nevertheless, based on the consistent decline of HAI incidence across all infection categories, it is unlikely that modifications in case definition can explain the remarkable decrease in HAI trends.

Substantial variation exists for causative pathogens of HAI across the three countries. This variability could be due to a number of factors, including baseline characteristics of participating hospitals and ICUs, variation in diagnostic standards and case definitions, geography and climate, and IPC practices. For example, Japan's BSI was dominated by staphylococci (39.9%) possibly because its reports were limited to device-associated modules in BSI. An interesting variation that is likely not attributable to systemic differences was noted for *A. baumannii*, which was isolated commonly from Taiwan and Korea but rarely from Japan. Results from HAI-net seem to support this notion, with higher proportions of HAI caused by *Acinetobacter spp.* in some countries [13].

Our study showed a general decrease in isolates of important AMR species: MRSA, CRPA and CRAB even though the number of participating ICUs has expanded from 2008 to 2015. This downward trend is likely due to hand hygiene to prevent cross-transmission of AMR pathogens, care bundles to prevent device- or procedure-associated infections, and antimicrobial stewardship programs to mitigate the selection pressure implemented in these countries [7, 18–20, 29]. A recent meta-analysis reported that antimicrobial stewardship programs in Asia reduced overall antimicrobial consumption by 9.74% and incidence density of important AMR pathogens such as MRSA by 0.9 to 1.4 isolates per 1000 patient-days [19]. Expenditure associated with antimicrobial prescription and hospitalization were also found to decrease by a range of 9.7 to 58.1%. These findings highlight the efficacy and importance of antimicrobial stewardship programs in combating the rise of AMR pathogens.

While surveillance of HAI may provide important feedback for IPC efforts, the high costs in establishing and maintaining the system may preclude many countries from undertaking such an ordeal. Introducing information technology in surveillance systems may help reduce labor intensive and increase the efficiency of surveillance [30–33]. In Asia, National Taiwan University Hospital has established a web-based real-time surveillance system based on algorithms for AMR pathogens, UTI and BSI. The surveillance system is sophisticated in its ability to integrate and analyse several data sources [32, 33]. Their studies and a recent

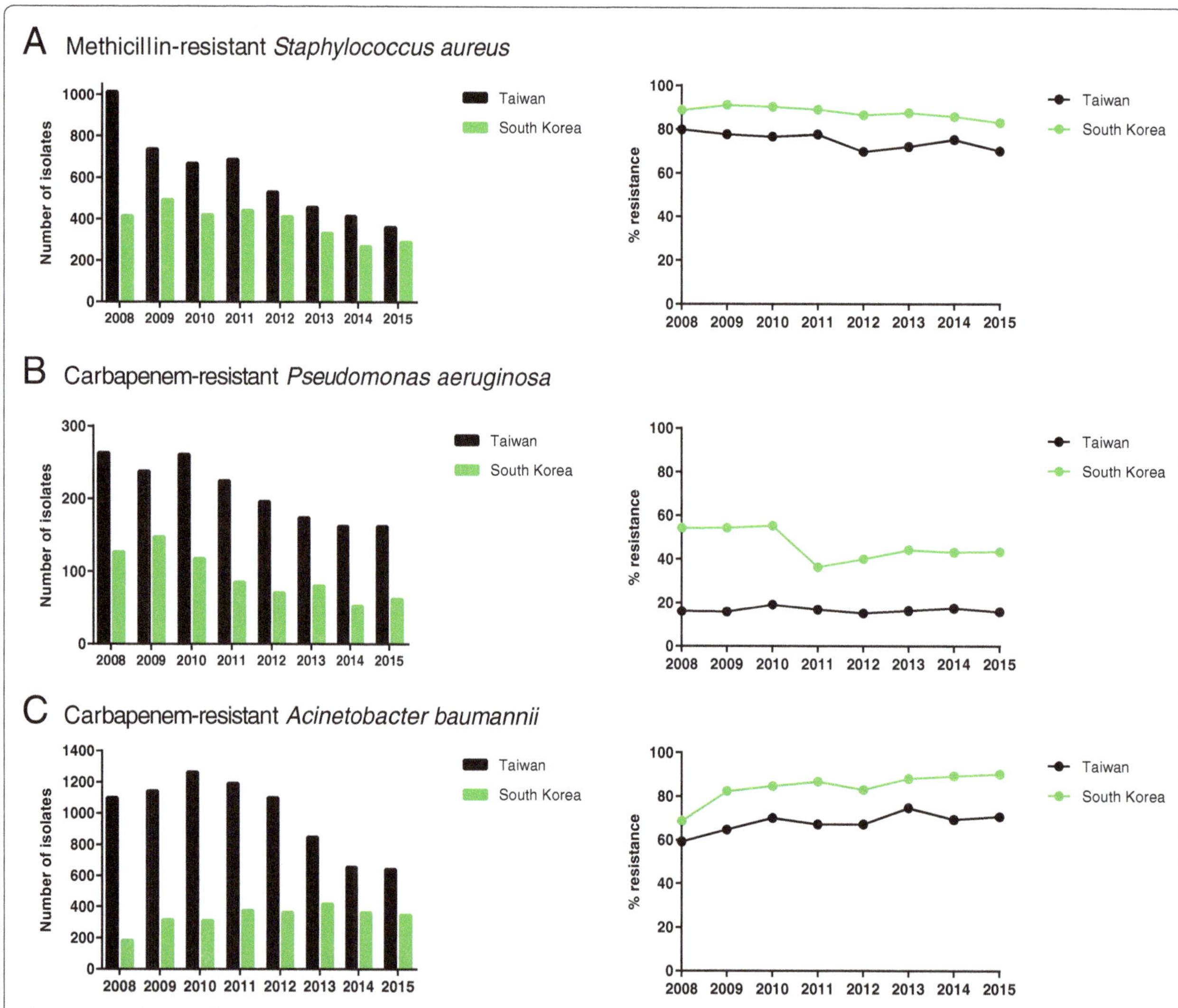

Fig. 3 Trends of the numbers and the proportions of antimicrobial resistance in selected bacteria causing healthcare-associated infections in the intensive care units in Taiwan and South Korea. Note: The proportions of antimicrobial resistance in selected pathogens were calculated as numbers of antimicrobial-resistant isolates divided by the total numbers of isolates of the same species. Japan's data included non-ICU patients and were not shown. **a** Methicillin-resistant *Staphylococcus aureus*; **b** Carbapenem-resistant *Pseudomonas aeruginosa*; **c** Carbapenem-resistant *Acinetobacter baumannii*

systematic review of the literature demonstrated that adopting electronic surveillance software yields considerable time savings pertaining to case findings, data collection, case ascertainment and classification while maintaining high levels of sensitivity and specificity [31–33]. Thus, information technology may represent an opportunity for countries seeking to establish HAI surveillance and overcome the gaps of human resources.

Our study provides a framework for other countries to establish or improve surveillance and IPC programs. Further studies on cost-effectiveness of these strategies will be helpful to relevant stakeholders as they allocate and prioritize budget for infection control. Our work also serves as the foundation for possible regional collaborations in East Asia or in greater Asia. Standardization of protocols will allow inter-country comparison and benchmarking. For Europe, the similarities and differences in HAI trends between our study and the HAI-net re-affirmed the need for continual surveillance and IPC efforts.

The strengths of this study were our ability to obtain an overview of the surveillance and IPC programs of Taiwan, Korea, and Japan that were seldom described in past reports. We were also able to obtain comprehensive HAI data from their surveillance systems and compare these data with Western developed countries and developing countries worldwide. The limitations were the need to use open access datasets. This restricted our ability to assess and compare HAI epidemiology comprehensively across the three countries. JANIS only releases data on UTI, CLABSI, and VAP in its surveillance reports. Information on the other infection modules: CAUTI, BSI, and HAP were unavailable. We were unable to comprehensively

Table 3 Comparison of healthcare-associated infections in intensive care units across different geographic regions

Countries/Regions (surveillance system)	Data source or type of study	Year	Overall[a]	Site-specific HAI (per 1000 patient-days)			Device-associated HAI (per 1000 device-days)		
				UTI [b]	BSI	HAP	CAUTI[b]	CLABSI	VAP
Taiwan (TNIS)	National surveillance	2015	5.0 (8514/1692998)	2.1	2.1	0.8	3.0	3.7	1.1
South Korea (KONIS)	National surveillance	2015	2.8[c] (2608/945605)	0.8	1.3	0.7	0.9	2.2	1.0
Japan (JANIS)	National surveillance	2015	2.7[d] (952/347386)	0.5	–	–	–	0.7[e]	1.5[e]
USA (NHSN) [12]	National surveillance	2012	1.6[f] (37872/23344616)	–	–	–	2.1	1.1	1.4
Europe (HAI-net) [13]	National surveillance	2015	2.6 (15821/6177114)	1.1	2.0	4.0	3.6	3.6	10.0
Southeast Asia [2]	Meta-analysis[g]	2000–2012	20.0[h] (16.9450/26681)	–	–	–	8.9	4.7	14.7
Developing countries worldwide [14]	Meta-analysis[g]	1995–2008	47.9[h] (28.54250/148893)	–	–	–	9.8	11.3	22.9
Developing countries worldwide (INICC)[i] [15]	Multi-center study	2010–2015	–	–	–	–	5.1	4.1	13.1

Abbreviations: BSI bloodstream infections, *CAUTI* catheter-associated urinary tract infections, *CLABSI* central line-associated bloodstream infections, *HAI* healthcare-associated infections, *HAI-net* Healthcare-associated Infections Surveillance Network (Europe), *HAP* hospital-acquired pneumonia, *ICU* intensive care units, *INICC* International Nosocomial Infection Control Consortium (developing countries worldwide), *NHSN* National Healthcare Safety network (USA), *UTI* urinary tract infections, *VAP* ventilator-associated pneumonia

[a]Data are pooled mean of site-specific HAI such as UTI, BSI, and HAP or otherwise specified, and computed from raw data provided in the reports. Thus, all these data should be interpreted appropriately

[b]The NHSN CAUTI definition was updated in 2015 and excluded *Candida*, yeasts or molds as potential CAUTI pathogens. Nevertheless, TNIS, KONIS and JANIS kept these pathogens and data are provided

[c]Data were collected during July 2015–June 2016

[d]Data are pooled means of UTI, CLABSI and VAP

[e]Data were calculated by episodes/1000 patient-day

[f]Data are pooled means of CAUTI, CLABSI and VAP

[g]Infection frequencies reported in high-quality studies were greater than those from low-quality studies

[h]Weights were given to different studies to compute the final data. Unweighted raw data were derived from the original article and denoted in parenthesis

[i]Data were prospectively collected from 861,284 patients in 703 ICUs from 50 countries

describe the complete pathogen rankings and AMR profiles for each country, because these data were unavailable on some surveillance systems. There are differences in protocols employed by each surveillance system, such as JANIS, which calculated device-associated infections differently. Standardization of protocols should allow for inter-country comparison. Furthermore, we need to include antibiotic use in future studies because of their critical impact on development of resistance. Finally, there were differences in the types of the hospitals enrolled in the three systems, wide variation of hospital participation rates (6.8% in Japan and 100% in Taiwan), and thus, discrepancies in hospital coverage rates (1.9% in Japan and 21.2% in Taiwan). Therefore, data presented here cannot be generalized to the entire 3 countries.

Conclusions

We found that national surveillance data obtained from Taiwan, South Korea, and Japan from 2008 to 2015 was associated with a 53.0% reduction in HAI in surveyed ICUs. There were differences among the countries in surveillance protocols, hospital coverage rates, national IPC programs, distribution of invading microorganisms and antibiotic resistance. The overall decrease in HAI appears to be due to improved surveillance coupled with a series of interventions in each country. We propose that a regional HAI network be established in East Asia similar to Europe's HAI-net. Such a coordinated effort should enable greater regional collaborations and development of joint strategies as we learn from one another.

Abbreviations

AMR: Antimicrobial resistance; AS: Antimicrobial stewardship; BSI: Bloodstream infection; CAUTI: Catheter-associated urinary tract infection; CLABSI: Central line-associated bloodstream infection; CRPA: Carbapenem-resistant *Pseudomonas aeruginosa*CRABCarbapenem-resistant *Acinetobacter baumannii*; FTE: Full-time equivalent; HAI: Healthcare-associated infections; HAI-net: European Healthcare-associated Infections Surveillance Network; HAP: Hospital-acquired pneumonia; IC: Infection control; ICD: Infection control doctor; ICN: Infection control nurse; ICP: Infection control personnel; ICU: Intensive care units; INICC: International Nosocomial Infection Control Consortium; IPC: Infection prevention and control; JANIS: Japan Nosocomial Infection Surveillance; KONIS: Korean National Healthcare-associated Infection Surveillance; MRSA: Methicillin-resistant *Staphylococcus aureus*; NHSN: National Healthcare Safety Network; TNIS: Taiwan Nosocomial Infection Surveillance; UTI: Urinary tract infection; VAP: Ventilator-associated pneumonia

Acknowledgements

We thank Calvin M. Kunin for his critical review of the manuscript.

Funding

No funding support.

Authors' contributions

Part of data were presented by CH Chiang at the International Conference on Prevention and Infection Control, 20–23 June 2017, Geneva, Switzerland. YC Chen coordinated and designed the study, and proofread the manuscript. CH Chiang, TS Yang and K Matsuda collected and analysed the data. SC Pan supervised statistical analysis. CH Chiang, SC Pan and YC Chen prepared the manuscript. FY Chang and SC Chang were involved in national infection control and prevention programs during the study period. HB Kim, YH Choi and other authors provided relevant information to consolidate the contents of the manuscript.

Consent for publication

Not applicable

Competing interests

The authors declare that they have no competing interests.

Author details

[1]College of Medicine, National Taiwan University, Taipei, Taiwan. [2]Department of Internal Medicine, National Taiwan University Hospital, Taipei, Taiwan. [3]Faculty of Medicine, Osaka University, Osaka, Japan. [4]Department of Internal Medicine, Seoul National University College of Medicine, Seoul, Republic of Korea. [5]Division of Infectious Diseases, Seoul National University Bundang Hospital, Seongnam, Republic of Korea. [6]Department of Infectious Diseases, Ajou University School of Medicine, Suwon, Republic of Korea. [7]Department of Infection Control Science, Juntendo University Faculty of Medicine, Tokyo, Japan. [8]Center for Infection Control, National Taiwan University Hospital, Taipei, Taiwan. [9]National Institute of Infectious Diseases and Vaccinology, National Health Research Institutes, Miaoli County, Taiwan. [10]Division of Infectious Diseases and Tropical Medicine, Department of Internal Medicine, Tri-Service General Hospital, National Defense Medical Center, Taipei, Taiwan.

References

1. European Centre for Disease Prevention and Control. Healthcare-associated Infections Surveillance Network. Available at: https://ecdc.europa.eu/en/about-us/partnerships-and-networks/disease-and-laboratory-networks/hai-net. Assessed 14 Apr 2018.
2. Ling ML, Apisarnthanarak A, Madriaga G. The burden of healthcare-associated infections in Southeast Asia: a systematic literature review and meta-analysis. Clin Infect Dis. 2015;60(11):1690–9.
3. Mehta Y, Jaggi N, Rosenthal VD, Kavathekar M, Sakle A, Munshi N, et al. Device-associated infection rates in 20 cities of India, data summary for 2004–2013: findings of the international nosocomial infection control consortium. Infect Control Hosp Epidemiol. 2016;37(2):172–81.
4. Tao L, Hu B, Rosenthal VD, Gao X, He L. Device-associated infection rates in 398 intensive care units in Shanghai, China: international nosocomial infection control consortium (INICC) findings. Int J Infect Dis. 2011;15(11):e774–80.
5. World Health Organization. Report on the burden of endemic health care-associated infection worldwide: clean care is safer care. Available at: http://apps.who.int/iris/bitstream/handle/10665/80135/9789241501507_eng.pdf;jsessionid=D87704F8824B725B0E90EBA22DE3BAAE?sequence=1. Accessed 14 Apr 2018.
6. Centers for Disease Control, R.O.C (Taiwan). Nosocomial Infections Surveillance System. Available at: http://www.cdc.gov.tw/english/info.aspx?treeid=00ed75d6c887bb27&nowtreeid=f0131176aa46d5db&tid=1A8C498AF5F8AF5D. Accessed 14 Apr 2018.
7. Tseng SH, Lee CM, Lin TY, Chang SC, Chuang YC, Yen MY, et al. Combating antimicrobial resistance: antimicrobial stewardship program in Taiwan. J Microbiol Immunol Infect. 2012;45(2):79–89.
8. Korean Society for Healthcare-associated Infection Control and Prevention. Korean Nosocomial Infections Surveillance System. Available at: http://www.koshic.org/main/main.html. Accessed 14 Apr 2018.
9. Choi JY, Kwak YG, Yoo H, Lee SO, Kim HB, Han SH, et al. Trends in the incidence rate of device-associated infections in intensive care units after the establishment of the Korean nosocomial infections surveillance system. J Hosp Infect. 2015;91(1):28–34.
10. Choi JY, Kwak YG, Yoo H, Lee SO, Kim HB, Han SH, et al. Trends in the distribution and antimicrobial susceptibility of causative pathogens of device-associated infection in Korean intensive care units from 2006 to 2013: results from the Korean nosocomial infections surveillance system (KONIS). J Hosp Infect. 2016;92(4):363–71.
11. Ministry of Health, Labour and Welfare, Japan. Japan Nosocomial Infections Surveillance. Available at: https://janis.mhlw.go.jp/report/icu.html. Accessed 14 Apr 2018.
12. Centers for Disease Control and Prevention, USA. National Healthcare Safety Network Reports. Available at: https://www.cdc.gov/nhsn/datastat/index.html. Accessed 14 Apr 2018.
13. European Centre for Disease Prevention and Control. Healthcare-associated infections acquired in intensive care units - Annual Epidemiological Report for 2015. Available at: https://ecdc.europa.eu/en/publications-data/healthcare-associated-infections-acquired-intensive-care-units-annual. Accessed 14 Apr 2018.
14. Allegranzi B, Bagheri Nejad S, Combescure C, Graafmans W, Attar H, Donaldson L, et al. Burden of endemic health-care-associated infection in developing countries: systematic review and meta-analysis. Lancet. 2011;377(9761):228–41.
15. Rosenthal VD, Al-Abdely HM, El-Kholy AA, AlKhawaja SAA, Leblebicioglu H, Mehta Y, et al. International nosocomial infection control consortium report, data summary of 50 countries for 2010-2015: device-associated module. Am J Infect Control. 2016;44(12):1495–504.
16. Haley RW, Culver DH, White JW, Morgan WM, Emori TG, Munn VP, et al. The efficacy of infection surveillance and control programs in preventing nosocomial infections in US hospitals. Am J Epidemiol. 1985;121(2):182–205.
17. Kim EJ, Kwak YG, Park SH, Kim SR, Shin MJ, Yoo HM, et al. Trends of device utilization ratios in intensive care units over 10-year period in South Korea: Device utilization ratio as a new aspect of surveillance. J Hosp Infect. 2017. doi: https://doi.org/10.1016/j.jhin.2017.10.007. [Epub ahead of print]. pii: S0195–6701(17)30547–9.
18. Price L, MacDonald J, Melone L, Howe T, Flowers P, Currie K, et al. Effectiveness of national and subnational infection prevention and control interventions in high-income and upper-middle-income countries: a systematic review. Lancet Infect Dis. 2018;18(5):e159–71.
19. Honda H, Ohmagari N, Tokuda Y, Mattar C, Warren DK. Antimicrobial stewardship in inpatient settings in the Asia Pacific Region: a systematic review and meta-analysis. Clin Infect Dis. 2017;64(suppl_2):S119–26.
20. Chen YC, Sheng WH, Wang JT, Chang SC, Lin HC, Tien KL, et al. Effectiveness and limitations of hand hygiene promotion on decreasing healthcare–associated infections. PLoS One. 2011;6(11):e27163.
21. Lai CC, Lee CM, Chiang HT, Hung CT, Chen YC, Su LH, et al. Implementation of a national bundle care program to reduce catheter-associated urinary tract infection in high-risk units of hospitals in Taiwan. J Microbiol Immunol Infect. 2017;50(4):464–70.
22. Lai CC, Cia CT, Chiang HT, Kung YC, Shi ZY, Chuang YC, et al. Implementation of a national bundle care program to reduce central line-associated bloodstream infections in intensive care units in Taiwan. J Microbiol Immunol Infect. 2017. doi: https://doi.org/10.1016/j.jmii.2017.10.001. [Epub ahead of print]. pii: S1684–1182(17)30231–1.
23. Eom JS, Lee MS, Chun HK, Choi HJ, Jung SY, Kim YS, et al. The impact of a ventilator bundle on preventing ventilator-associated pneumonia: a multicenter study. Am J Infect Control. 2014;42(1):34–7.
24. Umscheid CA, Mitchell MD, Doshi JA, Agarwal R, Williams K, Brennan PJ. Estimating the proportion of healthcare-associated infections that are reasonably preventable and the related mortality and costs. Infect Control Hosp Epidemiol 2011;32(2):101–1.
25. Organisation for Economic Co-operation and Development. Health at a Glance 2017 OECD Indicators. Available at: https://doi.org/10.1787/health_glance-2017-en. Accessed 14 Apr 2018.
26. Kwak YG, Lee SO, Kim HY, Kim YK, Park ES, Jin HY, et al. Risk factors for device-associated infection related to organisational characteristics of intensive care units: findings from the Korean nosocomial infections surveillance system. J Hosp Infect. 2010;75(3):195–9.
27. Sakamoto F, Sakihama T, Saint S, Greene MT, Ratz D, Tokuda Y. Health care–associated infection prevention in Japan: the role of safety culture. Am J Infect Control. 2014;42(8):888–93.
28. Healthcare Infection Control Practices Advisory Committee. Guideline for prevention of catheter-associated urinary tract infections 2009. Available at:

https://www.cdc.gov/infectioncontrol/pdf/guidelines/cauti-guidelines.pdf. Accessed 14 Apr 2018.
29. Krein SL, Greene MT, Apisarnthanarak A, Sakamoto F, Tokuda Y, Sakihama T, et al. Infection Prevention Practices in Japan, Thailand, and the United States: Results From National Surveys. Clin Infect Dis. 2017;64(suppl_2):S105–11.
30. Van Mourik MSM, Perencevich EN, Gastmeier P, Bonten MJM. Designing surveillance of healthcare-associated infections in the era of automation and reporting mandates. Clin Infect Dis. 2018;66(6):970–6.
31. Russo PL, Shaban RZ, Macbeth D, Carter A, Mitchell BG. Impact of electronic healthcare-associated infection surveillance software on infection prevention resources: a systematic review of the literature. J Hosp Infect. 2018;99(1):1–7. https://doi.org/10.1016/j.jhin.2017.09.002 Epub 2017 Sep 8.
32. Tseng YJ, Wu JH, Ping XO, Lin HC, Chen YY, Shang RJ, et al. A web-based multidrug-resistant organism surveillance and outbreak detection system with rule-based classification and clustering. J Med Internet Res. 2012;14(5):e131.
33. Tseng YJ, Wu JH, Lin HC, Chen MY, Ping XO, Sun CC, et al. A web-based, hospital-wide health care-associated bloodstream infection surveillance and classification system: development and evaluation. JMIR Med Inform. 2015; 3(3):e31.

Emergence of high drug resistant bacterial isolates from patients with health care associated infections at Jimma University medical center

Mulatu Gashaw[1,11*], Melkamu Berhane[2], Sisay Bekele[3], Gebre Kibru[1], Lule Teshager[1], Yonas Yilma[4], Yesuf Ahmed[5], Netsanet Fentahun[6], Henok Assefa[7], Andreas Wieser[8], Esayas Kebede Gudina[9] and Solomon Ali[1,10]

Abstract

Background: The rates of resistant microorganisms which complicate the management of healthcare associated infections (HAIs) are increasing worldwide and getting more serious in developing countries. The objective of this study was to describe microbiological features and resistance profiles of bacterial pathogens of HAIs in Jimma University Medical Center (JUMC) in Ethiopia.

Methods: Institution based cross sectional study was carried out on hospitalized patients from May to September, 2016 in JUMC. Different clinical specimens were collected from patients who were suspected to hospital acquired infections. The specimens were processed to identify bacterial etiologies following standard microbiological methods. Antibacterial susceptibility was determined in vitro by Kirby-Bauer disk diffusion method following Clinical and Laboratory Standards Institute guidelines.

Results: Overall, 126 bacterial etiologies were isolated from 118 patients who had HAIs. Of these, 100 (79.4%) were gram negative and the remaining were gram positive. The most common isolates were *Escherichia coli* 31(24.6%), *Klebsiella* species 30(23.8%) and *Staphylococcus aureus* 26 (20.6%). Of 126 bacterial isolates, 38 (30.2%), 52 (41.3%), and 24 (19%) were multidrug-resistant (MDR, resistant to at least one agent in three or more antimicrobial categories), extensively drug resistant (XDR, resistant to at least one agent in all but two or fewer antimicrobial categories (i.e. bacterial isolates remain susceptible to only one or two categories), pan-drug resistant (PDR, resistant to all antibiotic classes) respectively. More than half of isolated gram-negative rods (51%) were positive for extended spectrum beta-lactamase (ESBL) and/or AmpC; and 25% of gram negative isolates were also resistant to carbapenem antibiotics.

Conclusions: The pattern of drug resistant bacteria in patients with healthcare associated infection at JUMC is alarming. This calls for coordinated efforts from all stakeholders to prevent HAIs and drug resistance in the study setting.

Keywords: Antimicrobial agents, Drug resistant isolates, Multidrug resistance, Extensively resistance, Pandrug resistance, Carbapenem resistance, Extended spectrum beta-lactamase

* Correspondence: mulatugashaw@gmail.com; mulatu.gashaw@ju.edu.et
[1]School of Medical Laboratory Science, Jimma University, Jimma, Ethiopia
[11]Institute of Health, Jimma University, P.O. Box 1368, Jimma, Ethiopia
Full list of author information is available at the end of the article

Introduction

The emergence and rapid spread of multidrug resistant pathogenic bacteria is becoming a global health challenge [1]. Recent studies showed an increasing rate of bacterial resistance against available antibiotics. The problem is more pronounced in developing countries attributed to limited antibiotic option, irrational drug use, poor drug quality, poor sanitation, malnutrition, poor and inadequate health care systems, and lack of control for antibiotic use and stewardship program [2, 3].

In the past few decades, antimicrobial drugs have saved many lives and reduced the grief of many million people globally [3]. However, the extraordinary benefits of antimicrobials in reducing morbidity and mortality have been challenged by the emergence of drug resistant bacteria. The recent emergence and spread of these resistant bacteria have become a serious public health concern [4]. Especially, the spread of such bacteria in resource limited countries would have devastating consequences considering the health infrastructure, antibiotic options available and over all resource constraints observed in such countries [5].

In recent years, high dissemination of ESBL producing, carbapenem, and methicillin resistant bacteria are observed worldwide [6, 7]. It is described that the problem of ESBL-producing organisms is more intense in developing countries [8]. However, the magnitude of the problem is still probably underestimated due to inadequate or ineffective detection in some clinical settings [3, 7, 9]. ESBLs are a group of plasmid-mediated, diverse, complex and rapidly evolving enzymes which are capable of hydrolyzing penicillin's, broad-spectrum cephalosporin's and monobactam's [10]. Accordingly, ESBL enzyme producing bacteria have a capacity to resist the action of penicillin's, broad-spectrum cephalosporin's and monobactam's [11]. Furthermore, there is an evidence indicating that most of ESBL producing bacteria are also resistant for carbapenem antibiotics [12, 13]. ESBLs production is most commonly seen among Gram negative bacteria including *Escherichia coli, Klebsiella pneumoniae, Proteus mirabilis and Pseudomonas aeruginosa* [14].

Infections resulting from antibiotic resistant bacteria are more difficult and, in some instances, impossible to treat with current available antibiotics. Such infections lead to higher morbidity and mortality, imposing huge healthcare cost [15, 16]. In recent years, varieties of bacteria are becoming resistant against two or more classes of antibiotics as a result of selective pressure or horizontal gene transfer. For instance, the magnitude of resistance seen among *E. coli*, *S. aureus*, *Klebsiella* species, *P. aeruginosa*, *A. baumannii,* and *Enterobacter* species is more threatening as these bacteria are the commonest etiologies for commonly observed hospital and community acquired infections [17, 18].

In Ethiopia, the patterns of antibiotic resistance among commonly seen bacterial etiologies have been described previously in different settings [19–21]. However, most of these studies did not address the magnitude of ESBL producing and carbapenem resistance patterns comprehensively. It is also known that bacterial antibiotic resistance is a dynamic process. Resistance patterns seen in the past might not be representing the current situation due to the strong correlation between efficiency of antibiotic use and antibiotic resistance. As a result, information about the current antibiotic resistance pattern of bacteria is very vital to understand the dynamic and trend of resistance.

Clinical characteristics of patients with HAIs at Jimma University Medical Center have recently been published. The incidence and overall prevalence of HAIs at the hospital were 28.15 per 1000 patient days and 19.41% respectively [22]. In the current study, we aimed to determine the MDR, XDR, PDR, ESBL mediated and carbapenem resistance patterns of bacteria isolated from patients with HAIs at the hospital.

Methods and materials

Institution based cross-sectional study was carried out in all wards of JUMC from May, 2016 to September, 2016. Totally, 1015 patients were admitted, of these 197 patients had sign of healthcare associated infection during the study time and all were taken as study participants. Microbiological investigation was done for 192 participants suspected to have healthcare associated infection; no microbiological test was done for the other five cases due to inability to obtain proper specimen. Different clinical specimens (blood, urine, wound swab, pus, and sputum) were collected aseptically from the patients with signs of healthcare associated infection. Bacterial identification was performed by standard microbiological methods which are adopted from CLSI guideline.

Phenotypic determination of antibiotic susceptibility patterns

Antibacterial susceptibility of Penicillin (10 µg), Oxacillin (1 µg), Gentamycin (10 µg), Chloramphenicol (30 µg), Tetracycline (30 µg) Erythromycin (15 µg), Trimethoprim-sulfamethoxazole (1.25 g), Clindamycin (2 µg), Cefoxitin (30 µg), Ciprofloxacin (5 µg), Nitrofurantoin (300 µg), Norfloxacin (10 µg), Ampicillin (10 µg), Amoxicillin-clavulanic acid (10 µg), Ceftriaxone (30 µg), Ceftazidime (30 µg), Cefepime (30 µg), and Meropenem (10 µg), (Oxoid, UK) were determined in vitro by Kirby-Bauer disk diffusion method following Clinical and Laboratory Standards Institute guidelines [23].

ESBL and/or AmpC detection

The presence of an ESBL and/or AmpC was determined with Cefpodoxime (10 μg), Cefotaxime (30 μg), Cefepime (30 μg) and Ceftazidime (30 μg) containing antibiotic discs (Mast Group, UK) by disc diffusion confirmation test. After the discs were inserted on inoculated plates, then they were incubated at 35–37 °C for 18–24 h aerobically. Finally, zones of inhibition were read and recorded on excel sheet. The data from the excel sheet was transported to Mast group ESBL/AmpC and CARBA plus calculator spreadsheet (Mast group, UK) and reported as negative or positive for ESBL or/and AmpC and finally the results were recorded.

The results were registered as resistant, intermediate and susceptible; but for the sake of analysis intermediate and resistant isolates were grouped together as resistant. Classification of MDR, XDR and PDR were carried out according to Magiorakos et al, definitions [4]. All the antibiotic disks were from Oxoid (Oxoid, UK) and Mast discs (Mast group, UK). The inhibition zone diameter was measured using caliper and recorded on excel sheet.

Data quality control

Standard operating procedures (SOPs) were strictly followed while we did all bacteriological procedures starting from sample collection, isolation, identification and antibiotic susceptibility testing. Susceptible American Type Culture Collection (ATCC) 25,922 *E. coli* and ATCC 25923 *Staphylococcus aureus* were used as control strains and the test results were only accepted when the inhibition zone diameters of the above mentioned control strains were within performance ranges as described by CLSI [23]. ESBL positive ATCC 700603 *Klebsiella pneumoniae* and both ESBL and carbapenemase negative *E. coli* ATCC 25922 control strains were used in this study as positive and negative control respectively. To standardize the inoculum density of bacterial suspension for a susceptibility test, 0.5 McFarland standards, which is comparable with the approximate number of bacterial suspension (1.0×10^8 to $2.0\text{x}10^8$bacteria/mL), was used [23].

Data analysis and statistical tests

Data were double entered to Epi Data version 3.1 and transferred to SPSS version 20 and Microsoft Excel software for analysis and the results were presented as tables, pie-charts and graphs. *P*-values < 0.05 were considered as statistically significant.

Ethical consideration

The study was approved by the Institutional Review Board of Institute of Health, Jimma University. Informed written consent was also obtained from participants and/or guardians after explaining the objective of the study. All the laboratory results were communicated as early as possible with the treating physicians for better management of the patients.

Result

Socio-demography and background information of the participants

From 1015 patients who were enrolled in the study; only 197 admitted patients had developed sign of healthcare associated infection with in the study time. Of these, 118 (59.9%) patients had culture confirmed healthcare associated infections. Sociodemographic and clinical characteristics of study participants have recently been published. The incidence and overall prevalence of HAIs at the hospital were 28.15 per 1000 patient days and 19.41% respectively [22].

Isolation rate

Totally 240 clinical samples were obtained from 192 patients who were clinically diagnosed with healthcare associated infection. The most common sources of specimen were urine (55%) followed by wound swab/pus (24.2%), blood (15%), and sputum (5.8%). A total of 126 bacterial pathogens were isolated from 118 patient samples. A single organism was isolated from 110 (93.2%) patient samples, and two organisms were isolated from 8 (6.8%) patient samples who had been admitted to ICU. The overall culture positivity rate of participants was 118/192(61.5%). Most commonly isolated bacteria were *E. coli* 31(24.6%), *Klebsiella* species 30(23.8%) and *S. aureus* 26 (20.6%) (Fig. 1).

Drug resistance patterns of isolates to different classes of antibiotics

Antibiotic resistance patterns of the isolated pathogen of nosocomial origin are shown in Table 1. Half of *S. aureus* isolates were resistant to gentamicin 50.0% (13/26); and 53.84% (14/26) and 57.7% (15/26) of the isolates were resistant to methicillin /cefoxitin/oxacillin and ceftriaxone/chloramphenicol in vitro respectively; and all of *S. aureus* isolates were resistant against penicillin (Table 1). From a total of 26 *S. aureus* isolates, 3(11.5%), 10(38.5%) 10 (38.5%) and 3(11.6%) were MoDR, MDR, XDR and PDR respectively (Table 2).

From Gram negative bacteria, *E. coli* and *Klebsiella* species were the most frequent isolates. More than 90% of *E. coli* isolates were resistant against ampicillin, tetracycline and trimethoprim-sulfamethoxazole (Table 1). Conversely, only 16.1% of *E.coli* isolates were resistant against meropenem. Likewise, the resistance rate of *Klebsiella* species were 100% for ampicillin, 90% for tetracycline, 80% for trimethoprim

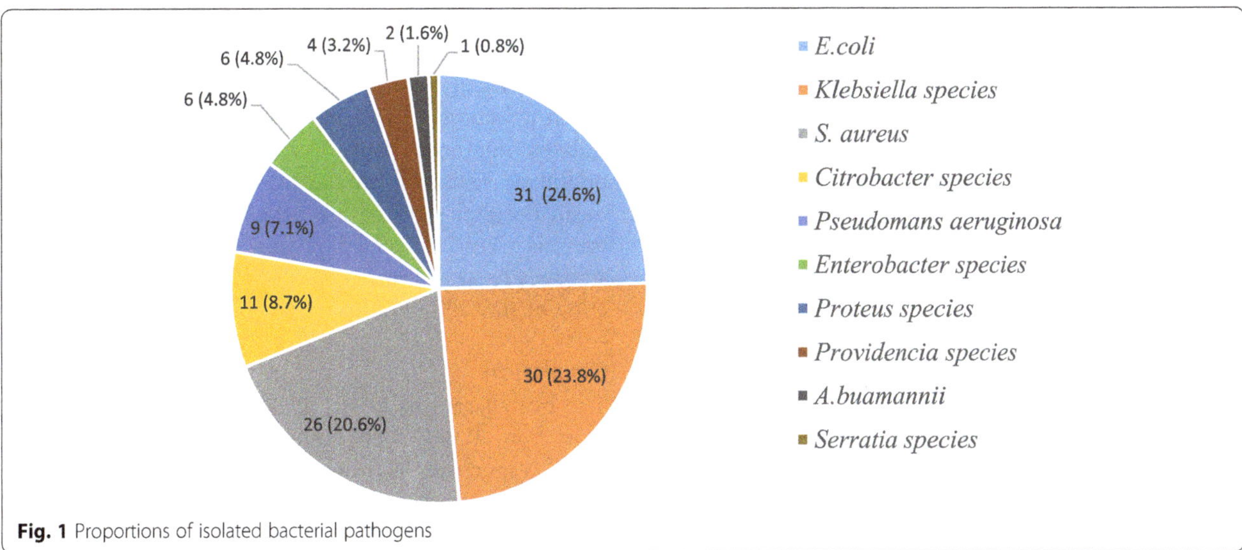

Fig. 1 Proportions of isolated bacterial pathogens

-sulfamethoxazole, 40% for ciprofloxacin and 30% for meropenem (Table 1).

Classification of isolates based on their drug resistance pattern

As shown in Table 2, among 126 bacterial isolates, 38 (30.2%), 52 (41.3%), and 24 (19%) were MDR, XDR, and PDR respectively. Eight of the isolates were resistant to a single antimicrobial class and only four *Klebsiella* isolates were susceptible to all classes of the antimicrobials. The predominant isolates (*E. coli*, *Klebsiella* species and *S. aureus)* showed very high antimicrobial resistance patterns. The overall MDR rate of the isolated bacteria was 30.16%. All bacteria isolated from ICU and pediatrics wards, 87.5% of bacteria isolated from Gynecology and obstetrics wards, 88% of bacteria isolated from Medical wards and 85.7% of bacteria isolated from surgical wards were MDR. The overall prevalence of PDR among all isolates was 19.0%. *Citrobacter species* (45.4%) and *Pseudomonas aeruginosa* (33.3%) have shown high pandrug resistance rate. On the

Table 1 Frequency of antimicrobial resistant bacterial isolates for selected antimicrobial classes

Antibiotic classes	Antibiotics	*S. aureus* (*n* = 26)	*E. coli* (*n* = 31)	*Klebsiella* species (*n* = 30)	*Citrobacter* species (*n* = 11)	*P. aeruginosa* (*n* = 9)	*Enterobacter* species (*n* = 6)	*Proteus* species (*n* = 6)	*Providencia* species (*n* = 4)	A. *buamannii* (*n* = 2)	*Serratia* species (*n* = 1)
Penecillins	Penicillin	26	–	–	–	–	–	–	–	–	–
3rd and 4th generation cephalosporins	Ampicillin	–	29	30	11	9	6	5	4	2	1
	Ceftriaxone	15	15	16	7	9	4	4	2	2	1
	Ceftazidime	–	16	17	8	8	5	4	2	2	1
	Cefepime	–	14	15	6	5	2	4	2	2	1
Anti-staphylococcal β-lactams	Oxacillin	14	–	–	–	–	–	–	–	–	–
Cephamycins	Cefoxitin	14	19	23	6	8	6	4	1	2	1
Aminoglycosides	Gentamycin	13	22	21	7	8	3	3	1	2	1
Phenicols	Chloramphenicol	15	19	20	8	9	1	3	3	2	1
Macrolides	Erythromycin	19	–	–	–	–	–	–	–	–	–
Lincosamides	Clindamycin	17	–	–	–	–	–	–	–	–	–
Tetracycline	Tetracycline	17	29	27	7	9	4	6	4	2	1
Folate pathway inhibitors	Trimethoprim-sulfamethoxazole	19	28	24	9	4	2	6	3	2	1
Fluoroquinolones	Ciprofloxacin	16	14	12	6	6	3	3	2	1	1
Carbapenems	Meropenem	–	5	9	2	4	1	0	1	2	1
Penecillins + β-lactamase inhibitors	Amoxicillin-clavulanic acid	–	28	29	9	9	6	6	4	2	1

Table 2 Frequency distribution of MultiS, MoDR, MDR, XDR, and PDR pattern of isolated bacteria

Isolated organisms	Total	MultiS	MoDR	MDR	XDR	PDR
S. aureus	26	0	3	10	10	3
E. coli	31	0	3	11	10	7
Klebsiella species	30	4	2	9	13	2
Citrobacter species	11	0	0	2	4	5
Enterobacter species	6	0	0	2	3	1
Proteus species	6	0	0	2	4	0
Providencia species	4	0	0	0	3	1
Pseudomonas aeruginosa	9	0	0	2	4	3
Acinetobacter baumannii	2	0	0	0	1	1
Serratia species	1	0	0	0	0	1
Total	126	4	8	38	52	24

MultiS, susceptible to all antibiotic classes; MoDR, resistant to single antibiotic class; MDR, resistant to at least one agent in three or more antimicrobial categories; XDR, resistant to at least one agent in all but two or fewer antimicrobial categories (i.e. bacterial isolates remain susceptible to only one or two categories); PDR, resistant to all antibiotic classes. Source: Based on definitions by Magiorakos et al. [4]

other hand, *Klebsiella* species (6.6%) and *S.aureus* (11.5%) have shown the least PDR rate. *E.coli* (22.6%) and *Enterobacter species* (16.7%) have also shown a moderate PDR rate.

Prevalence of ESBL, AmpC, and Carbapenemase producing isolates

Of the 1 hundred isolated gram-negative rods, 36 and 7% were positive for extended spectrum beta-lactamase (ESBL) and AmpC respectively. Eight percent of the isolates were positive for both extended spectrum beta-lactamase (ESBL) and AmpC. With regard to the proportion of carbapenemase producing isolates, 25% of gram negative isolates have shown carbapenem resistance (Table 3). To be precise, 16.1% of *E.coli* and 30.0% of *Klebsiella* species were carbapenem resistant isolates (Table 3).

Antimicrobial resistance pattern and impact on clinical outcome

Of 118 patients with culture confirmed healthcare associated infection, 13 patients (11.02%) died and all of the isolated microorganisms from these 13 patients were multidrug resistant (MDR) as shown in Table 4. The mean hospital stays of the patients infected with MDR bacteria were 15.4 ± 9.6 days (range 3–49 days). There is statistically significant association between mean duration of stay and infection with MDR bacteria (Table 4).

Discussion

The overall rate of MDR, XDR and PDR bacterial isolates from JUMC were found to be 30.16, 41.27 and 19.0% respectively. Furthermore, the observed MDR rate is significantly associated with prolonged hospital stay and all patients, who died, were infected with MDR bacterial species (even if, it is not statistically significant). On the other hand, the observed XDR and PDR rate at the hospital indicates that the problem of AMR is increasing at an alarming rate and pathogenic bacteria that circulate in JUMC are becoming more resistant to all available antibiotics. The occurrence of PDR pathogenic bacteria would also have huge potential threat and implications for patient care in the hospital and the community at large. As we are living in the era of very connected world, it is highly likely for these PDR bacteria to be disseminated to other parts of Ethiopia and other parts of the world as well.

To the best of our knowledge, there is no previous report from Ethiopia on the rate of XDR and PDR pathogenic bacteria to compare with this result. It is possible to list some reasons which might have contributed for this observed high XDR and PDR rate. The first reason might be associated with lack of AMR surveillance and stewardship program at JUMC and in Ethiopia in general. There is enough evidence that indicates AMR surveillance and stewardship program helps to understand

Table 3 Prevalence of ESBL, AmpC, and Carbapenem resistant isolates of gram negative rods

Isolated organisms	Total	ESBL & AmpC producing isolates				Carbapenemase resistance	
		Not ESBL & AmpC, N (%)	ESBL, N (%)	AmpC, N (%)	ESBL & AmpC, N (%)	Yes, N (%)	No, N (%)
E. coli	31	12(38.7)	14(45.2)	3 (9.7)	2 (6.5)	5 (16.1)	26 (83.9)
Klebsiella species	30	14 (46.7)	13 (43.3)	2 (6.7)	1 (3.3)	9 (30.0)	21 (70.0)
Citrobacter species	11	5	4	0	2	2	9
Enterobacter species	6	2	3	0	1	1	5
Proteus species	6	5	1	0	0	0	6
Providencia species	4	1	2	1	0	1	3
Pseudomonas aeruginosa	9	5	1	1	2	4	5
Acinetobacter baumannii	2	2	0	0	0	2	0
Serratia species	1	1	0	0	0	1	0
Total	100	49	36	7	8	25	75

Table 4 Antimicrobial resistance and associated factors

Variable	Non MDR ($N = 12$) (%)	MDR ($N = 106$) (%)	P
History of treatment[a]			
No	9 (75.0)	85 (80.19)	
Yes	3 (25.0)	21 (19.81)	0.672
Patient outcome			
Progress	12 (100)	93 (87.74)	
Died	0	13 (12.26)	0.198
Duration of stay in Hospital			
<=15 days	8 (66.6)	25 (23.58)	
> 15 days	4 (33.4)	81 (76.42)	0.002

Non-MDR: susceptible to all antibiotic classes/resistant to one/two antibiotic classes; MDR: resistant to at least one agent in three or more antimicrobial categories Magiorakos et al. [4]

[a] taking antibiotics in the last 3 months of the study period

the pattern of resistance and improve the utilization of antibiotics to prevent occurrence of antibiotic resistance.

The second reason might be associated with lack of comprehensive national antibiotic policies and problems in implementations of policies. In Ethiopia, there is no clear antibiotic policy and controlling mechanism about antibiotic usage. It is a common practice in Ethiopia to buy any antibiotic from private drug vendors and pharmacies without any prescription. This might have contributed for emergence and dissemination of antibiotic resistant bacteria at different settings. The third reason might be associated with lack of system to assess the quality and reliability of imported antibiotics in Ethiopia. For instance, one previous study which assessed the quality of anti-tuberculosis drugs in Ethiopia in 2013 has indicated that around 17% of anti TB drugs were fake drugs [24]. It is easy to imagine the role of these fake drugs on anti TB drug resistance. Likewise, though there is no previous research done in Ethiopia to assess the quality of antibiotics dispensed in private and government pharmacies, it is highly likely that some of them might be sub-standard, given that substantial proportion of the antibiotics in private pharmacies are supplied through unknown routes [25, 26].

The emergence of ESBL producing gram negative rods have become a rising concern in the developing world [27]. In this study, phenotypically, the most common ESBL producing microorganisms were *E. coli* and *Klebsiella* species which are 51.6% (16/31) and 46.7% (14/30) respectively; which is comparable with the studies done in Nigeria, Nepal and New Zealand in which ESBL producing *Enterobacteriaceae* were 44.3, 43.7 and 38.0% respectively [14, 28, 29]. However, the other studies done in India and Nepal showed that 30.18 and 18.4% of *Klebsiella pneumoniae* produce ESBL respectively which is lower than our report [30, 31]. Even though the prevalence of ESBLs is not well documented, in many parts of the world 10–40% of strains of *Escherichia coli* and *Klebsiella pneumoniae* are estimated to produce ESBLs [27]. High proportion of ESBL producing isolates was documented in the current study which might be due to the fact that our study participants were all hospitalized; since hospitalization was identified as the strongest independent risk factor to express ESBL [32].

Regarding to carbapenem resistance, 19 (21.4%), 4 (44.4%) and 2 (100%) of the *Enterobacteriaceae, P. aeruginosa* and *A. buamannii* were carbapenem resistant respectively which are found in the priority one list according to WHO classification [33]. In addition to that, 53.8% of the other commonly isolated *S. aureus* were methicillin resistant which also needs high attention. Therefore, high attention should be given to these pathogens which are considered as priority one and two according to WHO [33]. To compare with other similar studies, the rate of carbapenem resistance among *E.coli* (16.1%) and *Klebsiella* species (30%) is consistent with multinational study done in Europe [34]. In contrary, 25% carbapenem resistance rate observed in this study is lower than a report from Brazil which was 100% [35]. This could be explained by the difference in utilization of carbapenem antibiotics to treat different infections in the respective setups [36, 37]. The observed high carbapenem resistance rate can also be due to prescription of antibiotics without the knowledge of their susceptibility pattern, or introduction and dissemination of carbapenem resistant bacteria strains from other areas with high resistance rate might also be possible as JUMC is frequently visited by different European, Chinese and Korean nationalities due to different collaborative researches, training and service activities.

As reported by other studies, meropenem was the most effective antibiotic against most gram-negative rods [38]. To control high rate of antibiotic resistant isolates coordinated and urgent action is needed to prevent the development of drug resistance in the setting. Surveillance on antibiotic resistance will also be most useful to decide the correct empirical treatment and will help to control and prevent infections caused by resistant pathogens. Furthermore, our data suggest that the most effective antibiotics for gram-negative bacilli in vitro are meropenem followed by cefepime and for gram-positive organisms less resistance was observed against gentamycin.

Conclusion

In this study, high antimicrobial resistance rate was demonstrated. The observed high PDR, ESBL and carbapenem resistance rate is worrisome. Coordinated effort is needed from all stakeholders working in health system in Ethiopia to tackle this important public health problem. An immediate action should be taken at the hospital to start antibiotic stewardship program to reduce the observed antibiotic resistance and prevent further complications.

Abbreviations

HAI: Health care associated infection; MDR: Resistant to at least one agent in three or more antimicrobial categories; MoDR: Resistant to single antibiotic class; MultiS: Susceptible to all antibiotic classes; PDR: Resistant to all antibiotic classes; XDR: Resistant to at least one agent in all but two or fewer antimicrobial categories (i.e. bacterial isolates remain susceptible to only one or two categories)

Acknowledgements

We would like to thank Jimma University for funding this research and we would also like to thank all laboratory personnels working at Jimma University Medical Center, bacteriology laboratory for their unreserved support during data collection.

Funding

This project was funded by Jimma University through the Institute of Health, Research and Postgraduate Office.

Authors' contributions

MG, SA, EKG & MB conceived, designed, instrument development, supervision of data collection, analysis and manuscript writing. SB, GK, LT, YY, YA, NF, HA, and AW, participated in study design, development of instruments, supervision of data collection and editing and revision of the manuscript. All authors read and approved the final manuscript.

Consent for publication

Not applicable - This manuscript does not contain any individual person's data.

Competing interests

The authors declare that they have no competing interests.

Author details

[1]School of Medical Laboratory Science, Jimma University, Jimma, Ethiopia. [2]Department of Pediatrics and Child Health, Jimma University, Jimma, Ethiopia. [3]Department of Ophthalmology, Jimma University, Jimma, Ethiopia. [4]Department of Surgery, Jimma University, Jimma, Ethiopia. [5]Department of Obstetrics and Gynecology, Jimma University, Jimma, Ethiopia. [6]Department of Health Education and Behavioral Health, Jimma University, Jimma, Ethiopia. [7]Department of Epidemiology and Statistics, Jimma University, Jimma, Ethiopia. [8]Head of the parasitology laboratory and deputy head of the molecular diagnostics laboratory at the Max von Pettenkofer-Institute, Ludwigs-Maximilians-University (LMU), München, Germany. [9]Department of Internal Medicine, Jimma University, Jimma, Ethiopia. [10]WHO-TDR clinical research former fellow at AERAS Africa and Rockville, Rockville, MD, USA. [11]Institute of Health, Jimma University, P.O. Box 1368, Jimma, Ethiopia.

References

1. Chakraborty A, Pal NK, Sarkar S, Gupta MS. Antibiotic resistance pattern of Enterococci isolates from nosocomial infections in a tertiary care hospital in Eastern India. J Natl Sci Biol Med. 2015;6(2):394.
2. Colodner R, Rock W, Chazan B, Keller N, Guy N, Sakran W, et al. Risk factors for the development of extended-spectrum beta-lactamase-producing bacteria in nonhospitalized patients. Eur J Clin Microbiol Infect Dis. 2004; 23(3):163–7.
3. Ayukekbong JA, Ntemgwa M, Atabe AN. The threat of antimicrobial resistance in developing countries: causes and control strategies. Antimicrob Resist Infect Control. 2017;6(1):47.
4. Magiorakos AP, Srinivasan A, Carey R, Carmeli Y, Falagas M, Giske C, et al. Multidrug-resistant, extensively drug-resistant and pandrug-resistant bacteria: an international expert proposal for interim standard definitions for acquired resistance. Clin Microbiol Infect. 2012;18(3):268–81.
5. Lashinsky JN, Henig O, Pogue JM, Kaye KS. Minocycline for the Treatment of Multidrug and Extensively Drug-Resistant A. baumannii: A Review. Infect Dis Ther. 2017;6:1–13.
6. Bouchillon S, Johnson B, Hoban D, Johnson J, Dowzicky M, Wu D, et al. Determining incidence of extended spectrum β-lactamase producing Enterobacteriaceae, vancomycin-resistant enterococcus faecium and methicillin-resistant Staphylococcus aureus in 38 centres from 17 countries: the PEARLS study 2001–2002. Int J Antimicrob Agents. 2004;24(2):119–24.
7. Organization WH. Antimicrobial resistance: global report on surveillance: World Health Organization; 2014.
8. Pitout JD, Laupland KB. Extended-spectrum β-lactamase-producing Enterobacteriaceae: an emerging public-health concern. Lancet Infect Dis. 2008;8(3):159–66.
9. Fridkin S, Baggs J, Fagan R, Magill S, Pollack LA, Malpiedi P, et al. Vital signs: improving antibiotic use among hospitalized patients. MMWR Morb Mortal Wkly Rep. 2014;63(9):194–200.
10. Fernando M, Luke W, Miththinda J, Wickramasinghe R, Sebastiampillai B, Gunathilake M, et al. Extended spectrum beta lactamase producing organisms causing urinary tract infections in Sri Lanka and their antibiotic susceptibility pattern–a hospital based cross sectional study. BMC Infect Dis. 2017;17(1):138.
11. Tang SS, Apisarnthanarak A, Hsu LY. Mechanisms of β-lactam antimicrobial resistance and epidemiology of major community-and healthcare-associated multidrug-resistant bacteria. Adv Drug Deliv Rev. 2014;78:3–13.
12. Miriagou V, Cornaglia G, Edelstein M, Galani I, Giske C, Gniadkowski M, et al. Acquired carbapenemases in gram-negative bacterial pathogens: detection and surveillance issues. Clin Microbiol Infect. 2010;16(2):112–22.
13. Kumarasamy KK, Toleman MA, Walsh TR, Bagaria J, Butt F, Balakrishnan R, et al. Emergence of a new antibiotic resistance mechanism in India, Pakistan, and the UK: a molecular, biological, and epidemiological study. Lancet Infect Dis. 2010;10(9):597–602.
14. Ogefere HO, Aigbiremwen PA, Omoregie R. Extended-Spectrum Beta-lactamase (ESBL)–producing gram-negative isolates from urine and wound specimens in a tertiary health Facility in Southern Nigeria. Trop J Pharm Res. 2015;14(6):1089–94.
15. Kollef KE, Schramm GE, Wills AR, Reichley RM, Micek ST, Kollef MH. Predictors of 30-day mortality and hospital costs in patients with ventilator-associated pneumonia attributed to potentially antibiotic-resistant gram-negative bacteria. CHEST Journal. 2008;134(2):281–7.
16. Mauldin PD, Salgado CD, Hansen IS, Durup DT, Bosso JA. Attributable hospital cost and length of stay associated with health care-associated infections caused by antibiotic-resistant gram-negative bacteria. Antimicrob Agents Chemother. 2010;54(1):109–15.
17. Silvestri L, van Saene H. Hospital-acquired infections due to gram-negative bacteria. N Engl J Med. 2010;363(15):1482–6.
18. Finley RL, Collignon P, Larsson DJ, McEwen SA, Li X-Z, Gaze WH, et al. The scourge of antibiotic resistance: the important role of the environment. Clin Infect Dis. 2013;57(5):704–10.
19. Abera B, Kibret M, Mulu W. Extended-Spectrum beta (β)-lactamases and Antibiogram in Enterobacteriaceae from clinical and drinking water Sources from Bahir Dar City, Ethiopia. PloS one. 2016;11(11):e0166519.

20. Desta K, Woldeamanuel Y, Azazh A, Mohammod H, Desalegn D, Shimelis D, et al. High Gastrointestinal Colonization Rate with Extended-Spectrum β-Lactamase-Producing Enterobacteriaceae in Hospitalized Patients: Emergence of Carbapenemase-Producing *K. pneumoniae* in Ethiopia. PloS one. 2016;11(8):e0161685.
21. Mulualem Y, Kasa T, Mekonnen Z, Suleman S. Occurrence of extended spectrum beta (b)-lactamases in multidrug resistant Escherichia coli isolated from a clinical setting in Jimma university specialized hospital, Jimma, Southwest Ethiopia. East Afr J Public Health. 2012;9(2):58–61.
22. Ali S, Birhane M, Bekele S, Kibru G, Teshager L, Yilma Y, et al. Healthcare associated infection and its risk factors among patients admitted to a tertiary hospital in Ethiopia: longitudinal study. Antimicrob Resist Infect Control. 2018;7(1):2.
23. Wayne P. Clinical and laboratory standards institute. Perform Stand Antimicrob Susceptibility Testing. 2007;17.
24. Bate R, Jensen P, Hess K, Mooney L, Milligan J. Substandard and falsified anti-tuberculosis drugs: a preliminary field analysis. Int J Tuberc Lung Dis. 2013;17(3):308–11.
25. WHO. 1 in 10 medical products in developing countries is substandard or falsified. Geneva: World Health Organization; 2017.
26. WHO. Global Surveillance and Monitoring System for substandard and falsifed medical products. Geneva: World Health Organization; 2017. Licence: CC BY-NC-SA 3.0 IGO
27. Rupp ME, Fey PD. Extended spectrum β-lactamase (ESBL)-producing Enterobacteriaceae. Drugs. 2003;63(4):353–65.
28. Myat TO, Hannaway RF, Zin KN, Htike WW, Win KK, Crump JA, et al. ESBL-and carbapenemase-producing enterobacteriaceae in patients with bacteremia, Yangon, Myanmar, 2014. Emerg Infect Dis. 2017;23(5):857.
29. Parajuli NP, Acharya SP, Mishra SK, Parajuli K, Rijal BP, Pokhrel BM. High burden of antimicrobial resistance among gram negative bacteria causing healthcare associated infections in a critical care unit of Nepal. Antimicrob Resist Infect Control. 2017;6(1):67.
30. Shukla I, Tiwari R, Agrawal M. Prevalence of extended spectrum-lactamase producing Klebsiella pneumoniae in a tertiary care hospital. Indian J Med Microbiol. 2004;22(2):87.
31. Chaudhary P, Bhandari D, Thapa K, Thapa P, Shrestha D, Chaudhary H, et al. Prevalence of extended Spectrum Beta-lactamase producing Klebsiella Pneumoniae isolated from urinary tract infected patients. J Nepal Health Res Counc. 2016;14(33):111–5.
32. Bisson G, Fishman NO, Patel JB, Edelstein PH, Lautenbach E. Extended-spectrum β-lactamase–producing Escherichia coli and Klebsiella species: risk factors for colonization and impact of antimicrobial formulary interventions on colonization prevalence. Infect Control Hospital Epidemiol. 2002;23(5):254–60.
33. Organization WH. Global priority list of antibiotic-resistant bacteria to guide research, discovery, and development of new antibiotics. Geneva: World Health Organization; 2017.
34. Grundmann H, Glasner C, Albiger B, Aanensen DM, Tomlinson CT, Andrasević AT, et al. Occurrence of carbapenemase-producing Klebsiella pneumoniae and Escherichia coli in the European survey of carbapenemase-producing Enterobacteriaceae (EuSCAPE): a prospective, multinational study. Lancet Infect Dis. 2017;17(2):153–63.
35. Gonçalves IR, Ferreira M, Araujo B, Campos P, Royer S, Batistão D, et al. Outbreaks of colistin-resistant and colistin-susceptible KPC-producing Klebsiella pneumoniae in a Brazilian intensive care unit. J Hosp Infect. 2016;94(4):322–9.
36. Kebede HK, Gesesew HA, Woldehaimanot TE, Goro KK. Antimicrobial use in paediatric patients in a teaching hospital in Ethiopia. PLoS One. 2017;12(3):e0173290.
37. Yadesa TM, Gudina EK, Angamo MT. Antimicrobial use-related problems and predictors among hospitalized medical in-patients in Southwest Ethiopia: prospective observational study. PLoS One. 2015;10(12):e0138385.
38. Alexopoulou A, Vasilieva L, Agiasotelli D, Siranidi K, Pouriki S, Tsiriga A, et al. Extensively drug-resistant bacteria are an independent predictive factor of mortality in 130 patients with spontaneous bacterial peritonitis or spontaneous bacteremia. World J Gastroenterol. 2016;22(15):4049.

Beyond the hospital infection control guidelines: a qualitative study using positive deviance to characterize gray areas and to achieve efficacy and clarity in the prevention of healthcare-associated infections

Anat Gesser-Edelsburg[1,2*], Ricky Cohen[1], Adva Mir Halavi[1], Mina Zemach[3], Peter Vernon van Heerden[4], Sigal Sviri[4], Shmuel Benenson[4], Uriel Trahtemberg[4], Efrat Orenbuch-Harroch[4], Lior Lowenstein[5], Dan Shteinberg[6], Asher Salmon[4] and Allon Moses[4]

Abstract

Background: The literature is replete with attempts to design and promote customized guidelines to reduce infections during the care continuum. Paradoxically, these efforts sometimes result in gray areas where many staff members are unaware of what is required of them, which then leads to confusion, frustration, and uncertainty. We coined the phrase "gray areas" in this context to encompass the variety of situations on the care continuum that are not addressed in the accepted guidelines, and where staff members are unsure of how to proceed. The purpose of the present study was to characterize the gray areas that were reported by staff and to identify the practices of Positive Deviance (PD) individuals. We define to PD individuals as people who independently develop creative solutions to solve problems not identified by the majority in their community.

Methods: A qualitative constructivist research methodology was used that included personal interviews, observations and video recordings of identified PD practices to enhance infection control. The study was conducted January through March 2018, in two Intensive Care Units (ICU) units at Hadassah Hospital, Jerusalem, Israel. Personal interviews were conducted with 82 staff members from the General ICU (GICU) and Medical ICU (MICU).

Results: The study confirmed that guidelines cannot cover all the different situations that arise during the care continuum and can paradoxically result in the increased spread of hospital infections. Our study found there are numerous individuals who independently develop and implement solutions for gray areas. The creative and practical solutions of PD individuals can address the barriers and difficulties on the care continuum that were encountered by the staff in their communities. For example, inserting a central venous line is a complex practice in the general guidelines, while the PDs provided clear situation-specific solutions not covered in the guidelines.
(Continued on next page)

* Correspondence: ageser@univ.haifa.ac.il
[1]School of Public Health, University of Haifa, 199 Aba Khoushy Ave., Mount Carmel, 3498838 Haifa, Israel
[2]The Health and Risk Communication Research Center, University of Haifa, 199 Aba Khoushy Ave., Mount Carmel, 3498838 Haifa, Israel
Full list of author information is available at the end of the article

(Continued from previous page)

Conclusions: The recommendations of the present study are to encourage hospital personnel to create their own solutions for various situations on the care continuum, and to disseminate them within their units to achieve a bottom up change, in lieu of investing in new or specific written guidelines.

Keywords: Infection control guidelines, Positive deviance approach, Gray areas, Efficacy and clarity, Qualitative study

Background

Healthcare-associated infections (HAI) are one of the more complex problems in healthcare that no country or organization, despite multiple efforts, have managed to completely solve. The World Health Organization (WHO) claims that hundreds of millions of patients are affected by HAIs worldwide annually, which is not only a serious health issue, but also results in a financial drain on for the health system [1, 2].

Annually, approximately 4,544,100 infections and 37,000 fatalities are reported in the European Union (EU), and 2,000,000 infections and 100,000 fatalities in the United States (US), as a result of acquired infections transmitted through healthcare workers [3, 4]. A State Comptroller Report reported an estimated annual incidence of 40,000–100,000 HAI in Israel that resulted in 4000–6000 fatalities in 2012 [5].

HAI's can be reduced through infection prevention and control (IPC) practices based on evidence-based guidelines that are practical and feasible [6]. Guidelines and practices have been developed to help hospital workers reduce HAI. During the 1970's and 1980's, the Center for Disease Control and Prevention (CDC) produced guidelines, including instructions for hand washing with non-antimicrobial soap. The guidelines were appropriate, but hospitals lacked implementation policies for medical personnel not in direct contact with patients; such as technicians, laundry workers and hospital orderlies [7]. The guidelines were modified to clearly delineate different situations when hand washing was mandated, and the use of alcohol-based antiseptics for preventing contamination before and after contact with patients [8]. In 2004, the Institute for Healthcare Improvement (IHI) initiated a "100,000 Lives" campaign with six strategies to reduce morbidity and mortality in hospitalized patients, which included three HAI prevention methods to reduce central-line infections, surgical site infections and ventilator-associated pneumonia [9].

In 2009, updated hand hygiene (HH) guidelines were developed by the WHO, highlighting a new method called "My Five Moments for Hand Hygiene." The method includes systemwide changes, education and training, performance feedback, reminders in the workplace, and how to develop a safety climate. The vision was to develop guidelines that could be implemented at all income levels worldwide [10].

The latest WHO IPC guidelines, published in 2016, aim to improve practices with more effective and feasible guidelines, based on available resources, public health needs, and the local background. This includes the addition of water sanitation and hygiene (WASH), environmental and human factors, bed occupancy and staffing ratios, HH monitoring with feedback and the use of multi-modal strategies [11].

Very few studies in the literature have tried to analyze why, despite multiple efforts to make these guidelines operable, there remains a significant disparity between the guidelines and their implementation in the field. In one study Gurses et al. [12] tried to solve this problem and analyze its complexity. The research was conducted in 2006, in two separate teaching hospitals, in surgical ICUs. The study focused on four evidence-based guidelines: ventilator-associated pneumonia, central venous catheter-related bloodstream infections, surgical site infections, and catheter-associated urinary tract infections. Five subcategories of ambiguity relating to guideline discrepancies emerged from the study and included task, expectation, responsibility, method and exception ambiguity [12].

The gap between guidelines and maintaining them in the field has given rise to numerous intervention programs by public health workers. Despite the variety of interventions conducted for healthcare workers, the levels of compliance with HH still remain low at 50–60% [13–15]. A systematic review of intervention programs by Srigley et al. [16] concluded that interventions based on behavioral models were more successful in raising compliance with HH than interventions that only addressed knowledge and awareness.

According to Singhal [17] "the Positive Deviance (PD) approach is based on the premise that in every community there are certain individuals or groups whose uncommon behaviors and strategies enable them to find better solutions to problems than their peers, while facing worse challenges and having access to the same resources. However, these people are ordinarily invisible to others in the community." The PD approach differs from common approaches to problem-solving, as it seeks to identify and streamline existing resources that are derived from the staff within the unit, rather than import external "best practices". The approach focuses on the positive identification of solutions rather than problems. The PD approach identifies the behavioral practices of positively deviant individuals within the community and builds a social network to distribute and implement those practices over time [18, 19]. PD has been used to address the problem of hospital infections in the USA [20–23]. Global studies have shown that implementing the PD approach results in a significant and lasting improvement in staff compliance with guidelines for preventing infections, and a drop in the number of HAI's at healthcare centers. For example, a PD intervention was implemented across Veterans Affairs hospitals in the USA. The rate of healthcare-associated MRSA infections in ICUs before intervention was 1.64 infections per 1000 patient-days on October 2007, which was reduced to 0.62 infections per 1000 patient-days post-intervention on June 2010, a decrease of 62% ($P < 0.001$). The rate of HAI Methicillin-resistant *Staphylococcus aureus* (MRSA) infections in non-ICUs fell from 0.47 per 1000 patient-days to 0.26 infections per 1000 patient-days post intervention, a decrease of 45% (P < 0.001) [18, 20, 24].

Most studies to date have focused on evaluating the effectiveness of intervention programs with healthcare workers rather than identifying the reasons for the existing gaps between the written guidelines and their implementation, as Gurses et al. [12] pointed out in his study, we defined as "gray areas". "Gray areas" are the variety of situations on the care continuum that are not addressed by the accepted guidelines and where staff members were unsure how to proceed.

The purpose of the present study was to characterize the gray areas in the care continuum in ICUs where systematic guidelines are adhered to only partially by the staff, and where there are no practices of PD individuals that address these "gray areas" as reported by the staff.

Methods

Research design

A qualitative constructivist research method used personal interviews with staff members in different sectors, observations on the ground, and video recordings of identified positive behavioral practices to maintain hygiene. We also examined the gap between existing guidelines for hygiene maintenance and implementation in situ.

Sampling method and participant recruitment: The study was conducted January through March 2018, in two ICU's at Hadassah Hospital, Jerusalem, Israel. We chose to focus on ICU's where staff members are exposed to significant work stress, patient mortality, and feelings of professional frustration. These pressures increase the gap between the guidelines and their implementation [25–28]. Therefore, it is important to identify solutions and disseminate them in these units.

We used several sampling strategies during the study and interviewed over 90% of the staff in the GICU and MICU. In the first stage, intensive and heterogeneous sampling was used to include all representative sectors in the units (physicians, nurses, cleaning staff, etc.). In the second stage, we used snowball sampling [29] which is a method that identifies desired individuals (e.g. PDs) based on their colleagues' recommendations during the first interview. The advantage of snowball sampling is that information, usually hard to unveil, can be identified, especially when the behavior or lifestyle of the individual is an exception to the norm. In the third stage, we interviewed people identified as PDs by staff or the research team.

Study population

At Hadassah Hospital, a total of 82 participants were interviewed from the GICU and MICU: 47 nurses, 14 physicians, 5 nursing aides, 5 nursing students, 2 social workers, 2 physical therapists, 1 respiratory technician, 2 secretaries, 1 national service volunteer and 3 cleaning staff (Table 1).

Research tools

We triangulated the data obtained from different sources to bolster the study's validity: face-to-face interviews, observations and video. We also strengthened validity after the snowball sampling by obtaining confirmation from the Infection Control Unit (two physicians and an infection-control nurse) regarding the PD practices found. Interviews and observations were conducted alternatively in different day shifts for periods of several hours and PD behaviors were documented in detail in a field notes. Social Network Maps were produced using Social Network Visualizer 2.3 [30].

Interviews

Before each interview, staff members received an explanation about the study and its goals and signed an informed consent form. The semi-structured interview protocol (Additional file 1: Table S2) included questions regarding difficulties in maintaining infection control guidelines, risk perceptions of infectious diseases, norms, and the hospital's organizational culture. Interviewees were asked to name staff members they believed to be PD, defined as: persons who demonstrated positive deviant behaviors to maintain HH or who raised ideas for such practices. The interview protocol was based on Discovery & Action Dialogue (DAD) guidelines that are based on the PD approach [31]. The interviews elicited gray areas when we asked for situations lacking clear guidelines. Subsequently, interviewees were asked to identify staff who they thought had positive behavioral practices that addressed these "gray areas" effectively.

Observations

In the first stage, observations were made of all unit staff members' infection control maintenance practices of concern on the care continuum, as well as attitudes towards

Table 1 Interviewees: sociodemographic characteristics ($n = 82$)

Sociodemographic characteristics	Category	n (%)
Gender	Men	25 (30.5)
	Female	57 (69.2)
Age (years)	Mean (Max, Min, SD)	35.3 (67, 18, 11.3)
Ethnicity	Jewish	62 (75.6)
	Arab	20 (24.4)
Country of Origin	Israel	58 (74.4)
	Other	24 (29.3)
Tenure (years)	Mean (Max, Min, SD)	8.7 (40, 1, 8.6)
Position	Nurse	47 (57.3)
	Physician	14 (17.1)
	Nursing aide	5 (6.1)
	Nursing student	5 (6.1)
	Cleaning staff	3 (3.7)
	Other	8 (9.8)
Department	GICU	45 (54.9)
	MICU	37 (45.1)

procedures. In the second stage, we conducted focused observations only of PD individuals.

Video footage

Consenting staff members, identified in the interviews and observations as PD, were filmed performing the positive practices during their work. The use of this tool is based on Bandura's theory of social learning, which says that most human behavior is influenced and learned by observing the behavior of others [32]. The videos were important for designing and developing activities to spread the PD solutions, to help community members learn and practice the positive behaviors.

The data was first gathered via interviews, transcribed, observed and the main barriers and PD practices identified through content analysis. The data was then further analyzed using content analysis to find sub-themes derived from the main gray area themes, and to classify practices that stood out during the PD interviews. Throughout the study the researchers who collected the data via interviews and observations, reflexively examined themselves so as not to be judgmental or critical and to only focus on discovering positive practices.

The research processes

Stage I

Research documents were prepared, submitted and approved by the ethics committee of The Faculty of Social Welfare and Health Sciences at the University of Haifa (confirmation number 392/17) and by the Bnai Zion Medical Center Helsinki Committee (confirmation number 135–16-BNZ).

Stage II

A meeting was held with administration representatives from the Infection Control Unit, where the research goals, plan and PD approach were presented, and cooperation requested. After brainstorming and based on the hospitals' needs, the General and Medical ICU units were selected for the research.

Stage III

One meeting was held with multi-sectorial representatives (physicians, nurses, nurses' aides, orderlies and cleaning staff) in each unit, during which an explanation was provided about the research goals, framework and the PD approach.

Stage IV

The researchers entered the units with the unit head nurse and received a tour of the physical structure of the unit and introduction to shift staff. Subsequently they visited each unit twice a week, on different days, shifts and hours, during which general and direct observation was conducted of staff practices, and semi-structured protocol interviews were held. The interviews were recorded and transcribed by the researchers and all observations documented at the end of each observation. The researchers were trained to conduct interviews using the DAD method by the research supervisor, who is in an expert in qualitative studies.

Results

Classifying the PD's

It emerged from the interviews that not everyone who was perceived by their colleagues as a PD was in fact a PD individual. A staff member who is recommended as PD by their associates but who was not identified to be PD in the study, does not necessarily work inappropriately, but may work according to the guidelines without exhibiting unique positive behaviors. In the GICU (Fig. 1a), 20 individuals were found to be PDs (ten individuals who were found to be PDs by the researchers but had not been recommended by their colleagues, additional to another ten PDs who had been recommended). In the MICU (Fig. 1b), 13 individuals were found to be PDs (four individuals were identified as PD by the researchers who had not been recommended by their colleagues, in addition to nine found to be PD who had been recommended). The PD practices identified were often specific to a unit, yet some practices could be adopted by other units.

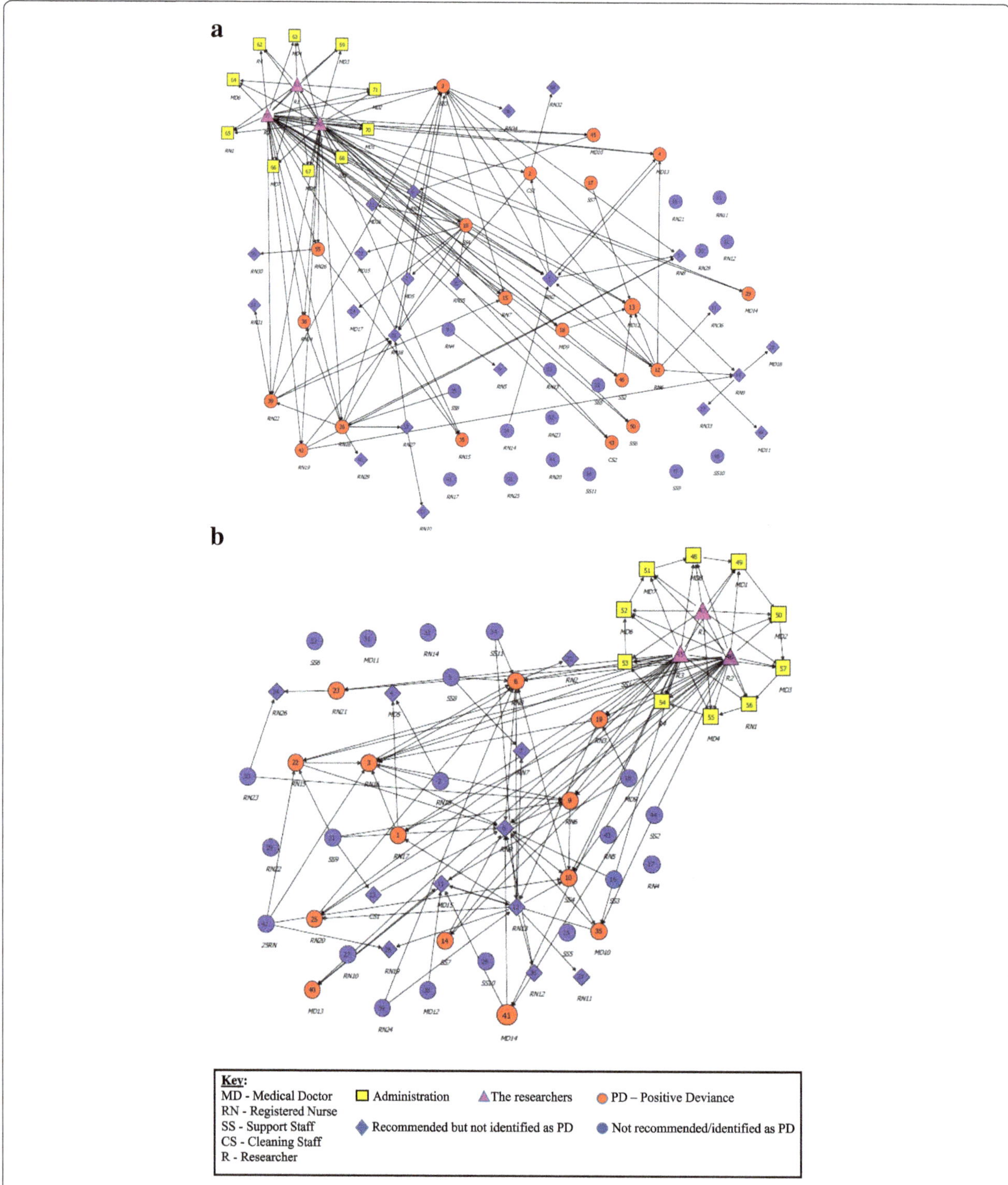

Fig. 1 **a** The Social Network - GICU at Hadassah Medical Center-Ein Kerem Hospital. **b** The Social Network - MICU at Hadassah Medical Center-Ein Kerem Hospital. Key relevant for both social network maps. Each map has separate staff members excluding yellow and pink staff. The maps present all the participants involved in the research (management, researchers and staff from all sectors). Each arrow indicates a participant's referral of another participant they recommended, or a participant identified by the researcher during the interviews and observations; sometimes the same team member was referred by several staff members. As shown by the maps, the research population was divided into three groups: (1) Red circles - the positive deviants (PDs) recommended by the staff and identified by the researchers; or identified only by the researchers, (2) Blue circles - staff not recommended and not identified as PDs., and (3) Blue diamonds – staff recommended but not identified as PDs

Gray areas on the care continuum

The interviews with representatives of the various sectors identified staff with obvious difficulties for staff, especially concerning care situations lacking clear guidelines and where a staff member interpreted or understood differently. Those issues are herewith designated "gray areas". Fifty-five out of the 85 interviewees (65%) of interviewees from the General and Medical ICUs spoke about gray area situations. Selected quotes related the gray areas from their comments about different situations on the care continuum are presented (Additional file 2: Table S3), and the solutions proposed by the PD (Additional file 3: Table S4).

The existing Israel Ministry of Health guidelines for HH are based on the WHO's Five Moments for Hand Hygiene, which refer to the main moments of patient care. However, there are many moments of contact on the care continuum that are not addressed by this model and where staff members were unsure how to proceed. Furthermore, because of the lack of training, specific guidelines or a clear definition of roles; staff members held different interpretations in different care situations. These conditions evoked feelings of confusion, uncertainty, and the perception of the procedures as incoherent. The gray areas on which the stakeholders focused addressed several themes as follows:

Lack of uniformity in infection control procedures

Some interviewees claimed the guidelines Hospital's specific infection control unit are stricter than those of the Israeli National Center for Infection Control, and conversely sometimes the National Center's guidelines are stricter than the hospital's, creating a lack of uniformity and confusion among staff. For example, a senior doctor mentioned that during the procedure of inserting a central line in a patient, the guidelines sequence steps do not address all the issues that occur in practice. During that specific procedure the neck area of the patient needs to be in a sterile field, and the ultrasound (US) probe has a cable that, when moved, can enter the sterile field, thus causing contamination. The doctor suggested fixing the probe in place to prevent movement and keep the field sterile. This exemplifies the gray areas that came to light during procedures that were not covered by the guidelines (see Additional files 2 and 3: Table S3 and S4). The guidelines are also unclear and interpreted differently by staff workers regarding cleaning a patient's room, washbasin and cleaning sinks (see Additional files 2 and 3: Table S3 and S4).

Vagueness in the guidelines concerning the extraction and sending of tests

Staff members repeatedly cited their confusion and uncertainty regarding obtaining, storing and submitting blood and urine samples. For instance, there is a lack of clarity about the correct way to remove samples from patients' rooms and how to put the sample into the dedicated bag before they are sent to the laboratory; without contaminating the bag, the vacuum collection tube system (designed to send the tests) and other areas (see Additional files 2 and 3: Table S3 and S4).

Uncertainty as to the definitions of "clean" or "contaminated" spaces around the unit, the location of equipment after use, and responsibility for performance and lack of guidelines concerning mobile equipment

Definition of spaces within the unit was mentioned mainly in relation to the space in front of the entrance to the patient's room. This space has a small table the staff uses for various purposes, such as: putting down disposable equipment (needles and syringes), writing instructions on monitoring pages, putting down tests and so on (see Additional files 2 and 3: Table S3 and S4). As arose from the interviews, there is confusion as to the definition of that space and the proper location of equipment and instruments within the unit after removal from the patient's room (after use or following a malfunction). It is not clear which equipment has been sterilized and cleaned and which has not, where equipment that needs to be removed should be placed so it is clear that it has not yet been sterilized, and who is responsible (see Additional files 2 and 3: Table S3 and S4). Another point is the absence of clear guidelines and disagreement concerning the use of mobile equipment and other items within a patient's room, such as stethoscope, cellphone, papers, stamp, etc. The staff members expressed uncertainty as to when to use, mark or disinfect these items and had different perspectives concerning the use of personal equipment in patients' rooms (see Additional files 2 and 3: Table S3 and S4).

Challenges in the transition from "clean" to "dirty" areas in the course of treatment and back

This issue was mentioned only by nurses, when they described how they operate when caring for patients. All of them knew how to explain the guiding principle of their work, which is to begin by treating the patient's "clean" areas (areas that do not involve excretions) and to end with the "dirty" areas (the digestive system), to avoid transferring bacteria from the dirty areas to the clean ones. However, the nurses described complex treatment situations that require them to move between areas: to remove gloves, sanitize hands and to continue the desired action (see Additional files 2 and 3: Table S3 and S4).

HH training and reminders

The issue of training was mentioned many times and in different contexts by staff members in different sectors. The physicians and nurses reported that on the one hand there are numerous training sessions, study days, and computer software teaching HH. However, they pointed to elements currently missing in the training that create confusion and deficiency. For example, the lack of customized training for each sector and for specialized work in the ICU. The interviews also raised the lack of training for staff not considered medical personnel such as cleaning staff and orderlies – who claimed that they never received systematic training regarding hygiene. The non-medical staff come in close contact with patients and their surroundings and intervening during their training process can help brake the chain of infection control (see Additional files 2 and 3: Table S3 and S4).

PD solutions for gray areas on the care continuum

Considering the gray areas mentioned in the interviews with the different sectors, 33 individuals were identified as "positive deviants," who, in contrast to the remaining 52 staff members who reported confusion and frustration, practiced behavioral practices that addressed the gray areas on the care continuum. A total of 14 practices that support maintenance of hygiene were discovered among the PD's, addressing different barriers to good hygiene in the gray areas such as the use of Tegaderm sticker to immobilize and cover the tape holding the tube in place, so it doesn't contaminate the sterile area, during insertion of a central line into the internal jugular vein (see Additional file 3: Table S4).

Discussion

The literature is replete with attempts to design and promote customized guidelines to reduce infections during the care continuum. However, the present study suggests that despite the importance of the written guidelines, they cannot cover all the different situations that arise during the care continuum that may result in the spread of hospital infections. The lack of solutions for different areas of the care continuum creates gray areas where some staff members do not know or are unaware of what is required of them, leading to confusion, frustration, and various interpretations by them. Gurses et al. [12] found that staff compliance with unit guidelines increases when they know the accepted norms and expectations of their unit and guidelines are less vague. It is also important to clearly define roles and responsibilities for performing specific tasks and meeting guidelines [12]. Two issues that arose from the present study and were discussed by Kim et al. [33] are adapting to changing medical situations and moving between clean and contaminated areas. Most staff members stated that existing infection control guidelines do not take into account for many medical conditions they encounter daily when priorities change, such as urgent resuscitation. Staff members also pointed to the need for HH solutions in situations such as bathing the patient, when staff members' hands go back and forth repeatedly between dirty areas (e.g. catheter) and clean areas such as the intubation tube.

Our findings indicate that written guidelines cannot be totally comprehensive as they fail to account for the dynamic nature of the work and therefore it is hard to translate them into the work environment, as guidelines cannot address all the gray areas on the care continuum. Srigley et al. [16] concurred and criticized the literature that has often focused on the planned behavior theory, whereas HH is usually an automatic, spontaneous, repetitive behavior affected by the perception of the context and environment. The movement of staff members between tasks is complex and identifying some of the specific situations when HH needs to be performed is a challenge. The study by Fuller et al. [34] tried to solve the complex continuous problems of the staff by creating hints to help the staff remember hygiene procedures. The study suggests that future interventions should be developed in cooperation with staff to build an "if then" program: "if X happens then I will do Y".

The PD approach we used in this study addresses the need to develop practices that arise from the professional community, follows the "if then" model, and provides responses in situ to gray areas on the care continuum. The study shows it is possible to identify staff members who found solutions, big and small, that are not written or recommended in the accepted "five moments" guidelines but address "problematic" and vague situations on the care continuum. One example is taking a blood sample from a patient in an isolation room. The guidelines focus on the order of actions to be followed while performing the task, but not what happens when the sample is removed from isolation room pending transfer to the laboratory via the vacuum tube collection system located in the middle of the unit. There is a lack of uniformity as to how staff members perform this action, and each tends to interpret it differently.

In one example, we observed a nurse PD take samples from a patient's room according to accepted procedure, then place the test tubes on a desk in the patient's room adjacent to the exit. The nurse removed her gloves and robe, performed HH, and obtained a special plastic bag for the samples. She then placed her hand inside the bag, returned to the room entrance and picked up the samples from the inside of the bag (without direct contact between the samples and her hand or the outside of the bag) and tied it at the top. Next, she placed the samples into the vacuum tube collection system without contaminating the environment, her hands or the laboratory technician. This example displays ingenuity and effectiveness, because it demonstrates how with one small action a long cascade of infection transfer is broken and that wisdom and expertise are in the hands of community members. This solution does not require special resources, is not written in the accepted guidelines, and is a simple behavior practice that is not considered a work method that most staff members use, that grew out of conditions on the ground and can be duplicated and learned by other staff.

Our study findings indicate that there are numerous individuals who find solutions to the gray areas. The creative and practical solutions of PDs can often address barriers and difficulties on the care continuum that were raised by the staff. Because these solutions come from the community, it is very likely that people within the system will be more open to adapting them [35]. The power of a solution that comes from the community also speaks to the issue of implementing guidelines. One of the barriers that arose in the present study is healthcare workers feeling that whoever wrote the guidelines is unfamiliar with the complexity of the work on the ground. We found that identifying PD staff members has a positive effect on the enthusiasm of the staff to participate in improving infection control. Furthermore, disseminating new ideas from staff members creates an environment of eagerness to find even more constructive ideas.

It is important to note that we are not suggesting ignoring existing guidelines, on the contrary, they are the scientific building blocks that need be used in practice. Our contribution is a tool kit that can be used to minimize the existing ambiguities between the written guidelines and work practices. The tool kit is composed of PD practices demonstrated through videos, face-to-face discussions and simulations. They are recommendations taught by the PD staff to their colleagues and thus diffused throughout the work environment. The findings that rise from this study are solutions from the ground (bottom up), an important resource that can help design community-based intervention programs customized to a hospital unit profile. The PD can be used to create "unwritten guidelines" that are derived from actual people and implemented in the medical unit's work environment. It stands to reason that this solution should be the easiest and best one to implement, since it makes sense both from a principled and practical point of view and is viewed by the staff as an efficient solution. Community involvement in building the infrastructure will lead to more openness and a multi-systemic effort to reduce infection rates in hospital units. Another study contribution is that it transfers the weight from focusing on the guidelines to focusing on practical solutions. Furthermore, as opposed to previous PD studies that focused only on the "how," this study focuses on the "why" – the staff's reasons and barriers; revealing the shortcomings of writing additional guidelines and structured programs and showing how the PD approach can address gaps. Previous studies focused on behaviors and less on the reasons for barriers, such as were pointed out during this research that could be resolved using the PD approach. The research contribution is also based on a variety of examples and adaptations that can be demonstrated through simulations to staff with different responsibilities in diverse units [20–23].

Limitations

From the staff members' interviews and observations, we found that hygiene and the prevention of HAI are considered sensitive subjects of great concern to unit staff, and even more so to hospital administrations. However, observing staff members can elicit feelings of resistance and stress and a tendency not to change behavior (the Hawthorne effect [36]). In our study we searched for the exceptional positive practices, and therefore, despite the social desire of the Hawthorne effect, it was not an issue since the staff won't try to "hide" or change behavior because mistakes were not observed\relevant. During our observations we emphasized that the research goal was to identify the gaps and the positive behaviors and not problems with staff, thereby reducing resistance. In addition, the interviews were in hospital ICUs that have their unique features and organizational culture, and we hope the study findings can be extrapolated to other units.

Conclusions

The present study characterized the gray areas in the care continuum that were explained by the staff, and where solutions were found through PD practices. Instead of investing in writing additional and specific guidelines for different situations and developing training programs for their implementation, it is important to encourage hospital personnel to create their own solutions for different situations on the care continuum, and to disseminate them in the units to achieve a bottom to top change.

Abbreviations

CDC: Center for Disease Control and Prevention; DAD: Discovery & action dialogue; EU: European union; GICU: General intensive care unit; HAI: Healthcare-associated infections; HH: Hand hygiene; ICU: Intensive care unit; IHI: Institute for healthcare improvement; IPC: Infection prevention and control; MICU: Medical intensive care unit; MRSA: Methicillin-resistant *Staphylococcus aureus*; PD: Positive Deviance; USA: United States of America; WASH: Water sanitation and hygiene; WHO: World health organization

Acknowledgements
The authors would like to thank all the participants of this study and the Israel National Institute for Health Policy Research for funding the research. In addition, the authors would like to thank Prof. Arvind Singhal for his ongoing consultancy to the research.

Funding
This research was funded by the Israel National Institute for Health Policy Research, grant number 2016\134\א.

Authors' contributions
AGE is the principal investigator and she has conceptualized the study, participated in the field research, written the manuscript and taken full responsibility for the study. RC is the research coordinator and assistance researcher together with AMH. Both RC and AMH participated in the field research, data analysis and written the manuscript. MZ is an external consultant, she was involved in conceptualized the study, preforming statistical analysis and read the manuscript draft and revised it critically for important intellectual content. PVvH, SS, SB, UT, EOH and AM were involved in the field research as being on Hadassah Hospital medical staff ICU's and Clinical Microbiology and Infectious Diseases unit. LL, DS and AS are the co-principal investigators of the study. They all read the manuscript draft and revised it critically for important intellectual content. All authors read and approved the manuscript.

Consent for publication
All the study participants gave their consent to publish the research.

Competing interests
The authors declare that they have no competing interests.

Author details
[1]School of Public Health, University of Haifa, 199 Aba Khoushy Ave., Mount Carmel, 3498838 Haifa, Israel. [2]The Health and Risk Communication Research Center, University of Haifa, 199 Aba Khoushy Ave., Mount Carmel, 3498838 Haifa, Israel. [3]Midgam Consulting & Research Ltd., 7 Metsada St, 5126112 Bnei Brak, Israel. [4]Hadassah University Medical Center. Ein Kerem, P.O. Box 12000, 9112001 Jerusalem, Israel. [5]Rambam Health Care Campus, P.O. Box 9602, 3109601 Haifa, Israel. [6]Bnai Zion Medical Center, 47 Golomb St, P.O.B. 4940, 3104802 Haifa, Israel.

References

1. Allegranzi B, Nejad SB, Pittet D. The burden of healthcare-associated infection. In: Pittet D, Boyce JM, Allegranzi B, editors. Hand hygiene: a handbook for medical professionals. 1st edition ed. hospital medicine: current concepts. Hoboken: Wiley; 2017. p. 1–7.
2. WHO. Health care-associated infections. In: Fact sheet; 2011.
3. Van Itterbeeck J, van Huis A. Environmental manipulation for edible insect procurement: a historical perspective. J Ethnobiol Ethnomed. 2012;8:3. https://doi.org/10.1186/1746-4269-8-3.
4. Zingg W, Cartier V, Walder B. No association between ultrasound-guided insertion of central venous catheters and bloodstream infection: a prospective observational study. J Hosp Infect. 2015;90(1):82. https://doi.org/10.1016/j.jhin.2015.01.007.
5. State Comptroller. Annual Control Report 63c for 2012 and for accounting for financial year 2011. Jerusalem: The State Comptroller and Ombudsman of Israel; 2013.
6. Storr J, Twyman A, Zingg W, Damani N, Kilpatrick C, Reilly J, et al. Core components for effective infection prevention and control programmes: new WHO evidence-based recommendations. Antimicrob Resist Infect Control. 2017;6:6. https://doi.org/10.1186/s13756-016-0149-9.
7. Eggimann P, Pittet D. Infection control in the ICU. Chest. 2001;120(6):2059–93.
8. Burke JP. Infection control - a problem for patient safety. N Engl J Med. 2003;348(7):651–6. https://doi.org/10.1056/NEJMhpr020557.
9. Berwick DM, Calkins DR, McCannon CJ, Hackbarth AD. The 100,000 lives campaign: setting a goal and a deadline for improving health care quality. JAMA. 2006;295(3):324–7. https://doi.org/10.1001/jama.295.3.324
10. Allegranzi B, Gayet-Ageron A, Damani N, Bengaly L, McLaws ML, Moro ML, et al. Global implementation of WHO's multimodal strategy for improvement of hand hygiene: a quasi-experimental study. Lancet Infect Dis. 2013;13(10):843–51. https://doi.org/10.1016/S1473-3099(13)70163-4.
11. WHO. Guidelines on Core Components of Infection Prevention and Control Programmes at the National and Acute Health Care Facility Level. Geneva; 2016. Contract No.: Report
12. Gurses AP, Seidl KL, Vaidya V, Bochicchio G, Harris AD, Hebden J, et al. Systems ambiguity and guideline compliance: a qualitative study of how intensive care units follow evidence-based guidelines to reduce healthcare-associated infections. Qual Saf Health Care. 2008;17(5):351–9. https://doi.org/10.1136/qshc.2006.021709.
13. Boyce JM, Pittet D. Healthcare infection control practices advisory C, force HSAIHHT. Guideline for hand hygiene in health-care settings. Recommendations of the healthcare infection control practices advisory committee and the HIPAC/SHEA/APIC/IDSA hand hygiene task force. Am J Infect Control. 2002;30(8):S1–46.
14. Erasmus V, Daha TJ, Brug H, Richardus JH, Behrendt MD, Vos MC, et al. Systematic review of studies on compliance with hand hygiene guidelines in hospital care. Infect Control Hosp Epidemiol. 2010;31(3):283–94. https://doi.org/10.1086/650451.
15. Whitby M, Pessoa-Silva CL, McLaws ML, Allegranzi B, Sax H, Larson E, et al. Behavioural considerations for hand hygiene practices: the basic building blocks. J Hosp Infect. 2007;65(1):1–8. https://doi.org/10.1016/j.jhin.2006.09.026.
16. Srigley JA, Corace K, Hargadon DP, Yu D, MacDonald T, Fabrigar L, et al. Applying psychological frameworks of behaviour change to improve healthcare worker hand hygiene: a systematic review. J Hosp Infect. 2015;91(3):202–10. https://doi.org/10.1016/j.jhin.2015.06.019.
17. Singhal A. The positive deviance approach to designing and implementing health communication interventions. In: Kim DK, Singhal A, Kreps GL, editors. Health communication strategies for developing Global Health programs. Health communication. New York: Peter Lang; 2013. p. 176.
18. Singhal A, Greiner K. Using the positive deviance approach to reduce hospital-acquired infections at the veterans administration healthcare system in Pittsburgh. In: Suchman AL, Sluyter DG, Williamson PR, editors. Leading change in healthcare: transforming organizations using complexity, positive psychology, and relationship-centered care. London: Radcliffe publishing; 2011. p. 177–209.
19. Maryland Patient Safety Center. MRSA Field Guide 2007.
20. Ellingson K, Muder RR, Jain R, Kleinbaum D, Feng PJ, Cunningham C, et al. Sustained reduction in the clinical incidence of methicillin-resistant Staphylococcus aureus colonization or infection associated with a multifaceted infection control intervention. Infect Control Hosp Epidemiol. 2011;32:1):1–8. https://doi.org/10.1086/657665.
21. Marra AR, Guastelli LR, de Araujo CM, dos Santos JL, Lamblet LC, Silva M Jr, et al. Positive deviance: a new strategy for improving hand hygiene compliance. Infect Control Hosp Epidemiol. 2010;31(1):12–20. https://doi.org/10.1086/649224.
22. Marra AR, Noritomi DT, Westheimer Cavalcante AJ, Sampaio Camargo TZ, Bortoleto RP, Durao Junior MS, et al. A multicenter study using positive deviance for improving hand hygiene compliance. Am J Infect Control. 2013;41(11):984–8. https://doi.org/10.1016/j.ajic.2013.05.013.
23. Marsh DR, Schroeder DG, Dearden KA, Sternin J, Sternin M. The power of positive deviance. BMJ. 2004;329(7475):1177–9. https://doi.org/10.1136/bmj.329.7475.1177.
24. Jain R, Kralovic SM, Evans ME, Ambrose M, Simbartl LA, Obrosky DS, et al. Veterans affairs initiative to prevent methicillin-resistant Staphylococcus aureus infections. N Engl J Med. 2011;364(15):1419–30. https://doi.org/10.1056/NEJMoa1007474.
25. Mealer M, Jones J, Moss M. A qualitative study of resilience and posttraumatic stress disorder in United States ICU nurses. Intensive Care Med. 2012;38(9):1445–51. https://doi.org/10.1007/s00134-012-2600-6.
26. Sharma P, Davey A, Davey S, Shukla A, Shrivastava K, Bansal R. Occupational stress among staff nurses: controlling the risk to health. Indian J Occup Environ Med. 2014;18(2):52–6. https://doi.org/10.4103/0019-5278.146890.
27. Shorter M, Stayt LC. Critical care nurses' experiences of grief in an adult intensive care unit. J Adv Nurs. 2010;66(1):159–67. https://doi.org/10.1111/j.1365-2648.2009.05191.x.
28. van Mol MM, Kompanje EJ, Benoit DD, Bakker J, Nijkamp MD. The prevalence of compassion fatigue and burnout among healthcare professionals in intensive care units: a systematic review. PLoS One. 2015;10(8):e0136955. https://doi.org/10.1371/journal.pone.0136955

29. Ulin PR, Robinson ET, Tolley EE. Qualitative methods in public health: a filed guide for applied research. San Francisco: Jossey-Bass; 2005.
30. Kalamaras J. SocNetV version 2.4. In: The social network visualizer project; 2018.
31. Lindberg C, Downham G, Buscell P, Jones E, Peterson P, Krebs V. Embracing collaboration: a novel strategy for reducing bloodstream infections in outpatient hemodialysis centers. Am J Infect Control. 2013;41(6):513–9. https://doi.org/10.1016/j.ajic.2012.07.015.
32. Bandura A. Social learning theory. Prentice-hall. Engelwood cliffs, NJ: 1977.
33. Kim YH, Jang TY. Clinical characteristics and therapeutic outcomes of patients with localized mucosal allergy. Am J Rhinol Allergy. 2010;24(4):e89–92. https://doi.org/10.2500/ajra.2010.24.3497.
34. Fuller C, Besser S, Savage J, McAteer J, Stone S, Michie S. Application of a theoretical framework for behavior change to hospital workers' real-time explanations for noncompliance with hand hygiene guidelines. Am J Infect Control. 2014;42(2):106–10. https://doi.org/10.1016/j.ajic.2013.07.019.
35. Singhal A, Buscell P, Lindberg C. Inspiring Change and Saving Lives the Positive Deviance Way. Bordentown: PlexusPress; 2014.
36. Monahan T, Fisher JA. Benefits of "observer effects": lessons from the field. Qual Res. 2010;10(3):357–76. https://doi.org/10.1177/1468794110362874.

Permissions

All chapters in this book were first published in AR&IC, by BioMed Central; hereby published with permission under the Creative Commons Attribution License or equivalent. Every chapter published in this book has been scrutinized by our experts. Their significance has been extensively debated. The topics covered herein carry significant findings which will fuel the growth of the discipline. They may even be implemented as practical applications or may be referred to as a beginning point for another development.

The contributors of this book come from diverse backgrounds, making this book a truly international effort. This book will bring forth new frontiers with its revolutionizing research information and detailed analysis of the nascent developments around the world.

We would like to thank all the contributing authors for lending their expertise to make the book truly unique. They have played a crucial role in the development of this book. Without their invaluable contributions this book wouldn't have been possible. They have made vital efforts to compile up to date information on the varied aspects of this subject to make this book a valuable addition to the collection of many professionals and students.

This book was conceptualized with the vision of imparting up-to-date information and advanced data in this field. To ensure the same, a matchless editorial board was set up. Every individual on the board went through rigorous rounds of assessment to prove their worth. After which they invested a large part of their time researching and compiling the most relevant data for our readers.

The editorial board has been involved in producing this book since its inception. They have spent rigorous hours researching and exploring the diverse topics which have resulted in the successful publishing of this book. They have passed on their knowledge of decades through this book. To expedite this challenging task, the publisher supported the team at every step. A small team of assistant editors was also appointed to further simplify the editing procedure and attain best results for the readers.

Apart from the editorial board, the designing team has also invested a significant amount of their time in understanding the subject and creating the most relevant covers. They scrutinized every image to scout for the most suitable representation of the subject and create an appropriate cover for the book.

The publishing team has been an ardent support to the editorial, designing and production team. Their endless efforts to recruit the best for this project, has resulted in the accomplishment of this book. They are a veteran in the field of academics and their pool of knowledge is as vast as their experience in printing. Their expertise and guidance has proved useful at every step. Their uncompromising quality standards have made this book an exceptional effort. Their encouragement from time to time has been an inspiration for everyone.

The publisher and the editorial board hope that this book will prove to be a valuable piece of knowledge for researchers, students, practitioners and scholars across the globe.

List of Contributors

Adebayo O. Shittu, Yewande O. Ajao, Mujibat O. Abiola and Ayodele O. Olatimehin
Department of Microbiology, Obafemi Awolowo University, Ile-Ife, Osun State 22005, Nigeria

Shima M. Abdulgader
Division of Medical Microbiology, Department of Pathology, Faculty of Health Sciences, University of Cape Town, Cape Town, South Africa

Mamadou Kaba
Division of Medical Microbiology, Department of Pathology, Faculty of Health Sciences, University of Cape Town, Cape Town, South Africa
Institute of Infectious Disease and Molecular Medicine, Faculty of Health Sciences, University of Cape Town, Cape Town, South Africa

Narbada Upreti and Megha Raj Banjara
Central Department of Microbiology, Tribhuvan University, Kirtipur, Nepal

Binod Rayamajhee
National College (Tribhuvan University), Khusibu, Kathmandu, Nepal
Department of Infectious Diseases and Immunology, Kathmandu Research Institute for Biological Sciences (KRIBS), Lalitpur, Nepal

Samendra P. Sherchan
Department of Global Environmental Health Sciences, School of Public Health and Tropical Medicine, Tulane University, New Orleans, LA, USA

Mahesh Kumar Choudhari
KIST Medical College and Teaching Hospital, Imadole, Lalitpur, Nepal

Stig Harthug
Department of Clinical Science, University of Bergen, Bergen, Norway
Norwegian Advisory Unit for Antibiotic Use in Hospitals, Department of Research and Development, Haukeland University Hospital, Jonas Lies vei 65, N-5021 Bergen, Norway

Jannicke Slettli Wathne
Department of Clinical Science, University of Bergen, Bergen, Norway
Norwegian Advisory Unit for Antibiotic Use in Hospitals, Department of Research and Development, Haukeland University Hospital, Jonas Lies vei 65, N-5021 Bergen, Norway
Department of Quality and Development, Hospital Pharmacies Enterprise in Western Norway, Bergen, Norway

Lars Kåre Selland Kleppe
Department of Infectious Diseases and Unit for Infection Prevention and Control, Department of Research and Education, Stavanger University Hospital,Stavanger, Norway

Hege Salvesen Blix
Department of Drug Statistics, Norwegian Institute of Public Health, Oslo, Norway

Roy M. Nilsen
Faculty of Health and Social Sciences, Western Norway University of Applied Sciences, Bergen, Norway

Esmita Charani
NHIR Health Protection Research Unit in Healthcare Associated Infections and Antimicrobial Resistance, Imperial College, London, UK

The Bergen Intervention Teams and Ingrid Smith
Innovation, Access and Use, Department of Essential Medicines and Health Products, World Health Organization (WHO), Avenue Appia 20, 1211 Geneva 27, Switzerland

Mohamed Abbas and Didier Pittet
Infection Control Programme and WHO Collaborating Centre on Patient Safety, Faculty of Medicine, University of Geneva Hospitals, Geneva, Switzerland

Tammam Aloudat
Médecins sans Frontières, Geneva, Switzerland

Javier Bartolomei
CAPPI Servette, Department of Mental Health and Psychiatry, Geneva University Hospitals, Genève, Switzerland

Manuel Carballo
International Centre for Migration, Health and Development, Geneva, Switzerland

Sophie Durieux-Paillard
Programme Santé Migrants, Department of Community Medicine, Primary Care and Emergency Medicine, Geneva University Hospitals, Geneva, Switzerland

Laure Gabus
Geneva, Switzerland

Alexandra Jablonka
Department of Clinical Immunology and Rheumatology, Hannover Medical School, Hannover, Germany
German Center for Infection Research (DZIF), PARTNER Site Hannover-Braunschweig, Hannover, Germany

Yves Jackson
Division of Primary Care Medicine, Geneva University Hospitals, Geneva, Switzerland
Institute of Global Health, Geneva University, Geneva, Switzerland

Kanokporn Kaojaroen
Department of Service Delivery and Safety, World Health Organization, Geneva, Switzerland

Daniel Koch
Division of Communicable Diseases, Federal Office of Public Health, Bern, Switzerland

Esperanza Martinez
Health Unit, International Committee of the Red Cross (ICRC), Geneva, Switzerland

Marc Mendelson
Division of Infectious Diseases and HIV Medicine, Department of Medicine, Groote Schuur Hospital, University of Cape Town, Cape Town, South Africa

Roumyana Petrova-Benedict
International Organization for Migration (IOM), Migration Health Division (MHD), Regional office (RO), Brussels, Belgium

Sotirios Tsiodras
4th Department of Medicine, Medical School, National and Kapodistrian University of Athens, Athens, Greece
Hellenic Centre for Disease Control and Prevention, Athens, Greece

Derek Christie
Division of environmental health, Institute of Global Health, Faculty of Medicine, University of Geneva, Geneva, Switzerland

Mirko Saam
Communication in Science, Geneva, Switzerland

Sally Hargreaves
Section of Infectious Diseases and Immunity, Department of Medicine, Imperial College London, Hammersmith Hospital, London W12 0HS, UK
The Institute for Infection and Immunity, St George's, University of London, London WC1E 7HU, UK

Marziyeh Tavakol, Hassan Momtaz and Elahe Tajbakhsh
Department of Microbiology, Shahrekord Branch, Islamic Azad University, Shahrekord, Iran

Parviz Mohajeri
Department of Microbiology, School of Medicine, Kermanshah University of Medical Sciences, Kermanshah, Iran
Nosocomial Infection Research Center, Kermanshah University of Medical Sciences, Kermanshah, Iran

Leili Shokoohizadeh
Department of Microbiology, School of Medicine, Hamadan University of Medical Sciences, Hamadan, Iran

Pinyo Rattanaumpawan, Chatiros Choorat, Teerawit Tangkoskul, Chakrapong Seenama and Visanu Thamlikitkul
Division of Infectious Diseases and Tropical Medicine, Bangkok, Thailand
Department of Medicine, Faculty of Medicine Siriraj Hospital, Mahidol University, 2 Wang Lang Rd., Bangkoknoi, Bangkok 10700, Thailand

Kanchanaporn Takonkitsakul
Department of Medicine, Faculty of Medicine Siriraj Hospital, Mahidol

University, 2 Wang Lang Rd., Bangkoknoi, Bangkok 10700, Thailand

Reza Ranjbar
Molecular Biology Research Center, Systems Biology and Poisonings Institute, Baqiyatallah University of Medical Sciences, Tehran, Iran

Farid Yadollahi Farsani
Molecular Biology Research Center, Systems Biology and Poisonings Institute, Baqiyatallah University of Medical Sciences, Tehran, Iran

Farhad Safarpoor Dehkordi
Young Researchers and Elites Club, Shahrekord Branch, Islamic Azad University, Shahrekord, Iran

Shraddha Siwakoti, Abhilasha Sharma, Ratna Baral, Narayan Raj Bhattarai and Basudha Khanal
Department of Microbiology, B. P. Koirala Institute of Health Sciences, Dharan 56700, Nepal

Asish Subedi
Department of Anaesthesiology and Critical care, B. P. Koirala Institute of Health Sciences, Dharan, Nepal

Teng-Ho Wang
Divison of Infection disease, Department of Internal Medicine, Taipei City Hospital, Zhongxiao Branch, Taipei, Taiwan
Graduate Institute of Bioengineering, Tatung University, Taipei, Taiwan
Division of Infection Control, Taipei City Hospital, Zhongxiao Branch, Taipei, Taiwan

Tsong-Rong Yan
Graduate Institute of Bioengineering, Tatung University, Taipei, Taiwan

Yi-Shing Leu
Division of Otolaryngology, MacKay Memorial Hospital, Taipei, Taiwan
Department of Medicine, MacKay Medical College, New Taipei City, Taiwan

Nai-Yu Wang
Department of Medical Research, MacKay Memorial Hospital, Taipei, Taiwan

Chang-Pan Liu
Department of Medical Research, MacKay Memorial Hospital, Taipei, Taiwan
Division of Infectious Diseases, Department of Internal Medicine, MacKay Memorial Hospital, Taipei, Taiwan
MacKay College of Medicine, Nursing and Management, Taipei, Taiwan
Infection Control Committee, MacKay Memorial Hospital, Taipei, Taiwan

Aina Gomila, Evelyn Shaw and Miquel Pujol
Department of Infectious Diseases, Hospital Universitari de Bellvitge, Institut Català de la Salut (ICS-HUB), Feixa Llarga s/n, L'Hospitalet de Llobregat, 08907 Barcelona, Spain
Spanish Network for Research in Infectious Diseases (REIPI RD12/0015), Instituto de Salud Carlos III, Madrid, Spain
Institut d'Investigació Biomèdica de Bellvitge (IDIBELL), Feixa Llarga s/n, L'Hospitalet de Llobregat, 08907 Barcelona, Spain

Jordi Carratalà
Department of Infectious Diseases, Hospital Universitari de Bellvitge, Institut Català de la Salut (ICS-HUB), Feixa Llarga s/n, L'Hospitalet de Llobregat, 08907 Barcelona, Spain
Spanish Network for Research in Infectious Diseases (REIPI RD12/0015), Instituto de Salud Carlos III, Madrid, Spain
Institut d'Investigació Biomèdica de Bellvitge (IDIBELL), Feixa Llarga s/n, L'Hospitalet de Llobregat, 08907 Barcelona, Spain
University of Barcelona, Barcelona, Spain

Cristian Tebé
Institut d'Investigació Biomèdica de Bellvitge (IDIBELL), Feixa Llarga s/n, L'Hospitalet de Llobregat, 08907 Barcelona, Spain

Leonard Leibovici and Noa Eliakim-Raz
Department of Medicine E, Beilinson Hospital, Rabin Medical Center, Petah Tikva; Sackler Faculty of Medicine, Tel Aviv University, Tel Aviv, Israel

Irith Wiegand, Christiane Vank, Ibironke Addy and Cuong Vuong
AiCuris Anti-infective Cures GmbH, Wuppertal, Germany

Laura Vallejo-Torres and Stephen Morris
UCL Department of Applied Health Research, University College London, London, UK

Joan M. Vigo
Informatics Unit, Fundació Institut Català de Farmacologia, Barcelona, Spain

Margaret Stoddart, Sally Grier and Alasdair MacGowan
Department of Medical Microbiology, Southmead Hospital, North Bristol NHS Trust, Bristol, UK

Nienke Cuperus and Leonard Van den Heuvel
Julius Center for Health Sciences and Primary Care, University Medical Center Utrecht, Utrecht, Netherlands

Poojan Shrestha and Philippe J. Guerin
Infectious Diseases Data Observatory, University of Oxford, Oxford, UK
Centre for Tropical Medicine and Global Health, Nuffield Department of Medicine, University of Oxford, Oxford, UK

Ben S. Cooper and Yoel Lubell
Centre for Tropical Medicine and Global Health, Nuffield Department of Medicine, University of Oxford, Oxford, UK
Mahidol Oxford Tropical Medicine Research Unit Faculty of Tropical Medicine, Mahidol University, 420/6 Rajvithi Road, Bangkok 10400, Thailand

Olivier Celhay
Mahidol Oxford Tropical Medicine Research Unit Faculty of Tropical Medicine, Mahidol University, 420/6 Rajvithi Road, Bangkok 10400, Thailand

Joanna Coast
School of Social and Community Medicine, University of Bristol, Bristol, UK

Raymond Oppong
Health Economics Unit, School of Health and Population Sciences, University of Birmingham, Birmingham, UK

Nga Do Thi Thuy
Oxford University Clinical Research Unit-Ha Noi, Ha Noi, Vietnam
National Hospital for Tropical Diseases, Hanoi, Vietnam

Heiman Wertheim
Oxford University Clinical Research Unit-Ha Noi, Ha Noi, Vietnam
Department of Medical Microbiology, Radboud Center of Infectious Diseases, Radboudumc, Nijmegen, Netherlands

Tuangrat Phodha
Faculty of Pharmacy, Mahidol University, Bangkok, Thailand

Maryam Raeispour and Reza Ranjbar
Molecular Biology Research Center, Systems Biology and Poisonings Institute, Baqiyatallah University of Medical Sciences, Tehran, Iran

Yeshwondm Mamuye GebreSilasie and Addisu Gize Yeshanew
Department of Microbiology, St. Paul's Hospital Millennium Medical College, Addis Ababa, Ethiopia

Kassu Desta Tullu
Department of Microbiology, School of Medical Laboratory Sciences, College of Health Science, Addis Ababa University, Addis Ababa, Ethiopia

Stefanie Kampmeier, Annelene Kossow, Larissa Monika Clausen and Alexander Mellmann
Institute of Hygiene, University Hospital Münster, Robert-Koch-Strasse 41, 48149 Münster, Germany

Dennis Knaack
Institute of Medical Microbiology, University Hospital Münster, Münster, Germany

Christian Ertmer, Antje Gottschalk and Hendrik Freise
Department of Anaesthesiology, Intensive Care and Pain Medicine, University Hospital Münster, Münster, Germany

Anna Camilla Birkegård and Kaare Græsbøll
Department of Applied Mathematics and Computer Science, Technical University of Denmark, Asmussens Allé Building 303B, 2800 Kgs. Lyngby, Denmark

Tariq Halasa and Nils Toft
Division of Diagnostics and Scientific Advice, Technical University of Denmark, Kemitorvet Building 204, 2800 Kgs. Lyngby, Denmark

Anders Folkesson
Department of Biotechnology and Biomedicine, Technical University of Denmark, Kemitorvet Building 204, 2800 Kgs. Lyngby, Denmark

Qiang Zhu, Jiewei Cui, Minghui Zhu, Liangan Chen, Zhen Yang and Zhixin Liang
Department of Respiratory Medicine, Chinese PLA General Hospital, Fuxing Road No. 28, Beijing 100853, China

Lichen Zhu
Department of Respiratory Medicine, Affiliated Hospital of Nantong Third People's Hospital, Qingnian Central Street No. 99, Jiangsu Province 226000, China

Yan Yue
The postgraduate department, Chinese PLA General Hospital, Beijing 100853, China

Hélène Mascitti, Clara Duran, Elisabeth-Marie Nemo, Ruxandra Câlin, Alexis Descatha, Benjamin Davido and Aurélien Dinh
Infectious disease unit, Raymond Poincaré University Hospital, AP-HP, Versailles Saint-Quentin University, 104 Bd R. Poincaré, 92380 Garches, France

Frédérique Bouchand
Pharmacy department, Raymond Poincaré University Hospital, AP-HP, Versailles Saint-Quentin University, 104 Bd R. Poincaré, 92380 Garches, France

Jean-Louis Gaillard and Christine Lawrence
Microbiological laboratory, Raymond Poincaré University Hospital, AP-HP, Versailles Saint-Quentin University, 104 Bd R. Poincaré, 92380 Garches, France

François Barbier
Intensive care unit, Orléans Hospital, 14 Avenue de l'Hôpital, 45067 Orléans, France

Susanne Barnett, Warren Rose, Theresa Emmerling and Keng Hee Peh
University of Wisconsin-Madison School of Pharmacy, 777 Highland Ave, Madison, WI 53705, USA

Laurel Legenza
University of Wisconsin-Madison School of Pharmacy, 777 Highland Ave, Madison, WI 53705, USA
University of the Western Cape School of Pharmacy, Robert Sobukwe, Cape Town 7535, South Africa

Renier Coetzee
University of the Western Cape School of Pharmacy, Robert Sobukwe, Cape Town 7535, South Africa

Nasia Safdar
University of Wisconsin School of Medicine and Public Health, 750 Highland Ave, Madison, WI 53726, USA

Noor Ul Ain, Anam Iftikhar, Syeda Sadia Bukhari, Samyyia Abrar, Shahida Hussain and Muhammad Hayat Haider
Department of Microbiology and Molecular Genetics, University of the Punjab, Lahore 5400, Pakistan

Saba Riaz
Department of Microbiology and Molecular Genetics, University of the Punjab, Lahore 5400, Pakistan
Citilab and Research Center, Lahore,Pakistan

Farhan Rasheed
Department of Pathology, Allama Iqbal Medical College, Lahore, Pakistan

Tobias Siegfried Kramer, Cornelius Remschmidt, Michael Behnke, Frank Schwab, Petra Gastmeier and Rasmus Leistner
Charité Universitätsmedizin Berlin, Institute of Hygiene and Environmental Medicine, Berlin, Germany
National Reference Center for the Surveillance of Nosocomial Infections, Berlin, Germany

Sven Werner
Department of Medical and Financial Controlling, Charité Universitätsmedizin Berlin, Berlin, Germany

Guido Werner
Robert Koch Institute, FG13 Nosocomial Pathogens and Antibiotic Resistance, Wernigerode, Germany
National Reference Centre for Staphylococci and Enterococci, Berlin, Germany

Sabiha Yusuf Essack
Antimicrobial Research Unit, School of Health Sciences, College of Health Sciences, University of KwaZulu-Natal, Durban 4000, South Africa

Raspail Carrel Founou
Antimicrobial Research Unit, School of Health Sciences, College of Health Sciences, University of KwaZulu-Natal, Durban 4000, South Africa
Department of Clinical Microbiology, Centre of Expertise and Biological Diagnostic of Cameroon, (CEDBCAM), Yaoundé, Cameroon

Luria Leslie Founou
Antimicrobial Research Unit, School of Health Sciences, College of Health Sciences, University of KwaZulu-Natal, Durban 4000, South Africa
Department of Food Safety and Environmental Microbiology, Centre of Expertise and Biological Diagnostic of Cameroon, (CEDBCAM), Yaoundé, Cameroon

Cong Cheng, Shunfei Lu and Wu Zhou
School of Medicine and Health, Lishui University, Lishui 323000, China

Junwan Lu, Jinfang Zhang, Lei Xu, Yabo Liu, Pingping Li, Tingyuan Zhu, Teng Xu, Huiguang Yi, Kewei Li, Peizhen Li and Qiyu Bao
School of Laboratory Medicine and Life Sciences/ Institute of Biomedical Informatics, Wenzhou Medical University, Wenzhou 325035, China

Liyan Ni
The Second Affiliated Hospital, Wenzhou Medical University, Wenzhou 325035, China

Jadwiga Wojkowska-Mach and Anna Rozanska
Department of Microbiology, Faculty of Medicine, Jagiellonian University Medical College, Czysta 18 Str., 31-121, Krakow, Poland

Brian Godman
Strathclyde Institute of Pharmacy and Biomedical Sciences, Strathclyde University, G4 ORE, Glasgow, UK
Health Economics Centre, Liverpool University Management School, Chatham Street, Liverpool, UK. Department of Laboratory Medicine, Division of Clinical Pharmacology, Karolinska Institute, Karolinska University Hospital Huddinge, SE-141 86 Stockholm, Sweden
Department of Public Health Pharmacy and Management, School of Pharmacy, Sefako Makgatho Health Sciences University, Garankuwa, South Africa

Amanj Kurdi
Strathclyde Institute of Pharmacy and Biomedical Sciences, Strathclyde University, G4 ORE, Glasgow, UK
Department of Pharmacology, College of Pharmacy, Hawler Medical University, Erbil, Iraq

Amanda Glassman
Center for Global Development, 2055 L Street NW, Washington, DC 20036, USA

Andrzej Pilc
Department of Neurobiology, Institute of Pharmacology, Polish Academy of Sciences, Krakow, Poland
Department of Drug Management, Faculty of Health Sciences, Jagiellonian University Medical College, Grzegorzecka 20 Str., 31-531, Krakow, Poland

Tomasz Bochenek
Department of Drug Management, Faculty of Health Sciences, Jagiellonian University Medical College, Grzegorzecka 20 Str., 31-531, Krakow, Poland

Szymon Skoczyński
Department of Pneumonology, School of Medicine in Katowice, Medical University of Silesia, Katowice, Poland

Marta Wałaszek
Department of Nursing, Institute of Health Sciences, State Higher Vocational School in Tarnów, Tarnów, Poland

Cho-Han Chiang and Tyan-Shin Yang
College of Medicine, National Taiwan University, Taipei, Taiwan

Shan-Chwen Chang
College of Medicine, National Taiwan University, Taipei, Taiwan
Department of Internal Medicine, National Taiwan University Hospital, Taipei,Taiwan

Jann-Tay Wang and Wang-Huei Sheng
College of Medicine, National Taiwan University, Taipei, Taiwan
Department of Internal Medicine, National Taiwan University Hospital, Taipei,Taiwan
Center for Infection Control, National Taiwan University Hospital, Taipei, Taiwan

Yee-Chun Chen
College of Medicine, National Taiwan University, Taipei, Taiwan
Department of Internal Medicine, National Taiwan University Hospital, Taipei,Taiwan
Center for Infection Control, National Taiwan University Hospital, Taipei, Taiwan
National Institute of Infectious Diseases and Vaccinology, National Health Research Institutes, Miaoli County, Taiwan

Sung-Ching Pan
Department of Internal Medicine, National Taiwan University Hospital, Taipei,Taiwan

Keisuke Matsuda
Faculty of Medicine, Osaka University, Osaka, Japan

Hong Bin Kim
Department of Internal Medicine, Seoul National University College of Medicine, Seoul, Republic of Korea
Division of Infectious Diseases, Seoul National University Bundang Hospital, Seongnam, Republic of Korea

Young Hwa Choi
Department of Infectious Diseases, Ajou University School of Medicine, Suwon, Republic of Korea

Satoshi Hori
Department of Infection Control Science, Juntendo University Faculty of Medicine, Tokyo, Japan

Feng-Yee Chang
10Division of Infectious Diseases and Tropical Medicine, Department of Internal Medicine, Tri-Service General Hospital, National Defense Medical Center, Taipei, Taiwan

Gebre Kibru and Lule Teshager
School of Medical Laboratory Science, Jimma University, Jimma, Ethiopia

Solomon Ali
School of Medical Laboratory Science, Jimma University, Jimma, Ethiopia
WHO-TDR clinical research former fellow at AERAS Africa and Rockville, Rockville, MD, USA

Mulatu Gashaw
School of Medical Laboratory Science, Jimma University, Jimma, Ethiopia
Institute of Health, Jimma University, Jimma, Ethiopia

Melkamu Berhane
Department of Pediatrics and Child Health, Jimma University, Jimma, Ethiopia

Sisay Bekele
Department of Ophthalmology, Jimma University, Jimma, Ethiopia

Yonas Yilma
Department of Surgery, Jimma University, Jimma, Ethiopia

Yesuf Ahmed
Department of Obstetrics and Gynecology, Jimma University, Jimma, Ethiopia

Netsanet Fentahun
Department of Health Education and Behavioral Health, Jimma University, Jimma, Ethiopia

Henok Assefa
Department of Epidemiology and Statistics, Jimma University, Jimma, Ethiopia

Andreas Wieser
Head of the parasitology laboratory and deputy head of the molecular diagnostics laboratory at the Max von Pettenkofer-Institute, Ludwigs-Maximilians-University (LMU), München, Germany

Esayas Kebede Gudina
Department of Internal Medicine, Jimma University, Jimma, Ethiopia

Ricky Cohen and Adva Mir Halavi
School of Public Health, University of Haifa, 199 Aba Khoushy Ave., Mount Carmel, 3498838 Haifa, Israel

Anat Gesser-Edelsburg
School of Public Health, University of Haifa, 199 Aba Khoushy Ave., Mount Carmel, 3498838 Haifa, Israel
The Health and Risk Communication Research Center, University of Haifa, 199 Aba Khoushy Ave., Mount Carmel, 3498838 Haifa, Israel

Mina Zemach
Midgam Consulting and Research Ltd., 7 Metsada St, 5126112 Bnei Brak, Israel

Peter Vernon van Heerden, Sigal Sviri, Shmuel Benenson, Uriel Trahtemberg, Efrat Orenbuch-Harroch, Asher Salmon and Allon Moses
Hadassah University Medical Center. Ein Kerem, 9112001 Jerusalem, Israel

Lior Lowenstein
Rambam Health Care Campus, 3109601 Haifa, Israel

Dan Shteinberg
Bnai Zion Medical Center, 47 Golomb St, 3104802 Haifa, Israel.

Index

M

P

R

S

T

V

W

www.ingramcontent.com/pod-product-compliance
Lightning Source LLC
Chambersburg PA
CBHW061314190326
41458CB00011B/3800
9781632426901